NSCA's Essentials of Training Special Populations

NSCA's Essentials of Training Special Populations

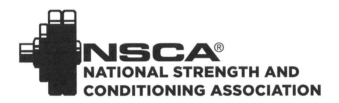

NSCA®
NATIONAL STRENGTH AND
CONDITIONING ASSOCIATION

Patrick L. Jacobs, PhD, CSCS,*D, FNSCA

Editor

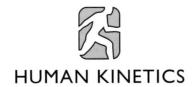

HUMAN KINETICS

Library of Congress Cataloging-in-Publication Data

Names: Jacobs, Patrick L., 1955- editor. | National Strength & Conditioning
  Association (U.S.), issuing body.
Title: NSCA's essentials of training special populations / National Strength
  and Conditioning Association ; Patrick L. Jacobs, editor.
Other titles: National Strength and Conditioning Association's essentials of
  training special populations | Essentials of training special populations
Description: Champaign, IL : Human Kinetics, [2017] | Includes
  bibliographical references and index.
Identifiers: LCCN 2017000180 (print) | LCCN 2017001698 (ebook) | ISBN
  9780736083300 (print) | ISBN 9781492546290 (e-book)
Subjects: | MESH: Physical Fitness | Resistance Training--methods | Disabled
  Persons--rehabilitation | Population Groups
Classification: LCC RA781 (print) | LCC RA781 (ebook) | NLM QT 256 | DDC
  613.7--dc23
LC record available at https://lccn.loc.gov/2017000180

ISBN: 978-0-7360-8330-0 (print)

The web addresses cited in this text were current as of March 2017, unless otherwise noted.

Acquisitions Editor: Roger W. Earle; **Senior Developmental Editor:** Christine M. Drews: **Managing Editor:** Kirsten E. Keller; **Copyeditor:** Joyce Sexton; **Indexer:** Susan Danzi Hernandez; **Permissions Manager:** Dalene Reeder; **Senior Graphic Designer**: Joe Buck; **Cover Designer:** Keith Blomberg; **Photographer (interior):** © Human Kinetics, unless otherwise noted; **Photo Asset Manager:** Laura Fitch; **Visual Production Assistant:** Joyce Brumfield; **Photo Production Manager:** Jason Allen; **Senior Art Manager:** Kelly Hendren; **Illustrations:** © Human Kinetics, unless otherwise noted; **Printer:** Walsworth

Printed in the United States of America   10 9 8 7 6 5 4 3 2

The paper in this book was manufactured using responsible forestry methods.

Human Kinetics
1607 N. Market Street
Champaign, IL 61820
USA

United States and International
Website: **US.HumanKinetics.com**
Email: info@hkusa.com
Phone: 1-800-747-4457

Canada
Website: **Canada.HumanKinetics.com**
Email: info@hkcanada.com.

E4822

Tell us what you think!
Human Kinetics would love to hear what we
can do to improve the customer experience.
Use this QR code to take our brief survey.

Contents

Chapter 5   Pulmonary Disorders and Conditions   145

Kenneth W. Rundell, PhD
James M. Smoliga, DVM, PhD, CSCS
Pnina Weiss, MD, FAAP

Chapter 6   Cardiovascular Conditions and Disorders   181

Ann Marie Swank, PhD, CSCS
Carwyn Sharp, PhD, CSCS,*D

Chapter 7   Immunologic and Hematologic Disorders   215

Don Melrose, PhD, CSCS,*D
Jay Dawes, PhD, CSCS,*D, NSCA-CPT,*D, FNSCA
Misty Kesterson, EdD, CSCS
Benjamin Reuter, PhD, ATC, CSCS,*D

Chapter 8 Neuromuscular Conditions and Disorders 267

Patrick L. Jacobs, PhD, CSCS,*D, FNSCA
Stephanie M. Svoboda, MS, DPT, CSCS
Anna Lepeley, PhD, CSCS

Chapter 9 Cognitive Conditions and Disorders 319

William J. Kraemer, PhD, CSCS,*D, FNSCA
Brett A. Comstock, PhD, CSCS
James E. Clark, MS, CSCS

Chapter 10 Cancer 341

Alejandro F. San Juan, PhD, PT
Steven J. Fleck, PhD, CSCS, FNSCA
Alejandro Lucia, MD, PhD

Preface

The benefits of engaging in an active lifestyle are extensive and apply across virtually all populations. However, many individuals are relatively inactive. Some are not active due to personal choices or perceived lack of time or resources or both. However, many individuals who could certainly profit from participation in exercise training do not do so because of their own particular characteristics. These individuals may require modifications to the general exercise recommendations for the apparently healthy adult population. With regard to exercise recommendations and training, these individuals can be considered members of various special populations. Persons with these special conditions commonly require specific exercise facility design and particular training equipment. Special populations may also require specific exercise programming supervised by exercise professionals with specialized training. It is the purpose of this book, *NSCA's Essentials of Training Special Populations,* to serve as a resource for exercise professionals working with special populations.

Special populations include individuals with chronic disease or disability and individuals who differ from the overall population with regard to recommendations for exercise training. Exercise training recommendations should also be modified, taking into account age (e.g., youth, persons who are elderly) or specific conditions related to sex (e.g., female athlete triad and pregnancy). The participation of special populations in regular exercise training is relatively low; this is related to deficiency in the access that persons with special conditions have to appropriate training opportunities. Historically, opportunities for exercise training for persons with special conditions were concentrated within clinical settings due to the specialized staffing in the medical model and the lack of appropriate opportunities in general exercise settings. Special populations should be provided opportunities for exercise conditioning in the least restrictive and most accessible and integrated settings possible. Limitations in suitable training environments include architectural accessibility and issues with general exercise equipment. Those factors aside, effective access to exercise opportunities is commonly limited by a lack of exercise professionals prepared in the specific issues related to exercise with special populations.

NSCA's Essentials of Training Special Populations was developed by the National Strength and Conditioning Association (NSCA) and was prepared by 26 expert contributors to provide specific recommendations for professionals regarding the training of persons with conditions that warrant specific programming modifications. This text is an indication of the dedication of the NSCA to providing appropriate preparatory materials and training for professionals who work with all members of our society.

NSCA's Essentials of Training Special Populations is intended to serve as a primary resource for the Certified Special Population Specialist (CSPS) certification examination. It can serve as a resource manual for commercial, community, and corporate health and fitness centers with clients who have special conditions. This text was also organized so as to serve as a textbook for university courses dedicated to the physical training of special populations.

This *Essentials* text provides evidence-based information on particular training protocols for particular special populations. While the training strategies recommended for special populations are based to a great degree on the established protocols for the general, apparently healthy population, specific training modifications are warranted for safe and effective training for each special condition. This text is organized to provide the reader with an understanding of the pathology and pathophysiology of the given condition. The known effects of various exercise programs in the particular special condition are discussed, with an emphasis on published controlled research investigations. Each chapter provides exercise recommendations particular to the special condition, with specific training modifications, precautions, and contraindications. Each chapter also discusses the medications commonly prescribed for each special condition, with emphasis on the potential effects of the medications on exercise responses and adaptations. A case study is provided as an example of the application of these recommendations within the given special condition.

The following outlines the topics covered in each chapter.

Chapter 1 addresses the benefits of exercise in general and the costs of inactivity at the individual and societal levels. Particular challenges to exercise training in special populations are discussed, with an emphasis on the need for appropriately trained exercise professionals.

Chapter 2 discusses the pivotal procedures of health appraisals and fitness assessments in regard to special populations. Medical clearance processes are specifically addressed.

Chapter 3 covers common musculoskeletal conditions and disorders and the respective recommendations for exercise training. Postural and low back pain issues are discussed as well as issues related to regeneration of muscular, skeletal, and joint structures.

Chapter 4 provides exercise recommendations for the most prevalent metabolic conditions and disorders. This chapter addresses some of the most common disease processes, including obesity, diabetes mellitus, and dyslipidemia. Other conditions discussed include hypothyroidism and hyperthyroidism, as well as chronic kidney disease.

Chapter 5 details pulmonary conditions and disorders that alter exercise recommendations from those for the general, apparently healthy adult population. Discussions specifically address the characteristics of, and exercise recommendations for, persons with asthma, chronic obstructive pulmonary disease, chronic restrictive pulmonary disease, and cystic fibrosis.

Chapter 6 deals with the characteristics of the most prevalent cardiovascular conditions and disorders. Condition-specific exercise recommendations are provided.

Chapter 7 offers recommendations for exercise professionals working with persons who have immunologic or hematologic conditions or disorders. The chapter provides information on such conditions as rheumatoid arthritis, lupus, chronic fatigue syndrome, fibromyalgia, HIV/AIDS, sickle cell disease, and hemophilia.

Chapter 8 discusses neuromuscular conditions and disorders, with specific recommendations for exercise training. Conditions covered include neuromuscular conditions that continue to progress over time, such as multiple sclerosis, Parkinson's disease, and muscular dystrophy, as well as conditions that generally do not progress, such as cerebral palsy, head injury, stroke, spinal cord injury, and epilepsy.

Chapter 9 provides information regarding cognitive disorders in relation to recommendations for exercise training. Developmental disorders covered in this chapter include autism spectrum disorder (ASD), Down syndrome, and intellectual disability (ID). The chapter also discusses the neurodegenerative diseases dementia and Alzheimer's disease.

Chapter 10 addresses characteristics of cancer and medical treatments. A review of exercise training studies in persons with cancer is provided, with professional recommendations for exercise training.

Chapter 11 covers children and adolescents, discussing physical development and physical activity levels. Age-specific recommendations for exercise training are provided.

Chapter 12 details the altered physiology with aging and discusses the effects of exercise in older adults. Specific exercise recommendations are provided for exercise professionals working with older adults.

Chapter 13 provides discussions of the physiology of particular female considerations that may alter recommendations for exercise. Discussions cover the female athlete triad and pregnancy and postpartum, as well as menopause and postmenopause.

This book is organized with a number of learning aids designed to assist the reader.

- Chapter objectives appear at the beginning of each chapter, providing the reader with an understanding of the expected reader outcomes.

- Key points summarize the important key concepts for the reader.

- Key terms are identified throughout the text in bold font. Each key term is defined near the first use of the term.

- Each chapter has one or more lists of recommended readings.

eBook
available at
HumanKinetics.com

Related specifically to the topics of the given chapters, these resources should be useful to readers wishing to learn more about a topic in general or specifically in preparation for the CSPS exam.

INSTRUCTOR AND PROFESSIONAL RESOURCES

To assist instructors and professionals using this text, these resources are available:

- *Instructor guide.* The instructor guide contains chapter objectives, chapter outlines, and key terms with definitions.
- *Presentation package and image bank.* This comprehensive resource, delivered in Microsoft PowerPoint, offers instructors and professionals a presentation package containing over 580 slides to help augment lectures and facilitate class discussions. In addition to outlines and key points, the resource contains more than 190 figures, tables, and photos from the textbook, which can be used as an image bank by instructors who need to customize their presentations. Easy-to-follow instructions help guide instructors on how to reuse the images within their own PowerPoint templates. The presentation package plus image bank is free to course adopters and is available online. For use outside of a college or university course, this presentation package plus image bank may be purchased separately at **US.HumanKinetics.com**
- *Test package.* The test package includes a bank of 130 multiple-choice questions, from which instructors can make their own tests and quizzes. Instructors can download Respondus or RTF files or files formatted for use in a learning management system.

Ancillary products supporting this text are free to adopting instructors. Contact your Sales Manager for details about how to access HK*Propel*, our ancillary delivery and learning platform.

Rationale and Considerations for Training Special Populations

Patrick L. Jacobs, PhD, CSCS,*D, FNSCA

After completing this chapter, you will be able to

- discuss the benefits of an active lifestyle,

- explain the negative consequences of leading an inactive lifestyle,

- list reasons commonly cited for not leading an active lifestyle and discuss which of these could be addressed by an exercise professional,

- discuss the characteristics of special populations with regard to exercise training and testing,

- explain the Americans with Disabilities Act with regard to exercise training,

- discuss the scope of practice of the exercise professional working with special populations, and

- describe how the concept of inclusive fitness differs from a traditional model of training special populations (rehabilitation settings).

Participation in structured exercise training is known to provide significant physical and psychological benefits. Exercise conditioning is now considered a viable means to enhance functional capacity and independence across different populations. Unfortunately, many persons who could benefit the most from increased daily activity do not do so. Various populations, due to their inherent characteristics, require specific exercise equipment and facility access compared to the general population. Because of their particular characteristics, these persons may also require specific exercise programming and therefore specially prepared exercise professional supervision. These groups can be considered **special populations** with regard to their particular requirements for safe and effective exercise training. Special populations include groups that differ from the overall population with regard to age (e.g., youth and people who are elderly) or specific conditions related to sex (e.g., female triad and pregnancy).

Special populations also include many persons with chronic disease or disability. Treatment of medical conditions has traditionally concentrated on disease curative efforts with emphasis on survival and life extension rather than on efforts to reduce the consequences of the disease processes (palliative). A shift to a more palliative emphasis and away from the purely curative approach is indicative of an increased emphasis on quality of life rather than the traditional concentration on quantity of life.

Members of many special populations may wish to engage in exercise training for a variety of reasons, which may be similar to or different from those of the general, apparently healthy population. Increased physical activity may increase physical work capacity, thereby enhancing quality of life and independence. Conversely, with a sedentary lifestyle, the negative consequences of the disease or disability processes may become more profound over time. Unfortunately, the participation of persons with these chronic conditions is quite low due to a lack of exercise training opportunities for persons with special conditions. Increased exercise training opportunities for these individuals necessitates appropriate access to, and supervision within, the exercise training environment.

BENEFITS OF EXERCISE

Active lifestyles, particularly those that include regular exercise, have been associated with numerous important health benefits as well as enhanced functional performance of daily activities. Consistent participation in a structured exercise plan and dietary control are components of most proven weight loss and weight maintenance programs. Increased activity can assist in the reduction of excessive body weight when applied with reduced caloric intake, can help prevent further weight gain, and has been shown to help support reduced body weight after the initial loss (16).

Increased physical activity reduces the chances of developing certain diseases while decreases in physical activity will increase the risk of diseases such as cardiovascular disease, diabetes mellitus, obesity, and hypertension (39). Many disease processes are associated with a number of risk factors, some of which are considered to be modifiable and are under an individual's control. For example, increased levels of physical activity may favorably influence high blood pressure (15) and detrimental blood lipid profiles (35), thereby reducing the chances of developing heart disease (39) or having a stroke (29). **Metabolic syndrome**, which is characterized by (a) overweight or obesity, (b) undesirable lipid profiles, (c) high blood pressure, and (d) high resting blood glucose levels, is well associated with the overall lack of physical activity (42). In contrast, physical activity, as part of a complete conditioning program, has been shown to be quite effective in reducing body weight (16) and blood pressure (15) with improvements in lipid levels (35) and resting sugar levels (3), thereby reducing the chances of developing metabolic syndrome (42) and diabetes (3).

Improvement in the performance of important daily activities with increased physical activity is commonly related to significant improvements in muscular strength and endurance with increased cardiovascular fitness (1, 5). For example, well-designed exercise programs have been shown to significantly reduce the risk of falls in the aging and middle-aged populations (8, 32). Reduced health risks tend to result in fewer medical complications, and this, combined with improved physical capacity, contributes to increased chances of longevity with greater levels of physical activity (6, 39).

Participation in regular physical activity is also known to provide enhancements in mental health while also increasing physical work capacity. Psychological improvements may include improvements in overall mood with reduced feelings of depression and anxiety (22).

Key Point

Increases in physical activity are associated with benefits including enhanced weight loss and improved weight maintenance, increased ability to perform important daily tasks, and improved psychological mood, with reduced chances of developing certain disease processes such as cardiovascular disease, diabetes mellitus, obesity, and hypertension.

It is important to note that active lifestyles, specifically participation in well-designed exercise programs, have been shown to provide significant benefits across populations regardless of chronological age, sex, training status, and current health condition. Whereas the benefits of exercise appear to be consistent across quite different groups (39), the actual exercise programming should be specifically selected or developed (or both) relative to the capabilities and goals of the individual. Thus, while exercise training will provide useful health and function advantages to the lives of most people, it is vital that the training programming be appropriate for the safe and effective participation of each individual. While the benefits of an active lifestyle are apparent and specific recommendations for exercise activity have been developed and made readily available, most Americans remain relatively inactive (13).

Key Point

While the benefits of increased activity levels are evident across sexes, ages, and health status, the training programs should be appropriate for the particular participant in order to provide safe and effective outcomes.

INACTIVITY AND COSTS TO INDIVIDUALS AND SOCIETY

The consequences of an inactive lifestyle are progressive, with significant consequences. Sedentary lifestyles are a leading cause of preventable death, with increasing risk of numerous disease processes including cardiovascular disease, diabetes, hypertension, obesity, osteoporosis, and lipid disorders (41). It appears that the adage "use it or lose it" accurately captures ongoing physical deterioration and declining function of many physiological systems during extended periods of physical inactivity (25). In general, the longer and more complete the period of inactivity, the greater the degree of systemic dysfunction (25). Approximately 50% of all U.S. adults have at least one chronic health condition, and about 25% have two or more of these disease processes (40).

The chronic diseases associated with inactivity are becoming increasingly prevalent and produce staggering economic effects. Obesity is now diagnosed in more than one-third of all American adults and in approximately 17% of children and adolescents aged 2 to 19 (31). The medical costs associated with obesity were estimated in 2008 at $147 billion annually (12). Approximately 12% of all U.S. adults are now diagnosed with diabetes, and another 37% are diagnosed with prediabetes, based on fasting glucose or A1C (glycated hemoglobin) levels (11). The total medical costs associated with diabetes in 2012 were estimated at $245 billion, which included both direct medical costs ($176 billion) and costs related to decreased productivity ($69 billion) (21). The average medical cost for each person with diabetes was calculated at $1,429 per year greater than the costs for a person of normal weight (17).

While the benefits of an active lifestyle and the health and functional risks of a sedentary way of life have been well established, the level of participation in an active lifestyle is relatively quite low. Only 15% to 20% of American adults, aged 18 years and above, regularly meet both the aerobic and strength training recommendations of the 2008 *Physical Activity Guidelines for Americans* (non-Hispanic whites, 21.3%; non-Hispanic blacks, 17.2%; Hispanics, 14.4%) (13).

WHY ARE PEOPLE INACTIVE?

The benefits of an active lifestyle (16, 39) and the negative consequences of a sedentary lifestyle (41) have been well established. However, less than one-fifth of all American adults meet basic exercise recommendations (13). The lack of activity has been related to changes in modern societies that reduce the physical nature of daily activities. Additionally, sedentary persons commonly report similar reasons for their inactive lifestyles, including time issues and a lack of opportunities within local communities.

Societal Issues

Several primary societal changes appear to have contributed substantially to the declining levels of physical activity exhibited over the past several decades. Significant technological advancements have dramatically reduced the amount of physical activity necessary in the performance of many daily tasks (37). Both work-related tasks and personal recreation pursuits (leisure interests) tend to involve less gross physical effort (37). There has been a shift from occupational duties relying on physical efforts of the individual toward work duties more commonly involving operating mechanized equipment. The percentage of non-farm workers in manufacturing positions was over 30% of the total U.S. workforce in 1950 but had declined to approximately 10% by 2007 (26). Most of this shift was matched by increased workers in the service sectors.

The automobile is now relied upon for virtually all transportation in the United States regardless of the distance involved (7). The shift in community development from smaller locally based units to extended suburban sprawl has dramatically reduced walking and cycling as realistic options for daily transportation (19). Unfortunately, the increased reliance on the automobile has been associated with the increasing incidence of obesity and other secondary medical complications (18).

The maturing of the "baby boomer" generation is projected to dramatically increase the segment the U.S. population aged 65 years and older from 13% in 2010 to approximately 19.3% by the year 2030 (38). This would represent an increase in the 65+ population by about 50% in a 20-year period. Unfortunately, as persons generally become less active with advancing age, particularly after retirement, this population shift is also creating a dramatic increase in the number of inactive persons (23).

The decline in physiological status that is generally associated with the aging processes is further compounded by reduced activity of the younger segments of our society. Decreased levels of physical activity in children and young adults limit peak development of bone and lean muscle mass during critical periods (27). The gradual decline in physiological status with aging may therefore be further compounded by lower peak levels of development. Reduced outdoor play activities and reductions in public school physical education programming often require participation in private extracurricular programming in order to achieve appropriate levels of physical activity (4).

Individual Issues

Reasons commonly reported by individuals for not being more physically active include perceived lack of time or convenience, lack of motivation or interest in exercise, lack of confidence to participate safely, lack of personal management skills or support systems or both, and perceived lack of suitable resources (10). These reported barriers to an active lifestyle are frequently cited by many persons despite their actual capacity and potential to live a more active lifestyle (10). Some of the commonly listed barriers are misperceptions based on individuals' incorrect beliefs concerning themselves and exercise. People who have been physically inactive for extended periods of time may feel that their level of physical deconditioning is too advanced to reverse. Others with limited exposure to physical exercise activities may not have the needed background in this area to understand the potential benefits of physical training despite their present status.

Many of the commonly cited barriers to increased participation in regular physical activity can be effectively addressed by an exercise professional who possesses the requisite background and knowledge to safely assess, design, and supervise training sessions on an individual basis. The exercise professional motivates and educates clients to guide them toward their specific goals.

Persons with physical disability or chronic disease have long been known to be less active than persons without disability or disease (20). These individuals may, in addition to the previously discussed perceived barriers to participation in physical activity programs, face actual substantial barriers to participation (33). For example, individuals may encounter limitations or restrictions in accessibility to exercise opportunities based on architectural accessibility issues or equipment selection (or both) in community training facilities. **Accessibility** to exercise opportunities certainly involves appropriate architectural and equipment issues but also appropriate training supervision. Barriers to participation in exercise activities may also be limited by a lack of community exercise professionals properly trained in the particular exercise issues related to the supervision of persons other than the healthy adult client.

SPECIFIC EXERCISE PROGRAMMING FOR SPECIAL POPULATIONS

Professional organizations have established general activity and exercise recommendations to provide guidance in planning and performance of exercise activities for the general population without chronic disease or disability. These guidelines are based on scientific evidence supporting the health and functional benefits of an active lifestyle. For example, the U.S. Department of Health and Human Services (DHHS) recommends that all healthy adults complete at least 2.5 hours of aerobic exercise weekly or complete at least 1.25 hours of vigorous aerobic exercise per week (13). Strength training is also recommended for all healthy adults at least two times weekly. While these recommendations were set forth by the DHHS for the general healthy adult population, specific recommendations were also established for particular populations. The 2008 *Physical Activity Guidelines for Americans* sets forth specific recommendations for activity in several populations known to be less active, including children, older adults, women who are pregnant, and persons with chronic disease or disability. These recommendations indicate that these special populations include individuals who, based on their specific characteristics, require particular condition-specific exercise programming in order to receive effective and safe training.

Key Point

Special populations are groups of individuals who, when considered with regard to exercise, differ from the general, apparently healthy adult population with respect to recommendations for exercise programming. These populations may exhibit characteristics that require condition-specific recommendations for exercise as well as appropriate precautions and contraindications to exercise in order to receive effective and safe training.

Professional recommendations for exercise training of the general adult population are based on known acute physiological responses to exercise activities as well as the established chronic adaptations to exercise stresses. Thus, the general recommendations for exercise in apparently healthy populations have been established for those individuals in whom the physiological systems generally respond in a standard manner. Changes in physiological functioning will presumably result in altered capacities for, and responses to, exercise in the acute setting, as well as potentially affecting the expected adaptations to exercise training over time. Thus, persons with some degree of physiological dysfunction may be considered as members of a special population who require specific programming in order to receive safe and effective exercise training.

The altered physiological functioning exhibited by special populations may be the result of a number of factors including chronic diseases and disabilities, as well as certain age- and sex-related issues. This text provides an overview of some of the most common special populations, with discussions of the pathology and pathophysiology of each condition, in order to provide the reader with a basic understanding of the unique physiological functioning of persons with the given condition (with emphasis on how this differs from that in the general, apparently healthy population). Specific recommendations for exercise activities as well as precautions and contraindications are provided for each condition.

Exercise training of special populations requires appropriate expertise and professional training of the exercise professionals involved, as well as provision of suitable training equipment and environments. The exercise professional needs to possess the background and education appropriate for the specialized training activities needed by the special population. Thus, this setting requires specialized knowledge and expertise related to the special population in addition to the professional proficiencies used with the general, apparently healthy population.

SCOPE OF PRACTICE OF THOSE WORKING WITH SPECIAL POPULATIONS

Various professions are licensed by governmental agencies (national, state, or both) in order to carry out the legally permitted procedures and processes. In these cases, the professional scope of practice is set forth by law. The licensing process involves specific education, experience, and demonstrated competency. Other professions do not have a governmental license but have standards of practice published by professional associations. Additionally, professional associations may administer specialized certifications that should also involve specific education and demonstration of competency.

The exercise professional is not licensed by a governmental agency, and there are no industry-wide standards. However, a number of allied professional organizations have published standards of care for the exercise professional. Likewise, numerous professional exercise associations offer various certifications that differ considerably. It is recommended that all exercise professionals fulfill a certification that involves assessment of both scientific concepts and practice competencies. Thus, the appropriate scope of practice for the exercise professional is determined by both

the industry-published standards of care and the particular certification process.

The scope of practice of the exercise professional involves designing and supervising safe and effective exercise programs in relation to the client's physiological status and goals. Assessment and training procedures are carried out, as well as provision of education and motivation during the training process. Exercise professionals must be aware of the limitations of their scope of practice and refer clients to suitable licensed health care professionals when appropriate.

The scope of practice of the exercise professional includes performing health appraisals in order to screen new clients for risk factors and symptoms of disease. The client should be referred to an appropriate health care professional when indicated by the health appraisal. Exercise professionals often encounter newly developed injuries or diseases with their existing clients. In such cases, the health appraisal (e.g., Par-Q) should be reapplied with adjustment of the training program or referral to a health care professional where appropriate.

Key Point

The scope of practice of the exercise professional includes conducting health appraisals and physical assessments as well as designing and supervising exercise training. The exercise professional should not engage in any activities that are presented as physical therapy or counseling but rather should refer clients to an appropriate licensed clinician.

For example, physical therapists commonly use therapeutic exercise as a means to address an injury or disease in terms of a patient's function. The scope of practice of physical therapy includes other interventions such as joint and soft tissue mobilization, neuromuscular education, gait training, and modalities. So while many of the therapeutic interventions applied in physical therapy may appear similar to those used by the exercise professional, it is vital that exercise professionals refrain from describing their services as physical therapy. Physical therapists are licensed health care professionals who diagnose and treat medical conditions (injuries and diseases) that limit function or cause pain. It is imperative that exercise professionals not present their services as physical therapy or as treating a disease or injury. Rather, it is recommended that the exercise professional refer clients who exhibit pain that limits motion, swelling of a joint or muscle, or limited range of motion to a medical or allied health professional for appropriate treatment.

The scope of practice of the exercise professional also does not include psychological services. Licensed health care professionals, such as mental health counselors and psychologists, have the appropriate background and training necessary for treatment of psychological issues. Just as it is inappropriate for exercise professionals to describe their services as "treating a disease" or as "injury rehabilitation," it is not acceptable for the exercise professional to provide counseling services directly related to disordered eating, body image, or other psychologically based issues.

Various populations have characteristics that require exercise programming differing from the recommendations offered for the general population (see table 1.1). It is vital that the exercise professional have the necessary knowledge base and training to fulfill these responsibilities with each client. Obviously, some clients require greater levels of professional expertise than others based on either their physiological status or their training goals.

The professional credential of Certified Special Population Specialist (CSPS) was established by the National Strength and Conditioning Association (NSCA) in order to provide a certification process specific to the exercise professional who seeks documentation of specialized advanced expertise with special populations. The CSPS certification provides the opportunity for the more experienced exercise professional to demonstrate, both to the potential client and to other professionals and institutions in the field, his advanced background in the area of training special populations. The NSCA defines the CSPS as follows (from www.nsca.com/Certification/CSPS/):

Certified Special Population Specialists (CSPSs) are fitness professionals who, using an individualized approach, assess, motivate, educate, and train special population clients of all ages regarding their health and fitness
needs, preventively, and in collaboration with healthcare professionals. Special populations include those with chronic and temporary health conditions.

CSPSs design safe and effective exercise programs, provide the guidance to help clients achieve their personal health/fitness goals, and recognize and respond to emergency situations. Recognizing their own areas of expertise, CSPSs receive referrals from and refer clients to other health care providers as appropriate.

PROFESSIONAL OPPORTUNITIES FOR THOSE TRAINING SPECIAL POPULATIONS

The exercise professional with expertise in the training of special populations (via formal education and professional certifications) is properly positioned to meet the growing need for professionals with appropriate background in this area. Various special populations are expected to grow in size with the increasing rate of inactivity in the general population compounded with specific growth in certain special populations. Almost one-half of all U.S. adults (117 million) have at least one chronic medical condition (e.g., hypertension, coronary heart disease, stroke, diabetes, cancer, arthritis), with more than two chronic conditions reported in over one-quarter of adults (60 million) (40). The current number of Americans over the age of 65 is calculated at over 40 million and is expected to increase to approximately 72 million persons by the year 2030. Because chronic conditions increase in prevalence in older populations, these figures indicate that an overwhelming number of persons in our society and a growing segment of our society will be classified as a part of special populations (9).

Health care costs associated with obesity and sedentary lifestyles are greater than $90 billion annually in the United States alone (28). These escalating costs place undue stress on both individual and employer health insurance systems. The medical system has made dramatic advances in the care of persons with disease, in particular in the area of emergency care. Survival and recovery

Table 1.1   Common Conditions, Disorders, or Diseases of Special Populations

Type of condition	Condition, disorder, or disease
Cardiovascular conditions	Myocardial infarction
	Angina
	Hypertension
	Peripheral vascular disease (e.g., deep vein thrombosis, peripheral artery disease)
	Congestive heart failure
	Valvular disorders
	Revascularizations
	Conduction defects or disorders (e.g., atrial fibrillation, pacemakers)
Pulmonary conditions	Chronic obstructive pulmonary disease (COPD) (e.g., emphysema, chronic bronchitis)
	Chronic restrictive pulmonary disease (CRPD) (e.g., fibrosis, sarcoidosis)
	Asthma
	Pulmonary hypertension
Metabolic conditions	Diabetes mellitus (types 1 and 2)
	Overfatness, obesity
	Metabolic syndrome
	Thyroid disorders (hypo- or hyperthyroidism)
	End-stage renal disease
Immunologic and hematologic conditions	AIDS/HIV (acquired immunodeficiency syndrome/human immunodeficiency virus)
	Chronic fatigue syndrome
	Fibromyalgia
	Anemia
	Autoimmune disorders (e.g., lupus, rheumatoid arthritis)
	Bleeding or clotting disorders
Musculoskeletal or orthopedic conditions	Osteoporosis and other low BMD (bone mineral density) conditions
	Limb amputations
	Osteoarthritis
	Lower back conditions
	Chronic musculoskeletal conditions (e.g., low back pain)
	Frailty
Joint disorders or conditions	Joint replacements
	Sarcopenia
	Posture conditions
	Cystic fibrosis
Neuromuscular conditions	Stroke or brain injury
	Spinal cord disabilities
	Multiple sclerosis
	Cerebral palsy
	Down syndrome
	Parkinson's disease
	Epilepsy
	Balance conditions
	Muscular dystrophy

Type of condition	Condition, disorder, or disease
Female-specific conditions	Pregnancy and postpartum Female athlete triad Menopausal or postmenopausal
Behavioral or psychological disorders	Disordered eating patterns Body image Depression Chemical dependency
Cancer	
Older adults	
Children and adolescents	

Note: Professionals working with individuals with any of these conditions need to do so within their proper scope of practice.

Adapted, by permission, from NSCA, 2012, *What is a special population?* Available: https://www.nsca.com/Education/Articles/What-is-a-Special-Population/

have significantly improved in many conditions considered to have questionable outcomes only a few decades ago. This dramatically extended life expectancy, from 66 years in males and 71.7 years in females in 1950 to 72.1 years in males and 79.0 years in females in 1990 (24). By the year 2009, the predicted life span from birth had grown to 76.0 years for men and to 80.9 years for women (2). Thus, during the same period of time in which length of life increased by approximately 10 years, our society became increasingly inactive. This has resulted in progressive extension of the length of life (quantity of life) with significant reductions in the level of functional independence during the later years of life (quality of life) (24).

The medical system may be an important referral source of new clients to the exercise professional with expertise with special populations. Chapter 2 of this text provides detailed discussions of the health appraisal process and the steps to determine the appropriateness of a medical clearance for a particular potential client. The medical clearance process establishes a means of communication between the exercise professional and a licensed health care professional. Medical clearance provides professional authorization for exercise testing and training in persons who exhibit particular risk factors. This process may also establish a line of communication between the exercise professional and the medical profes-

sionals with regard to future patients and their need to engage in purposeful exercise programming outside of the medical treatment environment.

Discharge plans from medical care, particularly physical therapy, usually involve some recommendations for activities and exercise strategies for the patient. Patients may have a limited background in exercise and active lifestyles, and their only experience in these areas may be the therapeutic activities in the rehabilitative setting. Thus, it is unlikely that they will seek to begin a structured exercise program with professional support even if this has been recommended by the clinician. It is recommended that the exercise professional establish working relationships with medical professionals in the community. In this way, the patient can be directly referred by the medical professional to an associated exercise professional who can provide the appropriate guidance and supervision.

Unfortunately, in many situations the rehabilitation plan must be carried out with time limitations related to the patient's medical insurance coverage. The therapeutic plan of care often must concentrate on the most vital skills of daily living in order to enhance the level of functional independence in the limited time available. Thus, many patients are discharged from the rehabilitation setting in a condition that warrants continued physical training. Exercise professionals with advanced background in training of special populations can certainly provide the needed assessment and training of these discharged patients, with clearance and recommendations from the clinician.

EXPECTATIONS IN THE TRAINING OF SPECIAL POPULATIONS

The benefits of engaging in an active lifestyle are extensive and apply across virtually all populations of persons regardless of age, sex, or social or racial group. As most persons will benefit from an appropriate exercise training program, it is the goal that opportunities for exercise training be available to all persons regardless of their particular characteristics.

Governmental legislation has addressed the issues related to the opportunities of persons with special needs to successfully enter into a more active lifestyle. Such legislation generally attempts to address the limitations to participation in exercise activities due to barriers and restraints associated with the exercise environment. The most notable of the legislative efforts is the **Americans with Disabilities Act** (ADA). The ADA prohibits discrimination of many types against persons with disabilities in different settings including the workplace, transportation, public accommodations, and governmental activities. This Act also addresses issues apparent in public and private settings for physical activity and exercise training. Governmental institutions (e.g., county parks) and larger recreation businesses are required by law to comply with the requirements of the ADA, while smaller individual recreation businesses are encouraged to comply to the extent possible that

Key Point

The Americans with Disabilities Act (ADA) specifically prohibits discrimination against persons with disabilities in the workplace, public accommodations, transportation, and governmental activities as well as public and private settings for physical activity and exercise training.

does not create undue financial hardships. While people commonly view the ADA as legislation that pertains only to architectural issues, other concerns relating to programming and staffing are also addressed.

The ADA asserts that as a matter of human rights, discrimination against persons with special needs is not acceptable. All persons are considered to possess certain rights and these rights can be expressed with respect to opportunities for an active, productive lifestyle. Specifically, the ADA addresses rights of individuals to pursue an active lifestyle, including the right to an integrated setting, the right to participate, the right to reasonable accommodations, the right to adaptive equipment, and the right to an assessment or evaluation (30). For example, the individual with a disability has the right to participate in any recreation or exercise activity offered to the general public. Participation should be offered in the least restrictive manner possible, and the opportunity to participate in an integrated setting should be made available. The individual should be able to participate with family, friends, and other community members regardless of the disability.

Traditionally, persons with disability or special needs were limited to exercise activities offered in the medical rehabilitation setting. While that environment usually provides appropriate professional supervision by staff that are familiar with the medical issues, the rehabilitation setting may not be integrated. It would be preferable to provide a more inclusive training environment in which the exercise activities, not the disabilities, are the common theme. **Inclusive fitness** is a growing approach to exercise training in which persons with special training needs are able to train in mainstream environments rather than in specialized secluded settings. There has been a shift in program delivery from the medical rehabilitation setting to the community-based recreation facility. Similarly, there has been a shift from prevention of secondary disabilities in persons with disability to health promotion and more recently to increasing physical work capacity as a means to enhance function, independence, and self-concept (34).

Key Point

Training of members of special populations should be carried out in the most inclusive, integrated, and accessible settings possible. As such, exercise training of special populations has shifted program delivery from specialized clinical settings to community-based recreation surroundings, while programming has moved from prevention of secondary disabilities to enhancement of physical work capacity as a means to improve function, independence, and self-concept.

APPROPRIATE ENVIRONMENTS FOR TRAINING SPECIAL POPULATIONS

Appropriate opportunities for all to participate in exercise activities require appropriate professional supervision and programming, as well as suitable training environments, in order to provide equal access to exercise training in a safe and effective environment. It would appear prudent to provide exercise facilities and equipment in accordance with both the recommendations established for the general training environment and also specific guidelines for special populations set forth by governmental agencies. Generalized recommendations for exercise facility design and equipment selection have been published in *NSCA's Essentials of Personal Training* (36). The reader is referred to that publication for a thorough discussion of the general requirements for exercise facilities and equipment.

The ADA was enacted in 1990 and addressed many issues that can be defined as "public accommodations." Similar to other businesses, exercise facilities have access considerations ranging from physical access through the front door and throughout the facility to bathroom access. However, smaller businesses with fewer than 15 employees are exempt from the requirement of the ADA. In 2010, the U.S. Department of Justice published the *ADA Standards for Accessible Design,* which sets forth standards for minimal accommodations in all new or altered governmental, public,

and commercial exercise facilities (14). Generally, these standards do not affect existing structures that are not undergoing new construction or alterations to existing facilities. However, certain topics included in the 2010 *Standards* but not specifically addressed in the original 1990 ADA standards, such as exercise standards, are absolute requirements without any "grandfather" options or release from requirements based on limited size of the business. Thus, all governmental, public, and commercial exercise facilities must comply with the 2010 *Standards* wherever possible.

Equal access to exercise training in a safe and effective environment necessitates appropriate physical access into and throughout the facility. Special populations may present physical characteristics that require particular considerations in order to access the training environment as independently and safely as possible. Standards for acceptable entry into and passage throughout the facility are usually based on the proven needs of the wheelchair user (14). Access into and throughout the exercise training facility must not limit entry with doors that require grasping of standard doorknobs or substantial pulling forces. Standard accommodations in this area include doorway lever handles and automated door opening systems (motion or large push button switches). A less preferable but acceptable accommodation would be a staff member assigned to open doors in a timely manner. Wheelchair users generally require greater space for travel routes. According to the 2010 *Standards,* facilities must provide a continuous path that is at least 36 inches (91 cm) wide, with recommendations for pathways to be at least 48 inches (122 cm) wide. Areas for wheelchair turnaround must be at least 60 inches (152 cm) in diameter.

Equal access to an exercise training facility must include appropriate access to the exercise machines for all, regardless of individuals' particular needs. Generalized recommendations for space requirements in exercise training areas usually call for 3-foot (0.9 m) distance between all exercise stations (36). Wheelchair users require more space than others, establishing a particular need for accessible routes to the exercise stations as well as greater space between exercise stations so that the wheelchair can safely navigate alongside the stations. There should be ample clear floor space to allow the wheelchair or other mobility device to be parked next to the exercise station without blocking access for other clients. The *2010 ADA Standards for Accessible Design* stipulates there must be an open floor space at least 3 by 4 feet (0.9 by 1.2 m) beside at least one of each type of exercise station (14). There may be an overlap between stations in open floor space. The exception to the open access requirements for the parked wheelchair alongside the device are exercise stations that allow direct use while in a wheelchair.

The *2010 Standards* also specifies that an option must be available for each type of training (e.g., strength, cardiovascular) for each special population. For example, if a facility has treadmills and stepper and elliptical exercise machines, then the facility must provide open access space next to at least one of each of those types of exercise devices. This also means that the exercise facility must provide a means of cardiovascular training accessible and usable by all potential clients, including those unable to participate in cardiovascular training with the legs. Therefore, the training facility should provide access to cardiovascular training with arms via such devices as arm cranking systems.

The use of specialized adaptive equipment and reasonable accommodations greatly enhances the participation of persons with special needs. Reasonable accommodations should be provided in order to facilitate participation and may include rule modifications or additional staffing to increase participation, as long as the accommodation does not provide an unfair competitive advantage. Similarly, adaptive equipment may provide a means to participate in exercise activities that would otherwise not be possible. For example, an adaptive apparatus to assist hand grasp may allow some persons to participate in a number of recreation and exercise activities requiring a firm, steady grasp of an implement or device.

In some cases, adaptations serve to make the use of generalized exercise equipment safer for someone with special needs. For example, a wheelchair user with limited leg and torso control will have sitting limitations in most exercise equipment due to lack of stability. The use of straps wrapped around the client and the torso provides increased stability in a manner similar to that with automobile seat belts and shoulder straps. Other basic adaptations include wrist straps and other assistance grasping devices to enable upper body training in clients without a strong grasp.

It is expected that persons with special needs be provided appropriate accessible exercise equipment. The individual should be able to position herself in the exercise device and independently operate the device without assistance. This may necessitate the use of specialized assistive equipment (e.g., lifting straps) or assistance from a staff member when needed.

It is important, for safety reasons and training efficacy, that the exercise equipment be appropriately sized for the client. In many cases, exercise equipment designed for use by adults is not appropriate for training children and persons of smaller dimensions. Similarly, general exercise equipment may not be suitable when training persons of larger than average dimensions. Larger-size individuals, such as those who are clinically obese, should be provided with comfortable seating in the exercise equipment (e.g., tractor-style seats), as they may not be able to comfortably position themselves in the seats of general equipment.

It is vital when training special populations to provide exercise equipment that allows training at the exercise intensity appropriate for the client. For example, numerous people with chronic conditions exhibit reduced walking pace, which is a limitation in the performance of many important daily activities. Treadmill walking may be an appropriate training activity for many clients, but it is imperative that the treadmill allow quite reduced speeds of walking for safety. Some special population clients may display reduced exercise capacity or aerobic endurance (or both). In such cases, it may be appropriate to provide seating (other than the exercise equipment) in the training area for recovery periods between exercise intervals.

The exercise training environment for special populations should provide a safe and effective setting for the performance of the client's training program. In some cases, this may involve the addition or modification of existing equipment and facilities for the general population. Other situations may call for reduction or elimination of some aspects within the generalized exercise training setting. For example, when working with individuals who have cognitive issues (e.g., Down syndrome, autism), it may be appropriate to train these individuals with reduced noise and visual distractions.

CONCLUSION

The benefits of leading an active lifestyle, including regular exercise training, are apparent across populations irrespective of age, sex, and current health condition. Unfortunately, many groups of persons that could benefit the most from supervised exercise training are unlikely to participate due to perceived and actual barriers. Many barriers to exercise can be effectively addressed by exercise professionals with the appropriate background and training.

Some groups of individuals can be considered special populations as they exhibit particular characteristics that require specific recommendations, precautions, and contraindications for exercise that may differ from those for the general, apparently healthy population. Exercise professionals working with special populations should possess the appropriate education and experience in order to provide safe and effective exercise training for these individuals. The Certified Special Population Specialist (CSPS) certification is awarded to exercise professionals who demonstrate the appropriate expertise necessary to safely and effectively train special population clients in exercise programming.

Exercise training of special populations should be carried out in the most inclusive manner possible. That is, whenever possible, persons with special needs should be able to exercise in the same environment as family, friends, and others in the community.

Key Terms

accessibility
Americans with Disabilities Act
inclusive fitness
metabolic syndrome
special populations

Study Questions

1. When treating chronic disease or disability, what would moving from curative efforts to palliative efforts represent?

    a. more emphasis on quality of life

    b. increased requirement for the number of medical professionals

    c. greater importance on disease survival

    d. more interest in increasing life span

2. Which of these barriers to exercise training currently represents a unique accessibility issue for those with physical disabilities or chronic diseases?

    a. lack of personal management skills or social support

    b. inadequate time to exercise

    c. inadequate financial resources

    d. lack of properly trained exercise professionals

3. Which of the following is a benefit of an exercise professional establishing a good relationship with medical professionals?

   a. provides an opportunity for the medical professional to suggest specific exercises

   b. allows the exercise professional to receive accurate advice in treating medical issues in clients

   c. makes direct referrals of clients to a qualified exercise professional more likely

   d. gives the exercise professional access to clients' medical records

4. All of the following describe the scope of practice of an exercise professional except

   a. assessing current health status

   b. assessing a client's physical goals

   c. designing an exercise program to meet a client's goals

   d. designing a stretching program to reduce joint pain and swelling

Health Appraisal and Fitness Assessments

John F. Graham, MS, CSCS,*D, RSCC*E, FNSCA

Malcolm T. Whitehead, PhD, CSCS

After completing this chapter, you will be able to

◆ describe the medical and health appraisal process;

◆ determine the need for medical clearance and medical supervision during exercise testing and training;

◆ administer specific tests that evaluate individual fitness parameters;

◆ evaluate the results of fitness tests;

◆ create SMART short-, medium-, and long-term goals; and

◆ understand the effective use of motivational and coaching techniques.

Before designing an exercise program for an individual who has a special need or condition, it is essential to review and evaluate the medical and health history. This analysis is an essential step before performing a safe and appropriate fitness assessment and developing an effective exercise program. This chapter identifies and outlines the medical and health history review process, explains the medical clearance process, clarifies the purposes and guidelines of safe and effective fitness assessments, provides detailed directions for common testing protocols and the interpretation of test results, and explains how an exercise professional can motivate a client to maximize success.

MEDICAL AND HEALTH HISTORY APPRAISAL

It is the responsibility of the exercise professional to provide each client with an evidence-based approach to assess, inform, and formulate short-, medium, and long-term plans regarding exercise needs and goals. A review of each client's medical and health history yields the information and data necessary to develop an effective and safe exercise program. It is also important to determine if the client needs to be referred to an appropriate health care professional for further evaluation and clearance before completing a fitness assessment and starting an exercise program. Therefore, this section focuses on assessing certain medical risks and determining health status as a precursor to performing a fitness assessment.

Preparticipation Screening

The purpose of the preparticipation screening process is to identify and classify any concerns related to participation in an exercise program, such as known or unknown chronic diseases or conditions that might limit exercise. This information may be obtained through the completion and review of a form that asks questions about medical and health history. A common component that nearly all questionnaires address relates to chronic disease. In the United States, chronic disease (or a related condition) afflicts as many as 117 million people (43) and contributes to a

large portion of mortality due to heart disease and cancer (11). As a result of the prevalence of chronic diseases, the screening process needs to be effective and efficient in order to determine limitations, reduce barriers to exercise, and reduce the risk to clients when initiating the exercise program (14, 29).

Preparticipation screening tools are a means by which valuable information can be collected and evaluated before a fitness assessment and exercise program implementation. These tools include the Physical Activity Readiness Questionnaire for Everyone (PAR-Q+) and the medical history questionnaire. These screening tools provide important information needed for determination of the appropriateness for medical clearance. It is important to point out that that everyone who will be exposed to clients' medical data needs to hold that information confidential in compliance with the Health Insurance Portability and Accountability Act (HIPAA).

Key Point

The exercise professional should use preparticipation screening as a tool to identify risks and limitations of each client before engaging in exercise testing or programming.

Physical Activity Readiness Questionnaire for Everyone

The Physical Activity Readiness Questionnaire for Everyone, commonly abbreviated as PAR-Q+, is a questionnaire (figure 2.1) developed in Canada that asks an individual to self-report signs and symptoms that may indicate the need for further medical-based screening before completing a fitness assessment or starting an exercise program (25, 42). The benefits of using the PAR-Q+ include cost-effectiveness and ease of administration. Further screening may be required to determine the appropriateness of submaximal or maximal exercise testing and whether the program can include moderate- or high-intensity exercise. While a client exercise readiness questionnaire such as the PAR-Q+ is an excellent initial screening tool, it does not identify all of an individual's medical and health concerns, so a further assessment may be needed.

Medical History Questionnaire

The medical history questionnaire (figure 2.2) is a tool complementary to the PAR-Q+ that more thoroughly recognizes existing diagnosed pathologies, orthopedic conditions, recent surgical procedures, self-reported medical history, and current medications. Sometimes one questionnaire covers both medical- and health-related issues, and other times there are two separate questionnaires; the specific form or forms depend on the preference of the exercise professional, type of facility where he works, common conditions of the clients he works with, or a combination of these factors. The information gathered from the PAR-Q+ and medical history questionnaire provides the exercise professional with the details necessary to identify specific health needs and risk factors and to determine the appropriateness of a fitness assessment and exercise program.

After all preparticipation screening forms are completed and all documentation has been thoroughly reviewed, it is necessary to evaluate the content of the information to identify any potential risks associated with the individual's present health status. This evaluation enables the exercise professional to refer people with existing disease or symptoms of disease to a health care professional for medical clearance.

Informed Consent Form

Before the administration of any exercise test or the initiation of a prescribed exercise program, it is the responsibility of the exercise professional to make certain that all procedures and exercises, benefits of participation, and risks and discomforts of each test, exercise, or program are explained to and understood by the client. Many professionals use an informed consent form (figure 2.3) to be sure that this task is adequately accomplished. The informed consent form contains details regarding the testing procedures and exercise programming and typically requires a signature from the client to indicate that she understands the procedures and exercises, acknowledges that participation in all activities is voluntary, and is aware that a test or exercise session can be stopped at any time without penalty. Any and all informed consent forms should be approved by administrators, legal counsel, or an institutional review board before use (22).

Medical Clearance Form

The exercise professional is responsible for screening clients to identify individuals who may be of increased exercise-related risk of serious cardiovascular events, such as myocardial infarction or sudden cardiac death. Professional guidelines have been established for referral of these individuals to a health care professional for clearance before initiating a fitness assessment or starting an exercise program (36). The medical clearance recommendation in no way relieves the exercise professional of the obligation to properly screen the client; rather it offers an opportunity for the health care professional and exercise professional to collectively ensure that the assessment and exercise program are implemented with the client's health and safety as a priority.

The medical clearance form allows the health care professional to identify specific medical concerns and, when appropriate, clearance (approval) for the individual to participate in exercise testing and programming. Additional information provided in the medical clearance form may include additional medical concerns or restrictions to exercise programming and the need for a client to have a diagnostic test before exercise.

After the client has been referred to a health care professional for medical clearance, the exercise professional must be sure that the medical clearance form is completed and returned to the exercise professional. There are many examples of this form; a comprehensive version is shown in figure 2.4.

Preparticipation Screening Review

The preparticipation screening tools (i.e., the PAR-Q+ form and the medical history questionnaire) allow the client to self-report known medical and health concerns. These tools address the client's medical history, current medications, surgical history, and orthopedic conditions, as well as diagnosed disease and signs of disease. The exercise professional should use the information derived from the screening tools to develop the client's fitness assessment and exercise program.

Figure 2.1

PAR-Q+

The Physical Activity Readiness Questionnaire for Everyone

The health benefits of regular physical activity are clear; more people should engage in physical activity every day of the week. Participating in physical activity is very safe for MOST people. This questionnaire will tell you whether it is necessary for you to seek further advice from your doctor OR a qualified exercise professional before becoming more physically active.

GENERAL HEALTH QUESTIONS

Please read the 7 questions below carefully and answer each one honestly: check YES or NO.	YES	NO
1) Has your doctor ever said that you have a heart condition ☐ OR high blood pressure ☐?	☐	☐
2) Do you feel pain in your chest at rest, during your daily activities of living, **OR** when you do physical activity?	☐	☐
3) Do you lose balance because of dizziness **OR** have you lost consciousness in the last 12 months? Please answer **NO** if your dizziness was associated with over-breathing (including during vigorous exercise).	☐	☐
4) Have you ever been diagnosed with another chronic medical condition (other than heart disease or high blood pressure)? **PLEASE LIST CONDITION(S) HERE:** _____	☐	☐
5) Are you currently taking prescribed medications for a chronic medical condition? **PLEASE LIST CONDITION(S) AND MEDICATIONS HERE:** _____	☐	☐
6) Do you currently have (or have had within the past 12 months) a bone, joint, or soft tissue (muscle, ligament, or tendon) problem that could be made worse by becoming more physically active? Please answer **NO** if you had a problem in the past, but it *does not limit your current ability* to be physically active. **PLEASE LIST CONDITION(S) HERE:** _____	☐	☐
7) Has your doctor ever said that you should only do medically supervised physical activity?	☐	☐

**If you answered NO to all of the questions above, you are cleared for physical activity.
Go to Page 4 to sign the PARTICIPANT DECLARATION. You do not need to complete Pages 2 and 3.**

- ▶ Start becoming much more physically active – start slowly and build up gradually.
- ▶ Follow International Physical Activity Guidelines for your age (www.who.int/dietphysicalactivity/en/).
- ▶ You may take part in a health and fitness appraisal.
- ▶ If you are over the age of 45 yr and **NOT** accustomed to regular vigorous to maximal effort exercise, consult a qualified exercise professional before engaging in this intensity of exercise.
- ▶ If you have any further questions, contact a qualified exercise professional.

If you answered YES to one or more of the questions above, COMPLETE PAGES 2 AND 3.

⚠ **Delay becoming more active if:**

You have a temporary illness such as a cold or fever; it is best to wait until you feel better.

You are pregnant - talk to your health care practitioner, your physician, a qualified exercise professional, and/or complete the ePARmed-X+ at **www.eparmedx.com** before becoming more physically active.

Your health changes - answer the questions on Pages 2 and 3 of this document and/or talk to your doctor or a qualified exercise professional before continuing with any physical activity program.

OSHF
Ontario Society for Health and Fitness

Copyright 2016 PAR-Q+ Collaboration   1/4
01-01-2016

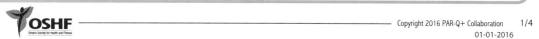
From NSCA, 2018, *NSCA's essentials of training special populations*, P. Jacobs (ed.), (Champaign, IL: Human Kinetics). Reprinted, by permission, from the PAR-Q+ Collaboration and the authors of the PAR-Q+ (Dr. Darren Warburton, Dr. Norman Gledhill, Dr. Veronica Jamnik, and Dr. Shannon Bredin).

PAR-Q+

FOLLOW-UP QUESTIONS ABOUT YOUR MEDICAL CONDITION(S)

1. **Do you have Arthritis, Osteoporosis, or Back Problems?**

If the above condition(s) is/are present, answer questions 1a-1c   If **NO** ☐ go to question 2

1a. Do you have difficulty controlling your condition with medications or other physician-prescribed therapies? (Answer **NO** if you are not currently taking medications or other treatments)   YES ☐ NO ☐

1b. Do you have joint problems causing pain, a recent fracture or fracture caused by osteoporosis or cancer, displaced vertebra (e.g., spondylolisthesis), and/or spondylolysis/pars defect (a crack in the bony ring on the back of the spinal column)?   YES ☐ NO ☐

1c. Have you had steroid injections or taken steroid tablets regularly for more than 3 months?   YES ☐ NO ☐

2. **Do you have Cancer of any kind?**

If the above condition(s) is/are present, answer questions 2a-2b   If **NO** ☐ go to question 3

2a. Does your cancer diagnosis include any of the following types: lung/bronchogenic, multiple myeloma (cancer of plasma cells), head, and neck?   YES ☐ NO ☐

2b. Are you currently receiving cancer therapy (such as chemotheraphy or radiotherapy)?   YES ☐ NO ☐

3. **Do you have a Heart or Cardiovascular Condition?** *This includes Coronary Artery Disease, Heart Failure, Diagnosed Abnormality of Heart Rhythm*

If the above condition(s) is/are present, answer questions 3a-3d   If **NO** ☐ go to question 4

3a. Do you have difficulty controlling your condition with medications or other physician-prescribed therapies? (Answer **NO** if you are not currently taking medications or other treatments)   YES ☐ NO ☐

3b. Do you have an irregular heart beat that requires medical management? (e.g., atrial fibrillation, premature ventricular contraction)   YES ☐ NO ☐

3c. Do you have chronic heart failure?   YES ☐ NO ☐

3d. Do you have diagnosed coronary artery (cardiovascular) disease and have not participated in regular physical activity in the last 2 months?   YES ☐ NO ☐

4. **Do you have High Blood Pressure?**

If the above condition(s) is/are present, answer questions 4a-4b   If **NO** ☐ go to question 5

4a. Do you have difficulty controlling your condition with medications or other physician-prescribed therapies? (Answer **NO** if you are not currently taking medications or other treatments)   YES ☐ NO ☐

4b. Do you have a resting blood pressure equal to or greater than 160/90 mmHg with or without medication? (Answer **YES** if you do not know your resting blood pressure)   YES ☐ NO ☐

5. **Do you have any Metabolic Conditions?** *This includes Type 1 Diabetes, Type 2 Diabetes, Pre-Diabetes*

If the above condition(s) is/are present, answer questions 5a-5e   If **NO** ☐ go to question 6

5a. Do you often have difficulty controlling your blood sugar levels with foods, medications, or other physician-prescribed therapies?   YES ☐ NO ☐

5b. Do you often suffer from signs and symptoms of low blood sugar (hypoglycemia) following exercise and/or during activities of daily living? Signs of hypoglycemia may include shakiness, nervousness, unusual irritability, abnormal sweating, dizziness or light-headedness, mental confusion, difficulty speaking, weakness, or sleepiness.   YES ☐ NO ☐

5c. Do you have any signs or symptoms of diabetes complications such as heart or vascular disease and/or complications affecting your eyes, kidneys, **OR** the sensation in your toes and feet?   YES ☐ NO ☐

5d. Do you have other metabolic conditions (such as current pregnancy-related diabetes, chronic kidney disease, or liver problems)?   YES ☐ NO ☐

5e. Are you planning to engage in what for you is unusually high (or vigorous) intensity exercise in the near future?   YES ☐ NO ☐

(continued)

From NSCA, 2018, *NSCA's essentials of training special populations*, P. Jacobs (ed.), (Champaign, IL: Human Kinetics). Reprinted, by permission, from the PAR-Q+ Collaboration and the authors of the PAR-Q+ (Dr. Darren Warburton, Dr. Norman Gledhill, Dr. Veronica Jamnik, and Dr. Shannon Bredin).

PAR-Q+

6. **Do you have any Mental Health Problems or Learning Difficulties?** *This includes Alzheimer's, Dementia, Depression, Anxiety Disorder, Eating Disorder, Psychotic Disorder, Intellectual Disability, Down Syndrome*

If the above condition(s) is/are present, answer questions 6a-6b   If **NO** ☐ go to question 7

6a.	Do you have difficulty controlling your condition with medications or other physician-prescribed therapies? (Answer **NO** if you are not currently taking medications or other treatments)	YES ☐ NO ☐
6b.	Do you have Down Syndrome and back problems affecting nerves or muscles?	YES ☐ NO ☐

7. **Do you have a Respiratory Disease?** *This includes Chronic Obstructive Pulmonary Disease, Asthma, Pulmonary High Blood Pressure*

If the above condition(s) is/are present, answer questions 7a-7d   If **NO** ☐ go to question 8

7a.	Do you have difficulty controlling your condition with medications or other physician-prescribed therapies? (Answer **NO** if you are not currently taking medications or other treatments)	YES ☐ NO ☐
7b.	Has your doctor ever said your blood oxygen level is low at rest or during exercise and/or that you require supplemental oxygen therapy?	YES ☐ NO ☐
7c.	If asthmatic, do you currently have symptoms of chest tightness, wheezing, laboured breathing, consistent cough (more than 2 days/week), or have you used your rescue medication more than twice in the last week?	YES ☐ NO ☐
7d.	Has your doctor ever said you have high blood pressure in the blood vessels of your lungs?	YES ☐ NO ☐

8. **Do you have a Spinal Cord Injury?** *This includes Tetraplegia and Paraplegia*

If the above condition(s) is/are present, answer questions 8a-8c   If **NO** ☐ go to question 9

8a.	Do you have difficulty controlling your condition with medications or other physician-prescribed therapies? (Answer **NO** if you are not currently taking medications or other treatments)	YES ☐ NO ☐
8b.	Do you commonly exhibit low resting blood pressure significant enough to cause dizziness, light-headedness, and/or fainting?	YES ☐ NO ☐
8c.	Has your physician indicated that you exhibit sudden bouts of high blood pressure (known as Autonomic Dysreflexia)?	YES ☐ NO ☐

9. **Have you had a Stroke?** *This includes Transient Ischemic Attack (TIA) or Cerebrovascular Event*

If the above condition(s) is/are present, answer questions 9a-9c   If **NO** ☐ go to question 10

9a.	Do you have difficulty controlling your condition with medications or other physician-prescribed therapies? (Answer **NO** if you are not currently taking medications or other treatments)	YES ☐ NO ☐
9b.	Do you have any impairment in walking or mobility?	YES ☐ NO ☐
9c.	Have you experienced a stroke or impairment in nerves or muscles in the past 6 months?	YES ☐ NO ☐

10. **Do you have any other medical condition not listed above or do you have two or more medical conditions?**

If you have other medical conditions, answer questions 10a-10c   If **NO** ☐ read the Page 4 recommendations

10a.	Have you experienced a blackout, fainted, or lost consciousness as a result of a head injury within the last 12 months **OR** have you had a diagnosed concussion within the last 12 months?	YES ☐ NO ☐
10b.	Do you have a medical condition that is not listed (such as epilepsy, neurological conditions, kidney problems)?	YES ☐ NO ☐
10c.	Do you currently live with two or more medical conditions?	YES ☐ NO ☐

PLEASE LIST YOUR MEDICAL CONDITION(S) AND ANY RELATED MEDICATIONS HERE: _____

_____

GO to Page 4 for recommendations about your current medical condition(s) and sign the PARTICIPANT DECLARATION.

Copyright 2016 PAR-Q+ Collaboration   3/4
01-01-2016

PAR-Q+

☑ **If you answered NO to all of the follow-up questions about your medical condition, you are ready to become more physically active - sign the PARTICIPANT DECLARATION below:**

▶ It is advised that you consult a qualified exercise professional to help you develop a safe and effective physical activity plan to meet your health needs.

▶ You are encouraged to start slowly and build up gradually - 20 to 60 minutes of low to moderate intensity exercise, 3-5 days per week including aerobic and muscle strengthening exercises.

▶ As you progress, you should aim to accumulate 150 minutes or more of moderate intensity physical activity per week.

▶ If you are over the age of 45 yr and **NOT** accustomed to regular vigorous to maximal effort exercise, consult a qualified exercise professional before engaging in this intensity of exercise.

⬤ **If you answered YES to one or more of the follow-up questions about your medical condition:**

You should seek further information before becoming more physically active or engaging in a fitness appraisal. You should complete the specially designed online screening and exercise recommendations program - the **ePARmed-X+ at www.eparmedx.com** and/or visit a qualified exercise professional to work through the ePARmed-X+ and for further information.

⚠ **Delay becoming more active if:**

✓ You have a temporary illness such as a cold or fever; it is best to wait until you feel better.

✓ You are pregnant - talk to your health care practitioner, your physician, a qualified exercise professional, and/or complete the ePARmed-X+ **at www.eparmedx.com** before becoming more physically active.

✓ Your health changes - talk to your doctor or qualified exercise professional before continuing with any physical activity program.

⬤ You are encouraged to photocopy the PAR-Q+. You must use the entire questionnaire and NO changes are permitted.
⬤ The authors, the PAR-Q+ Collaboration, partner organizations, and their agents assume no liability for persons who undertake physical activity and/or make use of the PAR-Q+ or ePARmed-X+. If in doubt after completing the questionnaire, consult your doctor prior to physical activity.

PARTICIPANT DECLARATION

⬤ All persons who have completed the PAR-Q+ please read and sign the declaration below.

⬤ If you are less than the legal age required for consent or require the assent of a care provider, your parent, guardian or care provider must also sign this form.

I, the undersigned, have read, understood to my full satisfaction and completed this questionnaire. I acknowledge that this physical activity clearance is valid for a maximum of 12 months from the date it is completed and becomes invalid if my condition changes. I also acknowledge that a Trustee (such as my employer, community/fitness centre, health care provider, or other designate) may retain a copy of this form for their records. In these instances, the Trustee will be required to adhere to local, national, and international guidelines regarding the storage of personal health information ensuring that the Trustee maintains the privacy of the information and does not misuse or wrongfully disclose such information.

NAME _____   DATE _____

SIGNATURE _____   WITNESS _____

SIGNATURE OF PARENT/GUARDIAN/CARE PROVIDER _____

───── **For more information, please contact** ─────
www.eparmedx.com
Email: eparmedx@gmail.com

Citation for PAR-Q+
Warburton DER, Jamnik VK, Bredin SSD, and Gledhill N on behalf of the PAR-Q+ Collaboration. The Physical Activity Readiness Questionnaire for Everyone (PAR-Q+) and Electronic Physical Activity Readiness Medical Examination (ePARmed-X+). Health & Fitness Journal of Canada 4(2):3-23, 2011.
Key References
1. Jamnik VK, Warburton DER, Makarski J, McKenzie DC, Shephard RJ, Stone J, and Gledhill N. Enhancing the effectiveness of clearance for physical activity participation; background and overall process. APNM 36(S1):S3-S13, 2011.
2. Warburton DER, Gledhill N, Jamnik VK, Bredin SSD, McKenzie DC, Stone J, Charlesworth S, and Shephard RJ. Evidence-based risk assessment and recommendations for physical activity clearance; Consensus Document. APNM 36(S1):S266-s298, 2011.

The PAR-Q+ was created using the evidence-based AGREE process (1) by the PAR-Q+ Collaboration chaired by Dr. Darren E. R. Warburton with Dr. Norman Gledhill, Dr. Veronica Jamnik, and Dr. Donald C. McKenzie (2). Production of this document has been made possible through financial contributions from the Public Health Agency of Canada and the BC Ministry of Health Services. The views expressed herein do not necessarily represent the views of the Public Health Agency of Canada or the BC Ministry of Health Services.

✝ **OSHF**
Ontario Society for Health and Fitness
This document has been adapted (with permission) for inclusion in *canfitpro* documents.

Copyright 2016 PAR-Q+ Collaboration   4/4
01-01-2016

Figure 2.2 Medical History Questionnaire

Demographic Information

Last name	First name	Middle initial
Date of birth	Sex	Home phone
Address	City, State	Zip code
Work phone	Family physician	

Section A

1. When was the last time you had a physical examination?

2. If you are allergic to any medications, foods, or other substances, please name them.

3. If you have been told that you have any chronic or serious illnesses, please list them.

4. Give the following information pertaining to the last 3 times you have been hospitalized.
   Note: Women, do not list normal pregnancies.

	Hospitalization 1	Hospitalization 2	Hospitalization 3
Reason for hospitalization	_____	_____	_____
Month and year of hospitalization	_____	_____	_____
Hospital	_____	_____	_____
City and state	_____	_____	_____

Section B

During the past 12 months

1. Has a physician prescribed any form of medication for you? ☐ Yes ☐ No

2. Has your weight fluctuated more than a few pounds? ☐ Yes ☐ No

3. Did you attempt to bring about this weight change through diet or exercise? ☐ Yes ☐ No

4. Have you experienced any faintness, light-headedness, or blackouts? ☐ Yes ☐ No

5. Have you occasionally had trouble sleeping? ☐ Yes ☐ No

6. Have you experienced any blurred vision? ☐ Yes ☐ No

7. Have you had any severe headaches? ☐ Yes ☐ No

8. Have you experienced chronic morning cough? ☐ Yes ☐ No

9. Have you experienced any temporary change in your speech pattern, such as slurring or loss of speech? ☐ Yes ☐ No

10. Have you felt unusually nervous or anxious for no apparent reason? ☐ Yes ☐ No

11. Have you experienced unusual heartbeats such as skipped beats or palpitations? ☐ Yes ☐ No

12. Have you experienced periods in which your heart felt as though it were racing for no apparent reason? ☐ Yes ☐ No

At present

1. Do you experience shortness or loss of breath while walking with others your own age? ☐ Yes ☐ No

2. Do you experience sudden tingling, numbness, or loss of feeling in your arms, hands, legs, feet, or face? ☐ Yes ☐ No

3. Have you ever noticed that your hands or feet sometimes feel cooler than other parts of your body? ☐ Yes ☐ No

4. Do you experience swelling of your feet and ankles? ☐ Yes ☐ No

5. Do you get pains or cramps in your legs? ☐ Yes ☐ No

6. Do you experience any pain or discomfort in your chest? ☐ Yes ☐ No

7. Do you experience any pressure or heaviness in your chest? ☐ Yes ☐ No

8. Have you ever been told that your blood pressure was abnormal? ☐ Yes ☐ No

9. Have you ever been told that your serum cholesterol or triglyceride level was high? ☐ Yes ☐ No

10. Do you have diabetes? ☐ Yes ☐ No
    If yes, how is it controlled?

    ☐ Dietary means ☐ Insulin injection ☐ Oral medication ☐ Uncontrolled

11. How often would you characterize your stress level as being high?

    ☐ Occasionally ☐ Frequently ☐ Constantly

12. Have you ever been told that you have any of the following illnesses? ☐ Yes ☐ No

    ☐ Myocardial infarction ☐ Arteriosclerosis ☐ Heart disease ☐ Thyroid disease

    ☐ Coronary thrombosis ☐ Rheumatic heart ☐ Heart attack ☐ Heart valve disease

    ☐ Coronary occlusion ☐ Heart failure ☐ Heart murmur

    ☐ Heart block ☐ Aneurysm ☐ Angina

13. Have you ever had any of the following medical procedures? ☐ Yes ☐ No

    ☐ Heart surgery ☐ Pacemaker implant

    ☐ Cardiac catheterization ☐ Defibrillator

    ☐ Coronary angioplasty ☐ Heart transplantation

Section C

Has any member of your immediate family been treated for or suspected to have had any of these conditions? Please identify their relationship to you (father, mother, sister, brother, etc.).

a. Diabetes

b. Heart disease

c. Stroke

d. High blood pressure

From NSCA, 2018, *NSCA's essentials of training special populations*, P. Jacobs (ed.), (Champaign, IL: Human Kinetics). Reprinted, by permission, from V.H. Heyward and A.L. Gibson, 2014, *Advanced fitness assessment and exercise prescription*, 7th ed. (Champaign, IL: Human Kinetics), 366, 367.

Figure 2.3   Informed Consent

In order to assess cardiovascular function, body composition, and other physical fitness components, the undersigned hereby voluntarily consents to engage in one or more of the following tests (check the appropriate boxes):

❏ Graded exercise stress test
❏ Body composition tests
❏ Muscle fitness tests
❏ Flexibility tests
❏ Balance tests

Explanation of the Tests

The graded exercise test is performed on a cycle ergometer or motor-driven treadmill. The workload is increased every few minutes until exhaustion or until other symptoms dictate that we terminate the test. You may stop the test at any time because of fatigue or discomfort.

The underwater weighing procedure involves being completely submerged in a tank or tub after fully exhaling the air from your lungs. You will be submerged for 3 to 5 seconds while we measure your underwater weight. This test provides an accurate assessment of your body composition.

For muscle fitness testing, you lift weights for a number of repetitions using barbells or exercise machines. These tests assess the muscular strength and endurance of the major muscle groups in the body.

For evaluation of flexibility, you perform a number of tests. During these tests, we measure the range of motion in your joints.

For balance tests, we will be measuring the amount of time you can maintain certain stances or the distance you are able to reach without losing balance.

Risks and Discomforts

During the graded exercise test, certain changes may occur. These changes include abnormal blood pressure responses, fainting, irregularities in heartbeat, and heart attack. Every effort is made to minimize these occurrences. Emergency equipment and trained personnel are available to deal with these situations if they occur.

You may experience some discomfort during the underwater weighing, especially after you expire all the air from your lungs. However, this discomfort is momentary, lasting only 3 to 5 seconds. If this test causes you too much discomfort, an alternative procedure (e.g., skinfold or bioelectrical impedance test) can be used to estimate your body composition.

There is a slight possibility of pulling a muscle or spraining a ligament during the muscle fitness and flexibility testing. In addition, you may experience muscle soreness 24 or 48 hours after testing. These risks can be minimized by performing warm-up exercises before taking the tests. If muscle soreness occurs, appropriate stretching exercises to relieve this soreness will be demonstrated.

Expected Benefits From Testing

These tests allow us to assess your physical working capacity and to appraise your physical fitness status. The results are used to prescribe a safe, sound exercise program for you. Records are kept strictly confidential unless you consent to release this information.

Inquiries

Questions about the procedures used in the physical fitness tests are encouraged. If you have any questions or need additional information, please ask us to explain further.

Freedom of Consent

Your permission to perform these physical fitness tests is strictly voluntary. You are free to stop the tests at any point, if you so desire.

I have read this form carefully and I fully understand the test procedures that I will perform and the risks and discomforts. Knowing these risks and having had the opportunity to ask questions that have been answered to my satisfaction, I consent to participate in these tests.

Date _____ Signature of patient _____

Date _____ Signature of witness _____

Date _____ Signature of supervisor _____

Figure 2.4 Medical Clearance Form Pertaining to a Fitness Assessment and Exercise Program

Dear Health Care Professional:

Your patient, _____, has contacted us regarding the fitness evaluation conducted by _____. The program is designed to evaluate the individual's fitness status before embarking on an exercise program. From this evaluation, an exercise prescription is formulated. In addition, other parameters related to a health improvement program are discussed with the participant. It is important to understand that this program is preventive and is not intended to be rehabilitative in nature.

The fitness testing includes: _____

_____

_____

A comprehensive consultation will be provided to the participant that serves to review the test results and explain recommendations for an individualized fitness program.

A summary of test results and our recommendations will be kept on file and may be made available to you upon request.

In the interest of your patient and for our information, please complete the following:

a. Has this patient undergone a physical examination within the last year to assess functional capacity to perform exercise? Yes ___ No ___

b. I consider this patient (please check one):

____ Class I: presumably healthy without apparent heart disease eligible to participate in an unsupervised program

____ Class II: presumably healthy with one or more risk factors for heart disease eligible to participate in a supervised program

____ Class III: patient not eligible for this program, and a medically supervised program is recommended

c. Does this patient have any preexisting medical/orthopedic condition(s) requiring continued or long-term medical treatment or follow-up? Yes ___ No ___

Please explain: _____

_____

d. Are you aware of any medical condition(s) that this patient may have or may have had that could be worsened by exercise? Yes ___ No ___

e. Please list any currently prescribed medication(s): _____

_____

_____

f. Please provide specific recommendations and/or list any restrictions concerning this patient's present health status as it relates to active participation in a fitness program.

_____

_____

Comments: _____

_____

Health Care Professional's signature: _____Date: _____

Client's name: _____

Phone (H): _____ Phone (W): _____

Address: _____

_____

AUTHORIZATION TO RELEASE MEDICAL INFORMATION

I consent to and authorize _____ to release any medical information concerning my ability to participate in an exercise program or fitness assessment. My authorization is not valid beyond one year of signature.

Patient's name (print) _____ Date _____

Patient's signature _____

Please return this form to:

Name _____

Street address _____

City, State, Zip _____

From NSCA, 2018, *NSCA's essentials of training special populations,* P. Jacobs (ed.), (Champaign, IL: Human Kinetics). Reprinted, by permission, from NSCA, 2013, *NSCA's essentials of personal training,* 2nd ed., J. Coburn and M. Malek (eds.), (Champaign, IL: Human Kinetics), 178.

Recognizing the risk factors for disease is vital for the accountability of the exercise professional and the reduction of health and safety risks incurred by clients. Additionally, it is the exercise professional's responsibility to identify signs and symptoms of cardiovascular, pulmonary, metabolic, immunologic, hematologic, orthopedic, neuromuscular, cognitive, psychological, and sensory disorders that require restrictions or modifications with exercise due to a potential exacerbation of an existing condition. Clients who have been diagnosed with or exhibit symptoms of disease may require modified assessment and programming guidelines, which are outlined for various conditions in subsequent chapters in this text.

The preparticipation screening affords data critical in the consideration for medical referral. Exercise professionals should apply established guidelines to determine the appropriateness of medical clearance before initiating an exercise program (36). The preparticipation tools include a self-report of the presence of disease, signs of disease, and training status, all of which determine the recommendations for medical clearance.

Medical Clearance Process

A fitness assessment should not be performed and an exercise program should not begin until the exercise professional has determined that the client does not exhibit or possess characteristics that potentially place the client at increased risk of a serious cardiovascular event. There are guidelines specifying the conditions that warrant referral of clients to a medical professional for clearance before the initiation of exercise testing or training (36). These recommendations are based on factors (e.g., current activity level, signs of potential disease, and known existence of disease) that increase the risk of a cardiovascular event during exercise and affect the parameters (e.g., intensity) of prescribed exercise.

It is known that persons who are physically inactive present a significantly greater risk of serious cardiovascular events as compared with physically active individuals (16). Regular physical activity has also been shown to be inversely related to the risk of a serious cardiovascular event during or immediately following intense exercise

(13). The relative risks of exercise-related cardiovascular events are known to be markedly greater from intense exercise than at rest; however, the absolute risk of a cardiac event during exercise is low (1). Finally, warning signs or symptoms of disease, particularly cardiovascular disease, are commonly exhibited before a serious cardiovascular event (41). Thus, the recommendations for medical referral are based on the known risks of exercise and include the client's current exercise training status, the presence of disease, signs or symptoms of disease, and the intensity of recommended exercise testing and training.

Recommendations for referral of clients for medical clearance is based to a great degree on the known presence of disease recognized to increase the risk of a serious exercise-related cardiovascular event. Diseases that should be considered in this regard include the following:

- Cardiovascular disease
  - Cardiac
  - Peripheral vascular disease
  - Cerebrovascular disease
- Metabolic disease
  - Type I and Type II diabetes
- Renal disease

The exercise professional should use the results of the PAR-Q+ and the medical history questionnaire to reveal any signs or symptoms that are suggestive of disease known to increase the risk of a cardiovascular event during exercise. Signs and symptoms of cardiovascular, renal, or metabolic disease include the following (2, 14, 18):

- Pain or discomfort in the arms, neck, chest, jaw, or other areas that could be indicative of **angina** or **ischemia** (impaired coronary artery blood flow)
- Shortness of breath during mild exertion or while resting
- Dizziness or **syncope** (fainting)
- **Orthopnea** (shortness of breath while lying supine) or paroxysmal dyspnea (shortness of breath that occurs while sleeping)
- Ankle **edema** (swelling or water retention)

- Heart palpations or tachycardia (elevated resting heart rate)
- Intermittent **claudication** (cramps in the lower leg)
- Heart murmur
- Unusual fatigue occurring with usual activities or shortness of breath with usual activities

Guidelines for the referral of clients for medical clearance are related to the prescribed intensity of the exercise program. Parameters for **light-intensity exercise**, **moderate-intensity exercise**, and **vigorous-intensity exercise** are the following (36):

- Light-intensity exercise:
  - 30% to <40% $\dot{V}O_2$ or heart rate reserve
  - 2 to <3 METs
  - 9-11 RPE (on 6- to 20-point Borg scale)
  - Intensity producing a slight increase in heart rate and respiration rate
- Moderate-intensity exercise:
  - 40% to <60% $\dot{V}O_2$ or heart rate reserve
  - 3 to <6 METs
  - 12-13 RPE (on 6- to 20-point Borg scale)
  - Intensity producing a noticeable increase in heart rate and respiration rate
- Vigorous-intensity exercise:
  - ≥60% to 90% $\dot{V}O_2$ or heart rate reserve
  - ≥6 METs
  - ≥14 RPE (on 6- to 20-point Borg scale)
  - Intensity producing a substantial increase in heart rate and respiration rate

Physically active clients who do not exhibit known disease or signs or symptoms of disease are not recommended to seek medical clearance and may continue with moderate- to vigorous-intensity training and may increase intensity as tolerated. Physically inactive clients without disease or signs of disease may start exercise training with light to moderate intensity without medical clearance, progressing intensity as tolerated.

Clients who are physically active and have history of cardiovascular, metabolic, or renal disease but are asymptomatic are not required to receive medical clearance for moderate-intensity exercise if they have received clearance in the previous 12-month period. Physically inactive clients who have a known disease but are asymptomatic should be referred to a medical professional for clearance prior to any exercise testing or training. Following medical clearance, these clients should begin with light- to moderate-intensity exercise with intensity gradually increased as tolerated.

Clients who develop new signs or symptoms of disease should be referred for medical clearance regardless of training status or the presence of disease. If the client is presently engaged in an exercise program, it must be discontinued and medical clearance should be obtained before recommencing any exercise program. Following medical clearance, inactive clients displaying symptoms of disease should initiate exercise at a light to moderate intensity level and progress as tolerated.

Program Supervision Recommendations

Medical clearance provides the exercise professional with approval and recommendations regarding specific concerns or restrictions to exercise testing and programming. Based on the medical evaluation and diagnosis, the physician or other health care professional will generally recommend either a supervised or medically supervised assessment and exercise program. A **supervised assessment and exercise program** is recommended for clients who have a medically identified condition or limitation but are still allowed to participate in a fitness assessment or exercise program (14). The assessment and programming need to be overseen by a certified fitness professional who can assess, monitor, and modify the testing or exercise session when necessary.

A **medically supervised assessment and exercise program** is recommended for high-risk clients who have medically identified participation restrictions related to assessment tests, exercise programming, or both (14). The assessments and programming are directed and monitored by a health care professional in a controlled clinical setting that offers immediate emergency care (14).

Key Point

Medical clearance provides the exercise professional with approval from a health care professional for the participation in either a supervised program or a medically supervised program. Exercise professionals should oversee the testing and training in supervised programs, while medically supervised programs should be managed by a health care professional.

FITNESS ASSESSMENT

After the medical and health history appraisal process, the exercise professional needs to assess the client's current level of functional fitness capacities before developing an exercise program. The decision regarding the battery of tests to perform requires consideration of the client's medical and health history and fitness-related goals, as well as the exercise professional's experience in conducting assessments on clients who have the specific needs or conditions presented by the client. Test selection is also influenced by the availability and necessity of the appropriate environment, facilities, and equipment.

After determining the tests, the exercise professional is responsible for administering the tests, recording and managing the data, and interpreting the results. These steps need to be completed before short-, medium-, and long-term goals can be established.

Rationale for and Benefits of Testing

Assessment (often simply called *testing*) is a critical component in the development of a safe and effective exercise program especially for clients who have a medical- or health-related condition. In all cases, the selected tests should be specific to each client and based on his needs.

The rationale for performing an assessment on a client includes the following (35):

- A baseline for future comparisons of improvement or rate of progress
- Identification of current levels of fitness that will contribute to the exercise program

- Establishment of appropriate exercise selection, frequency of exercise, intensity of exercise, and volume of exercise
- Development of short-, medium-, and long-term fitness goals
- Identification of a client's needs and limitations before exercise program initiation, as directed by a health care professional, and information received from client interaction
- A method of recording decisions regarding appropriate scope of practice in case the client experiences an injury or an exacerbation of a current medical or health condition after the program begins (21)

Assessment Goals

The exercise professional can use the results of an assessment in combination with information gathered from the medical and health history questionnaire and medical clearance form to design a proper exercise program. Understanding the client's current physical fitness, medical and health concerns, and well-being enables the exercise professional to create a program that is reasonable in frequency, intensity, time, and type of exercise to promote long-term participation. In conjunction, establishing program goals and objectives with the client as part of the assessment process is critical to adherence.

Assessment Standardization

One of the responsibilities of the exercise professional working with a client is to enhance physical fitness without causing harm to the client (21). Assessment test batteries should be standardized as much as possible, but some variation in test selection may be necessary to accommodate individual needs. All fitness assessment tests should be of high validity, reliability, and accuracy. Test administration should be standardized as much as possible, and the professional performing the assessments should be qualified and trained to administer each test.

Assessment Standards

The results obtained from fitness assessment tests can be compared to standards derived from **norm-referenced data**, from **criterion-referenced** standards, longitudinally to the results of the client, or from a combination of these approaches. Standards for fitness assessments based on norm-referenced data are used to compare the fitness level of like individuals (sex, age, and so on) on the same test. These results are usually reported as a percentile rank. In this type of system, results are often indicated as follows:

- 0% to 20% = well below average or poor
- 21% to 40% = below average
- 41% to 60% = average
- 61% to 80% = above average
- 81% to 100% = well above average or excellent

Criterion-referenced physical fitness tests have predetermined levels of acceptable minimal outcomes for performance. If the results of a criterion-referenced test exceed the minimal standard, then the client has successfully completed the test. A good example of a criterion-referenced fitness assessment is FitnessGram, which is a battery of tests that includes assessment of aerobic endurance, strength, flexibility, and body composition (44). The periodic and systematic collection of a client's longitudinal data allows for the observation of improvement in each fitness category over time. What is most critical for clients to observe with repeated assessments is a positive improvement in assessment scores from the baseline level, which highlights improvement and continuous movement toward the client's goals.

Currently, there are no general physical fitness standards based on normative or criterion-referenced data for diseased or disabled populations; therefore it is essential that the exercise professional establish realistic short-, medium-, and long-term goals for clients whose baseline scores place them below average or well below average for healthy individuals. The ability to set reasonable goals for improvements and progress levels for all clients who may not reach an average score based on norm-referenced standards is critical to exercise adherence for the client. Setting reasonable goals that can be attained provides a client with positive feedback upon attaining goals. Goal setting can be a valuable tool for enhancing participation in exercise programming (20). See the discussion of SMART goal setting later in this chapter.

Client Factors

In selecting a test, it is essential to evaluate factors that may positively and negatively influence a client's performance and subsequently affect the validity, reliability, and accuracy of the assessment results. It is incumbent on the exercise professional to recognize any condition that may result in the alteration of the standard assessment test battery and make adjustments according to the client's individual needs. For example, a client who has trouble walking should use an arm ergometer and not a treadmill as a testing mode during an assessment. Additionally, fatigue, whether a function of recent activities, insufficient nutrition or fluid intake, or the demands of the tests being administered, can affect assessment outcomes and as such should be accounted for when one is determining the timing and duration of test administration.

A client's maturity level and chronological age may also affect her test performance. For example, a treadmill test using the Bruce protocol may be considered an appropriate test for younger clients, but this protocol may need to be reduced in intensity for those with known disease or for older adult clients who have higher levels of risk.

Sex-specific physiological factors can affect assessment scores or the protocol of some assessments. Women generally have larger quantities of body fat and less muscle mass than men, as well as a smaller shoulder, hip, and knee structure that supports less muscle mass; as a result they have less of a mechanical advantage than their male counterparts (15). For example, the 30-second arm curl test requires different fixed loads for men (8 pounds [3.6 kg]) than for women (5 pounds [2.3 kg]), demonstrating the sex-specific differences related to client factors that an exercise professional needs to consider when selecting appropriate tests (38).

Key Point

The exercise professional needs to be aware that a client's maturity level and chronological age can both affect exercise test performance and the evaluation of the results.

Test Order

Assessment tests should generally be sequenced such that one test does not affect a subsequent test. For example, assessment of resting heart rate should precede assessments of cardiovascular endurance, as the cardiovascular endurance test will result in a heart rate that is elevated above resting levels. It is also important to always perform assessments in the same order so that comparisons can be made between assessments. The following list places assessment tests in an acceptable order (28):

1. Nonfatiguing tests such as height, weight, resting heart rate, resting blood pressure, flexibility, body composition, anthropometric measurements, and neuromuscular assessments

2. Tests of agility such as the T-test and hexagon test

3. Maximum muscular strength tests such as a one-repetition maximum (1RM) bench press

4. Local muscular endurance such as the partial curl-up test

5. Cardiovascular endurance such as the Bruce protocol or the arm ergometer test

FITNESS ASSESSMENT PROTOCOLS

Evaluating a client's fitness level requires preparation and organization to ensure valid, accurate, and reliable results and maintenance of client safety.

Proper and significant assessment outcomes are greatly affected by the ability of the exercise professional to prepare clients by educating them as to the measurement and assessment description, preparation guidelines, purpose and explanation of procedures, risks, benefits, and assessment expectations. Preparation to evaluate a client's fitness level requires preassessment measurements and selection of appropriate fitness assessments, which involves reviewing safety guidelines, calibrating equipment, and following documentation procedures.

Preassessment Measurements

A client's resting heart rate, resting blood pressure, weight, and height are commonly measured before more active fitness assessments when the person is resting and not subject to the rigors of an exercise test. These measurements help establish a baseline to measure progress and play a role in the design of the subsequent exercise program (e.g., resting heart rate needs to be known to calculate exercise heart rate using the Karvonen formula).

Assessment Protocol: Resting Heart Rate

Equipment

- Watch with a second hand
- Chair

Procedure

Have the client sit comfortably for 3 to 5 minutes. Palpate the radial pulse using the tips of the index and middle finger; do not use the thumb. Count the number of beats starting at 0 and count for 60 seconds.

Note: The exercise professional should not use the thumb to measure heart rate because the thumb has a pulse, which can cause inaccurate counting.

Assessment Protocol: Resting Blood Pressure

Blood pressure has two values: Systolic pressure is generated during left ventricular contraction, and diastolic pressure is generated when the left ventricle heart is relaxing and refilling during the cardiac cycle.

Equipment

- Mercury or aneroid *sphygmomanometer* (a blood pressure measuring device) with cuffs sized for children and adults
- Stethoscope
- Watch with a second hand
- Chair

Procedure

To obtain valid and reliable blood pressure measurements, the exercise professional should practice and become competent with this assessment before testing. Systolic and diastolic blood pressure can be measured according to the following protocol (see figure 2.5):

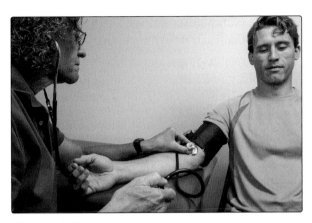

Figure 2.5 Body and equipment positions for measuring resting blood pressure.

- Position the client in an upright seated posture with the back supported and legs uncrossed.
- Select an appropriately sized cuff based on the circumference of the upper arm.
- Locate the brachial artery of the client.
- Securely place the cuff of the sphygmomanometer on the upper arm in a manner that covers the brachial artery and with the bottom of the cuff approximately 1 inch (2.5 cm) above the antecubital space.
- The cuff of the sphygmomanometer should be placed such that the dial or display is readily viewable by the exercise professional.
- When taking measurements, the bell of the stethoscope should be firmly placed directly over the antecubital space, and the client's arm should be level with the heart and in a horizontal position.
- Inflate the cuff rapidly to 160 mmHg or 20 mmHg above known resting systolic blood pressure (40).
- Begin to release the pressure from the cuff slowly (2-3 mmHg per second).
- Systolic blood pressure is recorded as the first audible Korotkoff sound.
- Diastolic pressure is recorded as the disappearance of all Korotkoff sounds.
- Record systolic and diastolic blood pressure in even numbers and to the nearest 2 mmHg (40).
- Consult table 2.1 near the end of the chapter for the blood pressure classifications for adults.

Note: The exercise professional should always select an appropriately sized blood pressure cuff for each client.

Assessment Protocol: Body Weight

Equipment

- Scale or balance that can be calibrated for accuracy

Procedure

Have the client empty his pockets and remove shoes and any other heavy articles of clothing (belts, jackets, heavy sweaters, shoes, and so on). Have the client stand on the measuring device until a stable measurement can be made, and report the weight (pounds or kilograms) to the precision allowed by the measuring device.

Assessment Protocol: Height

Equipment

- Medical stadiometer or a wall with a tape measure affixed to it

Procedure

Have the client remove her shoes and stand erect with the feet together in front of the stadiometer or facing away from the wall with the back of the heels touching the wall. Measure height as the vertical distance (inches or centimeters) from the floor to the crown on the top of the head to the precision allowed by the measuring device. If using a tape measure affixed to a wall, place a ruler (or similar object) on top of the client's head and, while keeping it level, extend it straight back to the tape measure.

Assessment Protocol: Lung Function

The forced expiratory volume (FEV_1) test is used to determine the volume of air exhaled in the first second following a maximal inhalation (3). This test can be used to determine a limitation in pulmonary flow rate.

Equipment

- Spirometer
- Nose clip

Procedure

The instructions for the specific spirometer being used for the test should be followed to obtain correct measurement of FEV_1. The exercise professional should use the nose clip to make certain that no air will come out of the nostrils during the test. The client is asked to perform a forced expiratory maneuver, which requires a maximal inhalation followed by a maximal exhalation while breathing into the spirometer.

Common Fitness Tests

There are eight types or categories of fitness assessments that are tied to the general components of overall fitness (30); commonly, at least one test from each of the following categories is performed:

1. Cardiovascular endurance assessments provide estimations of the client's maximal oxygen consumption ($\dot{V}O_2$max). Cardiovascular endurance tests employ a variety of testing modalities including the treadmill, stair stepper, recumbent stepper (6), cycle ergometer, and arm ergometer.

2. Muscular strength assessments determine the maximum force that a muscle or muscle group can exert in a single effort while maintaining proper technique. Muscular strength is typically assessed by the use of a one-repetition maximum (1RM) protocol.

3. Local muscular endurance assessments measure the ability of a muscle or muscle group to perform repeated submaximal contractions. Local muscle endurance assessments typically count the total number of repetitions per unit time, such as for the partial curl-up test.

4. Flexibility assessments measure the ability to move joints through a prescribed range of motion (ROM). Flexibility assessments include the sit-and-reach and back scratch tests.

5. Anthropometric assessments measure size, shape, and composition of the human body or body segments. Anthropometric assessments include body mass index (BMI), girth measurements, skinfold thicknesses, and bioelectrical impedance analysis (BIA).

6. Neuromuscular assessments measure the ability to do activities that require balance, coordination, skill, or a combination of these.

7. Functional performance assessments measure the ability to do specific physical activities of daily living. An example of a functional performance test is the 8-foot up-and-go test.

8. Assessments specific to clients who have a medical condition can be used in circumstances when other testing protocols may be inappropriate due to fitness or movement restrictions. These assessments include the 6-minute walk test, 2-minute step test, 30-second chair stand test, 30-second arm curl test, and the chair sit-and-reach test.

Cardiovascular Endurance Assessments

The ability to perform cardiovascular endurance exercise is important for completing activities of daily living and is commonly directly assessed in a laboratory setting through the use of a graded exercise test or a comparable field test. However, some clients with chronic disease or disabilities may not be able to achieve a true $\dot{V}O_2$max (30). Rather, they prematurely reach a point at which they cannot continue and are said to reach symptom-limited exhaustion, referred to as **peak $\dot{V}O_2$**. Many such people have a very low peak $\dot{V}O_2$; usually less than 25 ml · kg^{-1} · min^{-1} and often less than 20 ml · kg^{-1} · min^{-1} (30). Daily living activities, often taken for granted by those who are healthy and without disability, require oxygen consumption in the range of 12 to 30 ml · kg^{-1} · min^{-1}. Thus, some clients with chronic disease or disabilities may have a $\dot{V}O_2$max or peak $\dot{V}O_2$ below what is required for activities of daily living, employment, and maintenance of client independence, resulting in a reduced quality of life.

In general, reduced-intensity graded exercise test protocols (e.g., a RAMP protocol) are preferred for these populations over standard protocols (e.g., Bruce protocol). Many standard protocols increase work rate in relatively large, often nonlinear gradients and are effective only in screening for ischemic heart disease. In the management of chronic disease or disabilities, however, it is valuable to discern the exercise response in the submaximal range to best establish a proper exercise intensity for the client's exercise program. Ramp protocols can be superior in this regard because they indicate exercise responses at smaller increments, enabling the exercise professional to best determine the client's submaximal exercise capacity.

Another disadvantage of using a standard protocol is that the test cannot be individualized so that each client can complete the 8 to 10 minutes of exercise time recommended for an accurate assessment (26, 32, 33, 40). In other words, persons with chronic disease or disabilities may have low cardiovascular endurance exercise capacity and be unable to complete the test. Therefore, it is important for the exercise professional to know the client's approximate ability, estimate his peak exercise capacity, and design a test to yield three or four changes in work rates during an 8- to 10-minute test period (10).

Test Termination   The exercise professional must understand that a client can stop the exercise test at any time and for any reason. There are also test termination indicators that can be determined from observations of the client during a test; every exercise professional should be aware of these. An exercise test should be stopped immediately if any of the following occurs (22):

1. Client reports symptoms of angina.
2. Systolic blood pressure drops >10 mmHg from baseline with increasing work rate.
3. Extreme increase in blood pressure.
4. Systolic blood pressure >250 mmHg.
5. Diastolic blood pressure >115 mmHg.
6. Client experiences shortness of breath, wheezing, leg cramps, or other symptoms of claudication due to inadequate blood flow to the leg muscles.
7. Client experiences **ataxia** (loss of voluntary coordination of muscle movements), dizziness, **pallor** (pale skin color), **cyanosis** (blue or purple skin color due to a lack of oxygen in the blood), cold or clammy skin, nausea, or any other sign indicative of poor blood perfusion.
8. Failure of heart rate to increase with increasing work rate.
9. Change in heart rhythm.
10. Client requests to stop the test.
11. Physical or verbal indication of severe fatigue.
12. Malfunction of the testing equipment.

Exercise Test Modalities   The treadmill and cycle ergometer are the most commonly used devices for clinical exercise testing. Treadmill testing provides a more familiar form of physiological stress (because the client is walking or running), with clients more likely to attain a slightly higher oxygen consumption and peak heart rate than during cycle ergometer testing due to increased muscle mass utilization (3, 19, 34). The treadmill should have readily accessible handrails for clients to steady themselves; however, consistently holding the handrails can reduce the accuracy of exercise capacity and the quality of the heart rate recording and so should be discouraged. However, it may be necessary for some clients to hold the handrails lightly for balance. An emergency stop button should also be readily available to the client and supervising exercise professional.

Arm ergometry is an alternative method of exercise testing for clients who cannot perform leg exercise (e.g., due to a spinal cord injury) or for clients who primarily perform dynamic upper body work during occupational or leisure-time activities (4, 23). At the current time, no $\dot{V}O_2$max–peak normative data exist for comparing values derived from arm ergometry to the general population. Of additional concern is the impact of the smaller muscle mass used during arm ergometry, resulting in reports of $\dot{V}O_2$max–peak values that are approximately 20% to 30% lower than the values obtained during treadmill testing (4, 23). The real benefits of testing $\dot{V}O_2$max–peak using arm ergometry are to evaluate a client's progress and measure the effectiveness of a training program over time.

Testing Protocols   Many resources provide testing protocols for measuring cardiovascular endurance.

General guidelines for all cardiovascular endurance tests include the following recommendations (22):

- Heart rate and blood pressure should be taken immediately before the exercise test with the client in the same posture as will be used during the exercise test.
- Clients should be familiarized with the mode of exercise that will be used for the test.
- An adequate warm-up of approximately 2 to 3 minutes should be completed before an exercise test.
- Every protocol used should consist of approximately 3-minute exercise stages accompanied by appropriate increments in work rate.
- Heart rate should be measured a minimum of two times during each stage (near the end of the second and third minutes of each stage).
- Blood pressure should be measured during the last minute of each stage so the exercise professional is aware of an abnormal blood pressure response to increasing work rate.
- Ratings of perceived exertion (RPE) should be taken near the end of the last minute of each stage using an appropriate scale.
- The exercise professional should monitor the client for signs or symptoms to terminate the test, such as these:
  - Attainment of 70% HRR or 85% of age-predicted maximal heart rate
  - If the client fails to conform to the exercise test protocol
  - If the client requests to stop the test for any reason
  - If the client experiences an emergency situation
- An adequate cooldown at an intensity less than or equal to the work rate of the first stage should be completed after the test (if the test has not been terminated for an emergency). A passive cooldown should be implemented if the client has experienced signs of discomfort or if an emergency situation has occurred.
- Measurement of heart rate, blood pressure, and RPE should continue for a minimum of 5 minutes after the test. In the event of an abnormal response to the test, an extended postexercise test observation period may be warranted.

After estimating or calculating $\dot{V}O_2max$ from the various tests, consult table 2.2 near the end of the chapter for the cardiovascular endurance classifications for adults.

Key Point

The exercise professional should always remind the client that she can stop the exercise test at any time and for any reason.

Assessment Protocol: Treadmill Test

Equipment

- Treadmill with an emergency stop button
- Stopwatch
- Rating of perceived exertion chart

Procedure

The Bruce treadmill test remains the most commonly used protocol; however, it employs relatively large intensity increments (i.e., 1-3 METs [metabolic equivalents] per stage) every 3 minutes. Consequently, changes in physiological responses may be less uniform and exercise capacity may be markedly overestimated when it is predicted from exercise time or work rate. Protocols with larger intensity increments are better suited for screening younger or physically active clients, whereas protocols with smaller increments, such as Balke-Ware (i.e., 1 MET per stage or less), are preferable for clients with chronic disease or disabilities. Advantages of smaller incremental increases include the following (2):

- Avoidance of large and unequal increments in work rate
- Uniform increases in hemodynamic and physiological responses
- More accurate estimates of exercise capacity and ventilatory threshold
- Individualization of the test protocol (individualized incremental changes)
- Targeted test duration

Whichever exercise protocol is selected, it should be individualized so the treadmill speed and increments in grade are based on the client's capability. For example, increases in grade of 1% to 3% per stage, with constant belt speeds of 1.5 to 2.5 miles per hour (2.4-4 km/h), can be used for treadmill tests for clients with a chronic disease or other limitation.

Due to the fatiguing effect of cardiovascular endurance assessments, they should be administered after all other tests have been completed. During each stage of a treadmill test the exercise professional can obtain RPE and heart rate data that can be used to compare the level of fatigue to future tests on the same client. Protocols for the Bruce and Balke-Ware treadmill tests are presented next.

Bruce Treadmill Protocol

The Bruce treadmill test begins with a very slow speed but at a relatively steep incline, and every 3 minutes, both the speed and the percent grade are increased until volitional fatigue is attained by the client (9). See table 2.3 near the end of the chapter for the time and intensity assignments for each stage of the test.

Balke-Ware Treadmill Protocol

The Balke-Ware treadmill test begins at a speed of 3.4 miles per hour (5.5 km/h) and 0% grade. The speed of the treadmill does not change again during the test. At the beginning of the second minute, the grade is set to 2% and increases by 1% every minute until volitional fatigue is reached (5).

Scoring

To estimate $\dot{V}O_2$max for the Bruce and Balke-Ware treadmill tests, the exercise duration spent during the test should be used in one of the equations from table 2.4 near the end of the chapter. Exercise duration should be expressed as time in minutes and in decimal format; for example, 9 minutes and 15 seconds would equal 9.25 minutes.

Assessment Protocol: YMCA Step Test (40)

Equipment

- Box or bench 12 inches (30 cm) in height
- Metronome
- Stopwatch

Procedure

Set the metronome to 96 beats (24 steps) per minute and the stopwatch to 3 minutes. Instruct the client to keep pace with the metronome by stepping up on the box or bench with the right foot, then the left foot, and then stepping down with the right foot, then the left foot. The client should practice stepping in time to the metronome before doing the test.

Clients can measure their heart rate in one of two ways: either by locating their radial pulse (marking it with a felt tip pen) and taking it manually, or by wearing a heart rate monitor. Time starts when the client begins stepping.

Scoring

After time expires, have the client immediately sit down and take the pulse for 1 minute. The score for the test is the heart rate during this minute. Results from this test can be compared to the normative data found in table 2.5 near the end of the chapter.

Clients should stop the test if they can no longer keep up with the metronome or if they become too fatigued to continue. If this occurs, record the ending pulse rate and the amount of time completed. On the next test, the goal will be to complete the full 3 minutes, or at least a greater percentage of it than the last time.

Assessment Protocol: Recumbent Stepper (7)

Equipment

- Recumbent stepper
- Stopwatch
- Rating of perceived exertion chart

Procedure

Individuals are required to maintain a constant step rate of 100 steps per minute for the entire test. The work rate for stage 1 is the same for all clients (30 watts), and subsequent work rates are assigned based on the heart rate response from stage 1. Heart rate should be taken during the final 10 seconds of minutes 2 and 3 of each stage to determine if steady-state heart rate (a change of no more than ±5 beats per minute) has been attained. If steady-state heart rate has not been attained, then the current work rate should be maintained for an additional minute and heart rate should be taken again. Use the following information to determine appropriate work rates for stages 2 through 4:

Work Rates for the Recumbent Stepper Test

Stage 2
- Heart rate <80 beats/min: 125 watts (W)
- Heart rate 80-89 beats/min: 100 W
- Heart rate 90-100 beats/min: 75 W
- Heart rate >100 beats/min: 50 W

Stage 3
- Heart rate <80 beats/min: 150 W
- Heart rate 80-89 beats/min: 125 W
- Heart rate 90-100 beats/min: 100 W
- Heart rate >100 beats/min: 75 W

Stage 4
- Heart rate <80 beats/min: 175 W
- Heart rate 80-89 beats/min: 150 W
- Heart rate 90-100 beats/min: 125 W
- Heart rate >100 beats/min: 100 W

Adapted from Billinger et al., 2012.

Rating of perceived exertion should be measured during the final minute of each work rate and recorded. The test should continue until volitional fatigue or achievement of 85% age-predicted maximal heart rate.

Scoring

The following equation was developed to estimate $\dot{V}O_2$ max from the work rate ($watts_{end\ submax}$) and heart rate in the final stage (7):

$$\dot{V}O_2 \text{ peak (in } ml \cdot kg^{-1} \cdot min^{-1}) = 125.707 - (0.476)(\text{age in years}) + (7.686)(\text{sex } [0= \text{female}; 1= \text{male}]) - (0.451)(\text{weight in kg}) + (0.179)(watts_{end\ submax}) - (0.415)(HR_{end\ submax})$$

▶ Assessment Protocol: YMCA Cycle Ergometer Test (17)

Equipment

- Cycle ergometer
- Stopwatch
- Rating of perceived exertion chart

Procedure

Clients are required to maintain a constant pedal rate of 50 rpm (using a 6 m per revolution flywheel) for the entire test. The work rate for stage 1 is the same for all clients—150 kgm/min (a 0.5-kg workload)—and subsequent work rates are assigned based on the heart rate response from stage 1. Heart rate should be taken during the final 30 seconds of minutes 2 and 3 of each stage to determine if steady-state heart rate (±5 beats per minute) has been attained. If steady-state heart rate has not been attained, then the current work rate should be maintained for an additional minute and heart rate should be taken again. Rating of perceived exertion should be measured during the final minute of each work rate and recorded. The test should continue until volitional fatigue or achievement of 85% age-predicted maximal heart rate. Use the information in table 2.6 near the end of the chapter to determine appropriate work rates for stages 2 through 4.

Scoring

To estimate $\dot{V}O_2$max from the YMCA cycle ergometer test, the exercise professional must extrapolate estimated maximal work rate from the heart rate and work rate data obtained from the submaximal test. Plot each heart rate obtained for every work rate from the test. Draw a diagonal line through the data points that extends to the age-predicted maximal heart rate (220 − age). Extend a line downward to the horizontal axis of the graph. The estimated maximal work rate is the value obtained where this line bisects the horizontal axis.

Figure 2.6 shows an example based on a 38-year-old individual who had an exercise heart rate at the end of stage 1 (150 kgm/min), stage 2 (450 kgm/min), and stage 3 (600 kgm/min) of 91, 130, and 155 beats/min, respectively.

Using the following formula, the exercise professional can use the estimated maximal work rate to calculate $\dot{V}O_2$max:

$$\dot{V}O_2\text{max} = [(1.8 \times \text{estimated maximal work rate in kgm/min)} / \text{body mass in kg}] + 7$$

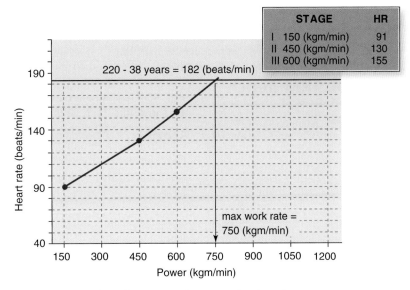

Figure 2.6 Plotting heart rate and work rate to estimate maximal work rate.

Reprinted, by permission, from V.H. Heyward and A.L. Gibson, 2014, *Advanced fitness assessment and exercise prescription*, 7th ed. (Champaign, IL: Human Kinetics), 105.

Assessment Protocol: Arm Ergometer Test (4)

Equipment

- Upper body ergometer or a cycle ergometer with the pedals replaced by handgrips
- Stopwatch
- Rating of perceived exertion chart

Procedure

The protocol for the arm ergometry tests requires that clients be seated in an upright position, with the feet flat on the ground, and the center of the axis of rotation of the crank arms adjusted to approximately shoulder height. The elbows should remain slightly flexed during the range of motion for every revolution of the crank arms. A crank arm speed of 75 to 80 rpm must be maintained for the duration of the test. Beginning work rate is 10 watts, and this work rate should be increased an additional 10 watts every 2 minutes until volitional fatigue or until 75 rpm cannot be maintained.

Scoring

First, one converts watts to kgm/min by multiplying watts by 6.12; then, using the following formula, use the maximal work rate attained during the test to calculate $\dot{V}O_2$max:

$\dot{V}O_2$max (in ml · kg^{-1} · min^{-1}) = [(3 × work rate in kgm/min) / body mass in kg] + 3.5

Muscular Strength Assessments

Muscle strength testing can reveal several important aspects of strength, including maximal force, the smoothness of contraction and relaxation (lack of spasticity), balance of strength between extensor and flexor muscle groups, symmetry between left and right sides of the body, and resistance to fatigue (40).

Muscular strength is defined as the force that a muscle or muscle group can exert in a single maximal effort—a 1RM—while maintaining proper form (28). Muscular strength is an important component of fitness, as a minimal level of muscular strength is necessary to conduct functions of daily living and participate in recreational activities (14).

Assessment Protocol: 1RM Bench Press (28)

Equipment

- Bench press bench
- Barbell
- Weight plates
- Barbell clips or locks
- Spotter

Procedure

The client should perform an exercise-specific warm-up of 5 to 10 repetitions using a light to moderate load first. Then the client should perform at least two additional heavier warm-up sets of two to five repetitions at approximately 60% to 80% of the estimated 1RM. The resistances should be progressively increased in a conservative manner, and the client should attempt to perform one repetition at each increment in resistance. Following each attempt, allow a recovery period of 2 to 4 minutes. Increase and decrease the load until the client can complete only one repetition with proper technique and no assistance from the spotter. The client's 1RM should be attained within three to five total trials.

Scoring

The 1RM must be divided by the client's body weight in order to compare to normative values in table 2.7 near the end of the chapter.

Assessment Protocol: 1RM Leg Press (22)

Equipment

- Leg press machine

Procedure

Before testing begins, the exercise professional should adjust the seat, foot platform, or both (depending on the design of the machine) so that when the client is in the bottom (or most forward) position of the leg press, his thighs are parallel to the foot platform. The result of this adjustment

is that the movement is performed through a standardized range of motion. To perform the test, follow the same procedure as for the 1RM bench press test, though the loads that are lifted are usually heavier than for the 1RM bench press test, so the load increases in each trial set will be greater (28).

Scoring

The 1RM must be divided by the client's body weight in order to compare to normative values in table 2.8 near the end of the chapter.

Local Muscular Endurance Assessments

Local muscular endurance is the ability of muscles or groups of muscles to perform repeated submaximal contractions (28). Tests that evaluate local muscle endurance typically count the total number of repetitions per unit time.

Assessment Protocol: Partial Curl-Up Test (22)

Equipment

- Metronome
- Ruler
- Adhesive tape
- Exercise mat

Procedure

The client lies supine on an exercise mat, arms by the sides, elbows extended, palms flat on the mat, and knees flexed to 90°. Place a piece of tape at the tip of the fingers of each hand and a second piece of tape parallel to the first piece 10 cm (4 in.) away (see figure 2.7). Set the metronome to 50 beats per minute and have the client curl forward and upward, lifting the shoulder blades off of the exercise mat by flexing the trunk to 30° in time with the metronome (25 curl-ups per minute). Clients should avoid flexing the neck and perform as many curl-ups as possible in 1 minute without pausing until they can no longer reach the distant piece of tape at the end of the curl-up or until they complete a maximum of 25 repetitions.

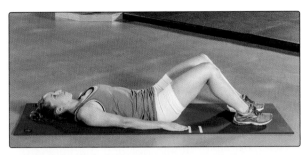

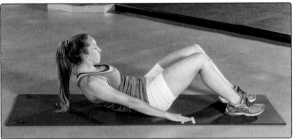

Figure 2.7 Starting and ending positions for the partial curl-up test.

Scoring

The score is the total number of curl-ups completed; see table 2.9 near the end of the chapter for norms for this test.

Flexibility Assessments

Flexibility is defined as the range of motion (in degrees) that can be performed by a joint of the body (28). Maintaining flexibility of all joints facilitates optimal movement and function; in contrast, when an activity moves the structures of a joint beyond a joint's range of motion, tissue damage can occur. The degree of flexibility of a joint depends on the distensibility of the joint capsule, appropriate warm-up, muscle viscosity, and compliance of connective tissues such as ligaments and tendons. Flexibility is joint specific, and as a result, no single test of flexibility exists that can be used to evaluate total body flexibility.

Assessment Protocol: Sit-and-Reach Test (22)

The sit-and-reach test has been used commonly to assess low back and hip joint flexibility since low back pain affects a significant number of people in their lifetime (40). The relative importance of hamstring flexibility to activities of daily living and sport performance also suggests the inclusion of the sit-and-reach test for health-related fitness testing.

Equipment

- Sit-and-reach box or adhesive tape
- A measuring tape or stick

Procedure

Whether using a sit-and-reach box or a measuring tape or stick, the client should first warm up with exercises that engage the hamstrings and lower back, such as walking or jogging for 3 to 5 minutes. This should be followed by several repetitions of alternating between flexing forward and reaching toward the toes with the knees extended in a standing or sitting position, then reaching upward toward the ceiling in a smooth continuous motion (without jerking). Make a note of the warm-up routine used by the client so it can be replicated for future testing to assist in reliability of the test results.

When using a sit-and-reach box, the client should be in a seated position facing the box with the shoes off. The knees should be fully extended with the feet placed on the base of the box and the medial edges of the feet 6 inches (15 cm) apart. The client should keep the knees fully extended during the duration of the test, arms fully extended, and hands overlapped, with the palm of one touching the dorsal surface of the other. The client should then reach forward slowly, flexing at the hips, and push the fingertips over the scale on the box in a controlled manner. When full extension is obtained, the client should hold this position for approximately 2 seconds. To maximize the best stretch, ask the client to exhale when reaching forward.

When using a measuring tape or stick, first tape it to the floor; then place one piece of tape 24 inches (61 cm) long across and at a right angle to the measuring stick at the 15-inch (38 cm) mark. After warming up, the client should sit without shoes in a position with the measuring stick between the legs and its zero end toward the body. The feet should be approximately 12 inches (30 cm) apart, toes pointed upward, and heels touching the edge of the taped line at the 15-inch (38 cm) mark. Clients should keep the knees fully extended during the duration of the test, arms fully extended, and hands overlapped with the palm of one touching the dorsal surface of the other. The client should then be instructed to reach forward in a controlled manner with both hands as far as possible on the

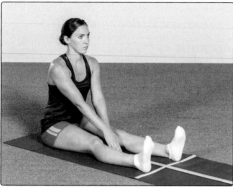

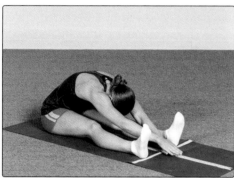

Figure 2.8 Starting and ending positions for the sit-and-reach test using a measuring tape or stick.

measuring stick. When full extension is obtained, the client should hold this position for approximately 2 seconds with the fingertips remaining in contact with the measuring stick (see figure 2.8). To maximize the best stretch, ask the client to exhale when reaching forward. The exercise professional may hold the client's knees down, if necessary, to keep them straight.

Scoring

The client is allowed three trials, with the highest taken as the score to the closest 0.25 inch (1 cm). See table 2.10 near the end of the chapter for norms for this test.

Assessment Protocol: Back Scratch Test (38)

Equipment

- Yardstick (meterstick)

Procedure

The client should stand and place her preferred hand over the same-side shoulder with the palm down and fingers fully extended. The client should then reach down the middle of the back as far as

possible. The elbow should be pointed up toward the ceiling. The client should then place the opposite arm around her back with the dorsal surface of the hand touching the back. With this hand, the client should reach up the back as far as possible in an attempt to touch or overlap the extended middle fingers of both hands. Practice attempts are allowed in order to determine the preferred position. Clients should not grip the fingers of opposite hands together and pull.

Scoring

Clients are allowed two practice trials in the preferred position before administration of two test trials. Record both scores to the nearest 0.5 inch or 1 cm, measuring the distance of overlap or distance between the tips of the middle fingers, with the higher of the two values recorded as the overall score. Clients are awarded one of the following scores:

- Minus (–) score if the middle fingers do not touch
- Zero (0) score if the middle fingers just barely touch
- Plus (+) score if the middle fingers overlap

Anthropometric and Body Composition Assessments

Measurements of limbs and body segments—typically the largest circumference of those areas—are commonly performed by an exercise professional before a client begins an exercise program, especially if the goal is to lose body fat or gain muscle tissue. Those assessments do not determine the body composition of a client, however. Commonly, measurements of skinfold thicknesses at three to seven anatomical sites or a bioelectrical impedance analysis (BIA) test is performed to give better insight into the client's fat weight and lean body mass.

Assessment Protocol: Body Mass Index (BMI)

Equipment

- Scale or balance that can be calibrated for accuracy
- Medical stadiometer or a wall with a tape measure affixed to it

Procedure

Measure the client's height and weight (refer to the "Preassessment Measurements" section).

Scoring

Determine the client's BMI by using one of the following formulas:

BMI (in kg/m^2) = [body weight in pounds / (height in inches × height in inches)] × 703

BMI (in kg/m^2) = [body weight in kg / (height in meters) × (height in meters)]

Based on the client's BMI, he is then placed into one of the following classifications:

- Normal: between 18.5 and 24.9 kg/m^2
- Overweight: between 25 and 29.9 kg/m^2
- Obese: 30 kg/m^2 or more

Assessment Protocol: Waist-to-Hip Girth Ratio

Equipment

- Gulick or other nonelastic measuring tape

Procedure

Measure the circumference of the waist (the narrowest portion of the abdomen) and the hip (maximum protrusion of the buttocks) in either inches or centimeters. Apply adequate tension to the measuring tape to promote an accurate measurement of circumference, but the tape should not be tight enough to indent the skin. Make certain the measuring tape is horizontal and parallel to the floor before taking measurement readings.

Scoring

Determine the client's waist-to-hip girth ratio by dividing the waist circumference by the hip circumference; see table 2.11 near the end of the chapter for norms for this test.

Assessment Protocol: Skinfold Measurements

A caliper is used to measure the thickness of a double fold of skin at various anatomical sites. The test relies on the observation that within any population a certain fraction of the total body fat lies just under the skin (subcutaneous fat), and that if one could obtain a representative sample of the fat, overall body fat (density and composition) could be predicted. The thicknesses of the skinfolds at various sites (depending on the formula used based on the client's demographic) are used to estimate body density and calculate the client's percentage of body fat. The body density equations for men and women typically use the sum of three or seven skinfolds. To be accurate and valid, the exact skinfold techniques that were used to derive the equations must be applied, and appropriate levels of training and experience of the exercise professional should be observed.

Equipment

- Skinfold caliper that is valid and reliable and can be calibrated for accuracy
- Gulick or other nonelastic measuring tape
- Marking pen

Procedure

Skinfold measurements should be made on dry skin, before exercise, on the right side of the body. The skin should be firmly pinched with the thumb and index finger, and the caliper arms should be placed 1 to 2 cm (0.4 to 0.8 in.) away from the thumb and finger, perpendicular to the skinfolds, and halfway between the crest and base of the fold. Wait 1 to 2 seconds (maximum) before reading the caliper, and keep the skin pinched while reading the caliper. Take duplicate measurements at each site and retest if duplicate measurements are not within 10%. Rotate through measurement sites or allow time for skin to regain normal texture and thickness before taking the duplicate measurement and any additional retests. Average the two closest measurements to the nearest 0.5 cm.

Based on the formula selected to estimate body density (see table 2.12 near the end of the chapter), choose the number and location of the sites for measuring the skinfolds using the following techniques (40):

- Chest: A diagonal fold one-half of the distance between the anterior axillary line and the nipple for men
- Midaxillary: A vertical fold on the midaxillary line at the level of the xiphoid process of the sternum (an alternate method is a horizontal fold taken at the level of the xiphoid–sternal border in the midaxillary line)
- Triceps: A vertical fold on the posterior midline of the upper arm, halfway between the acromion and olecranon processes, with the

arm held relaxed to the side of the body in the anatomical position

- Subscapular: A diagonal fold (at a 45° angle) extending from the vertebral border to a point 1 to 2 cm (0.4 to 0.8 in.) below the inferior angle of the scapula
- Abdomen: A vertical fold 2 cm (0.8 in.) to the right side of the umbilicus
- Suprailiac: A diagonal fold in line with the natural angle of the iliac crest taken in the anterior auxiliary line immediately superior to the iliac crest
- Thigh: A vertical fold on the anterior midline of the thigh, midway between the proximal border of the patella and the inguinal crest (hip)
- Calf: A vertical fold at the maximum circumference of the calf on the midline of its medial border

Photographs of the common sites are shown in figure 2.9.

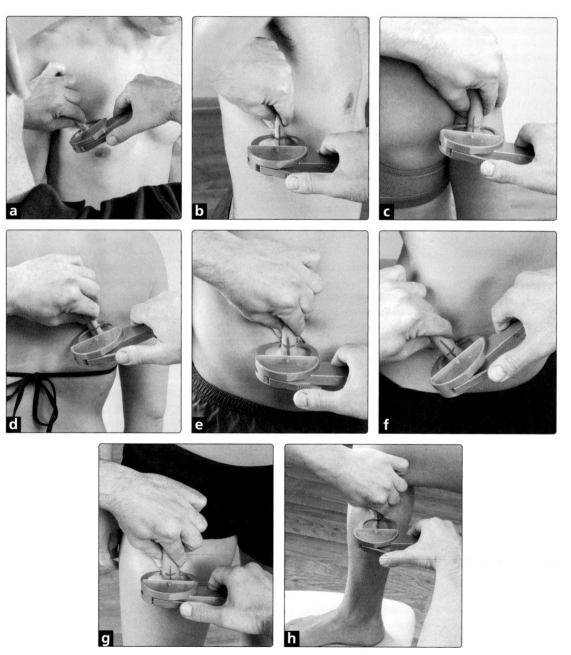

Figure 2.9 Skinfold measurements: *(a)* chest skinfold, *(b)* midaxilla skinfold, *(c)* triceps skinfold, *(d)* subscapula skinfold, *(e)* abdomen skinfold, *(f)* suprailium skinfold, *(g)* thigh skinfold, and *(h)* medial calf skinfold.

Scoring

Use the appropriate formula from table 2.12 to estimate body density (Db) and then use the Siri equation (% body fat = 495 / Db − 450) where needed to calculate estimated percent body fat. Percent body fat standards for adults, children, and physically active adults are presented in table 2.13 near the end of the chapter.

Assessment Protocol: Bioelectrical Impedance

Bioelectrical impedance analysis is a simple, quick, noninvasive method that can be used to estimate percentage of body fat. This technique requires that a small electrical current be sent through the body. This current is undetectable to the person being tested and is based on the assumption that tissues high in water content (e.g., skeletal muscle) will conduct electrical currents with less resistance than those with little water (e.g., adipose tissue) (22). Because adipose tissue contains little water, fat will impede the flow of electrical current.

There are several types of commercially available BIA devices. Some place electrodes on the hand and foot; some are handheld devices; and others, which look much like bathroom scales, have contact points at the bottom of the feet. Whatever the design of the machine, as the introduced current passes through the body, voltage decreases. This voltage drop (impedance) is used to calculate percentage of body fat. Typically, other information such as sex, height, and age is used in conjunction with impedance to predict percentage of body fat.

Bioelectrical impedance analysis has gained wide use in the fitness industry because it is easy to use, relatively inexpensive, and noninvasive. The accuracy of this technique depends on the type of equipment and equations used; however, a standard error of approximately ±4% commonly is reported (22). In other words, the percentage of body fat value from BIA is typically within 4% of that obtained using hydrostatic weighting, considered the gold standard for body composition. One problem with the use of BIA is that the relationship between impedance and percentage of body fat varies among populations. This means that the best equation to predict percentage of body fat depends on the person being tested and the corresponding equation used.

It is recommended that people with implanted defibrillators avoid BIA assessment until the safety of BIA with these clients has been determined (22). Also, any substance that alters the body's hydration state such as alcohol or diuretics, including caffeine (for clients who do not ingest it on a regular basis), should be avoided for at least 48 hours before the test. (Note that diuretics taken under a physician's direction should not be stopped, however.) Exercise should be avoided for 12 hours before the test, and clients should avoid eating and should drink only enough to maintain hydration during the final 4 hours before the test (22). A client's menstrual cycle phase should be noted for future testing because of its ability to alter hydration level.

Procedure

Remove any oil and lotion from the skin with alcohol before placing the electrodes on the skin, if necessary. Place the electrodes precisely as directed by the manufacturer of the impedance device used. Incorrect electrode placement greatly reduces the accuracy of the test.

Scoring

Percent body fat standards for adults, children, and physically active adults are presented in table 2.13.

Neuromuscular Assessments

Neuromuscular tests assess balance, coordination, and skill and are most useful for testing clients with a neuromuscular disability or deficits and those who are severely debilitated from chronic disease or are frail, therefore needing specific assessment and programming (30).

Assessment Protocol: Balance Assessment (37)

The Balance Error Scoring System (BESS) is used to evaluate a client's static postural stability on hard and soft surfaces.

Equipment

- Hard floor surface
- Medium-density foam balance pad (45 cm² × 13 cm [~18 in.² × 5 in.] thick with a density of 60 kg/m³ and a load deflection of 80-90)
- Stopwatch

Procedure

Static postural stability is evaluated while the client stands in three defined positions on a hard floor surface and a foam balance pad for a total of six evaluation positions. The foot positions for the BESS are as follows:

- Double-leg support with the feet together and parallel to each other
- Single-leg support while standing only on the nondominant foot with the knee of the dominant leg flexed to approximately 90°.
- Tandem with the dominant foot in the front and the nondominant foot in the back, with the toes of the nondominant foot touching the heel of the dominant foot

Scoring

While standing in each position, the client must close her eyes and place hands on hips while attempting to remain as steady as possible for 20 seconds. If the client loses her balance, the exercise professional should instruct her to attempt to regain the initial position as quickly as possible. Clients are assessed 1 point for each of the following errors:

- Lifting hands off the hips
- Opening the eyes
- Stepping, stumbling, or falling
- Moving the hip into more than 30° of flexion or abduction
- Lifting the forefoot or heel
- Remaining out of the test position for more than 5 seconds

A trial is counted as incomplete if the client cannot maintain the position a minimum of 5 seconds, and for each incomplete position the client receives a maximum of 10 points. During each trial the exercise professional counts the total number of errors and awards 1 point for each error up to a maximum of 10 errors per trial. The total number of errors from all six trials is counted as the overall score. Normative data for the BESS test are provided in table 2.14 near the end of the chapter.

Functional Performance Assessments

A wide array of tests and test batteries have been developed to assess various aspects of functional performance. These test batteries vary in their total number of tasks, but typically the tasks are timed or ranked using a simple scale. Many functional performance measures have components that relate directly to the mobility and strength of an individual. These can be important assessment tools since, as an example, independent-living individuals who barely surpass these functional thresholds of mobility and strength are at risk for future disability (30).

Assessment Protocol: 8-Foot Up-and-Go Test (38)

Equipment

- Stopwatch
- Folding chair with a 17-inch (43 cm) seat height
- Tape measure
- Cone

Procedure

The chair should be placed against a wall and be facing the cone. The cone should be placed 8 feet (2.4 m) away from the front edge of the chair. The client should be instructed to sit upright in the middle of the chair with his feet flat on the floor and with hands on knees. When the exercise professional says "go," the client gets up from the chair and walks as quickly as possible around the cone and back to the chair and returns to a seated position. The exercise professional should start the stopwatch on the "go" signal regardless of whether or not the client has begun moving. The stopwatch should be stopped as soon as the client has returned to the seated position. The client is allowed practice trials before being scored.

Scoring

The exercise professional should administer two test trials and record both times to the nearest tenth of a second. The faster of the two trials is recorded as the score. Standards for the test are presented in table 2.15 near the end of the chapter.

Assessments Specific to Clients With a Limited Ability or Restrictions

Although most assessments can be performed by clients who have a wide range of fitness levels, some have limited physical ability to complete a test or have a medical condition that restricts them from even beginning a test. In either case, there are valid assessments an exercise professional can use that apply reduced stress on a client when other procedures are not appropriate or recommended.

Assessment Protocol: 6-Minute Walk Test (38)

Equipment

- Long measuring tape
- Two stopwatches
- Four cones
- Masking or painter's tape
- Felt tip marker
- 12 to 15 lap markers per person (ice pop sticks or index cards and pencils to keep track of laps walked)

Procedure

The area for the test is a rectangle 5 yards (4.6 m) by 20 yards (18 m). The long sides should be marked off in 5-yard (4.6 m) segments identified by strips of tape, and a cone should be placed at each corner. The cumulative distance of each segment should be written on the piece of tape. A skilled exercise professional can test up to 12 people at once, using partners to assist with scoring, but 6 at a time is more manageable. To keep the clients motivated, two or more persons should be tested at a time.

On the "go" signal, the exercise professional starts the two stopwatches and the clients begin walking counterclockwise as fast as possible (not running) around the course, covering as much distance as possible in the 6-minute time limit. To keep track of the distance walked, the exercise professional gives a lap marker to each client every time a lap of the course is completed. Clients should be made aware of the time remaining in the test and be provided with verbal encouragement. At the end of the 6-minute test period, clients should stop, stand next to the closest 5-yard (4.6 m) segment tape marker on their right, and keep moving in place for a 1-minute cooldown.

Scoring

Record the score of each client as total yards (or meters) walked in the 6-minute time period. Each lap marker represents 50 yards (46 m), with the distance of the final partial lap added to the product of the lap markers × 50 (or × 46 for total meters). For example, if a client has collected eight lap markers (representing eight laps) and stopped next to the 45-yard (41 m) marker, the score would be a total of 445 yards (407 m). Only one trial should be administered per day. Standards for the test are shown in table 2.16 near the end of the chapter.

Assessment Protocol: 2-Minute Step Test (38)

Equipment

- Stopwatch
- Measuring tape or a piece of string or cord approximately 30 inches (76 cm) long
- Masking or painter's tape
- Tally counter

Procedure

Determine the minimum step height for each client by finding the midway point between the patella (kneecap) and the front of the hip (iliac crest). The midway point can be found using a tape measure or stretching a piece of string or cord from the middle of the patella to the iliac crest and then folding in half. This midway point on the thigh can be temporarily marked with a piece of tape. To monitor step height, have the client stand next to a wall, and transfer the marking tape from the thigh to the wall at the same height as it was on the thigh. On the "go" signal the client begins stepping in place and continues for the 2-minute time period. Use the tally counter to count the number of times that the right knee reaches the height of the tape on the wall. If the knee cannot be lifted to the height of the tape, the client can be asked to slow down (decrease step rate), or to stop to momentarily rest so the client can resume lifting the knee to the right height (but do not stop the stopwatch).

Scoring

The score is the number of high enough steps completed with the right leg in 2 minutes. Only one trial should be administered per day. Standards for the test are shown in table 2.17 near the end of the chapter.

▶ Assessment Protocol: 30-Second Chair Stand Test (38)

Equipment

- Stopwatch
- Chair with a seat height of approximately 17 inches (43 cm) and preferably with legs that angle forward to prevent tipping

Procedure

Place the chair securely against a wall to avoid movement during testing. Instruct the client to sit in the middle of the chair with the back straight, feet flat on the floor, and arms crossed at the wrists and held against the chest. On the signal "go," the client rises to a fully standing position without using the hands, and then returns to a fully seated position. Encourage the client to complete as many full stands as possible in the 30 seconds. Before testing, demonstrate proper form, then at a faster pace, to show that the object is to do as many repetitions as one can within safety limits; then have the client practice one or two stands to learn and then reinforce proper form.

Safety Tips

- Brace the chair against the wall or have someone hold it steady.
- Watch for balance problems.
- Stop the test immediately if the client complains of pain or dizziness.

If clients are unable to perform even one stand without using their hands, allow them to push off their legs or the chair, or use a cane or walker, if necessary. If an adaptation such as this is needed, be sure to describe it on the testing sheet. Although the recorded test score is zero for purposes of comparing to normative standards, indicate the adapted score so that performance changes can be evaluated from one test time to the next.

Scoring

The score is the total number of stands completed in 30 seconds. If a client is more than halfway up at the end of 30 seconds, it counts as a full stand. Administer only one test trial per day. Standards for the test are shown in table 2.18 near the end of the chapter.

▶ Assessment Protocol: 30-Second Arm Curl Test (38)

Equipment

- Stopwatch
- Straight-back or folding chair with no arms
- 5-pound (2.3 kg) dumbbell for women
- 8-pound (3.6 kg) dumbbell for men

Procedure

The client should be seated upright on the chair with her feet flat on the floor. The dominant side of the client's body should be located close to the edge of the seat to allow unimpeded movement of the dumbbell. The dumbbell should be held at the side in the dominant hand using a neutral (handshake) grip with the elbow fully extended. On the signal "go," the client curls the dumbbell up to a supinated (palms facing up) position and then lowers the dumbbell to the starting position. Encourage the client to complete as many arm curls as possible in the 30 seconds. Before testing, demonstrate proper form and have the client practice one or two repetitions without the dumbbell to learn and then reinforce proper form.

Scoring

The score is counted as the total number of repetitions in 30 seconds. If the client's elbow is more than halfway flexed at the end of the 30 seconds, it counts as the final repetition. Only one trial should be administered per day. Standards for the test are shown in table 2.19 near the end of the chapter.

▶ Assessment Protocol: Chair Sit-and-Reach Test (38)

Equipment

- Chair with a seat height of approximately 17 inches (43 cm) and preferably with legs that angle forward to prevent tipping
- 18-inch (46 cm) ruler or half of a yardstick or meterstick

Procedure

Place the chair securely against a wall in order to avoid movement during testing. The assessment begins with the client sitting on the edge of the chair so that the buttocks are even with the front edge of the chair. The knee of one leg should be flexed with that foot flat on the floor and the knee of the other leg fully extended. The heel of the extended leg should be placed on the floor with the foot flexed to approximately 90°. The client should exhale while slowly flexing forward at the waist toward the toes. While flexing forward, the arms should be outstretched with the hands overlapping. If the extended knee starts to flex, the client should be asked to move slowly back until the knee is fully extended again. The score is recorded as the maximum distance reached and held for 2 seconds. The client should stretch only to the point where slight discomfort from muscle tension is experienced and never to the point of pain. This test should not be administered to individuals with osteoporosis or lower back pain caused by forward flexion of the back. The client should attempt the test with both legs and determine which is preferred, and only the preferred leg is used for test scoring purposes.

Scoring

The client is allowed two practice trials, and then two test trials are administered. The higher of the two trials is recorded as the score for the test. The exercise professional measures the distance from the tips of the middle fingers to the top of the shoe (to the nearest half-inch or 1 cm). The midpoint at the top of the shoe represents the zero point. If the reach is short of this point, record the distance as a negative (–) score. Standards for the test are shown in table 2.20 near the end of the chapter.

SMART GOAL SETTING

As an exercise professional starts to work with a participant (typically after the exercise professional is hired and under contract), the participant becomes a client. One of the most important steps to take after the fitness assessment is completed and the results are compared to norms or standards is to set goals based on the deficiencies that are revealed from testing.

Exercise professionals use goals in an effort to clearly define the purpose of an exercise program or a specific exercise session. Goals can affect exercise program outcomes by providing direction and motivation for exercise and stimulating and enhancing a client's adherence to the program (27).

An exercise professional should assist a client in setting short-, medium-, and long-term goals. The goals of each client vary based on his desired training outcomes and individual limitations. The acronym SMART can be used to guide the goal-setting process; it is commonly defined in this way (8):

S: Specific

M: Measurable

A: Action oriented (or achievable)

R: Realistic (or relevant)

T: Time-bound (or timed)

Another way to characterize goal setting is to say that each goal set should demonstrate the seven practical principles of effective goal setting (20):

1. Make goals specific, measurable, and observable.
2. Clearly identify time constraints.
3. Set moderately difficult goals.
4. Record goals and monitor progress.
5. Diversify process, performance, and outcomes.
6. Set short-range goals to achieve medium- and long-range goals.
7. Make sure goals are internalized (clients should participate in setting them or should set their own goals).

Using a combination of these approaches and guidelines, the exercise professional should work with each client to define goals for an exercise program.

MOTIVATIONAL AND COACHING TECHNIQUES

Motivation is the drive that directs a client's behavior (39). The exercise professional plays a key role in influencing and encouraging a client's motivation. Addressing the three basic needs of clients—competence, autonomy, and relatedness—will result in an effective outcome (39):

- Competence is typically met when a person feels successful.
- Autonomy is met when the person feels that the decision to participate is made without outside pressure or influence.
- Relatedness is achieved when the person feels connected to and appreciated by others.

If the exercise professional can positively influence these three factors, the client is in the best position to succeed.

CONCLUSION

The proper screening and assessment of clients with chronic disease or disabilities is a critical starting point before testing or implementing an exercise program because it enables the exercise professional to educate, train, and motivate clients. Before developing an exercise program for an individual with a chronic disease or disability, the exercise professional needs to gather relevant information and documentation that will be used to assess current levels of health, potential medical risks, and need for medical clearance. Tests and assessments can be used to evaluate current levels of functional fitness and areas in need of improvement, provide baseline measurements for developing an exercise program, and establish a baseline for comparisons to future assessments. To evaluate assessment quality, exercise professionals must understand validity, reliability, and accuracy. Test selection should be based on the client's level of functional capacity, chronic disease or disability status, and fitness goals. Exercise professionals must always remain keenly aware of potential risks during the assessment process, including risk of falls, and be attentive to signs and symptoms of possible health problems that require medical referral. Consistent and effective test preparation is essential, and accordingly the assessment process should be well structured and implemented using the appropriate protocols. Following testing, it is important that the exercise professional present the results and explain how those results compare to established norms so that SMART short-, medium-, and long-term goals can be set and reached through the effective use of motivational and coaching techniques.

Key Terms

angina	moderate-intensity exercise
ataxia	norm-referenced data
claudication	orthopnea
criterion-referenced standards	pallor
cyanosis	peak $\dot{V}O_2$
edema	sphygmomanometer
ischemia	supervised assessment and exercise program
light-intensity exercise	syncope
medically supervised assessment and exercise program	vigorous-intensity exercise

Study Questions

1. An exercise professional is responsible for using which of the following forms for referring clients who may be of increased exercise-related risk of a serious cardiovascular event?

   a. PAR-Q+

   b. informed consent

   c. medical history

   d. medical clearance

2. When performing assessments in a single session, what is the appropriate test order after nonfatiguing measurements have been performed?

   a. maximum muscle strength, agility, local muscle endurance, cardiovascular endurance

   b. cardiovascular endurance, local muscle endurance, agility, maximum muscle strength

   c. agility, maximum muscle strength, local muscle endurance, cardiovascular endurance

   d. local muscle endurance, maximum muscle strength, agility, cardiovascular endurance

3. Which of the following statements reflects proper procedure for the back scratch test?

   a. No practice trial is allowed.

   b. Both hands are palms up on the back.

   c. Score the test by measuring the distance or overlap between the hands.

   d. Both hands should go over the top of the shoulder and attempt to touch in the middle of the back.

4. For a client with extremely limited cardiovascular endurance, which of the following is the most appropriate test for cardiovascular endurance?

   a. YMCA step test

   b. 6-minute walk test

   c. Bruce treadmill test

   d. YMCA cycle ergometer test

Table 2.1   Classification of Blood Pressure for Adults

Blood Pressure Classification	SBP (mmHg)	DBP (mmHg)
Normal	<120	and <80
Prehypertension	120-139	or 80-89
Stage 1 Hypertension	140-159	or 90-99
Stage 2 Hypertension	≥160	or ≥100

SBP, systolic blood pressure; DBP, diastolic blood pressure

Reprinted from National Institutes of Health/National Heart, Lung, and Blood Institute, 2004, *The seventh report of the Joint National Committee on prevention, detection, evaluation, and treatment of high blood pressure* (Washington, DC: U.S. Department of Health and Human Services), 12.

Table 2.2   Cardiovascular Endurance Classifications for Adults (in ml · kg^{-1} · min^{-1})

Age (years)	Poor	Fair	Good	Excellent	Superior
Women					
20-29	≤35	36-38	40-43	44-48	49+
30-39	≤33	34-36	37-41	42-46	47+
40-49	≤32	33-35	36-38	39-44	45+
50-59	≤28	29-31	32-35	36-40	41+
60-69	≤26	27-28	29-32	33-36	37+
70-79	≤25	26-27	28-29	30-36	37+
Men					
20-29	≤41	42-45	46-49	51-55	56+
30-39	≤40	41-43	44-47	48-53	54+
40-49	≤37	38-41	42-45	46-52	53+
50-59	≤34	35-38	39-42	43-48	49+
60-69	≤31	32-34	35-38	39-44	45+
70-79	≤28	29-31	32-35	36-42	43+

Reprinted, by permission, from V.H. Heyward and A.L. Gibson, 2014, *Advanced fitness assessment and exercise prescription*, 7th ed. (Champaign, IL: Human Kinetics), 81; Data from Cooper Institute for Aerobics Research 2005.

Table 2.3   Time and Intensity Assignments for the Bruce Treadmill Test

Stage	Time (min)	Speed (mph)	Speed (km/h)	METs	Grade (%)
1	1-3	1.7	2.7	4.6	10
2	3-6	2.5	4.0	7.0	12
3	6-9	3.4	5.5	10.2	14
4	9-12	4.2	6.8	12.1	16
5	12-15	5.0	8.0	14.9	18
6	15-18	5.5	8.9	17.0	20

References: (9, 22)

Table 2.4 Equations for Estimating $\dot{V}O_2$max from the Bruce and Balke-Ware Treadmill Tests

Protocol	Population	Reference	Equation
Bruce[a]	Active and sedentary men	Foster et al. (1984)	$\dot{V}O_2$max $= 14.76 - 1.379(\text{time}) + 0.451(\text{time}^2) - 0.012(\text{time}^3)$ $r = 0.98$, $SEE = 3.35$ (ml · kg^{-1} · min^{-1})
	Active and sedentary women	Pollock et al. (1982)	$\dot{V}O_2$max $= 4.38(\text{time}) - 3.90$ $r = 0.91$, $SEE = 2.7$ (ml · kg^{-1} · min^{-1})
	Cardiac patients and elderly persons[b]	McConnell and Clark (1987)	$\dot{V}O_2$max $= 2.282(\text{time}) + 8.545$ $r = 0.82$, $SEE = 4.9$ (ml · kg^{-1} · min^{-1})
Balke	Active and sedentary men	Pollock et al. (1976)	$\dot{V}O_2$max $= 1.444(\text{time}) + 14.99$ $r = 0.92$, $SEE = 2.50$ (ml · kg^{-1} · min^{-1})
	Active and sedentary women[c]	Pollock et al. (1982)	$\dot{V}O_2$max $= 1.38(\text{time}) + 5.22$ $r = 0.94$, $SEE = 2.20$ (ml · kg^{-1} · min^{-1})

[a]For use with the standard Bruce protocol; cannot be used with modified Bruce protocol.

[b]This equation is used only for treadmill walking while holding the handrails.

[c]For women, the Balke protocol was modified: speed 3.0 mph; initial workload 0% grade for 3 min, increasing 2.5% every 3 min thereafter.

SEE = standard error of estimate.

Reprinted, by permission, from V.H. Heyward and A.L. Gibson, 2014, *Advanced fitness assessment and exercise prescription*, 7th ed. (Champaign, IL: Human Kinetics), 92.

Table 2.5 Norms for the YMCA Step Test (Recovery Heart Rate in beats/min)

Rating	AGE (YEARS)					
	18-25	26-35	36-45	46-55	56-65	66+
Male						
Excellent	70-78	73-79	72-81	78-84	72-82	72-86
Good	82-88	83-88	86-94	89-96	89-97	89-95
Above average	91-97	91-97	98-102	99-103	98-101	97-102
Average	101-104	101-106	105-111	109-115	105-111	104-113
Below average	107-114	109-116	113-118	118-121	113-118	114-119
Poor	118-126	119-126	120-128	124-130	122-128	122-128
Very poor	131-164	130-164	132-168	135-158	131-150	133-152
Female						
Excellent	72-83	72-86	74-87	76-93	74-92	73-86
Good	88-97	91-97	93-101	96-102	97-103	93-100
Above average	100-106	103-110	104-109	106-113	106-111	104-114
Average	110-116	112-118	111-117	117-120	113-117	117-121
Below average	118-124	121-127	120-127	121-126	119-127	123-127
Poor	128-137	129-135	130-138	127-133	129-136	129-134
Very poor	142-155	141-154	143-152	138-152	142-151	135-151

Reprinted, by permission, from J.R. Morrow et al., 2011, *Measurement and evaluation in human performance*, 4th ed. (Champaign, IL: Human Kinetics), 200.

Table 2.6 Work Rates for the YMCA Cycle Ergometer Test

Stage	Heart rate <80 beats/min	Heart rate 80-89 beats/min	Heart rate 90-100 beats/min	Heart rate >100 beats/min
Stage 2	750 kgm/min (2.5 kg)	600 kgm/min (2.0 kg)	450 kgm/min (1.5 kg)	300 kgm/min (1.0 kg)
Stage 3	900 kgm/min (3.0 kg)	750 kgm/min (2.5 kg)	600 kgm/min (2.0 kg)	450 kgm/min (1.5 kg)
Stage 4	1,050 kgm/min (3.5 kg)	900 kgm/min (3.0 kg)	750 kgm/min (2.5 kg)	600 kgm/min (2.0 kg)

Reference: (17)

Table 2.7 Body Weight-to-Strength Ratio Norms for the 1RM Bench Press

Percentile rankings* for men	AGE (YEARS)					
	20-29	30-39	40-49	50-59	60+	
90	1.48	1.24	1.10	0.97	0.89	
80	1.32	1.12	1.00	0.90	0.82	
70	1.22	1.04	0.93	0.84	0.77	
60	1.14	0.98	0.88	0.79	0.72	
50	1.06	0.93	0.84	0.75	0.68	
40	0.99	0.88	0.80	0.71	0.66	
30	0.93	0.83	0.76	0.68	0.63	
20	0.88	0.78	0.72	0.63	0.57	
10	0.80	0.71	0.65	0.57	0.53	
Percentile rankings* for women	**AGE (YEARS)**					
	20-29	30-39	40-49	50-59	60+	70+
90	0.54	0.49	0.46	0.40	0.41	0.44
80	0.49	0.45	0.40	0.37	0.38	0.39
70	0.42	0.42	0.38	0.35	0.36	0.33
60	0.41	0.41	0.37	0.33	0.32	0.31
50	0.40	0.38	0.34	0.31	0.30	0.27
40	0.37	0.37	0.32	0.28	0.29	0.25
30	0.35	0.34	0.30	0.26	0.28	0.24
20	0.33	0.32	0.27	0.23	0.26	0.21
10	0.30	0.27	0.23	0.19	0.25	0.20

*Descriptors for percentile rankings: 90 = well above average; 70 = above average; 30 = below average; 10 = well below average.

Data for women provided by the Women's Exercise Research Center, The George Washington University Medical Center, Washington, DC, 1998.

Data for men provided by The Cooper Institute for Aerobics Research, *The Physical Fitness Specialist Manual,* Dallas: The Cooper Institute, 2005.

Reprinted, by permission, from V.H. Heyward and A.L. Gibson, 2014, *Advanced fitness assessment and exercise prescription,* 7th ed. (Champaign, IL: Human Kinetics) 162.

Table 2.8 Body Weight-to-Strength Ratio Norms for the 1RM Leg Press

Percentile rankings* for men	AGE (YEARS)					
	20-29	30-39	40-49	50-59	60+	
90	2.27	2.07	1.92	1.80	1.73	
80	2.13	1.93	1.82	1.71	1.62	
70	2.05	1.85	1.74	1.64	1.56	
60	1.97	1.77	1.68	1.58	1.49	
50	1.91	1.71	1.62	1.52	1.43	
40	1.83	1.65	1.57	1.46	1.38	
30	1.74	1.59	1.51	1.39	1.30	
20	1.63	1.52	1.44	1.32	1.25	
10	1.51	1.43	1.35	1.22	1.16	

Percentile rankings* for women	AGE (YEARS)					
	20-29	30-39	40-49	50-59	60+	70+
90	2.05	1.73	1.63	1.51	1.40	1.27
80	1.66	1.50	1.46	1.30	1.25	1.12
70	1.42	1.47	1.35	1.24	1.18	1.10
60	1.36	1.32	1.26	1.18	1.15	0.95
50	1.32	1.26	1.19	1.09	1.08	0.89
40	1.25	1.21	1.12	1.03	1.04	0.83
30	1.23	1.16	1.03	0.95	0.98	0.82
20	1.13	1.09	0.94	0.86	0.94	0.79
10	1.02	0.94	0.76	0.75	0.84	0.75

*Descriptors for percentile rankings: 70 = above average; 50 = average; 30 = below average; 10 = well below average.

Data for women provided by the Women's Exercise Research Center, The George Washington University Medical Center, Washington, DC, 1998.

Data for men provided by The Cooper Institute for Aerobics Research, *The Physical Fitness Specialist Manual,* Dallas: The Cooper Institute, 2005.

Reprinted, by permission, from V.H. Heyward and A.L. Gibson, 2014, *Advanced fitness assessment and exercise prescription,* 7th ed. (Champaign, IL: Human Kinetics) 163.

Table 2.9 Norms for the Partial Curl-Up Test

	AGE (YEARS)					
	15-19	20-29	30-39	40-49	50-59	60-69
Men						
Excellent	25	25	25	25	25	25
Very good	23-24	21-24	18-24	18-24	17-24	16-24
Good	21-22	16-20	15-17	13-17	11-16	11-15
Fair	16-20	11-15	11-14	6-12	8-10	6-10
Needs improvement	≤15	≤10	≤10	≤5	≤7	≤5
Women						
Excellent	25	25	25	25	25	25
Very good	22-24	18-24	19-24	19-24	19-24	17-24
Good	17-21	14-17	10-18	11-18	10-18	8-16
Fair	12-16	5-13	6-9	4-10	6-9	3-7
Needs improvement	≤11	≤4	≤5	≤3	≤5	≤2

Source: Canadian Physical Activity, Fitness & Lifestyle Approach: CSEP-Health & Fitness Program's Appraisal and Counselling Strategy, 3rd edition, © 2003. Reprinted with permission from the Canadian Society for Exercise Physiology.

Table 2.10   Norms for the Sit-and-Reach Test*

	AGE (YEARS)					
	15-19	**20-29**	**30-39**	**40-49**	**50-59**	**60-69**
Men						
Excellent	≥39	≥40	≥38	≥35	≥35	≥33
Very good	34-38	34-39	33-37	29-34	28-34	25-32
Good	29-33	30-33	28-32	24-28	24-27	20-24
Fair	24-28	25-29	23-27	18-23	16-23	15-19
Needs improvement	≤23	≤24	≤22	≤17	≤15	≤14
Women						
Excellent	≥43	≥41	≥41	≥38	≥39	≥35
Very good	38-42	37-40	36-40	34-37	33-38	31-34
Good	34-37	33-36	32-35	30-33	30-32	27-30
Fair	29-33	28-32	27-31	25-29	25-29	23-26
Needs improvement	≤28	≤27	≤26	≤24	≤24	≤22

*Distance measured in centimeters using a sit-and-reach box with the zero point at 26 cm. If using a box with the zero point at 23 cm, subtract 3 cm from each value in this table.

Source: Canadian Physical Activity, Fitness & Lifestyle Approach: CSEP-Health & Fitness Program's Appraisal and Counselling Strategy, 3rd edition, © 2003. Reprinted with permission from the Canadian Society for Exercise Physiology.

Table 2.11   Norms for Waist-to-Hip Girth Ratio

		RISK			
	Age	**Low**	**Moderate**	**High**	**Very high**
Men					
	20-29	<0.83	0.83-0.88	0.89-0.94	>0.94
	30-39	<0.84	0.84-0.91	0.92-0.96	>0.96
	40-49	<0.88	0.88-0.95	0.96-1.00	>1.00
	50-59	<0.90	0.90-0.96	0.97-1.02	>1.02
	60-69	<0.91	0.91-0.98	0.99-1.03	>1.03
Women					
	20-29	<0.71	0.71-0.77	0.78-0.82	>0.82
	30-39	<0.72	0.72-0.78	0.79-0.84	>0.84
	40-49	<0.73	0.73-0.79	0.80-0.87	>0.87
	50-59	<0.74	0.74-0.81	0.82-0.88	>0.88
	60-69	<0.76	0.76-0.83	0.84-0.90	>0.90

Reprinted, by permission, from V.H. Heyward and A.L. Gibson, 2014, *Advanced fitness assessment and exercise prescription,* 7th ed. (Human Kinetics) 257; Data from G.A. Bray and D.S. Gray, 1988, "Obesity - Part I - Pathogenesis," *The Western Journal of Medicine* 149:429-441.

Table 2.12   Body Composition Skinfold Prediction Equations

SKF sites	Population subgroups	Equation	Reference
Σ7SKF (chest + abdomen + thigh + triceps + subscapular + suprailiac + midaxilla)	Black or Hispanic women, 18-55 years	Db (g·cc^{-1})^a = 1.0970 − 0.00046971(Σ7SKF) + 0.00000056(Σ7SKF)^2 − 0.00012828(age)	Jackson et al. (1980)
	Black men or male athletes, 18-61 years	Db (g·cc^{-1})^a = 1.1120 − 0.00043499(Σ7SKF) + 0.00000055(Σ7SKF)^2 − 0.00028826(age)	Jackson and Pollock (1978)
Σ4SKF (triceps + anterior suprailiac + abdomen + thigh)	Female athletes, 18-29 years	Db (g·cc^{-1})^a = 1.096095 − 0.0006952(Σ4SKF) + 0.0000011(Σ4SKF)^2 − 0.0000714(age)	Jackson et al. (1980)
Σ3SKF (triceps + suprailiac + thigh)	White or anorexic women, 18-55 years	Db (g·cc^{-1})^a = 1.0994921 − 0.0009929(Σ3SKF) + 0.0000023(Σ3SKF)^2 − 0.0001392(age)	Jackson et al. (1980)
Σ3SKF (chest + abdomen + thigh)	White men, 18-61 years	Db (g·cc^{-1})^a = 1.109380 − 0.0008267(Σ3SKF) + 0.0000016(Σ3SKF)^2 − 0.0002574(age)	Jackson and Pollock (1978)
Σ3SKF (abdomen + thigh + triceps)	Black or white collegiate male and female athletes, 18-34 years	%BF = 8.997 + 0.2468(Σ3SKF) − 6.343(gender^b) − 1.998(race^c)	Evans et al. (2005)
Σ2SKF (triceps + calf)	Black or white boys, 6-17 years Black or white girls, 6-17 years	%BF = 0.735(Σ2SKF) + 1.0 %BF = 0.610(Σ2SKF) + 5.1	Slaughter et al. (1988)

ΣSKF = sum of skinfolds (mm).

[a]Use population-specific conversion formulas to calculate %BF (percent body fat) from Db (body density).

[b]Male athletes = 1; female athletes = 0.

[c]Black athletes = 1; white athletes = 0.

Table 2.13 Percent Body Fat Standards for Adults, Children, and Physically Active Adults

		RECOMMENDED %BF* LEVELS FOR ADULTS AND CHILDREN			
	NR*	Low	Mid	High	Obesity
Males					
6-17 years	<5	5-10	11-25	26-31	>31
18-34 years	<8	8	13	22	>22
35-55 years	<10	10	18	25	>25
55+ years	<10	10	16	23	>23
Females					
6-17 years	<12	12-15	16-30	31-36	>36
18-34 years	<20	20	28	35	>35
35-55 years	<25	25	32	38	>38
55+ years	<25	25	30	35	>35
		RECOMMENDED %BF LEVELS FOR PHYSICALLY ACTIVE ADULTS			
		Low	Mid	Upper	
Males					
18-34 years		5	10	15	
35-55 years		7	11	18	
55+ years		9	12	18	
Females					
18-34 years		16	23	28	
35-55 years		20	27	33	
55+ years		20	27	33	

*NR = not recommended; %BF = percent body fat.

Data from Lohman, Houtkooper, and Going 1997.

Reprinted, by permission, from V.H. Heyward and A.L. Gibson, 2014, *Advanced fitness assessment and exercise prescription*, 7th ed. (Champaign, IL: Human Kinetics), 220.

Table 2.14   Norms for the Balance Error Scoring System (BESS) Test

Classification[a]	Superior	Above average	Broadly normal	Below average	Poor	Very poor
Men						
20-29 years[b]	0-4	5-6	7-14	15	16-21	22+
30-39 years	0-4	5-6	7-15	16-18	19-26	27+
40-49 years	0-5	6-7	8-16	17-20	21-27	28+
50-54 years	0-6	7	8-17	18-23	24-28	29+
55-59 years	0-7	8-10	11-20	21-28	29-34	35+
60-64 years	0-8	9-11	12-21	22-27	28-35	36+
65-69 years	0-12	13-14	15-23	24-33	34-39	40+
Women						
20-29 years[b]	0-5	6-7	8-14	15-19	20-25	26+
30-39 years	0-4	5-6	7-15	16-19	20-27	28+
40-49 years	0-5	6-7	8-15	16-20	21-29	30+
50-54 years	0-7	8-9	10-20	21-24	25-35	36+
55-59 years	0-8	9-10	11-21	22-28	29-39	40+
60-64 years	0-9	10-12	13-22	23-31	32-43	44+
65-69 years[b]	0-13	14	15-24	25-27	28-38	39+

[a]These classification ranges correspond to the following percentile ranks: superior: >90th percentile; above average: 76th to 90th percentile; broadly normal: 25th to 75th percentile; below average: 10th to 24th percentile; poor: 2nd to 9th percentile; very poor: <2nd percentile.

[b]Unusually small sample sizes limit the usefulness of these normative reference values.

Adapted from G.L. Iverson and M.S. Koehle, 2013, "Normative data for the balance error scoring system in adults," *Rehabilitation Research and Practice* 1-5. Copyright © 2013 Grant L. Iverson and Michael S. Koehle. This is an open access article distributed under the Creative Commons Attribution License 3.0.

Table 2.15a Standards for the 8-Foot Up-and-Go Test for Women (in Seconds)

Percentile rank	AGE (YEARS)						
	60-64	65-69	70-74	75-79	80-84	85-89	90-94
95	3.2	3.6	3.8	4.0	4.0	4.5	5.0
90	3.7	4.1	4.0	4.3	4.4	4.7	5.3
85	4.0	4.4	4.3	4.6	4.9	5.3	6.1
80	4.2	4.6	4.7	5.0	5.4	5.8	6.7
75	4.4	4.8	4.9	5.2	5.7	6.2	7.3
70	4.6	5.0	5.2	5.5	6.1	6.6	7.7
65	4.7	5.1	5.4	5.7	6.3	6.9	8.2
60	4.9	5.3	5.6	5.9	6.7	7.3	8.6
55	5.0	5.4	5.8	6.1	6.9	7.6	9.0
50	5.2	5.6	6.0	6.3	7.2	7.9	9.4
45	5.4	5.8	6.2	6.5	7.5	8.2	9.8
40	5.5	5.9	6.4	6.7	7.8	8.5	10.2
35	5.7	6.1	6.6	6.9	8.1	8.9	10.6
30	5.8	6.2	6.8	7.1	8.3	9.2	11.1
25	6.0	6.4	7.1	7.4	8.7	9.6	11.5
20	6.2	6.6	7.3	7.6	9.0	10.0	12.1
15	6.4	6.8	7.7	8.0	9.5	10.5	12.7
10	6.7	7.1	8.0	8.3	10.0	11.1	13.5
5	7.2	7.6	8.6	8.9	10.8	12.0	14.6

Table 2.15b Standards for the 8-Foot Up-and-Go Test for Men (in Seconds)

Percentile rank	AGE (YEARS)						
	60-64	65-69	70-74	75-79	80-84	85-89	90-94
95	3.0	3.1	3.2	3.3	4.0	4.0	4.3
90	3.0	3.6	3.6	3.5	4.1	4.3	4.5
85	3.3	3.9	3.9	3.9	4.5	4.5	5.1
80	3.6	4.1	4.2	4.3	4.9	5.0	5.7
75	3.8	4.3	4.4	4.6	5.2	5.5	6.2
70	4.0	4.5	4.6	4.9	5.5	5.8	6.6
65	4.2	4.6	4.8	5.2	5.7	6.2	7.0
60	4.4	4.8	5.0	5.4	6.0	6.5	7.4
55	4.5	4.9	5.1	5.7	6.2	6.9	7.7
50	4.7	5.1	5.3	5.9	6.4	7.2	8.1
45	4.9	5.3	5.5	6.1	6.6	7.5	8.5
40	5.0	5.4	5.6	6.4	6.9	7.9	8.8
35	5.2	5.6	5.8	6.6	7.1	8.2	9.2
30	5.4	5.7	6.0	6.9	7.3	8.6	9.6
25	5.6	5.9	6.2	7.2	7.6	8.9	10.0
20	5.8	6.1	6.4	7.5	7.9	9.4	10.5
15	6.1	6.3	6.7	7.9	8.3	9.9	11.1
10	6.4	6.6	7.0	8.3	8.7	10.5	11.8
5	6.8	7.1	7.4	9.0	9.4	11.5	12.9

Reprinted, by permission, from R.E. Rikli and C. J. Jones, 2013, *Senior fitness test manual,* 2nd ed. (Champaign, IL: Human Kinetics), 160.

Table 2.16a Standards for the 6-Minute Walk Test for Women (in Yards)

Percentile rank	AGE (YEARS)						
	60-64	65-69	70-74	75-79	80-84	85-89	90-94
95	741	734	709	696	654	638	564
90	711	697	673	655	612	591	518
85	690	673	650	628	584	560	488
80	674	653	630	605	560	534	463
75	659	636	614	585	540	512	441
70	647	621	599	568	523	493	423
65	636	607	586	553	508	476	406
60	624	593	572	538	491	458	388
55	614	581	561	524	477	443	373
50	603	568	548	509	462	426	357
45	592	555	535	494	447	409	341
40	582	543	524	480	433	394	326
35	570	529	510	465	416	376	308
30	559	515	497	450	401	359	291
25	547	500	482	433	384	340	273
20	532	483	466	413	364	318	251
15	516	463	446	390	340	292	226
10	495	439	423	363	312	261	196
5	465	402	387	322	270	214	150

Table 2.16b Standards for the 6-Minute Walk Test for Men (in Yards)

Percentile rank	AGE (YEARS)						
	60-64	65-69	70-74	75-79	80-84	85-89	90-94
95	825	800	779	762	721	710	646
90	792	763	743	716	678	659	592
85	770	738	718	686	649	625	557
80	751	718	698	661	625	596	527
75	736	700	680	639	604	572	502
70	722	685	665	621	586	551	480
65	710	671	652	604	571	532	461
60	697	657	638	586	554	512	440
55	686	644	625	571	540	495	422
50	674	631	612	555	524	477	403
45	662	618	599	539	508	459	384
40	651	605	586	524	494	442	366
35	638	591	572	506	477	422	345
30	626	577	559	489	462	403	326
25	612	562	544	471	444	382	304
20	597	544	526	449	423	358	279
15	578	524	506	424	399	329	249
10	556	499	481	394	370	295	214
5	523	462	445	348	327	244	160

Reprinted, by permission, from R.E. Rikli and C. J. Jones, 2013, *Senior fitness test manual*, 2nd ed. (Champaign, IL: Human Kinetics), 156.

Table 2.17a Standards for the 2-Minute Step Test for Women (in Steps)

Percentile rank	AGE (YEARS)						
	60-64	65-69	70-74	75-79	80-84	85-89	90-94
95	130	133	125	123	113	106	92
90	122	123	116	115	104	98	85
85	116	117	110	109	99	93	80
80	111	112	105	104	94	88	76
75	107	107	101	100	90	85	72
70	103	104	97	96	87	81	69
65	100	100	94	93	84	79	66
60	97	96	90	90	81	76	63
55	94	93	87	87	78	73	61
50	91	90	84	84	75	70	58
45	88	87	81	81	72	67	55
40	85	84	78	78	69	64	53
35	82	80	74	75	66	61	50
30	79	76	71	72	63	59	47
25	75	73	67	68	60	55	44
20	71	68	63	64	56	52	40
15	66	63	58	59	51	47	36
10	60	57	52	53	46	42	31
5	52	47	43	45	37	39	24

Reprinted, by permission, from R.E. Rikli and C. J. Jones, 2013, *Senior fitness test manual,* 2nd ed. (Champaign, IL: Human Kinetics), 157.

Table 2.17b Standards for the 2-Minute Step Test for Men (in Steps)

Percentile rank	AGE (YEARS)						
	60-64	65-69	70-74	75-79	80-84	85-89	90-94
95	135	139	133	135	126	114	112
90	128	130	124	126	118	106	102
85	123	125	119	119	112	100	96
80	119	120	114	114	107	95	91
75	115	116	110	109	103	91	86
70	112	113	107	105	99	87	83
65	109	110	104	102	96	84	79
60	106	107	101	98	93	81	76
55	104	104	98	95	90	78	72
50	101	101	95	91	87	75	69
45	98	98	92	87	84	72	66
40	96	95	89	84	81	69	62
35	93	92	86	80	78	66	59
30	90	89	83	77	75	63	55
25	87	86	80	73	71	59	52
20	83	82	76	68	67	55	47
15	79	77	71	63	62	50	42
10	74	72	66	56	56	44	36
5	67	67	67	47	48	36	26

Reprinted, by permission, from R.E. Rikli and C. J. Jones, 2013, *Senior fitness test manual,* 2nd ed. (Champaign, IL: Human Kinetics), 157.

Table 2.18a Standards for the 30-Second Chair Stand Test for Women (Number of Repetitions)

Percentile rank	AGE (YEARS)						
	60-64	65-69	70-74	75-79	80-84	85-89	90-94
95	21	19	19	19	18	17	16
90	20	18	18	17	17	15	15
85	19	17	17	16	16	14	13
80	18	16	16	16	15	14	12
75	17	16	15	15	14	13	11
70	17	15	15	14	13	12	11
65	16	15	14	14	13	12	10
60	16	14	14	13	12	11	9
55	15	14	13	13	12	11	9
50	15	14	13	12	11	10	8
45	14	13	12	12	11	10	7
40	14	13	12	12	10	9	7
35	13	12	11	11	10	9	6
30	12	12	11	11	9	8	5
25	12	11	10	10	9	8	4
20	11	11	10	9	8	7	4
15	10	10	9	9	7	6	3
10	9	9	8	8	6	5	1
5	8	8	7	6	4	4	0

Table 2.18b Standards for the 30-Second Chair Stand Test for Men (Number of Repetitions)

Percentile rank	AGE (YEARS)						
	60-64	65-69	70-74	75-79	80-84	85-89	90-94
95	23	23	21	21	19	19	16
90	22	21	20	20	17	17	15
85	21	20	19	18	16	16	14
80	20	19	18	18	16	15	13
75	19	18	17	17	15	14	12
70	19	18	17	16	14	13	12
65	18	17	16	16	14	13	11
60	17	16	16	15	13	12	11
55	17	16	15	15	13	12	10
50	16	15	14	14	12	11	10
45	16	15	14	13	12	11	9
40	15	14	13	13	11	10	9
35	15	13	13	12	11	9	8
30	14	13	12	12	10	9	8
25	14	12	12	11	10	8	7
20	13	11	11	10	9	7	7
15	12	11	10	10	8	6	6
10	11	9	9	8	7	5	5
5	9	8	8	7	6	4	3

Reprinted, by permission, from R.E. Rikli and C. J. Jones, 2013, *Senior fitness test manual,* 2nd ed. (Champaign, IL: Human Kinetics), 154.

Table 2.19a Standards for the 30-Second Arm Curl Test for Women (Number of Repetitions)

Percentile rank	AGE (YEARS)						
	60-64	65-69	70-74	75-79	80-84	85-89	90-94
95	24	22	22	21	20	18	17
90	22	21	20	20	18	17	16
85	21	20	19	19	17	16	15
80	20	19	18	18	16	15	14
75	19	18	17	17	16	15	13
70	18	17	17	16	15	14	13
65	18	17	16	16	15	14	12
60	17	16	16	15	14	13	12
55	17	16	15	15	14	13	11
50	16	15	14	14	13	12	11
45	16	15	14	13	12	12	10
40	15	14	13	13	12	11	10
35	14	14	13	12	11	11	9
30	14	13	12	12	11	10	9
25	13	12	12	11	10	10	8
20	12	12	11	10	10	9	8
15	11	11	10	9	9	8	7
10	10	10	9	8	8	7	6
5	9	8	8	7	6	6	5

Table 2.19b Standards for the 30-Second Arm Curl Test for Men (Number of Repetitions)

Percentile rank	AGE (YEARS)						
	60-64	65-69	70-74	75-79	80-84	85-89	90-94
95	27	27	26	24	23	21	18
90	25	25	24	22	22	19	16
85	24	24	23	21	20	18	16
80	23	23	22	20	20	17	15
75	22	21	21	19	19	17	14
70	21	21	20	19	18	16	14
65	21	20	19	18	18	15	13
60	20	20	19	17	17	15	13
55	20	19	18	17	17	14	12
50	19	18	17	16	16	14	12
45	18	18	17	16	15	13	12
40	18	17	16	15	15	13	11
35	17	16	15	14	14	12	11
30	17	16	15	14	14	11	10
25	16	15	14	13	13	11	10
20	15	14	13	12	12	10	9
15	14	13	12	11	12	9	8
10	13	12	11	10	10	8	8
5	11	10	9	9	9	7	6

Reprinted, by permission, from R.E. Rikli and C. J. Jones, 2013, *Senior fitness test manual*, 2nd ed. (Champaign, IL: Human Kinetics), 155.

Table 2.20a Standards for the Chair Sit-and-Reach Test for Women (in Inches)

Percentile rank	AGE (YEARS)						
	60-64	65-69	70-74	75-79	80-84	85-89	90-94
95	8.7	7.9	7.5	7.4	6.6	6.0	4.9
90	7.2	6.6	6.1	6.1	5.2	4.6	3.4
85	6.3	5.7	5.2	5.2	4.3	3.7	2.5
80	5.5	5.0	4.5	4.4	3.6	3.0	1.7
75	4.8	4.4	3.9	3.7	3.0	2.4	1.0
70	4.2	3.9	3.3	3.2	2.4	1.8	0.4
65	3.7	3.4	2.8	2.7	1.9	1.3	−0.1
60	3.1	2.9	2.3	2.1	1.4	0.8	−0.7
55	2.6	2.5	1.9	1.7	1.0	0.4	−1.2
50	2.1	2.0	1.4	1.2	0.5	−0.1	−1.7
45	1.6	1.5	0.9	0.7	0.0	−0.6	−2.2
40	1.1	1.1	0.5	0.2	−0.4	−1.0	−2.7
35	0.5	0.6	0.0	−0.3	−0.9	−1.5	−3.3
30	0.0	0.1	−0.5	−0.8	−1.4	−2.0	−3.8
25	−0.6	−0.4	−1.1	−1.3	−2.0	−2.6	−4.4
20	−1.3	−1.0	−1.7	−2.0	−2.6	−3.2	−5.1
15	−2.1	−1.7	−2.4	−2.8	−3.3	−3.9	−5.9
10	−3.0	−2.6	−3.3	−3.7	−4.2	−4.8	−6.8
5	−4.0	−3.9	−4.7	−5.0	−5.0	−6.3	−7.9

Table 2.20b Standards for the Chair Sit-and-Reach Test Men (in Inches)

Percentile rank	AGE (YEARS)						
	60-64	65-69	70-74	75-79	80-84	85-89	90-94
95	8.5	7.5	7.5	6.6	6.2	4.5	3.5
90	6.7	5.9	5.8	4.9	4.4	3.0	1.9
85	5.6	4.8	4.7	3.8	3.2	2.0	0.9
80	4.6	3.9	3.8	2.8	2.2	1.1	0.0
75	3.8	3.1	3.0	2.0	1.4	0.4	−0.7
70	3.1	2.4	2.4	1.3	0.6	−0.2	−1.4
65	2.5	1.8	1.8	0.7	0.0	−0.8	−1.9
60	1.8	1.1	1.1	0.1	−0.8	−1.3	−2.5
55	1.2	0.6	0.6	−0.5	−1.4	−1.9	−3.0
50	0.6	0.0	0.0	−1.1	−2.0	−2.4	−3.6
45	0.0	−0.6	−0.6	−1.7	−2.6	−2.9	−4.2
40	−0.6	−1.1	−1.2	−2.3	−3.2	−3.5	−4.7
35	−1.3	−1.8	−1.8	−2.9	−4.0	−4.0	−5.3
30	−1.9	−2.4	−2.4	−3.5	−4.6	−4.6	−5.8
25	−2.6	−3.1	−3.1	−4.2	−5.3	−5.2	−6.5
20	−3.4	−3.9	−3.9	−5.0	−6.2	−5.9	−7.2
15	−4.4	−4.8	−4.8	−6.0	−7.2	−6.8	−8.1
10	−5.5	−5.9	−5.9	−7.1	−8.4	−7.8	−9.1
5	−7.3	−7.5	−7.6	−8.8	−10.2	−9.3	−10.7

Reprinted, by permission, from R.E. Rikli and C. J. Jones, 2013, *Senior fitness test manual,* 2nd ed. (Champaign, IL: Human Kinetics), 158.

3

Musculoskeletal Conditions and Disorders

Carwyn Sharp, PhD, CSCS,*D

After completing this chapter, you will be able to

◆ describe the pathophysiology of low back pain, posture conditions, osteoporosis and osteopenia, osteoarthritis, joint disorders, joint replacements, frailty, and sarcopenia;

◆ understand the major medication groups and their effects on individuals and the exercise response for those with these musculoskeletal conditions and disorders;

◆ explain the effects of different exercise modalities on individuals with low back pain, posture conditions, osteoporosis and osteopenia, osteoarthritis, joint disorders, joint replacements, frailty, and sarcopenia; and

◆ recognize appropriate exercise programming, precautions, and contraindications for individuals with low back pain, posture conditions, osteoporosis and osteopenia, osteoarthritis, joint disorders, joint replacements, frailty, and sarcopenia.

This chapter describes a number of significant musculoskeletal limitations to healthy movement, physical activity, and exercise participation, which in turn affect overall health, morbidity, and mortality. The underlying causes and risk factors of these conditions are outlined to provide the exercise professional with an understanding of the roles of exercise in the prevention, management, and treatment of symptoms. How the exercise professional can develop and implement effective and safe training programs for these individuals is then discussed. Included in this chapter are low back pain, posture conditions, osteoporosis and osteopenia, osteoarthritis, joint disorders, joint replacements, frailty, and sarcopenia. As with other diseases and disabilities described in this text, when developing a training program for individuals with one or more of these conditions, the exercise professional must not only understand the given disorder, but also be aware of and address other comorbidities that may be present and their accompanying treatment plans.

DISORDERS OF THE SPINE AND ASSOCIATED MUSCULATURE

Disorders of the spine and associated musculature are relatively common in Western countries such as the United States. However, they are complex and varied in onset, cause(s), and symptomatology between individuals and the disorders themselves, often leading to the disorders being defined based on general features. The difficulties in determining the exact etiology and symptoms result in largely individualized approaches to treatment, with exercise prescription recommendations that reflect an integrated team strategy encompassing medical, health, and exercise professionals. The conditions discussed next, low back pain and posture disorders, are examples of the more common afflictions described in the literature; thus the exercise professional is more likely to see individuals suffering from these versus others over their career.

Low Back Pain

Low back pain has a complex and often individualized etiology, making a specific and universally accepted clinical definition challenging. Thus **low back pain (LBP)** is generally defined as "pain and discomfort, localized below the costal margin and above the inferior gluteal folds, with or without leg pain" (157) (figure 3.1). Low back pain may be the result of a known trauma or pathology, or more commonly, may have an idiopathic (i.e., unknown cause or origin) etiology, which is referred to as nonspecific LBP. In conjunction, nonspecific LBP is characterized by the duration of persistent symptoms: acute (<6 weeks); subacute (6 to 12 weeks); or chronic (12+ weeks) (157).

The prevalence of LBP in developed countries is pervasive, with an estimated lifetime prevalence of 58% to 70% (111, 144, 161); prevalence rates increase with advancing age (45, 66). The direct and indirect economic costs of LBP in the United States have been estimated as $12.2 to $90.6 billion and $7.4 to $28.17 billion per year, respectively (40). The wide variance in these estimates has been attributed to the methodological differences employed by the various researchers, which may be further confounded by a lack of an accepted definition (40). It is important to note, however, that the costs associated with LBP are substantial and include a combination of medical office visits, diagnostic tests, medications, surgery, travel costs to medical appointments, and lost wages and productivity. Thus the high prevalence of this condition and its costs to the individual and society are significant.

Pathophysiology of Low Back Pain

Low back pain and nonspecific LBP in particular often have a complex, highly variable etiology, which has been associated with a number of factors including, but not limited to, age, sex, height, weight, low physical fitness, smoking, and poor general health (140). In conjunction, studies have shown that various occupational factors such as high physical demands, lifting and forceful movements, and whole-body vibration may contribute 28% to 50% of reported low back issues (140). Differences in pathophysiology or spinal abnormalities—affecting one or more spinous structures, various intervertebral joints or discs, musculature, or neural components leading to inflammation, swelling, and pain in one or more of these areas—can also contribute to the

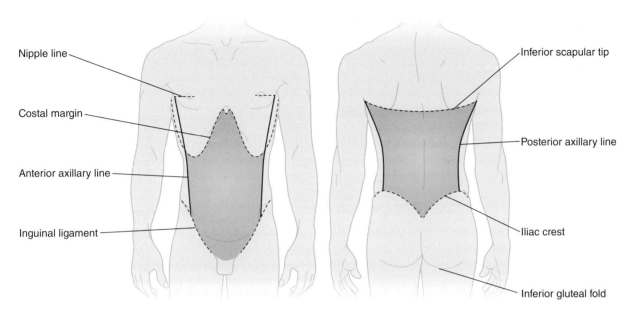

Figure 3.1 Low back pain is generally defined as a localized pain or ache below the costal margin and above the inferior gluteal folds.

development of LBP and the high degree of variability in symptom severity and recurrence (141).

Key Point

Low back pain is highly variable and complex in etiology and is most commonly of unknown cause or origin. Symptom severity and recurrence are also highly variable, making an individualized treatment plan essential.

Common Medications Given to Individuals With Low Back Pain

Various over-the-counter (OTC) and prescription medications are prescribed for and used by individuals with LBP (see medications table 3.1 near the end of the chapter) (1, 157). Over-the-counter nonsteroidal anti-inflammatory drugs (NSAIDs) such as ibuprofen (e.g., Advil and Motrin) and naproxen (e.g., Aleve) may reduce inflammation, swelling, and mild pain. Over-the-counter nonopioid analgesics such as acetaminophen (e.g., Tylenol) are mild to moderate pain relievers that are also often used by those with LBP. If used as directed, both NSAIDs and nonopioid analgesics have minimal side effects and impact on the acute

responses to physical activity (1, 140) but may impair the postexercise skeletal muscle protein synthetic response (153). Ingestion of NSAIDs can also result in gastrointestinal (GI) irritation or bleeding if they are taken for prolonged periods or at higher than recommended doses; acetaminophen may similarly cause GI discomfort such as stomach pain and in rare cases may lead to GI bleeding or negatively affect hepatic and renal functioning (159). It should also be noted that in 2015 the U.S. Food and Drug Administration (FDA) updated and strengthened its warning that the use of NSAIDs increases the risk of heart attack and stroke and that these risks increase with high doses and longer use (158). Topical capsicum plasters, another OTC medication, may also provide pain relief for individuals with LBP and appear to have no impact on exercise capacity (1).

Individuals with LBP may also use antispasmodic muscle relaxants such as Valium in conjunction with or in isolation from other medications and may suffer from dizziness and drowsiness as a result. This class of medication is typically prescribed to be taken before sleep and should have little effect on exercise capacity the following day, but communication with clients to verify is essential. Those individuals prescribed antidepressants, the most common class of which is selective serotonin reuptake inhibitors (SSRIs) (e.g., Prozac, Zoloft, and Paxil), may experience numerous side effects such as nausea, dizziness, drowsiness, and headaches; however, these are less severe than with other classes and do not appear to affect the response to exercise (112). People who experience these side effects should talk with their physician about timing, such as in the evening before sleep, so as to facilitate engagement in a physical activity program during the day.

Few research studies are available on whether oral opiates to treat the symptoms of nonspecific LBP have any negative effects on exercise capacity; however, some evidence suggests that opiates may affect hand–eye coordination (2), and this should be taken into account. Long-term use of SSRIs and opiates is not recommended, as the list of side effects increases as does their physiological impact.

Exercise professionals should also be aware that normal aging affects pharmacodynamics and that older adults with LBP are at a greater risk than others for side effects from medications taken for this condition; this may be further complicated by other medications that are being taken concomitantly (30).

Effects of Exercise in Individuals With Low Back Pain

Low back pain and nonspecific LBP often result in a reduction in levels of physical activity, which may or may not be a result of physical impairment or disability (88). As such, a key aspect in the treatment of this condition is education regarding the efficacy of physical activity in both the treatment and management of the condition, as well as improving general health and physical functioning. The research examining the roles of exercise for individuals with LBP has focused on either a biomedical impairment or a general conditioning model (140). The biomedical impairment model reflects the assumption that the condition is a function of insufficient trunk strength, mobility, or both, whereas the general conditioning model assumes that deconditioning is a significant underlying contributor. However, while trunk strength, trunk mobility, and aerobic conditioning are common modalities for chronic nonspecific LBP treatment, systematic reviews of the scientific literature have failed to show strong correlations or predictive capacity between these proposed causes and the condition itself (140). These findings may be a product of the high variability in the methodologies employed in the research of this area or the highly variable and individualized nature of symptoms. In any case, what is currently evident is that exercise is more efficacious than rest, so in the absence of specific guidelines, it is recommended that exercise professionals refer to the generally accepted guidelines adopted by the U.S. Department of Health and Human Services (DHHS) in 2008 for developing exercise workouts and programs for adults with LBP (156). However, the exercise prescription must be individualized in its implementation and progression to reflect the limitations, strengths, weaknesses, and goals of the client for successful development of health, fitness, and function.

Exercise Recommendations for Clients With Low Back Pain

With this in mind, testing and assessment for trunk strength, muscular endurance, and mobility, as well as general aerobic capacity, may be considered before initiating a training program. In conjunction, a medical clearance should be required before testing to ensure there are no structural limitations to exercise.

Program design guidelines for clients with LBP are summarized in table 3.1. The recommendations for a resistance training program to improve overall muscular strength and endurance, and in particular abdominal and lumbar extensor strength, are two to four sets (one set if the client is sedentary or low in conditioning) of 8 to 12 repetitions per exercise at an initial light to moderate intensity, one or two times per week (156). Flexibility training should aim to increase trunk, hip flexor, and extensor mobility via three repetitions of 10-second static hold for each exercise (141). Recommendations for aerobic exercise (e.g., brisk walking) are to engage large muscle groups at an initial light to moderate intensity for at least 10 minutes three or more times per day on three or more days per week, progressing to at least 300 minutes of moderate or 150 minutes of vigorous (or an equivalent combination of both intensities) per week. Exercise should cease immediately if there is an increase in lower back pain, with possible referral to a physician or other health care professional depending on the severity and duration of the increased pain.

Table 3.1 Program Design Guidelines for Clients With Low Back Pain

Type of exercise	Frequency	Intensity	Volume
Resistance training			
	Begin with one or two sessions per week	Begin with light to moderate intensity (40-80% one repetition maximum [1RM]), using multijoint exercises to engage all major muscle groups	Start with 1 set per exercise of 8-12 reps
	Increase to two or more sessions per week as tolerated	Progress to moderate to high intensity with 1-2 min rest between sets	Increase to 2-4 sets per exercise as appropriate
Aerobic training			
Modes: walking, jogging, running, swimming, other aquatic exercise	Begin with at least three sessions per week	Begin with light to moderate intensity (30% to <60% $\dot{V}O_2$ or heart rate reserve or 55% to <75% maximal heart rate [MHR], or RPE of 9-13 on Borg 6- to 20-point scale)	Begin with at least 10 min per session three or more times per day
	Progress to four or more sessions a week OR Three or more sessions a week	Moderate intensity (40% to <60% $\dot{V}O_2$ or heart rate reserve or 65% to <75% MHR, or RPE of 12-13 on Borg 6- to 20-point scale) / Vigorous intensity (≥60% $\dot{V}O_2$ or heart rate reserve or ≥75% MHR, or RPE of ≥14 on Borg 6- to 20-point scale)	300 min per week / 150 min per week

Reference: (156)

Case Study

Low Back Pain

Mr. Y, 41 years old, has had persistent dull pain on the left aspects of his lower back for 14 weeks. He is an office administrator who sits at his desk for almost 8 hours each day. The onset of pain occurred while he was play wrestling with his four children, when he felt a sharp pain in his lower back. He was able to stand but with considerable pain and stiffness. Mr. Y has taken acetaminophen intermittently for pain relief ever since and uses a heating pad for relief also. Flexion of the spine, such as in picking up his children, heightens the pain; and although the

(continued)

Low Back Pain *(continued)*

pain has subsided it is still present, sometimes radiating down his left leg. Before his injury Mr. Y had been inconsistently running and doing resistance exercise a total of one or two times per week over the past year.

With this medical and fitness history, and following clearance from Mr. Y's physician or other health care professional, his exercise professional altered the resistance training program to light to moderate intensity and added a second abdominal and lower back and gluteal activa-

tion exercise, for an initial four-week phase. The exercise professional also added trunk, hip flexor, and extensor mobility exercises before each resistance and aerobic session, which Mr. Y had not been doing previously. After this initial phase, the exercise professional will reassess symptoms, trunk strength, muscular endurance, and mobility, as well as general aerobic capacity, to determine the efficacy of these training program modifications.

Recommended Readings

Airaksinen, O, Brox, JI, Cedraschi, C, Hildebrandt, J, Klaber-Moffett, J, Kovacs, F, Mannion, AF, Reis, S, Staal, JB, Ursin, H, and Zanoli, G. Chapter 4. European guidelines for the management of chronic nonspecific low back pain. *Eur Spine J* 15(suppl 2):S192-S300, 2006.

van Tulder, M, Becker, A, Bekkering, T, Breen, A, Gil del Real, MT, Hutchinson, A, Koes, B, Laerum, E, and Malmivaara, A. Chapter 3. European guidelines for the management of acute nonspecific low back pain in primary care. *Eur Spine J* 15(suppl 2):S169-S191, 2006.

Posture Conditions

The term **posture** generally refers to the position of a person's head, neck, trunk, and limbs in space or when standing, seated, or lying down. "Good posture," then, may be seen as alignment of the musculoskeletal system that allows maximum efficiency of body movement and functions and does not place pathological stress on the muscular, skeletal, or nervous systems (22). In order to assess whether someone's posture allows for optimal health and functioning, testing should be undertaken under both static and dynamic conditions to reflect daily conditions that are static (e.g., sitting and standing) and those that are dynamic (e.g., walking) (22, 79). The roles of the spine in posture are significant, and various spinal conditions exist that lead to postural dysfunctions, pain, and discomfort, such as excessive scoliosis. The spine has a natural shape and curvature expressed as the forward convex (i.e., **lordotic**) cervical curve, the forward concave (i.e.,

kyphotic) thoracic curve, and the lordotic lumbar curve (figure 3.2). This curvature assists in maintaining a balanced and efficient upright posture during standing and locomotion (22). However, certain medical and nonmedical conditions exist that can lead to **hyperlordosis** (i.e., excessive lordosis of the cervical or more commonly the lumbar spine), **hyperkyphosis** (i.e., excessive kyphosis of the thoracic spine), and **scoliosis** (i.e., mediolateral curvature of the spine), all of which negatively affect optimal posture.

The prevalence of these spinal conditions varies greatly depending on the population studied, environmental factors, methodology for spinal measurement, and age (19, 22, 47, 71, 131, 135, 171). However, the National Scoliosis Foundation estimates that 2% to 3% of the U.S. population, or approximately 7 million people, have scoliosis. The highest incidence of scoliosis is between 10 to 15 years, with females being eight times more likely than males to have a curvature that requires treatment (104). This prevalence, and the

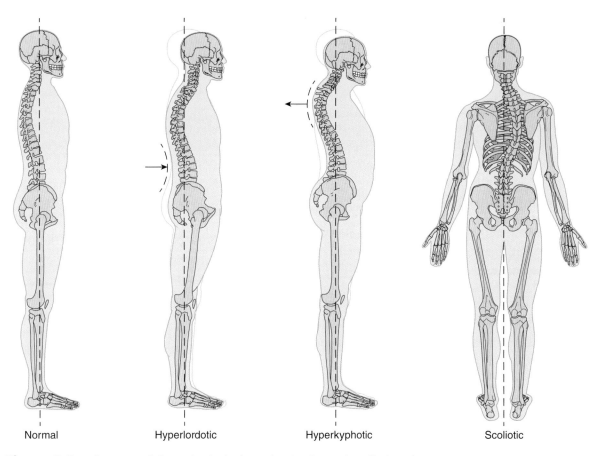

Figure 3.2 The normal, hyperlordotic, hyperkyphotic, and scoliotic spine.

potential for long-term and chronic health issues if the opportunities for early intervention are missed, may result in adverse personal and societal health impacts.

Pathophysiology of Posture Conditions

The spine undergoes a variety of changes throughout the life span that alter the susceptibility to adverse spinal curvature and subsequent postural dysfunction (22). In general, the causes of lumbar hyperlordosis, hyperkyphosis, and scoliosis are unknown (i.e., idiopathic); however, a number of risk factors have been identified. Physical and psychological stress, trauma, sporting activities, occupational behaviors such as prolonged sitting, slouching, and wearing high heels have been associated with increased risks (22). Lumbar hyperlordosis has also been associated with conditions such as cerebral palsy, muscular dystrophy, obesity, osteoar-thritis, and in some cases pregnancy, as well as from shortened (i.e., "tight") hip flexor muscles or weak abdominal, lower back, hamstring or gluteus maximus musculature (17, 22). Lumbar hyperlordosis can lead to LBP and increased risk of lumbar injury. Hyperkyphosis (also called "humpback," "hunchback," or "dowager's hump") may occur as the result of osteoarthritis, osteoporosis, or trauma to the thoracic spine. Severe hyperkyphosis can lead to impaired lung capacity and function, nerve impingement, and pain (39). While the majority of scoliosis cases are largely idiopathic (104), they may still be categorized as structural (e.g., a deformity in the vertebrae) or functional scoliosis (which is reversible and the result of either disparity in leg lengths, pain, or muscle spasm). Scoliosis can lead to compromised movement patterns, pain, reduced physical functioning, and impaired respiratory functions (166).

Common Medications Given to Individuals With Posture Conditions

Treatment for spinal deformities depends on the severity, location, age of diagnosis, and concomitant conditions. Severe curvature and resulting symptoms may require bracing or corrective surgery such as disc replacement, kyphoplasty, or spinal fusion. Mild lumbar hyperlordosis, hyperkyphosis, and scoliosis, on the other hand, may be treated with exercise or medications such as NSAIDs (e.g., ibuprofen), or both, and nonnarcotic analgesics (e.g., acetaminophen) for pain, inflammation, and swelling (see medications table 3.1 near the end of the chapter). As mentioned previously, caution is advised with NSAIDs, as their use increases the risk of heart attack and stroke, and these risks increase with high doses and longer use (158).

Effects of Exercise in Individuals With Posture Conditions

Exercise is commonly recommended as a means to treat or manage certain posture conditions and their symptoms (13, 57, 134). However, individuals who have more than mild severity of any of these conditions should be referred to a physician or other health care professional for treatment, including corrective exercise programming. The goals of an exercise program for clients with posture conditions are typically to improve flexibility and range of motion and build muscular strength to support and maintain optimum posture. This is true also for those experiencing one or more of these conditions during pregnancy or postpartum. In conjunction, reducing body fat in individuals for whom this is a contributing factor may also be a goal of an exercise program.

Exercise Recommendations for Clients With Posture Conditions

Meta-analysis of the existing literature has not yielded a consensus on specific exercise prescription to attenuate or reverse posture conditions. This appears largely due to variance in the methodologies, populations, and exercise prescription, as well as the preponderance of idiopathic diagnoses. As such, guidelines and goals are general and include increased strength of the weakened muscles and increased flexibility and range of motion of the tight and shortened muscles, which may have contributed to the condition.

- For those with mild lumbar hyperlordosis, inclusion of exercises that increase flexibility of the hip flexors, hamstrings, and erector spinae, plus those that strengthen the abdominal, lower back, and gluteal muscles and hamstrings, are recommended.

- Mild hyperkyphosis exercise programming should include stretching the cervical and thoracic vertebral flexors (e.g., isometric and dynamic neck retraction) and strengthening the thoracic vertebral extensors. It should also be noted that hyperkyphosis can make it difficult to complete overhead exercises such as a military press.

- For clients with mild scoliosis, include stretching for the concave side and strengthening exercises for the convex side. If vertebral column rotation is also present, these clients should first be referred to a physician or other health care professional for further testing to ensure there is no risk of nerve impingement.

Program design guidelines for clients with posture conditions are summarized in table 3.2. The recommended initial prescription for improving strength for beginner or deconditioned adults with mild posture conditions is one to three sets of 6 to 12 repetitions at approximately 60% to 80% of estimated 1RM, two or three times per week, with the goal of progressing (over 12 or more months of consistent training) to an advanced program of two to six sets of up to six repetitions at ≥85% of 1RM and 2 to 5 minutes rest between sets four or more times per week (105, 156). To increase flexibility and range of motion, it is recommended that clients initially complete static stretches three to seven times per week of all major muscle groups and hold each stretch for 15 to 30 seconds (105). An increased

Key Point

Individuals who have a posture condition of more than mild severity should be referred to a medical professional for treatment.

number of repetitions (typically two or three initially) should be incorporated for those areas specific to the posture condition of the client as identified earlier in this section.

Table 3.2 Program Design Guidelines for Clients With Mild Posture Conditions

Type of exercise	Frequency	Intensity	Volume
Resistance training			
Modes: weight training machines, free weights, or both, body weight, elastic tubing	Begin with 2-3 sessions per week	Initially moderate intensity (60-80% 1RM), using multijoint exercises to engage all major muscle groups	Start with 1-3 sets per exercise of 6-12 reps and 2-5 min rest between sets
	Progress to ≥4 sessions per week	Progress to high intensity (>80% 1RM)	Increase to 2-6 sets of ≤6 repetitions per exercise and 2-5 min rest between sets
Flexibility training			
	3-7 times per week	Stretches should be held at the point of mild discomfort (i.e., not painful)	Each stretch held for 15-30 s

References: (105, 156)

Case Study

Posture Conditions

Mrs. P is a 79-year-old retiree who has been diagnosed by her physician with mild thoracic hyperkyphosis. Assessment by the exercise professional has also highlighted that she has poor lower and upper body mobility and muscular weakness. The exercise professional has developed a training program that initially includes resistance training two days per week, and because Mrs. P is a novice with risk of falling, has prescribed a total body circuit weight training format on machines, including two exercises to strengthen the thoracic vertebral extensors (e.g., supermans and back extension if tolerated), with one to three sets of six repetitions. Before and after each training session (i.e., weight training and aerobic sessions) Mrs. P will complete upper and lower body static stretching and mobility exercises for 5 to 10 minutes with particular emphasis on dynamic neck retraction to stretch the cervical flexors, as well as stretches for the thoracic spine flexors.

Recommended Readings

Bansal, S, Katzman, WB, and Giangregorio, LM. Exercise for improving age-related hyperkyphotic posture: a systematic review. *Arch Phys Med Rehabil* 95(1):129-140, 2014.

Britnell, SJ, Cole, JV, Isherwood, L, Stan, MM, Britnell, N, Burgi, S, Candido, G, and Watson, L. Postural health in women: the role of physiotherapy. *J Obstet Gynaecol Can* 27(5):493-510, 2005.

Kritz, MF and Cronin, CJ. Static posture assessment screen of athletes: benefits and considerations. *Strength Cond J* 30(5):18-27, 2008.

DISORDERS OF THE SKELETAL SYSTEM

The adult human skeleton consists of approximately 206 bones as well as associated cartilage, ligaments, and tendons; it functions to provide leverage, support, protection, blood cell production, endocrine functions, and energy metabolism and also acts as a reservoir for calcium and phosphorus. However, bone is not a static material. Rather, it is highly dynamic and responds to stimuli such as muscular contractions, which result in movement around joints and locomotion, and the lack of stimuli, resulting in loss of bone mass and strength. Disorders of the skeletal system such as osteoporosis and osteopenia, osteoarthritis, and joint disorders can have profound direct and indirect impacts on an individuals' health, well-being, and fitness. Due to these concerns and the prevalence and incidence of these diseases and disorders, as well as the ability of exercise to posi-

tively affect them, exercise professionals should be knowledgeable of their pathophysiology, medical treatments, and optimal exercise interventions.

Osteoporosis

The World Health Organization (WHO) defines **osteoporosis** as a bone mineral density (BMD) at the hip or spine greater than or equal to 2.5 standard deviations (SD) below the "young normal" adult score (clinically referred to as T-score ≤2.5 SD), as measured by dual-energy x-ray absorptiometry (DXA) (164). The National Institutes of Health further defines osteoporosis functionally as a reduction in bone strength resulting in an increased risk of fracture (75). Bone is a dynamic tissue with active and mature cells involved in bone deposition and resorption (figure 3.3), so bone mass at any point in time is a function of the net effects of bone formation and resorption mechanisms. Osteoporosis then is the result of cumulative net bone resorption.

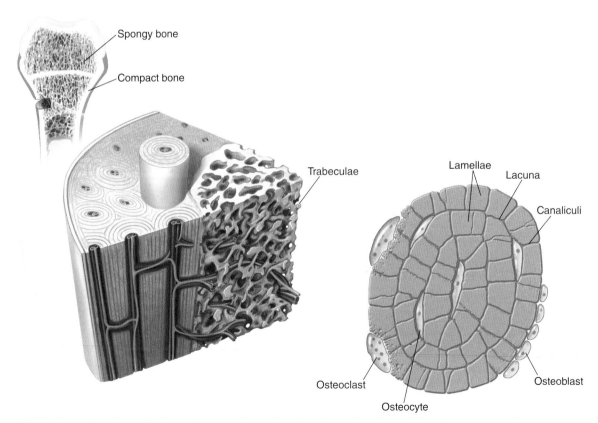

Figure 3.3 Bone is a dynamic tissue that consists of active deposition (osteoblasts), resorption (osteoclasts), and mature bone cells (osteocytes).

In 2014, osteoporosis was estimated to affect 10.2 million adults 50 years and older in the United States (169), contributing to approximately 2 million bone fractures per year and other physical and psychological effects (169). A further 43.4 million are estimated to have low bone density (i.e., osteopenia), which increases the risk for osteoporosis. Significant sex differences in osteoporosis have been observed, with women eight times more likely to have type 1 and two times more likely to have type 2 osteoporosis (see next section for subtype clarification) (169). The estimated prevalence of osteoporosis in the United States also differs among racial and ethnic groups, affecting an estimated 7.7 million non-Hispanic white, 0.5 million non-Hispanic black, and 0.6 million Mexican American adults (169). The increase in mortality and morbidity associated with osteoporosis is highlighted by the approximately 24% of individuals over the age of 50 with hip fractures who die within one year after the fracture (146). In addition, the financial cost of osteoporosis and associated fractures in the United States in 2008 was estimated at $22 billion (18), making it a significant health concern.

Pathophysiology of Osteoporosis

Osteoporosis may be classified as either primary or secondary. **Primary osteoporosis**, often called age-related osteoporosis, is the most common and represents the cumulative loss of bone associated with aging in both females and males (155). This is in part a consequence of declining activity of osteoblasts (i.e., bone-forming cells) after the age of 35 years, resulting in a small but natural loss of bone mass each year thereafter (146). Primary osteoporosis may be subclassified as type 1 or type 2. **Type 1 osteoporosis**, also referred to as **postmenopausal osteoporosis**, generally occurs from 50 to 65 years of age, resulting in accelerated bone resorption and decreased bone formation due to the loss of estrogen binding to its receptors on bone (155). This accelerated phase of bone loss appears to last from 4 to 10 years, resulting in an estimated loss of 5% to 10% and 20% to 30% of cortical and trabecular bone, respectively (35, 121). This is followed by a continued but slower

phase of loss (i.e., **type 2 [senile] osteoporosis**, which is evident after 70 years of age), resulting in a further 20% to 25% loss of cortical and trabecular bone in both men and women before the end of life. Type 2 osteoporosis is thought to be caused by a combination of factors in both men and women, including decreased renal vitamin D production and subsequent calcium absorption, decreased nutrient intake including calcium and vitamin D, decreased physical activity, and decreased estrogen and testosterone activity (121, 155). In men, while testosterone positively affects bone formation, estrogen is a more potent stimulator; and as testosterone levels decrease with aging, so too does the amount of testosterone available to be converted by the aromatase enzyme to estrogen (121, 122). In conjunction, aging men experience an increase in sex hormone-binding globulin, produced by the liver, which binds both testosterone and estrogen, thus further reducing bioavailability and negatively affecting bone mass and strength (62).

Secondary (type 3) osteoporosis is a consequence of another disease state (e.g., cystic fibrosis, anorexia nervosa, Crohn's disease) or medication use (e.g., glucocorticoid-induced osteoporosis) (155). However, other risk factors for osteoporosis have been identified, including hypogonadism, inactive lifestyle, smoking, alcohol abuse, and excessive protein, sodium, and caffeine intake (73).

Osteoporosis is a significant health concern because it not only increases the risk of bone fracture and health disorders such as progressive spinal deformity (e.g., thoracic kyphosis) in older adults, but also increases morbidity and mortality rates (155). However, much can be done to prevent and treat this disease especially if it is diagnosed and treated early.

Common Medications Given to Individuals With Osteoporosis

Several medications have been shown to be effective at improving BMD in osteoporotic individuals via antiresorptive and bone-forming mechanisms (see medications table 3.2 near the end of the chapter). **Hormone therapy** (previously known as **hormone replacement therapy, HRT**) using estrogen, progesterone, or both was formerly the most prescribed antiresorption treatment for osteoporosis; however, evidence for a concomitant decreased risk of heart disease with HRT has recently been questioned, as several long-term clinical trials have shown an increased risk for breast cancer, blood clots, stroke, and heart attacks (91). Thus it is recommended that cardiovascular risk factors be examined when HRT is being considered as a treatment for osteoporosis. (Note that progesterone is added to estrogen to reduce the risk of endometrial cancer.)

Selective estrogen receptor modulators (SERMs) are also classified as agents that reduce bone resorption. These include raloxifene, which is approved for use in postmenopausal women (146), and tamoxifen citrate, the first commercially available SERM, which is also used to treat metastatic breast cancer. Oral amino bisphosphonates such as alendronate are commonly prescribed to reduce the resorption of bone; however, a common side effect of this class of drugs is GI irritation (146). A number of synthetic analogues of the thyroid hormone calcitonin exist and may be used to decrease bone resorption by inhibiting the actions of the bone-resorbing osteoclasts and increasing osteoblast activity (32). From a nonpharmaceutical standpoint, the National Osteoporosis Foundation also recommends 1,200 mg per day of calcium for adults more than 50 years of age and not taking estrogen.

Effects of Exercise in Individuals With Osteoporosis

The National Osteoporosis Foundation of the United States recommends the implementation of regular weight-bearing and muscle-strengthening exercise to both prevent and treat osteoporosis (38). While moderate- to high-intensity weight-bearing exercise with a cyclical movement pattern has been shown to be more beneficial (100), light-intensity physical activity is a viable option for those whose bones are too fragile or who have another condition that precludes high intensity (146). Increasing muscular strength improves bone mass and strength through the transfer of mechanical stress to the bone via ten-

dons. In conjunction, improvements in muscular strength also assist in reducing the risk of falls (100). Regular aerobic exercise has also been shown to provide sufficient stimulus to improve markers of bone synthesis and breakdown (124). In conjunction, activities that improve balance and proprioception should also be included to reduce the risk of falls and fractures (100).

Key Point

Resistance training can reduce the risk of fractures not only by increasing bone strength and density, but the resultant increases in muscle strength can reduce the risk of falls.

Exercise Recommendations for Clients With Osteoporosis

As part of the preexercise screening process for those with osteoporosis, it is important to be aware of (1) any exercise limitations due to previous fractures (e.g., reduced locomotion capacity due to hip fracture), (2) muscle weaknesses or imbalances, (3) balance or proprioceptive issues, (4) the presence of other chronic diseases (e.g., cardiovascular disease, osteoarthritis), and (5) associated medications. The severity and location of osteoporosis are also important, as clients who are severely osteoporotic should avoid high-impact weight-bearing activity, despite the evidence of its efficacy, due to their increased risk of fracture.

Exercise testing can be undertaken with those who have osteoporosis to establish baseline values and determine exercise tolerance to assist in prescription; however a physician or other health care professional's clearance should be obtained before testing, and fall mitigation procedures should be implemented and maintained at all times. The validity of such tests may be compromised in clients with a fear of falling, so appropriate education about the mitigation procedures may improve test results.

Program design guidelines for clients with osteoporosis are summarized in table 3.3. Clients with osteoporosis are likely to be deconditioned, and thus initial use of light-intensity training is recommended (146).

- Aerobic exercise for those with mild to moderate osteoporosis (T-score <3) should include weight-bearing, large muscle mass activities such as running or walking at light to moderate intensity, 30 to 60 minutes per session, three to five days per week (i.e., ≥150 minutes per week) (146).

- Aerobic exercise in clients with severe osteoporosis, which may be represented as multiple fractures in recent years or noticeable spinal changes (e.g., kyphosis), should follow the same guidelines for duration and frequency but use light-intensity and low-impact exercises such as walking or swimming in the exercise program.

- Resistance training of two or three sets of 8 to 10 repetitions at 60% to 80% 1RM, two or three days per week, is also recommended (146). Using free weights with clients who are conditioned to do so safely will increase proprioceptive and balance demands. Again, for those with severe osteoporosis, a more conservative approach should be taken to reduce or avoid high-impact, twisting, and any activity resulting in bone or joint pain.

- Also recommended is flexibility training to increase mobility and range of motion, particularly at the hip, knee, and pectoral girdle, consisting of three stretches per muscle group, holding each stretch for up to 30 seconds, at a frequency of five to seven days per week (146). Avoid excessive twisting, flexion, and extension of the spine for anyone diagnosed as severely osteoporotic or with a history of fractures.

- Functional training that specifically aims to increase balance and proprioception is recommended two to five days per week.

In order to achieve the frequency of prescription, it may be necessary to complete more than one training modality in a single session, for example, flexibility exercises before and after resistance training.

Table 3.3 Program Design Guidelines for Clients With Osteoporosis

Type of exercise	Frequency	Intensity	Volume
Resistance training			
Modes: weight training machines or free weights or both, body weight, elastic tubing	Two or three sessions per week	Moderate intensity (60-80% 1RM), using multijoint exercises to engage all major muscle groups	2-3 sets per exercise of 8-10 repetitions and 2-5 min rest between sets
Aerobic training			
Mild to moderate osteoporosis (T-score <3)	3-5 days/week	Light to moderate (40-70% HRpeak), weight-bearing, large muscle mass activities such as running or walking	30-60 min per session (150 min per week)
Severe osteoporosis	3-5 days/week	Light to moderate (40-50% HRpeak), low- or no-impact weight-bearing, large muscle mass activities such as walking or swimming	30-60 min per session (150 min per week)
Flexibility training			
	5-7 days/week	Stretches should be held at the point of mild discomfort (i.e., not painful)	Three stretches per muscle group; hold each stretch for 15-30 s

Case Study

Osteoporosis

Ms. L is a 61-year-old woman who has recently been having pain in her hips and back when she walks or stands for long periods of time. She thought this might be arthritis, which "runs in her family," but she fell on the ice this past winter and the pain has worsened. X-rays showed a vertebral compression fracture, and follow-up DXA showed that she had a T-score of –2.6 SD.

Ms. L's initial treatment for the vertebral compression fracture involved two weeks of rest and NSAIDs for pain management followed by two months of wearing a brace. After her recovery phase, her physician provided clearance and encouragement for her to participate in a resistance exercise program; she received directions to avoid direct spinal loading from exercises such as squats and avoid exercises that encourage or require excessive spinal flexion or extension. To mitigate her osteoporosis, the exercise professional prescribed resistance training of three sets of 8 to 10 repetitions at 75% 1RM two days per week using free weights, as well as limited range of motion back extension and abdominal flexion on machines. Ms. L already walked seven days per week for 60 minutes; however, she did not stretch before or after. So, her exercise professional added static range of motion exercises for 5 to 10 minutes before and for 5 minutes afterward (avoiding excessive vertebral flexion, extension, and rotation) and intermittent periods of higher intensity during her walks.

Recommended Readings

Clarke, BL and Khosla, S. Physiology of bone loss. *Radiol Clin North Am* 48(3):483-495, 2010.

Moreira, LD, Moreira, LDF, Oliveira, MLD, Lirani-Galvão, AP, Marin-Mio, RV, Santos, RND, and Lazaretti-Castro, M. Physical exercise and osteoporosis: effects of different types of exercises on bone and physical function of postmenopausal women. *Arq Bras Endocrinol Metabol* 58(5):514-522, 2014.

Mosti, MP, Carlsen, T, Aas, E, Hoff, J, Stunes, AK, and Syversen, U. Maximal strength training improves bone mineral density and neuromuscular performance in young adult women. *J Strength Cond Res* 28(10):2935-2945, 2014.

Mosti, MP, Kaehler, N, Stunes, AK, Hoff, J, and Syversen, U. Maximal strength training in postmenopausal women with osteoporosis or osteopenia. *J Strength Cond Res* 27(10):2879-2886, 2013.

Osteopenia

Osteopenia is defined by the WHO as a BMD of 1.0 to 2.5 SD below that of a "young normal" adult (i.e., T-score –1.0 to –2.5 SD) (164) and has been estimated to affect approximately 43.4 million individuals in the United States (169). These individuals are at a significantly increased risk of osteoporosis and associated negative health concerns.

Pathophysiology of Osteopenia

The pathophysiology of osteopenia is generally the same as that already described for osteoporosis; however, the loss of bone mass and strength has not progressed to the same degree. It should be noted that osteopenia is not a condition exclusive to postmenopausal women but rather is present in younger women as a result of various factors, which may include hypothalamic amenorrhea, anorexia nervosa, limited calcium intake, or vitamin D insufficiency (61, 74). Individuals diagnosed with osteopenia should ensure that they have an appropriate intake of readily bioavailable calcium and vitamin D and rule out malabsorption from conditions such as celiac disease and Crohn's disease or the effect of medications such as cholestyramine and neomycin, among others. In conjunction, assessment of current and previous physical activity and exercise training programs can provide insight into whether afflicted individuals have been exposed to sufficient bone-forming stimuli throughout their lifetime. Diagnosis of osteopenia before osteoporosis allows for the implementation of interventions that increase the likelihood of reversing or slowing the rate of this disease.

Key Point

Osteopenia is not just a condition of postmenopausal women, but can be present in younger women as a result of a variety of factors including certain medical conditions, insufficient nutrient intake, or the side effect of a medication.

Common Medications Given to Individuals With Osteopenia

All medications have risks for side effects, and because the absolute risk of fracture for someone with osteopenia is relatively low, medications are generally not recommended until lifestyle (i.e., diet and exercise) and underlying conditions have been investigated as potential contributors. Those who are deemed to have a high risk for fractures—that is, they have other risk factors including

the presence of osteopenia—may be prescribed medications such as those for osteoporosis (see medications table 3.2 near the end of the chapter).

Effects of Exercise in Individuals With Osteopenia

The positive effects of various resistance training and aerobic exercise protocols to treat and manage osteopenia have been demonstrated (20, 101, 102) and reflect those for osteoporosis. These protocols typically place high cyclical strain on bone, which appears to be most effective at increasing BMD and strength.

Exercise Recommendations for Clients With Osteopenia

Due to the shared pathophysiology and progressive nature of osteopenia in relation to osteoporosis, the exercise recommendations for osteopenia are the same as those for osteoporosis (see exercise recommendations for osteoporosis earlier in the chapter), with the exception that in most cases of osteopenia, the absolute risk of fracture is lower than that of osteoporosis, so the high-impact or high-intensity exercise may be included. Note that consultation with the client's physician to determine fracture risk should be undertaken as part of the assessment phase of developing an exercise program.

Case Study

Osteopenia

Mrs. A is a 34-year-old executive who has a sedentary job but is an active triathlete. She is conscious of her diet and has been gluten and dairy free for 10 years. She has been having pain in her shins when she runs and has found that she has multiple stress fractures in both tibia. Further testing showed that she has celiac disease, resulting in calcium and vitamin D malabsorption. Subsequent DXA illustrated that she has a BMD T-score of –1.4 SD.

To improve Mrs. A's BMD and strength, her physician recommended that she start calcium and vitamin D supplementation. She was also asked to refrain from running but to maintain

her swimming and cycling until her stress fractures healed (six to eight weeks) and then gradually reintroduce running. In addition it was recommended that she incorporate and maintain high-intensity resistance training to improve muscle strength and bone stress to further increase her bone density.

Because Mrs. A had no experience in resistance training and knew she would struggle to slowly reintroduce running into her program, she hired an exercise professional to assist her. She began her resistance training with two sessions per week at 75% of her predicted 1RM, with three sets per exercise of 8 to 10

(continued)

Osteopenia *(continued)*

repetitions and 2 minutes rest between sets. Her exercise professional included core multijoint exercises such as the squat and deadlift to engage all major muscle groups and to maximize the bone deposition stimulus. Mrs. A also started a walking program of 30 minutes five days per week and progressed to three days of running at 70% of her peak heart rate and two days of walking. Her exercise professional prescribed flexibility training before and after all training sessions, with three repetitions of each stretch, and 30 seconds of holding each postexercise static stretch. Given that specialized nutrition guidance and prescription and clinical psychology were outside her exercise professional's scope of practice, it was recommended that Mrs. A meet and work with a sport dietician in conjunction with her sport psychologist to optimize her short- and long-term success.

Recommended Readings

Bolton, KL, Egerton, T, Wark, J, Wee, E, Matthews, B, Kelly, A, Craven, R, Kantor, S, and Bennell, KL. Effects of exercise on bone density and falls risk factors in post-menopausal women with osteopenia: a randomised controlled trial. *J Sci Med Sport* 15(2):102-109, 2012.

Kim, YI, Park, JH, Lee, JS, Kim, JW, Yang, SO, Jeon, DJ, Kim, MC, Jeong, TH, Lee, YG, and Rhee, BD. Prevalence and risk factors of the osteoporosis of perimenopausal women in the community population. *Korean J Med* 62(1):11-24, 2002.

Mosti, MP, Kaehler, N, Stunes, AK, Hoff, J, and Syversen, U. Maximal strength training in postmenopausal women with osteoporosis or osteopenia. *J Strength Cond Res* 27(10):2879-2886, 2013.

Roghani, T, Torkaman, G, Movasseghe, S, Hedayati, M, Goosheh, B, and Bayat, N. Effects of short-term aerobic exercise with and without external loading on bone metabolism and balance in postmenopausal women with osteoporosis. *Rheumatol Int* 33(2):291-298, 2013.

DISORDERS OF JOINT STRUCTURES

Joints are a key component of the musculoskeletal system and not only play a central role in movement of the human body and body segments (e.g., appendages), but also must support the weight of the various limbs and the entire body (e.g., vertebral joints). Thus the health and viability of joints are integral to movement and subsequently to health. The structural components of the body's joints undergo various normal and sometimes degenerative changes due to aging and are also susceptible to injury, infection, disease, and other conditions that can have negative impacts on the ability of joints to function optimally. This in turn can often lead to decreases in movement and physical activity and thereby a plethora of well-known associated negative health consequences. However, physical activity can also provide a positive stimulus for joint health and, as previously discussed, is important to overall health.

This section examines a number of the more common conditions associated with joints (i.e., osteoarthritis, joint sprains and dislocations, and joint replacements) that the exercise professional is most likely to encounter in clients. Exercise professionals should be knowledgeable regarding the pathophysiology, medical treatments, and considerations and the roles of exercise interventions that can support individuals' physical activity and health even with these joint structure disorders.

Osteoarthritis

Osteoarthritis (OA) is a degenerative joint disease affecting the cartilage, joint lining, ligaments, and bone, leading to pain, swelling, and stiffness of the affected joint(s) (figure 3.4). Osteoarthritis most

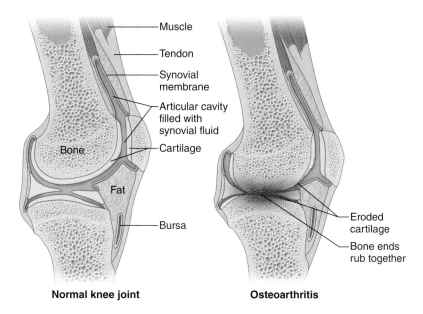

Figure 3.4 Osteoarthritis is a degenerative joint disease affecting the cartilage, joint lining, ligaments, and bone of the affected joint.

commonly affects the knees, hips, hands, and spine and is associated with decreased physical activity and increased morbidity and mortality (108, 130). Osteoarthritis is the most common form of arthritis and joint disorder in the United States (106, 172), affecting approximately 13.9% or 26 million adults over the age of 25 years (82). Females are at higher risk than males, especially after the age of 50 years (25), and there is an increased incidence with aging for both sexes that plateaus at approximately 80 years (25). As such, with an expanding older population, the prevalence of OA is expected to concomitantly increase. In terms of financial impact, the direct and indirect costs of OA were estimated in excess of $40 billion in 2009 (103).

Pathophysiology of Osteoarthritis

The American Academy of Orthopedic Surgeons defines OA as quantifiable joint deterioration (cartilage, bone, and joint space) by x-ray or DXA, symptoms of deterioration (i.e., pain, swelling, inflammation, and stiffness of the joint), or a combination of the two (5). The progressive degeneration of cartilage and underlying bone changes with OA can be substantial and may result in bone articulating directly with bone. The symptoms of OA typically begin at 40 years of age and increase

in severity and range with aging (85).

The specific cause(s) of OA are currently unknown, and while a genetic association has been proposed, other risk factors for the development of OA have been identified (72, 118, 147); these include sex, age, race, excess body mass, prior joint trauma, physically demanding occupation, structural misalignment, muscle weakness, and estrogen deficiency. Progression of the disease can be influenced by improper loading patterns that place repetitive stress on areas of the joint cartilage and associated structures that are suboptimally suited to accommodating such loads (159). With these risk factors in mind, OA is classified by its etiology and is generally regarded as **idiopathic localized**, **idiopathic general**, or **secondary osteoarthritis** (i.e., associated with known trauma, neuropathic, or other identifiable medical condition).

Key Point

The progression of osteoarthritis can be influenced by improper loading patterns that place repetitive stress on areas of the joint cartilage; therefore, it is essential that proper exercise technique and movement patterns be taught and demonstrated before increasing training load or volume.

Common Medications Given to Individuals With Osteoarthritis

Currently there is no cure for OA, and thus the goal of treatment options is to reduce pain, inflammation, and other symptoms as well as progression of the disease, thereby increasing function. This may be achieved, depending on the risk factors present with each individual, by a combination of education, weight reduction, gait modification, exercise, medication, or surgery (e.g., arthroscopy, osteotomy, joint fusion, and joint replacement) (see medications table 3.3 near the end of the chapter). The American College of Rheumatology (ACR) recommends a combination of pharmacological and nonpharmacological measures to improve the effectiveness of the treatments (65).

A number of OTC and prescription medications are used by individuals in the management and treatment of symptoms of OA (see medications table 3.3 near the end of the chapter) (9). Over-the-counter NSAIDs such as ibuprofen (e.g., Advil and Motrin) and naproxen (e.g., Aleve) may reduce inflammation, swelling, and mild pain. Over-the-counter nonopioid analgesics such as acetaminophen (e.g., Tylenol) are mild to moderate pain relievers that are also often used by those with LBP. Over-the-counter dietary supplements such as glucosamine (hydrochloride and sulfate) and chondroitin sulfate individually and in combination have been extensively researched as nutraceuticals to assist in relieving pain and inflammation and stimulating net cartilage production (48). Current reviews of the literature are equivocal in humans; however, a limitation in some studies is the use of nonpharmaceutical-grade ingredients that may affect potency; more research is needed to determine their efficacy (48, 64, 113). (Note that the U.S. FDA does not test or analyze dietary supplements, as they are not regulated in the same manner as pharmaceuticals. People should always consult their physician or other health care professional before consuming dietary supplements.) Various topical pain relievers with ingredients such as capsaicin, menthol, comfrey, and salicylates (e.g., Aspercreme, Bengay, Capzasin-P, and Icy Hot) are also available OTC; however, they appear to have equivocal beneficial effects on OA pain (3, 27, 148), and further research to elucidate their effectiveness is needed.

Nonsteroidal anti-inflammatory drugs including ibuprofen (e.g., Advil) and aspirin, which can help reduce inflammation, swelling, and associated pain, are common nonprescription medications taken by those with OA. If taken as directed in low doses for short periods of time, OTC NSAIDs have relatively few and minor side effects. However, they can result in GI irritation or bleeding, and their use can increase the risk of heart attack and stroke; these risks increase if they are taken for prolonged periods or at higher than recommended doses (158). Nonopioid analgesics such as acetaminophen (e.g., Tylenol) are mild to moderate pain relievers that are also commonly taken by those with OA. They have relatively few side effects when taken as directed. The known side effects include GI discomfort such as stomach pain, headache, and in rare cases GI bleeding, or negative effects on hepatic and renal functioning.

If the pain or swelling from OA is moderate to severe, the physician may prescribe one or more medications such as cyclooxygenase-2 (COX-2) enzyme inhibitors. These drugs are a subclass of NSAIDs but act selectively on COX-2 enzymes to reduce inflammation, with reduced risk of stomach irritation. However, as with other cyclooxygenase inhibitors, there is an increased risk of heart attack and stroke with longer duration of use.

Corticosteroids, powerful anti-inflammatory agents that are injected directly into the joint (e.g., betamethasone, cortisone acetate, and prednisone), may also be used in isolation or conjunction with other medications depending on the individual's symptoms. Despite the name, corticosteroids are not in fact steroids but rather are synthetic drugs that structurally resemble cortisol. Corticosteroids are prescribed for moderate to severe joint pain or inflammation after NSAIDs have been found to be ineffective. In general, corticosteroids are considered safe; however, potential side effects associated with large doses taken over prolonged periods (i.e., months or years) include heart attack, stroke, and stomach bleeding. Another known potential side effect of use of corticosteroids is osteoporosis, as they can both reduce osteoblast activity and increase bone resorption. Viscosupplements are agents injected into the joint cavity of patients with OA to increase joint lubrication and cushioning. Hyaluronic acid (e.g., Euflexxa, Hyalgan) is one such agent that is naturally found in joint fluid (149) and has been shown to be safe and efficacious as a treatment and may be given as a weekly injection (149).

For severe joint pain, powerful prescription analgesics (i.e., narcotic pain relievers) may be used for short-term treatment (e.g., Darvocet, morphine, Oxycontin, Percocet, and Vicodin). Unlike NSAIDs, which act as anti-inflammatory agents and have a mild analgesic effect, narcotic pain relievers have no anti-inflammatory effects. The most common side effects are constipation, drowsiness, dry mouth, and sometimes difficulty urinating. Caution should be taken with their use, as there is a risk of developing a tolerance, dependency, or addiction.

Effects of Exercise in Individuals With Osteoarthritis

While activities that cause or exacerbate pain in individuals with OA should be avoided, the benefits of exercise are well documented and may reduce joint pain for many (81, 123). Those with OA who are overweight or obese can also benefit from physical activity and exercise-induced fat loss as this reduces the pressure on weight-bearing joints. Exercise may also increase joint stability, muscle strength, coordination, balance, proprioception, and joint mobility (11).

Exercise Recommendations for Clients With Osteoarthritis

Program design guidelines for individuals with OA are summarized in table 3.4. The American College of Rheumatology recommends that clients with OA engage in range of motion, resistance, and aerobic exercise.

- Aerobic exercise that uses large muscle mass such as swimming, cycling, or walking should be undertaken three to five days per week at a light to moderate intensity (i.e., 55 to <75% maximal heart rate [MHR] or an RPE of 9 to 13) for 20 to 30 minutes (10).

- Resistance training, two or three times per week at a moderate intensity for six to eight repetitions and two or three sets per exercise, in a progressive overload manner is also recommended (10).

- Exercise to increase flexibility and mobility should be initiated three to seven days per week, with three sets of one to five repetitions per muscle group, and held for 5 to 30 seconds, according to initial flexibility and comfort levels.

Table 3.4 Program Design Guidelines for Clients With Osteoarthritis

Type of exercise	Frequency	Intensity	Volume
Resistance training			
Modes: weight training machines, free weights or both, body weight, elastic tubing	Two or three sessions per week	Moderate intensity (60-80% 1RM), using multijoint exercises to engage all major muscle groups	2-3 sets per exercise of 6-8 repetitions and 2-3 min rest between sets
Aerobic training			
	3-5 days/week	Light to moderate (55-75% MHR), RPE 9-13) weight-bearing, large muscle mass activities such as swimming, cycling, or walking	20-30 min per session (goal of at least 150 min per week)
Flexibility training			
	3-7 days/week	Stretches should be held at the point of mild discomfort (i.e., not painful)	3 sets of one to five stretches per muscle group; hold each stretch for 5-30 s

Case Study

Osteoarthritis

Mrs. J is 58 years old, physically active, 5 feet, 6 inches tall (1.68 m), and 135 pounds (61 kg). She is a manager for a temporary staffing agency and has had progressively increasing pain and swelling in both knees for the past 12 months. Initially in the morning her knees are stiff until she has been moving for 10 to 15 minutes. She has had to reduce her running to walking, and recently even walking more than 20 minutes has become painful. She has been taking ibuprofen daily for nine months to reduce swelling and pain, and while her self-selected dosage has steadily increased, it is no longer effective at managing her pain. X-rays of her lower back, hips, and knees reveal that Mrs. J has narrowing of the joint spaces, an indication of cartilage loss, and mild increased density of the subchondral bone consistent with OA. Due to the ineffectiveness of ibuprofen, her physician has prescribed celecoxib (Celebrex), a COX-2 inhibitor, even in light of the FDA's recent warning that COX-2 inhibitors may increase the risk of heart attack and stroke. This was in conjunction with recommending a modified aerobic training program, adding resistance training and mobility to improve overall joint health and function, as well as addressing any potential issues of bone and muscular strength, which are both important at Mrs. J's age.

Due to the continuing decline in her exercise abilities in the past year and the long-term medical and health implications, Mrs. J hired an exercise professional with certification and experience working with OA clients. With her reduced ability to run, her exercise professional prescribed aerobic sessions on a bicycle three to five days per week at a moderate intensity (RPE of 12-13) for a duration as long as she was pain-free or her pain was tolerable. On days when her symptoms are low, Mrs. J was encouraged to walk, as this is what she prefers and enjoys. Her exercise professional also initiated a resistance training program twice a week again at a moderate intensity, given her athletic background, engaging in two sets of six to eight repetitions of predominantly multijoint exercises while remaining in a pain-free range of motion. However, to accommodate the cartilage loss in her lower back, hips, and knees, Mrs. J's exercise professional implemented low step-ups, leg press, and lying hamstring curls instead of squats and deadlifts, and asked her to limit her range of motion by her symptoms. Her exercise professional also started her on a progressive flexibility program of static stretches three days per week, repeating each stretch three times and holding for up to 30 seconds.

Recommended Readings

Buckwalter, JA, Saltzman, C, and Brown, T. The impact of osteoarthritis: implications for research. *Clin Orthop Relat Res* Oct(427 suppl):S6-S15, 2004.

Roddy, E, Zhang, W, Doherty, M, Arden, NK, Barlow, J, Birrell, F, Carr, A, Chakravarty, K, Dickson, J, Hay, E, and Hosie, G. Evidence-based recommendations for the role of exercise in the management of osteoarthritis of the hip or knee—the MOVE consensus. *Rheumatology (Oxford)* 44(1):67-73, 2005.

Vincent, KR, Conrad, BP, Fregly, BJ, and Vincent, HK. The pathophysiology of osteoarthritis: a mechanical perspective on the knee joint. *PM R* 4(5 suppl):S3-S9, 2012.

Joint Disorders

The joints of the human body are made up of primary and supporting structures including cartilage, ligaments, bone, bursa, joint cavity, synovial fluid, muscle, tendons, blood vessels, and nerves. Joints, and the various structures that make up a joint, are susceptible to disorders of varying etiology, for example, genetics, disease, trauma, and aging. Two of the most common joint disorders are sprains (figure 3.5) and dislocations (figure 3.6).

The American Academy of Orthopaedic Surgeons (AAOS) defines a **joint sprain** as a stretch or tear (or both) of a ligament (8). Typical acute symptoms of a sprain include tenderness or pain at the joint, bruising, inflammation, swelling, and joint laxity or stiffness. The joints most susceptible to sprains are the ankles, knees, and wrists. From 2002 to 2006 there were an estimated 3,140,132 ankle sprains in the United States (162), with the incidence higher in females compared with males, children compared with adolescents, and adolescents compared with adults (46). Lateral ankle sprains were the most common ankle sprain cited (46), with nearly half of all ankle sprains reported during athletic activity. Basketball, football, and soccer were associated with the highest percentages of ankle sprains at 41.1%, 9.3%, and 7.9%, respectively (162).

Joint dislocation (i.e., luxation), on the other hand, is an abnormal separation of the joint surfaces. Common acute symptoms of a dislocation include pain at the joint especially during movement, limited range of motion, numbness or tingling, swelling, and bruising. The joint may be visibly misshapen, particularly in the case of complete dislocation; however this is not always the case, as with partial dislocations. The shoulder is the most commonly reported joint dislocation, with 71.8% of cases occurring in males and with a peak incidence for those aged 20 to 29 years (170).

The risks of joint sprains or dislocation with participation in exercise and physical activity are evident, with almost half of the reported injuries occurring during sport activity or recreation (170). Thus, since all children and adults are encouraged to engage in daily physical activity to improve and maintain health, exercise professionals should be knowledgeable about these conditions.

Pathophysiology of Joint Disorders

Sprains are caused by direct or indirect trauma such as a fall (e.g., landing on outstretched arms and hands while falling, causing wrist sprain), excessive joint movement (e.g., "rolling an ankle" on a rock while walking), or a blow to the body or joint (e.g., tackling an opponent at the knee, causing sprain of the medial collateral ligament of the knee). The

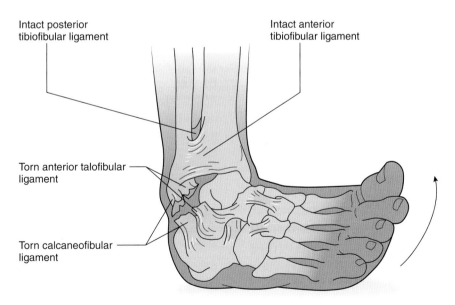

Intact posterior tibiofibular ligament

Intact anterior tibiofibular ligament

Torn anterior talofibular ligament

Torn calcaneofibular ligament

Figure 3.5 Joint sprain is one of the most common joint disorders and involves a stretch or tear of a ligament.

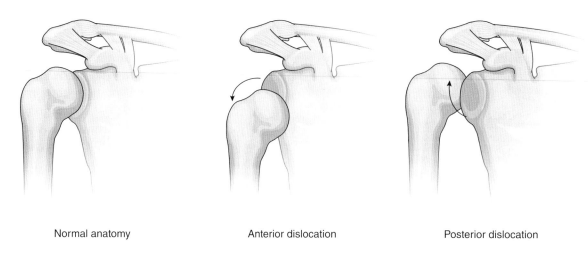

Normal anatomy   Anterior dislocation   Posterior dislocation

Figure 3.6 Joint dislocation is one of the most common joint disorders and is categorized in terms of the degree of separation and extent of the injuries to the associated structures.

latter forces the joint beyond its functional range of motion, stretching ligament(s) farther than their normal length. This excessive movement results in overstretch, tear, or complete rupture of one or more ligaments that support the joint.

Sprains are categorized by (1) the degree of stretch or tearing of the ligament's collagen fibers and (2) the resulting degree of joint instability. A **grade 1 sprain** (i.e., mild) is identified as minimal tenderness and swelling with overstretch of the ligament, no significant tear of fibers, and no apparent joint instability. A **grade 2 sprain** (i.e., moderate) has moderate degrees of tenderness and swelling, with tearing of some fibers but not the entire ligament, and possible mild joint instability. **Grade 3 sprain** (i.e., severe) is a complete rupture of the ligament with concomitant joint instability, significant swelling, and tenderness.

Similar to the situation with sprains, the primary cause of joint dislocation is sudden impact caused by either a blow to a joint or associated structure(s) or a fall. In the case of shoulder dislocation, aside from the previously mentioned risk factors of sex, age, and sport participation, genetics is also a risk factor for individuals with hypermobile joints due to loosened ligaments (142). A previous dislocation is also a risk factor for further injury to the joint, as the trauma from dislocation often does irreparable damage and joints are more loose after each dislocation (77).

Dislocation is categorized in terms of the degree of separation, **partial** or **complete**, and extent of the associated injuries: **simple dislocation** (no major bone trauma), **complex dislocation** (significant bone and ligament trauma), or **severe dislocation** (damage includes trauma to blood vessels and nerves associated with the joint) (4).

Common Medications Given to Individuals With Joint Disorders

Medications commonly prescribed in the acute recovery phase of sprains and dislocations include ibuprofen and other OTC NSAIDs to reduce inflammation, swelling, and mild pain, or acetaminophen or other nonopioid analgesics for mild to moderate pain. Both NSAIDs and nonnarcotic analgesics have few side effects, which are typically mild if they are used for short periods of time and in low doses. However, as mentioned previously, these drugs can impair skeletal muscle protein synthetic response (153). It is also worth emphasizing that caution is advised with NSAIDs as high doses and longer use have been associated with increases in the risk of heart attack and stroke (158).

Effects of Exercise in Individuals With Joint Disorders

According to the American Physical Therapy Association, there is some evidence that supports the inclusion of weight-bearing functional exercises and single-limb balance activities in the postacute rehabilitation period to improve strength and mobility for ankle sprains (93). In addition, there is evidence that sport-related training may reduce the risk of recurring ankle sprains (93).

According to the AAOS, treatment for grade 1 sprains includes strengthening, range of motion, and flexibility as tolerated, but should be initiated only after a physician or other health care professional's clearance has been obtained and the initial healing phase (typically two or three days), denoted by lack of pain and swelling, is complete (8). Note that complete healing may take four to six weeks. The treatment of grade 2 and 3 sprains requires immobilization and physical therapy treatment and as such is outside the scope of practice for exercise professionals. As with rehabilitation for sprains, the goals of rehabilitation for dislocation are to optimize joint range of motion and strength. The treatment of partial and complete dislocations typically requires immobilization and physical therapy and is outside the scope of practice of exercise professionals.

Key Point

While the goals of rehabilitation for sprains and dislocations are to optimize joint range of motion and strength, exercise professionals should ensure the client has been released by a physician, physical therapist, or other health care professional before initiating a training program.

Exercise Recommendations for Clients With Joint Disorders

For ankle sprains, the AAOS recommends an initial one-week phase of rest and repair, followed by a second phase of one to two weeks to restore range of motion, flexibility, and strength, with a subsequent final phase of several weeks to months of progressive modified training with no turning or twisting of the ankle (8). The specific exercises and programming depend on the severity of the injury and speed of recovery. It should be noted that exercise programming for postrecovery sprains and dislocations should be undertaken after consultation and clearance from the client's physician or other health care professional, and exercise should cease if there is any pain. A final-phase program for an ankle sprain might include flexibility training sessions of an initial low-impact dynamic warm-up of 5 to 10 minutes such as walking or stationary bicycle, then completion of three or four low-intensity stretches for the musculature that supports the joint, holding each stretch for 30 seconds, with two sets of 10 repetitions, six or seven days per week (6). This final phase of strengthening should also include two to four bodyweight strengthening and balance–coordination exercises (e.g., calf raise for ankle sprain) of one or two sets of 5 to 10 repetitions through full joint range of motion, again six or seven days per week, and one resisted exercise of three sets of 10 repetitions with a frequency of three times per week (6).

The AAOS also provides exercise guidelines for those having suffered a shoulder injury such as dislocation (7). Guidelines are similar to those for joint sprain. The initial postrecovery program is typically four to six weeks in duration. For each exercise session, after an initial warm-up of 5 to 10 minutes of walking or stationary cycling, the client should complete three or four low-intensity stretches for the musculature that supports the shoulder (i.e., the deltoids, rotator cuff muscles, trapezius, rhomboids, biceps, and triceps) with one or two sets of 4 to 10 repetitions, with each stretch held for 30 seconds, five to seven days per week. This is followed by three to six initial light-resistance (e.g., bands or lightweight dumbbells) strengthening and stabilization exercises in each plane, with one to three sets of 5 to 20 repetitions through full joint range of motion, three times per week. Intensity and volume should follow a progressive overload model from an initial low intensity and volume. Program design guidelines for individuals with joint disorders are summarized in table 3.5.

Table 3.5 Postrecovery Exercise Program Guidelines for Clients With Joint Sprain or Dislocation

Type of exercise	Frequency	Intensity	Intensity
Ankle joint sprain (6)			
Resistance training: bodyweight strengthening and balance–coordination	Six or seven sessions per week	Light to moderate intensity	1-2 sets of 5-10 repetitions per exercise for the affected joint
Resistance training: external resistance	Three sessions per week	Light to moderate intensity	3 sets of 10 repetitions
Flexibility training	6-7 days per week	Light intensity	2 sets of 10 repetitions of three or four stretches per muscle group associated with the injured joint; hold each stretch for 30 s
Shoulder joint dislocation (7)			
Resistance training: bands or light dumbbells	Three sessions per week	Light intensity	1-3 sets of 5-20 repetitions of three to six exercises for the shoulder musculature
Flexibility training	5-7 days per week	Light intensity	1-2 sets of 4-10 repetitions of three or four stretches per muscle group of the shoulder joint; hold each stretch for 30 s

Note: Exercise programming for postrecovery sprains and dislocations should be undertaken only after consultation and clearance from the client's physician or other health care professional, and exercise should cease immediately if there is any pain.

Case Study

Joint Disorders

Mrs. S (35-year-old married mother of three young children) presented to the exercise professional on Tuesday at her local health club after spraining her right ankle playing a game of soccer with her children in her backyard on Friday night. Her ankle rolled over, and it was instantly very painful, with significant swelling and bruising starting to show shortly thereafter. Mrs. S went to the emergency room, and an x-ray confirmed that there was no fracture. She elevated and rested her foot over the weekend and on Monday at work elevated as much as possible. She met with her primary care physician on Monday, who confirmed there was no fracture and cleared her for walking and light exercise to mobilize the joint. While bruising is still present, she is no longer experiencing tenderness and there is virtually no swelling. Mrs. S is currently taking 400 mg of acetaminophen as directed by her physician.

Mrs. S had been working out consistently for several months with continued weight loss for an upcoming class reunion and would like to continue to train. Her exercise professional asked her to warm up on the stationary bicycle and maintain a low intensity for 5 minutes. With no pain during warm-up, Mrs. S's exercise professional directed her through low-intensity stretches as normal but with one extra calf stretch (for a total of three), then bodyweight calf raises and banded ankle dorsiflexion and plantarflexion. The exercise professional initially modified her existing program to reduce stresses on her ankle, for example using knee extension and hamstring curl machines instead of squats and deadlifts for her lower body to avoid extra pressure on her ankle, and using bench press and lat pulldown instead of physioball dumbbell press and one-arm bent-over row, respectively. She also avoids planks (supine, prone, and side) due to the increased stress on her ankles.

Recommended Readings

American Academy of Orthopaedic Surgeons. Foot and ankle conditioning program. 2012. http://orthoinfo. aaos.org/topic.cfm?topic=A00667. Accessed January 6, 2017.

American Academy of Orthopaedic Surgeons. Rotator cuff and shoulder conditioning program. 2012. http://orthoinfo.aaos.org/topic.cfm?topic=A00663. Accessed January 6, 2017.

Doherty, C, Delahunt, E, Caulfield, B, Hertel, J, Ryan, J, and Bleakley, C. The incidence and prevalence of ankle sprain injury: a systematic review and meta-analysis of prospective epidemiological studies. *Sports Med* 44(1):123-140, 2014.

Joint Replacements

Joint replacement surgery (also known as **arthroplasty**) involves replacement of part (e.g., articular cartilage) or all of a damaged or arthritic joint with a metal, plastic, or ceramic prosthesis in order to return the joint to normal pain-free movement (figure 3.7). While total hip and knee replacements are the most common, other joints are also replaced, including, but not limited to, shoulder, elbow, and ankle (63). In 2011 approximately 1.4 million joint replacement surgeries were performed in the United States, including over 640,000 knee and 300,000 hip total joint replacements. The cumulative number of individuals living in the United States with knee replacements is estimated at over 4 million (165), with a higher prevalence in females than males (165) and overall prevalence increasing with age. The financial cost of joint replacements was estimated at approximately $16 billion in the United States in 2006 and was projected to rise with the increasing aging population and prevalence of obesity (167).

Pathophysiology of Joint Replacements

Several risk factors leading to joint replacement have been identified; these include age, sex, body mass index, developmental disorders, fractures, injury, and diseases leading to degeneration of one or more aspects of the joint. However, both primary and secondary OA was the principal

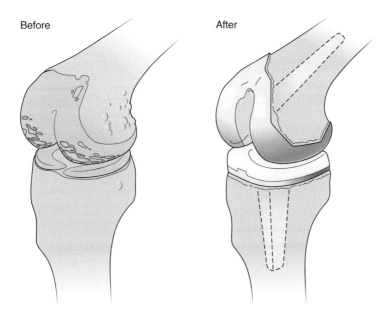

Before   After

Figure 3.7 Joint replacement surgery (arthroplasty) involves replacement of part or all of a damaged joint with a metal, plastic, or ceramic prosthesis in order to return the joint to normal pain-free movement.

diagnosis for 85.3% and 97.3% of hip and knee total replacement surgeries, respectively, in the United States in 2011 (63).

Common Medications Given to Individuals With Joint Replacements

Arthroplasty is an invasive procedure, and the medications commonly associated with the surgery include anesthesia, sedatives, intravenous prescription opioid pain relievers (e.g., morphine, fentanyl, oxycodone), and antibiotics. Once the individual is released from the hospital following surgery and acute recovery, various OTC and prescription medications are prescribed (see medications table 3.4 near the end of the chapter). Over-the-counter medication for mild to moderate pain relief (e.g., acetaminophen [Tylenol]) and reducing inflammation (e.g., ibuprofen [Advil]) may be taken for up to several weeks postsurgery; however, as noted earlier, caution is advised as NSAIDs increase the risk of heart attack and stroke with higher doses and longer use. Prescription oral opioid pain relievers may be prescribed for those with more severe pain; however, extended use of these drugs is not recommended because they are highly addictive. Oral antibiotics are also typically prescribed to prophylactically prevent infections, and while side effects are not common, they may include nausea, vomiting, GI distress, or allergic reaction. Oral anticoagulants such as warfarin (Coumadin) are also commonly prescribed because surgery increases the risk of blood clots.

Effects of Exercise in Individuals With Joint Replacements

Postoperative physical activity and exercise to stimulate leg blood flow are encouraged to reduce the risk of blood clots such as deep vein thrombosis and pulmonary embolism, which are strikingly common; 40% to 60% of total hip and total knee arthroplasty patients who did not receive antithrombosis treatment had a confirmed postoperative diagnosis (59).

Exercise Recommendations for Clients With Joint Replacements

Recovery and rehabilitation following joint replacement are highly individualized, as the healing and pain associated with the surgery can last weeks to months, as can the adjustment to the new joint and its movement. During this period of reduced activity, loss of muscle strength will accrue and should be considered and addressed. Initially the client's physician and physical therapist direct the exercise prescription to restore normal and healthy movement patterns and strengthen the joint and associated structures and musculature.

Due to the invasive nature of the surgery, the various types of joint replacement (i.e., partial or total), individualized responses to recovery and rehabilitation, and inconsistencies in the literature, specific exercise prescription is highly individualized. Following the initial recovery and rehabilitation phase, evidence of functionally stable and painless movement patterns of the affected joint is necessary before the client begins a strength and conditioning program. General guidelines for such a program include the following (95, 160):

- A period of six months is recommended before engaging in vigorous exercise.
- An initial period of low-impact aerobic exercises (i.e., those that combine cyclic low limb movement patterns with low rotational and minimal impact forces) is highly recommended. This includes cycling, swimming, walking, low-impact aerobics, weight training, and cross-country skiing.
- High-impact activities and contact sports should be avoided.
- Exercise and physical activity that include frequent jumping or plyometrics are contraindicated in most cases but should be evaluated individually.

Key Point

Postoperative physical activity is encouraged in individuals with joint replacements to stimulate leg blood flow and reduce the risk of blood clots. Clearance to exercise from a physician or other health care professional should be obtained prior to initiating exercise.

- The client's prior exercise and sporting experience should be considered in these recommendations, as this may indicate an increased tolerance for those activities.

In conjunction it is recommended that exercise professionals refer to the generally accepted guidelines adopted by the U.S. DHHS for developing exercise sessions and programs for adults with joint arthroplasty (156), while ensuring that the exercise prescription is individualized in its implementation and progression to reflect the limitations, strengths, weaknesses, and goals of the client. The recommendations for a resistance training program are to improve overall muscular strength and endurance; however, a loss of muscle mass may also have occurred, and if so should be addressed. Initial recommendations are two to four sets (one set if the client is sedentary or low in conditioning) of 8 to 12 repetitions per exercise at an initial light to moderate intensity, one or two times per week (156). To increase flexibility and range of motion it is recommended that clients initially complete static stretches three to seven times per week of all major muscle groups and hold each stretch for 15 to 30 seconds (105). Recommendations for aerobic exercise are to engage large muscle groups (e.g., brisk walking) at an initial light to moderate intensity for at least 10 minutes three or more times per day, three or more days per week, progressing to at least 300 minutes of moderate or 150 minutes of vigorous (or an equivalent combination of both intensities) per week. Exercise should cease immediately if there is any pain, with referral to a physician or other health care professional. Program design guidelines for clients with joint replacements are summarized in table 3.6.

Table 3.6 Exercise Program Guidelines for Clients With Joint Replacement (Arthroplasty)

Type of exercise	Frequency	Intensity	Volume
Resistance training			
Modes: weight training machines, free weights, or both; body weight, elastic tubing	Begin with one or two sessions per week	Initial light to moderate intensity (40-80% 1RM), using multijoint exercises to engage all major muscle groups	Start with 1 set per exercise of 8-12 reps
	Increase to at least two sessions per week as tolerated	Progress to moderate to high intensity (after 6 months) with 1-2 min rest between sets	Increase to 2-4 sets per exercise as appropriate
Aerobic training			
Modes: walking, jogging, running, swimming, cycling	3-7 days per week	Begin with light to moderate intensity (30% to <60% $\dot{V}O_2$ or heart rate reserve or 55% to <75% MHR, or RPE of 9-13 on Borg 6- to 20-point scale)	Begin with at least 10 min 3 or more times per day
		Moderate intensity (40% to <60% $\dot{V}O_2$ or heart rate reserve or 65% to <75% MHR, or RPE of 12-13 on Borg 6- to 20-point scale)	300 min per week
		Vigorous intensity (≥60% $\dot{V}O_2$ or heart rate reserve or ≥75% MHR, or RPE of ≥14 on Borg 6- to 20-point scale)	150 min per week
Flexibility training			
	3-7 times per week	Stretches should be held at the point of mild discomfort (i.e., not painful)	Each stretch held for 15-30 s

References: (105, 156)

Case Study

Joint Replacements

Mr. D, a 66-year-old retired school teacher and prior semiprofessional rugby player, was diagnosed with obesity, diabetes, hypertension, and OA of both knees and right shoulder. Mr. D experienced increasing knee pain, swelling, and stiffness with concomitant decreased range of motion and functional ability over several years. After initial NSAID medication use, he was prescribed a COX-2 inhibitor and weekly hyaluronic acid injections for five weeks. At that time, due to continuing pain, Mr. D underwent a bilateral total knee arthroplasty with no complications or infection. He started an inpatient rehabilitation and recovery program due to the bilateral nature of his surgeries and progressed well with minimal narcotic pain medication use. He also participated in nutritional counseling and weight loss exercise programming. Following nine months of outpatient and at-home rehabilitation, Mr. D lost a significant amount of weight (predominantly fat mass but also some muscle mass based on DXA) and was more active and pain-free than he had been in many years. He swims three times per week, participates in progressive resistance training twice a week with an exercise professional, and plays with his four grandchildren as often as possible.

Recommended Readings

Geerts, WH, Bergqvist, D, Pineo, GF, Heit, JA, Samama, CM, Lassen, MR, and Colwell, CW. Prevention of venous thromboembolism: American College of Chest Physicians Evidence-Based Clinical Practice Guidelines (8th Edition). *Chest* 133(6 suppl):381S-453S, 2008.

Helmick, CG and Watkins-Castillo, S. United States Bone and Joint Initiative: The Burden of Musculoskeletal Diseases in the United States (BMUS). 2014. www.boneandjointburden.org. Accessed May 25, 2015.

Mayer, F and Dickhuth, H. FIMS Position Statement: Physical activity after total joint replacement. *Int SportMed J* 9(1):39-43, 2008.

DISORDERS OF THE MUSCULAR SYSTEM

Skeletal muscle mass plays a central role in an individual's health both directly and indirectly via metabolic functions, whole-body protein metabolism, and the production of locomotion, muscular endurance, strength, and power. Consequently, conditions that negatively affect the muscular system, such as injury, disease, aging, and disuse, can have significant effects on an individual's health and fitness. This section examines two disorders of the muscular system associated with aging: frailty and sarcopenia.

Frailty

Frailty is a commonly used term in the health and medical communities, yet there is currently no consensus definition (14, 58, 90). While frail health may occur at any time in one's life (14), frailty is generally associated with older adults who experience a syndrome of poor health, reduced muscle strength, and reduced ability to participate in physical and functional activities, including activities of daily living, leading to further increased vulnerability to negative health conditions, morbidity, and mortality (24, 42, 119, 152). Evidence suggests that the prevalence of frailty increases with age and varies from 4% to

59% in older adults, with approximately 20% to 50% of those aged 85 years of age or older being frail (31, 36). And as the older adult population (i.e., 65 years of age and older) is estimated to double in the next 25 years (29), there are growing concerns about the expanding individual, societal, and economic impacts of this syndrome.

Pathophysiology of Frailty

Disagreement among researchers and practitioners exists on the precise etiology of frailty, but frailty is generally considered the result of a multifactorial interaction of age-related deficits in various physiological and psychological systems, in conjunction with nutritional and environmental stressors (24, 152). It is associated with other chronic diseases (14), and risk increases after the age of 65 years (14). Older adults are particularly prone to frailty, as many older individuals are susceptible to a negative cycle of disease and disuse (i.e., lack of weight-bearing activities), which further exacerbates the frailty condition. For example, inadequate caloric or dietary protein intake can contribute to sarcopenia (age-related loss of skeletal muscle mass and strength). This may in turn contribute to osteoporosis and increased risk of falling—with potential hospitalization and bed rest to treat a fracture leading to further muscle and bone density loss during immobilization, making the individual even more frail. Frailty also increases the risk of and recovery from other health issues, exacerbating an already negative perpetuating cycle (14). Due to the multifactorial aspects of frailty and lack of agreement on its definition, multiple diagnostic tools and tests exist to diagnose this syndrome (24, 69).

Common Medications Given to Individuals With Frailty

The multifactorial etiology of frailty and the potential presence of one or more comorbidities result in treatment with multiple medications (51, 68, 116). The exercise professional therefore must become aware of these medical conditions and medications via completion of prescreening medical, health, and activity history questionnaires, as well as their effects individually and in combination on exercise capacity and phys-

iological responses to exercise (e.g., β-blockers can attenuate the normal rise in heart rate with increasing exercise intensity and duration). The side effects of these medications individually and in combination should also be known for safety and exercise prescription reasons. For example, β-blockers and diuretics can cause fatigue and weakness, while diuretics and certain antidepressants may cause postural hypotension, and the same class of antidepressants can also cause dizziness (14). See medications table 3.5 near the end of the chapter for more detail.

Effects of Exercise in Individuals With Frailty

Exercise of varying modes, intensity, and duration has been shown to be efficacious in frail populations in improving balance, performance in activities of daily living, gait speed, fall prevention, and other markers of functional capacity (33, 34, 139). Goals for an exercise program to address the multifaceted contributors to frailty, depending on individual deficits, may include (14):

1. Increase functional capacity

2. Increase neuromuscular coordination to improve balance and reduce risk of falls

3. Increase muscular strength, power, and mass to reduce the risk of falling, increase functional capabilities, and attenuate sarcopenia and its related negative health impacts

4. Improve cardiovascular functioning to attenuate cardiovascular disease and other comorbidities

Exercise Recommendations for Clients With Frailty

Frailty is complicated by the existence of multiple conditions and a complex etiology in older clients; thus health, medical, and activity prescreening should be used to (a) stratify risks, such as cardiovascular and orthopedic risks, and (b) obtain a full and comprehensive list of all medications and supplements. The exercise professional should consider tests that assess potential neuromuscular, proprioceptive, balance, muscular strength, and flexibility–mobility deficits, as well as reflecting activities of daily living. To determine aerobic exercise intensity and duration tolerance before the onset of negative symptoms, medical supervision of a cardiorespiratory exercise test is also recommended due to the high risk of falls and other adverse events in this population.

Program design guidelines for frail older clients are summarized in table 3.7. In order to increase functional capacity and independence, aerobic exercise that recruits large muscle mass such as walking, cycling, swimming, and chair exercises is recommended three to five days per week for 5 to 60 minutes per session (14). Light-intensity resistance exercise three days per week and progressing to moderate intensity is also recommended (14). Moderate- to high-intensity resistance exercise has been shown to be well tolerated and to have positive effects on functional capacity, muscle mass, and strength; however, this should proceed in a progressive fashion based on individual responses (52, 138). Flexibility and mobility training is encouraged on most or all days in order to promote healthy movement patterns, continued independence, and activities of daily living (110). Neuromuscular exercises that increase coordination, balance, and gait are also recommended within a comprehensive training program to reduce the risk of falls and associated increased morbidity and mortality. These may be functionally based exercises such as chair stand, one-foot stand, or tandem gait (14).

Insufficient nutritional intake (i.e., total calories and protein) is common in older adults, and referral to a registered dietician or nutritionist is recommended so that dietary recall or blood tests (or both) can be undertaken to determine nutritional status, as well as counseling regarding the importance of nutrition for health and optimal adaptations to exercise (145). Older frail clients have an increased risk of overhydration and dehydration; it is important to appreciate this throughout training sessions, as it can adversely affect health, training adaptations, recovery, and consistency of training (97).

Case Study

Frailty

Mrs. R, an 87-year-old widow living alone, is 5 feet, 1 inch (1.55 m) tall, weighing 104 pounds (47 kg). She has been prompted repeatedly by her sons to join a fitness facility and work with an exercise professional to get stronger and become more active. She admits being fatigued a great deal and has various muscular and joint aches. Mrs. R has slow ambulation and jerky gait movement patterns with a wide stance and is slow to rise from a chair, often requiring assistance due to poor strength and balance. She agreed to go to a fitness facility, and her oldest son, who pays for the sessions, drives her to the facility and helps her get from the car to inside the facility.

Mrs. R takes multiple medications, including Benazepril (an angiotensin-converting enzyme [ACE] inhibitor for high blood pressure), Coumadin to reduce her risk of blood clots and stroke, Celebrex for her OA, and Lipitor (a statin for lowering her cholesterol). She also had osteoporotic fractures of the right wrist and proximal hip from slipping on the ice last winter.

Mrs. R is on a fixed income and often does not have an appetite so she eats infrequent small meals with very little protein content. Mrs. R has unintentionally lost 10 pounds of mass in the past two years. Low nutrient consumption may have affected her calcium, magnesium, and protein intake.

Her exercise professional prescribed a total body program incorporating seated upper body exercises using light dumbbells and low resistance bands, and sit-to-stand and standing knee flexion for the lower body to improve muscular strength, balance, and tension on bone. Recumbent cycle ergometer for aerobic conditioning in the temperature-controlled environment was also included, and each session starts and finishes with flexibility and mobility exercises.

Recommended Readings

Evans, WJ and Campbell, WW. Sarcopenia and age-related changes in body composition and functional capacity. *J Nutr* 123(2 suppl):465-468, 1993.

Fiatarone, MA, Marks, EC, Ryan, ND, Meredith, CN, Lipsitz, LA, and Evans, WJ. High-intensity strength training in nonagenarians. Effects on skeletal muscle. *JAMA* 263(22):3029-3034, 1990.

Fielding, RA, Vellas, B, Evans, WJ, Bhasin, S, Morley, JE, Newman, AB, van Kan, GA, Andrieu, S, Bauer, J, Breuille, D, and Cederholm, T. Sarcopenia: an undiagnosed condition in older adults. Current consensus definition: prevalence, etiology, and consequences. International working group on sarcopenia. *J Am Med Dir Assoc* 12(4):249-256, 2011.

Smit, E, Winters-Stone, KM, Loprinzi, PD, Tang, AM, and Crespo, CJ. Lower nutritional status and higher food insufficiency in frail older US adults. *Br J Nutr* 110(1):172-178, 2013.

Table 3.7 Program Design Guidelines for Frail Older Clients

Type of exercise	Frequency	Intensity	Volume
Resistance training			
Modes: body weight, elastic tubing, machines or free weights or both	Three sessions per week	Initial light to moderate intensity (40-80% 1RM), using multijoint exercises to engage all major muscle groups	Start with 1 set per exercise of 8-12 reps; increase to 2-4 sets per exercise as appropriate
Aerobic training			
Modes: walking, cycling, swimming, and chair exercises	3-5 days per week	Initially light to moderate intensity (30% to <60% $\dot{V}O_2$ or heart rate reserve or 55% to <75% MHR, or RPE of 9-13)	Begin with 5 min 3 or more times per day, up to 60 min per session
Flexibility training			
	3-7 times per week	Stretches should be held at the point of mild discomfort (i.e., not painful)	Each stretch held for 15-30 s

References: (14, 52, 105, 110, 138, 156)

Sarcopenia

Sarcopenia is the multifactorial loss of skeletal muscle mass, strength, power, and functional capacity with aging (23, 50, 53, 98, 120, 125, 126). Sarcopenia appears to begin at approximately 20 to 35 years of age depending on various factors, and it results in a loss of 30% of one's muscle mass by 80 years (16, 56, 163) as well as increased morbidity and mortality rates (99). In 2001 it was estimated that the cost of sarcopenia in the United States was $18.4 billion per year (70). It is also estimated that more than 250,000 deaths a year in the United States are the result of inactivity, a risk factor for sarcopenia (76). Sarcopenia is a current and considerable health concern, particularly in light of the projected doubling of the population aged 65 years and older from 2010 to 2040 (29).

Pathophysiology of Sarcopenia

Research has shown that sarcopenia has multiple contributing factors, including physical inactivity or disuse, chronic diseases, inflammation, insulin resistance, motor unit remodeling—functional muscle denervation, altered endocrine function and decreased anabolic hormone levels, decreased muscle protein synthesis, and nutritional deficiencies including inadequate protein and energy intake (43, 80, 107, 127-129, 158, 168). Due to the number of contributing risk factors and the increasing older adult population, a significant amount of research investigating various interventions is currently being undertaken.

Key Point

> While various factors may contribute to sarcopenia, the integrated roles of resistance training and adequate nutrition, particularly protein and energy intake, have been shown to be highly efficacious.

Common Medications Given to Individuals With Sarcopenia

Physicians and researchers have implemented a number of interventions to address the primary symptoms of reduced muscle mass and strength for those with sarcopenia. Currently the most prevalent treatments for sarcopenia are nutrition (e.g., increasing protein, amino acid, or total caloric intake or some combination of these, as well as vitamin D), resistance exercise (e.g., training to increase muscular strength, power, or both), and hormonal therapies. Hormonal therapy to attenuate or reverse sarcopenia has included the administration of testosterone and other androgens such as dehydroepiandrosterone sulphate (DHEA), with some evidence that they may increase skeletal muscle mass and satellite cells; however, effects on muscle strength and function are mixed (26, 60, 89, 132). In conjunction, the side effects of testosterone supplementation (e.g., increased prostate size, fluid retention, polycythemia [i.e., elevated hematocrit], and sleep apnea [26]) have meant that this is an ongoing area of research that is not universally implemented in those with sarcopenia. Growth hormone and insulin-like growth factor 1 (IGF-1) also act to increase skeletal muscle mass and stimulate satellite cells, and like testosterone, they decline with aging; thus supplementation has been investigated as a treatment option. Equivocal results have been obtained to date in the

literature as a whole, with a relatively high incidence of side effects (e.g., fluid retention, orthostatic hypotension, and carpal tunnel syndrome); however, some studies have shown increases in muscle mass and strength, and further research is ongoing (26, 132).

Other interventions such as creatine, myostatin, and angiotensin-converting enzyme (ACE) inhibitors are also undergoing study as potential treatment options (26, 132). See medications table 3.6 near the end of the chapter for a summary of common medications used for treatment of sarcopenia.

Effects of Exercise in Individuals With Sarcopenia

Unfortunately, it is estimated only 10% of older adults participate in resistance training programs (137). While numerous barriers to exercise participation by older adults have been identified, many studies cite poor health, injury, and pain as the major barriers (94, 136). Resistance training has been shown extensively to improve skeletal muscle mass, strength, and power in older individuals via improved neuromuscular functioning, plasma hormone concentrations, and skeletal muscle protein synthesis, thus attenuating the effects of sarcopenia (28, 41, 44, 49, 137, 154). More recent evidence indicates that muscular power, the ability to rapidly produce force, may affect daily physical performance more than strength (15, 67, 87, 92). Further, there is evidence that muscular power may be lost at a greater rate than muscle strength in older individuals (143, 151). There is evidence that **Type II muscle fibers**, those responsible for high force and rate of force development, experience selective atrophy with advancing age (83, 87). Due to this accelerated loss of Type II fibers, an exercise intervention to ameliorate or reverse sarcopenia should target these fibers by requiring the individual to generate high levels of force at higher speeds. Sayers found that peak muscle power was experienced at high resistances of 80% to 90% of maximum (133), and Peterson and colleagues obtained similar results in a variety of populations for developing maximum strength (114).

Exercise Recommendations for Clients With Sarcopenia

Older adults with sarcopenia often have comorbidities, which the exercise professional should be aware of, as both the comorbidities and the condition of sarcopenia can be barriers to exercise. With this in mind, it is recommended that a health and activity questionnaire be completed by all clients with sarcopenia to identify potential risk factors for cardiovascular disease and orthopedic conditions. Clients with two or more risk factors should be referred to their physician or other health care professional for clearance before starting an exercise program.

Program design guidelines for clients with sarcopenia are summarized in table 3.8. For clients who are cleared to exercise, it is recommended that they engage in a progressive resistance training program, completing one to three sets of 10 to 15 repetitions per muscle group of 8 to 10 multijoint exercises at a light to moderate intensity (12, 115) and advance to higher-intensity training if and when appropriate (96). It is recommended that 1RM or similar high-intensity testing be avoided in clients with sarcopenia due to the risk of injury or aggravating any other existing condition (115). A frequency of two resistance training sessions per week is recommended; however, the optimal frequency for the mature and frail adult has not been definitively established. It should be noted that maintenance of strength in older adults has been achieved with as little as one session per week (115).

Aerobic exercise capacity declines with aging, and inclusion of aerobic training has been shown to improve skeletal muscle and cardiovascular function in older adults (54). It is recommended that clients with sarcopenia engage in aerobic exercise that recruits large muscle mass such as walking, cycling, or swimming, three to five days per week, for 20 to 60 minutes per session at light to moderate intensity.

Flexibility and mobility training in order to promote healthy movement patterns and reduce mortality (110), as well as neuromuscular exercises that increase coordination and balance, is also recommended five to seven days per week.

Table 3.8 Program Design Guidelines for Clients With Sarcopenia

Type of exercise	Frequency	Intensity	Volume
Resistance training			
Modes: body weight, elastic tubing, machines or free weights or both	Two to three sessions per week	Initial light to moderate intensity	1-3 sets per exercise of 10-15 reps of 8 to 10 multijoint exercises
Aerobic training			
Modes: walking, cycling, swimming, and chair exercises	3-5 days per week	Initially light to moderate intensity (30% to <60% $\dot{V}O_2$ or heart rate reserve or 55% to <75% MHR, or RPE of 9-13)	20-60 min per session
Flexibility training			
	5-7 days per week	Stretches should be held at the point of mild discomfort (i.e., not painful)	Each stretch held for 15-30 s

References: (12, 54, 110, 115)

Case Study

Sarcopenia

Mr. C, age 72, is a retired university professor who has been referred to an exercise professional by his physician to start a resistance training program after a fall resulted in a fractured scaphoid and four fractured ribs. Mr. C's physician diagnosed him with sarcopenia. Mr. C appears otherwise relatively healthy for his age, although he takes Lipitor for high cholesterol and Tamsulosin for an enlarged prostate.

Based on discussion with an exercise professional about his health, activity, and nutritional habits, it appeared that Mr. C was chronically hypocaloric and consumed insufficient dietary protein. This was confirmed by a follow-up consultation with a registered dietician. The exercise professional started Mr. C on a machine-based total body circuit workout at moderate intensity for 8 to 12 weeks, with the goal to move to free weights and higher intensities depending on how quickly he adapted. The dietician also initially recommended that Mr. C consume the recommended 0.8 gram protein per kilogram body weight per day and that they meet again to discuss ways to implement recommendations for his total calorie intake and other nutritional needs.

Recommended Readings

Porter, MM. The effects of strength training on sarcopenia. *Can J Appl Physiol* 26(1):123-141, 2001.

Roth, SM, Ferrell, RF, and Hurley, BF. Strength training for the prevention and treatment of sarcopenia. *J Nutr Health Aging* 4(3):143-155, 2000.

Sayers, SP. High-speed power training: a novel approach to resistance training in older men and women. A brief review and pilot study. *J Strength Cond Res* 21(2):518-526, 2007.

Vandervoot, AA and Symons, TB. Functional and metabolic consequences of sarcopenia. *Can J Appl Physiol* 26(1):90-101, 2001.

CONCLUSION

The important theme of this chapter for the exercise professional is that while musculoskeletal disorders and conditions are often associated with varying levels of pain, may be seen as pervasive across the age span, and have various etiologies, appropriate individualized exercise, even in the presence of medications, offers the opportunity to provide symptom relief and improved functionality for the vast majority of clients. Accordingly, exercise professionals need to be aware of the pathophysiology, medications, symptoms, and issues associated with each condition, as well as how they may limit and interact to influence the exercise response, in order to guide their clients safely and effectively. Exercise programming must be individualized, and in certain circumstances such as daily variations in pain, the exercise professional must be flexible in programming to support individuals with muscular disorders and conditions so that they may reach their goals of health, fitness, and functionality.

Key Terms

arthroplasty
complete dislocation
complex dislocation
frailty
grade 1 sprain
grade 2 sprain
grade 3 sprain
hormone therapy
hormone replacement therapy (HRT) (see
    hormone therapy)
hyperkyphosis
hyperlordosis
idiopathic general osteoarthritis
idiopathic localized osteoarthritis
joint dislocation
joint sprain
kyphotic
lordotic

low back pain (LBP)
osteoarthritis (OA)
osteopenia
osteoporosis
partial dislocation
posture
primary osteoporosis
sarcopenia
scoliosis
secondary osteoarthritis
secondary osteoporosis (type 3
    osteoporosis)
severe dislocation
simple dislocation
type 1 osteoporosis (postmenopausal
    osteoporosis)
type 2 osteoporosis (senile osteoporosis)
Type II muscle fibers

Study Questions

1. Which of the following terms refers to an excessive forward convex curvature of the lumbar spine?

    a. scoliosis

    b. hyperlordosis

    c. kyphosis

    d. hyperkyphosis

2. The usage of topical capsicum plasters to treat low back pain

    a. can cause drowsiness or dizziness

    b. may cause long-term liver function problems

    c. does not appear to have an impact on exercise capacity

    d. works by inhibiting inflammation in the affected tissue

3. Osteoarthritis affects women more than men, but at what age does the risk plateau for women and men?

    a. 50

    b. 60

    c. 70

    d. 80

4. All of the following are goals for an exercise program to improve frailty except

    a. reduce the risk of falling

    b. increase functional capacity

    c. lessen the effects of sarcopenia

    d. decrease neuromuscular coordination

Medications Table 3.1　Common Medications Used to Treat Musculoskeletal Disorders

Drug class and names	Mechanism of action	Most common side effects	Effects on exercise
Nonsteroidal anti-inflammatory drugs (NSAIDs)			
ibuprofen (Advil, Motrin), naproxen (Aleve, Anaprox), celecoxib (Celebrex)	Inhibit cyclooxygenase enzymes 1 and 2 (COX-1, COX-2), thereby inhibiting the inflammation pathways	Possible GI irritation or bleeding if taken in high doses or for prolonged periods; increased risk of heart attack and stroke, which increases with high doses and with longer use	None; may impair postexercise skeletal muscle protein synthesis
Nonnarcotic analgesics			
acetaminophen (Tylenol)	Block cyclooxygenase enzyme in the central nervous system (CNS)	Possible GI discomfort or headache; in rare cases GI bleeding or impaired hepatic and renal function	None; may impair postexercise skeletal muscle protein synthesis
Muscle relaxants			
carisoprodol (Soma), cyclobenzaprine (Flexeril), diazepam (Valium)	Act centrally to induce total body muscle relaxation	Dry mouth, dizziness, drowsiness, urinary retention	None; for safety, should not exercise when dizzy or drowsy
Antidepressants			
selective serotonin reuptake inhibitors (SSRIs): fluoxetine (Prozac), sertraline hydrochloride (Zoloft), paroxetine hydrochloride (Paxil)	Block serotonin uptake in the brain, leading to enhanced mood	Nausea, dizziness, fatigue, drowsiness, tremors, headaches	None; for safety, should not exercise when dizzy or drowsy
Short-term oral opiates			
hydrocodone (Vicodin), oxycodone (Oxycontin, Percocet), codeine, morphine	Bind to opioid receptors in brain and spinal cord (and GI tract), thereby suppressing the CNS	Nausea, drowsiness, constipation, urinary retention	None; for safety, should not exercise when dizzy or drowsy

References: (84, 112, 153)

Medications Table 3.2 Common Medications Used to Treat Osteoporosis and Osteopenia

Drug class and names	Mechanism of action	Most common side effects	Effects on exercise
Hormone therapy			
estrogen (Cenestine), estrogen and progesterone (Femhrt)	Reduce bone resorption	Increased risk for breast cancer, blood clots, stroke, and heart attacks	None
Selective estrogen receptor modulators (SERMs)			
raloxifene (Evista), tamoxifen citrate (Nolvadex)	Reduce bone resorption by binding to estrogen receptors on bone	Fatigue, hot flashes, mood swings	Fatigue may affect motivation and ability to train at high intensity or for prolonged duration
Amino bisphosphonates			
alendronate (Fosamax), ibandronate (Boniva), risedronate (Actonel)	Reduce bone resorption	GI irritation; long-term use may increase risk of fracture in femur shaft	GI irritation may be avoided if these are taken upon waking with a full glass of water, and at least 30 min before any food, beverage, or medication
Calcitonin			
nasal calcitonin (Fortical, Miacalcin)	Reduce bone resorption	Runny nose, dry nose, nasal irritation, headache, dizziness, nausea, allergic response	None

References: (21)

Medications Table 3.3   Common Medications and Supplements Used to Treat Osteoarthritis

Drug class and names	Mechanism of action	Most common side effects	Effects on exercise
Over-the-counter dietary supplements			
glucosamine (hydrochloride and sulfate) and chondroitin sulfate	Proposed anti-inflammatory, analgesic, and cartilage regeneration	None	None
Over-the-counter topical pain relievers			
capsaicin (Capzasin-P); trolamine salicylate (Aspercreme); methyl salicylate and menthol (Bengay); combination of menthol, camphor, and methyl salicylate (Icy Hot)	Capsaicin stimulates vanilloid receptor subtype 1 (VR1) receptor to mimic pain, which is interpreted as heat and ultimately decreases the sensation of pain; salicylates may act as a counterirritant to mask pain	Skin irritation, burning sensation	None
Nonsteroidal anti-inflammatory drugs (NSAIDs)			
ibuprofen (Advil, Motrin), naproxen (Aleve, Anaprox), celecoxib (Celebrex)	Inhibit cyclooxygenase enzymes 1 and 2 (COX-1, COX-2), thereby inhibiting the inflammation pathways	Possible GI irritation or bleeding if taken in high doses or for prolonged periods; increased risk of heart attack and stroke, which increases with high doses and with longer use	None; may impair postexercise skeletal muscle protein synthesis
COX-2 inhibitors			
celecoxib (Celebrex, Celebra) *Note:* rofecoxib (Vioxx) and valdecoxib (Bextra) no longer available due to increased risk of heart attack and stroke with long-term use	Inhibit cyclooxygenase enzyme 2 (COX-2), thereby inhibiting the inflammation pathway	Possible GI irritation, nausea, or diarrhea; headache; insomnia; may increase risk of heart attack and stroke with longer use	None; may impair postexercise skeletal muscle protein synthesis
Nonnarcotic analgesics			
acetaminophen (Tylenol)	Block cyclooxygenase enzyme in the central nervous system (CNS)	Possible GI discomfort or headache; in rare cases GI bleeding or impaired hepatic and renal function	None; may impair postexercise skeletal muscle protein synthesis
Corticosteroids			
betamethasone (Celestone Soluspan), cortisone acetate (Cortone), prednisone (Rayos), triamcinolone (Azmacort)	Anti-inflammatory	Drowsiness	Drowsiness may affect motivation to train and ability to train at high intensity or for prolonged duration
Viscosupplement			
hyaluronic acid (Orthovisc)	Joint lubricant and cushioning	May cause allergic reaction in rare cases	None
Opioid (narcotic) pain relievers			
acetaminophen and propoxyphene (Darvocet), oxycodone (Oxycontin), acetaminophen and oxycodone (Percocet), acetaminophen and hydrocodone (Vicodin)	Bind to opioid receptors in the CNS to reduce sensations of pain	Constipation, drowsiness, dry mouth, and difficulty urinating	Drowsiness may affect motivation to train and ability to train at high intensity or for prolonged duration

References: (153)

Medications Table 3.4   Common Medications Used to Treat Joint Replacement (Arthroplasty)

Drug class and names	Mechanism of action	Most common side effects	Effects on exercise
Nonsteroidal anti-inflammatory drugs (NSAIDs)			
ibuprofen (Advil, Motrin), naproxen (Aleve, Anaprox), celecoxib (Celebrex)	Inhibit cyclooxygenase enzymes 1 and 2 (COX-1, COX-2), thereby inhibiting the inflammation pathways	Possible GI irritation or bleeding if taken in high doses or for prolonged periods; increased risk of heart attack and stroke, which increases with high doses and with longer use	None; may impair postexercise skeletal muscle protein synthesis
Nonnarcotic analgesics			
acetaminophen (Tylenol)	Block cyclooxygenase enzyme in the central nervous system (CNS)	Possible GI discomfort or headache; in rare cases GI bleeding or impaired hepatic and renal function	None; may impair postexercise skeletal muscle protein synthesis
Short-term oral opiates			
hydrocodone (Vicodin), oxycodone (Oxycontin, Percocet), codeine, morphine	Bind to opioid receptors in brain and spinal cord (and GI tract), thereby decreasing pain transmission at both sites	Nausea, drowsiness, constipation, urinary retention	None known
Oral anticoagulants			
warfarin (Coumadin)	Inhibit the formation of vitamin K-dependent clotting factors, thereby decreasing the ability to form blood clots	Less common side effects include increased risk of severe bleeding, dizziness, weakness, diarrhea, vomiting	May increase bleeding (internal and external) in response to injury; avoid high-impact and contact activities

References: (55, 153)

Medications Table 3.5 Common Medications Used to Treat Frailty

Drug class and names	Mechanism of action	Most common side effects	Effects on exercise
β-blockers			
metoprolol (Lopressor)	Reduce blood pressure by competitively binding to β-adrenergic receptors on the heart, blood vessels, and lungs	Fatigue, dizziness, headache, GI distress, constipation, diarrhea, nausea, vomiting	Inhibit the exercise-induced increases in heart rate and blood pressure; thus use of RPE to measure intensity is important
Thiazide diuretic			
hydrochlorothiazide (Esidrix, Microzide)	Impairs sodium (salt) and water resorption in the kidneys, thus increasing urine output and lowering total body water volume and blood pressure	May cause symptoms of allergic reaction, dry mouth, thirst, nausea, vomiting, fatigue, dizziness, fast or uneven heartbeat, muscle pain or weakness	None; however, fatigue, muscle weakness, and dizziness may impair ability to exercise
Antidepressants			
sertraline (Zoloft)	Increase serotonin levels in the brain	Fatigue, muscle weakness, dizziness, nausea, vomiting, diarrhea	Fatigue, muscle weakness, and dizziness may impair ability to exercise
Angiotensin-converting enzyme (ACE) inhibitors			
enalapril (Vasotec)	Decrease blood pressure by inhibiting the activity of ACE, thereby reducing the production of angiotensin II, which causes blood vessel dilation	Orthostatic intolerance, unusual weakness, blurred vision, confusion	None
Oral anticoagulants			
warfarin (Coumadin)	Inhibit the formation of vitamin K-dependent clotting factors, thereby decreasing the ability to form blood clots	Increased risk of severe bleeding, dizziness, weakness, diarrhea, vomiting	May increase bleeding (internal and external) in response to injury; avoid high-impact and contact activities
Cholesterol-lowering agent (statin)			
simvastatin (Zocor)	Inhibits 3-hydroxy-3-methyl-glutaryl-coenzyme A (HMG-CoA) reductase enzyme in the liver, thereby decreasing cholesterol production	Dizziness, headache, fainting, fast or irregular heartbeat	May reduce strength and aerobic exercise tolerance; may increase muscle damage associated with eccentric exercise

References: (55, 78, 117, 150)

Medications Table 3.6   Common Medications Used to Treat Sarcopenia

Drug class and names	Mechanism of action	Most common side effects	Effects on exercise
Androgens			
testosterone (Depo-Testosterone), dehydroepiandrosterone sulphate [DHEA] (Fidelin)	Increase muscle protein synthesis and satellite cells	Increased prostate size, fluid retention, polycythemia, sleep apnea	No effects on acute exercise response; chronic injections increase muscle mass and may improve muscle strength in frail adults
Mitogen			
human growth hormone (Genotropin)	Increases insulin-like growth factor (IGF-1) and stimulates satellite cell fusion	Dizziness, headache, bradycardia or tachycardia, blurred vision, nervousness	No effects on acute exercise response; can increase lean muscle mass but no effect on aerobic capacity; for safety, should not exercise when dizzy or drowsy
Dietary supplement			
creatine, creatine monohydrate; creatine hydrochloride (Con-Cret)	Increases intracellular creatine stores, thus extending or increasing ATP resynthesis	GI distress, diarrhea, water retention	May increase muscle mass and strength, may improve short high-intensity and anaerobic exercise performance
Angiotensin-converting enzyme (ACE) inhibitors			
enalapril (Vasotec)	Decrease blood pressure by inhibiting the activity of ACE, thereby reducing the production of angiotensin II, which causes blood vessel dilation	Orthostatic intolerance, unusual weakness, blurred vision, confusion	None

References: (37, 86, 109, 117)

4

Metabolic Conditions and Disorders

Thomas P. LaFontaine, PhD, CSCS, NSCA-CPT

Jeffrey L. Roitman, EdD

Paul Sorace, MS, CSCS

After completing this chapter, you will be able to

◆ understand the underlying causes and prevalence of obesity, type 1 and type 2 diabetes, dyslipidemia, hyper- and hypothyroidism, and chronic kidney disease;

◆ recognize the most common medications prescribed in the management of these conditions and their basic mechanisms of action and side effects;

◆ explain the benefits of exercise in the prevention and management of these metabolic conditions; and

◆ understand the essential principles of exercise programming, including precautions, for clients with obesity, type 1 and type 2 diabetes, dyslipidemia, hyper- and hypothyroidism, and chronic kidney disease.

Numerous studies have shown that chronic metabolic disorders including obesity, dyslipidemia, hypertension, and type 2 diabetes are largely preventable (1, 32, 188). Evidence (88, 154) is strong that persons who adhere to a low-risk lifestyle have a 72% to 90% lower risk for diseases such as type 2 diabetes compared to persons with a high-risk lifestyle (table 4.1). Unfortunately, only 3% to 8% of persons in the United States practice a low-risk lifestyle (14, 65, 66, 124, 188). This chapter addresses the role of exercise in the prevention and management of four common metabolic disorders: obesity, type 2 diabetes mellitus, type 1 diabetes mellitus, and dyslipidemia. In addition, a brief discussion of exercise and hypothyroidism, hyperthyroidism, and chronic kidney disease is presented.

OBESITY

Obesity is a term that reflects excess adipose tissue. Obesity develops and progresses in humans and animals due to an imbalance of calorie intake and expenditure in which intake exceeds expenditure over an extended period of time. A genetic component is present, but the exact contribution and magnitude of genetics are uncertain (32a, 101a). However, it appears that obesity is rarely solely due to genetic abnormalities.

Epidemiology of Obesity

Over the past 30 years, obesity in the United States has reached epidemic proportions (157). The prevalence of overweight and obesity combined in the U.S. adult population was almost 70% in 2010 (157), and recent data from the Centers for Disease Control and Prevention showed that self-reported obesity prevalence among U.S. adults was 30.4% (34). Also, 18% of youth between ages 6 and 19 are classified as obese (156). The terms **overweight** and **obesity** are defined in various ways, but in this chapter they are defined as follows:

- *Overweight* refers to a body mass index (BMI) between 25 and 29.9. The health risk of being overweight is less definitive than that for being obese.
- *Obesity* refers to a BMI over 30.
  - Stage 1 obesity: 30.0 to 34.9
  - Stage 2 obesity: 35.0 to 39.9
  - Stage 3 obesity: ≥40.0

Pathophysiology of Obesity

Many chronic diseases including obesity appear to have a similar underlying pathophysiology. The cluster of conditions includes a systemic, subclinical inflammation, vascular and metabolic dysfunction, and hormonal irregularities (81, 116). Adipose tissue was previously thought of as simple fat storage depots. It is now clear that adipose tissue is metabolically active; it produces substances called **adipokines** (i.e., adiponectin and leptin) and other hormone-like substances that promote inflammation, metabolic dysfunction, and increased deposition of adipose tissue

Table 4.1 Definition of Low-Risk Versus High-Risk Lifestyles

Lifestyle component	Low risk	High risk
Exercise habits	30 min or more, 5 days per week (optimally 4-7 h per week) of aerobic exercise; 2-3 h per week of resistance training; regular flexibility exercise	Sedentary (no regular physical activity or exercise)
Diet quality	Low fat, high fiber, higher fish intake, low meat intake, moderate nut intake, high intake of fruits and vegetables, low-glycemic whole grains and legumes, and low-fat dairy	High fat, low fiber, high in cholesterol, meats, and high-fat dairy, low in fish, low intake of fruits and vegetables, high-glycemic whole grains
Smoking	Nontobacco user	Uses tobacco, 1 pack/day
BMI (body mass index)	18.9-24.9	>30
Alcohol intake (no. of drinks)	1/day in women, 1-2 in men	0 or 3+ per day

References: (60, 124, 173)

(122). The inflammation that accompanies excess adipose tissue results from an imbalance between pro- and anti-inflammatory adipokines. Proinflammatory adipokines facilitate metabolic, immune, and vascular dysfunction, as well as abnormal glucose and fat metabolism, excess insulin secretion, insulin resistance, and other pathophysiological changes (25, 81, 122).

The initial factor responsible for accumulation of adipose tissue is a positive net caloric balance. Therefore the effects of dietary pattern and specific macronutrients on pathophysiology are pertinent to this discussion. Consumption of excess dietary fat, particularly saturated and trans fat, processed meats, and refined simple and processed carbohydrate, causes variable degrees of inflammation and vascular, metabolic, and immune system dysfunction (123). These foods are prevalent in excess within the American or "Western" dietary pattern (121, 202, 213). Table 4.2 provides a comparison of a Western animal-based versus a plant-based dietary pattern (a Mediterranean diet, for example). Low levels of physical activity and long bouts of sitting add to the inflammation and metabolic dysfunction (73, 174).

Key Point

Consumption of saturated and trans fat, processed meats, and refined simple and processed carbohydrate is linked with inflammation and vascular, metabolic, and immune system dysfunction.

Finally, the neurohormonal and physiological control of appetite is influenced both by the central nervous system and by adipokines. One example is the neurohormone leptin, a protein produced in fat cells that circulates in blood and alerts the brain that there is enough stored energy. Persons with obesity often have high levels of leptin but their brains are not receiving the message that they have adequate energy (127). This has been described as leptin resistance and is similar to insulin resistance. The pathophysiology associated with obesity includes excess plasma leptin, increased hunger, and decreased fatty acid catabolism promoting accumulation of adipose. Resistance, aerobic, and combined training have been shown to improve leptin resistance (20, 57, 110).

Table 4.2   Characteristics of the Western Animal-Based Diet Versus a Plant-Based Diet

Dietary component	Western animal-based diet	Plant-based diet
Fat intake (% of kcal)	High (30-45%)	Moderate-low (10-30%)
Saturated fat (% of kcal)	High (10-15%)	Low (<7%)
Trans fat (% of kcal)	High (2-5%)	Low (<1%)
Polyunsaturated and monounsaturated fat (% of kcal)	High (20-25%)	Moderate to low (15-20%)
Protein intake (% of kcal)	High (25-50%)	Moderate to low (15-25%)
Carbohydrate intake (% of kcal)	Low to moderate (30-50%)	Moderate to high (55-65%)
Simple–processed (% of kcal)	High (>10%)	Low (≤5%)
Complex high fiber (g/day)	Low (10-20)	High (30-45+)
Meat intake	High	Low
Processed meat intake	Moderate to high	Low
Fruit and vegetable intake (servings per day)	Low (<4)	High (6-9)
Whole-grain intake (servings per day)	Low (0-3)	High (4-8)
Bean, legume intake (servings per week)	Low (0-2)	High (4-7)
Nut intake (servings per week)	Low (0-2)	High (4-7)

References: (173, 202, 222)

Common Medications Given to Individuals With Obesity

Numerous efforts have been made to develop an effective antiobesity medication. The optimal medication obviously would result in a sustained and significant weight loss (i.e., perhaps greater than 10%) with minimal side effects and contraindications. Considering the multifactorial genetic and environmental causes of obesity, it is not surprising that a "magic bullet" has not been discovered (172). It also is essential that any medication used to promote weight loss be prescribed in conjunction with a progressive resistance and aerobic exercise training program and a healthy lower-calorie diet. See medications table 4.1 near the end of the chapter for information on Food and Drug Administration–approved medications for obesity.

Effects of Exercise in Individuals With Obesity

This section discusses weight loss programs and research on exercise, daily physical activity, diet, and weight loss. It is particularly pertinent to emphasize that individual preference and situations are extremely important in guiding successful long-term sustainable weight loss programs. Exercise professionals must be aware of the needs and goals of clients in achieving successful weight management outcomes.

Energy Balance

It is rare that either food restriction or increased physical activity alone can produce significant long-term weight loss in persons with obesity (86, 187). Thus the optimal strategy for weight loss and prevention of weight regain uses a combination of exercise and calorie restriction to create a daily negative caloric balance (4, 5, 48, 64, 68, 83, 137). For example, combining 250 kcal/day in exercise-related energy expenditure with 250 kcal/day in calorie restriction produces an energy deficit of 500 kcal/day. Theoretically, based on the assumption that a negative caloric balance of 3,500 kcal is equivalent to 1 pound (0.5 kg) of adipose fat, this approach should produce a weight loss of approximately 1 pound/week. Though this seems logical, individual physiological, biochemical, and genetic variations affect the real-life application of this principle; thus weight loss does not necessarily happen "as calculated" (83, 86). However, this principle works in the long term and is key to an effective weight loss program or a weight regain prevention program.

Hill and colleagues (86), in a review article, summarized the concept of energy balance and weight loss. A positive energy balance, in which calorie intake exceeds energy expenditure, leads to excess adiposity and obesity. Energy balance is regulated through three components of energy expenditure: resting metabolic rate (RMR), the thermic effect of the digestion and assimilation of food (TEF), and the thermic effect of activity (EE_{PA}). Obesity is the result of an imbalance in one or more of these components. Some experts suggest that a reduced calorie expenditure in physical activity (85, 86) may be the most critical factor. From a societal perspective in the United States, since the 1970s, observed increases in food intake and decreases in daily physical activity and exercise (structured physical activity) have resulted in an imbalance in calorie intake and output leading to the present epidemic of obesity (85). Pontzer (167) has suggested that the relationship between EE_{PA} and total energy expenditure (TEE) is more complex than the current additive model (TEE = RMR + TEF + EE_{PA}). Rather than EE_{PA} increasing in a linear dose–response relationship, ecological and experimental data from several species suggest that TEE is constrained with respect to EE_{PA} (i.e., TEE is maintained homeostatically within a narrow range and the body adapts to long-term increases in EE_{PA} by reducing energy expenditure in other systems such as RMR and TEF [167]).

In general, if a person increases energy intake above energy expenditure over an extended period of time without increasing energy output, weight gain results. As much as 60% to 80% of this weight gain can be body fat (86). Conversely, if energy expenditure exceeds energy intake, a negative energy balance is achieved and weight loss occurs. As much as 60% to 80% of this loss is body fat (86). Studies have shown that energy balance and thus body weight are best regulated at high rather than low levels of EE_{PA} (86, 129). Food restriction is a common strategy to produce weight loss, often without concomitant increased physical activity. This strategy results in a loss of as much as 20% to 40% of lean body mass, which leads to a reduction in RMR and EE_{PA}.

A certain level of physical activity (EE_{PA}) is required to maintain a healthy body weight and an even higher level to lose nonlean mass. The EE_{PA} is the most variable of the three components—it accounts for about 15% to 30% of our daily calorie expenditure and can be manipulated upward relatively easily. Thus, increasing physical activity through exercise and nonexercise physical activity is critical to weight loss. Also if lean body mass is lost, more physical activity is required to maintain the loss of fat mass and to prevent weight regain.

Finally, it has been established that it is easier to prevent weight gain than to lose weight over the long term (85, 86, 187). Calorie intake was more equally matched with higher levels of physical activity than with decreased levels of food consumption (86). Thus, efforts to prevent weight gain in the general population should be as assertive as those to facilitate weight loss.

Diet and Weight Loss

Countless weight loss and fad diets are available (205). Consumers may be unaware of the drawbacks, dangers, and disadvantages of these diets. Many are based on false scientific premises while others were developed on the basis of valid scientific information that is inappropriately interpreted. Some are scientifically and behaviorally valid but virtually impossible to maintain and adhere to over long periods and therefore are not practical for most people.

Weight loss diets can be classified into four broad categories:

- **Low-calorie balanced diets:** Characterized by caloric restriction of around 1,200 kcal per day for women and 1,400 to 1,500 kcal per day for men. The quality of foods and the number of calories consumed are extremely important. In general, these diets are composed of low caloric density foods such as fruits and vegetables, beans, legumes, and in general a plant-based dietary pattern.
- **Low-fat (high-carbohydrate) diets:** Characterized by restriction of daily calories from fat.

Often 15% to 20% and sometimes as few as 10% of kilocalories come from fat. Attention must be given to the type of fat consumed; that is, monounsaturated and polyunsaturated should be predominant in these diets. This diet also is generally a plant-based diet and should be focused on complex, high-fiber carbohydrate and lean sources of animal and vegetable protein. It can also be vegetarian.
- **Low-carbohydrate (high-fat, high-protein, or both) diets:** Restriction of carbohydrate to 50 to 150 g per day (212) or 20% to 40% of total caloric intake (69) although it may be as low as less than 10% of total daily calories. Strict limitations on refined carbohydrate (processed grains used in white pasta, white bread, processed cereals, and sugar) along with moderate to high protein and, sometimes, high fat are common characteristics of these diets. Some of these dietary plans gradually increase carbohydrate but generally are restricted to less than 150 g per day. Fat intake in some of these diets is not controlled or limited.
- **Low-carbohydrate, low-fat (high protein) diets:** These diets restrict both carbohydrate and fat while emphasizing high amounts of protein, usually of animal origin. In general, nuts, seeds, berries, and tuber plant foods are allowed, but the emphasis is on a large amount of lean meat intake.

Although there are many variations of these broad categories, this is a convenient way to look at the dietary patterns promoted for weight loss. There are also very low calorie diets (VLCD)—less than 800 kcal per day—that are implemented under medical supervision in order to enhance safety and effectiveness and therefore outside the realm of this book.

The basic principles of creating a negative energy balance include the following:

- **The total change in energy balance, called** *energy flux,* **may be important to the effectiveness of creating a negative energy balance.** A greater energy flux may ensure more success than a smaller energy flux. Those individuals with the greatest energy flux (induced by a combination of reduced calorie intake and increased energy expenditure) may be more able to lose weight. Higher levels of physical activity and exercise may allow persons to regulate energy intake more effectively. On the other hand, individuals with a low energy flux (small changes in energy balance) may not be able to restrict kilocalories enough to successfully lose weight or prevent weight regain.

- **Dietary pattern may variably affect weight loss depending on whether a person is in negative, positive, or equivalent energy balance.** Studies show that specific macronutrient intake makes little difference in weight loss. In other words, a calorie is a calorie, and the type of calorie makes little if any difference. This appears to be particularly true over the long periods of time—years and decades—during which most adults gain weight. Hall and colleagues (82) found that subjects on a low-fat but relatively high-sugar diet achieved more fat loss than those on an equal-calorie, low-carbohydrate diet. Hall concluded, "We can definitely reject the claim that carbohydrate restriction is required for body fat loss" (82). In another study among young adults who were overweight and obese, isocaloric feeding after a 10% to 15% weight loss resulted in decreases in resting and total energy expenditure that were the greatest with the low-fat diet, moderate with the low glycemic index diet, and the least with the very-low-carbohydrate diet (58).

- **When a negative energy balance is present, there is little difference in weight loss associated with high-protein, low-fat, or low-carbohydrate diets** (71). However, a healthy dietary pattern that is plant based has been shown to predict successful weight loss maintenance (10, 104, 220).

- It seems possible that moderate increases in physical activity (30 minutes per day) can prevent weight gain over the long term, but that relatively large increases in physical activity (60-90 minutes per day) are necessary to prevent weight regain (220).

- **The challenge of maintaining a weight loss is more difficult because losing weight causes decreased energy requirements both at rest and during exercise.** Therefore, after a weight loss, maintaining that loss may require increased energy expenditure (48, 219, 220).

- **Systematic changes in the environment are needed for weight loss and to prevent weight gain.** Both the food and the exercise or activity environments that support sustained healthy eating practices and physical activity are critical to weight loss and preventing weight regain (85, 202).

In conjunction with these basic principles, it is worth noting that some people may be genetically prone to obesity (2); thus there are difficulties using traditional methods of producing a negative energy balance for intake and expenditure with food and exercise.

Exercise Recommendations for Clients With Obesity

An important factor to consider when planning exercise for weight loss is that persons with obesity are likely to be less tolerant of weight-bearing exercise and prone to exercise-related injuries. Furthermore, the prescribed intensity, duration, and frequency interact to exacerbate the injury rate such that initially lower frequency, duration, and intensity are strongly encouraged (5, 48). In many cases, initially using 5- to 15-minute intermittent bouts two or three times a day is recommended. The importance of a positive initial engagement with an exercise program cannot be overstated. Experts recommend gradual progression in duration from 30 to 60 minutes per session and from 150 to 300 minutes or more per week for weight loss, to prevent weight regain, and to reduce associated chronic disease risk factors (4, 48). The National Weight Control Registry (220) suggests that 60 to 90 minutes of exercise per day may be required to prevent weight regain.

The role of resistance training as an independent contributor to weight loss or prevention of weight regain is less clear. It does not appear that including resistance training in a weight loss exercise program increases the loss of fat mass or prevents the reduced resting energy expenditure that accompanies significant weight loss (48, 91). As with aerobic exercise, resistance training alone does not appear to promote significant weight loss independent of caloric restriction. However, combining resistance training and aerobic exercise has been shown (176, 218) to be similar to aerobic exercise for bodyweight and fat loss while resistance training promotes an increase in fat-free mass. Resistance training also may improve visceral obesity and systemic inflammation (192).

Arguably the most effective programs address increased nonexercise physical activity (NEPA) and leisure-time physical activity (LTPA) and reduced sitting time. Leisure-time physical activity refers to energy expended while engaging in recreational physical activities, and NEPA describes energy expended due to engaging in activities of daily living or non–LTPA-related activities. Prescribed increases in LTPA along with decreased sitting time can make significant contributions to the increased calorie expenditure necessary to create a negative caloric balance (105, 118). Finding ways for clients who are obese and overweight to increase daily physical activity and LTPA and to decrease sitting time appears to be critical to weight loss and prevention of weight regain. The most effective program will include regular daily exercise (300+ kcal per day), increased NEPA and LTPA, and decreased sitting time (61, 118).

There is little question that increased physical activity and reduced calorie intake are both necessary to establish the negative energy balance required to achieve successful weight loss. Research demonstrates that weight loss programs using activity alone are not as effective as weight loss programs using diet alone. However, in both of these types of programs the total amount of weight loss is only a few pounds (~1 kg) over the long term (12 months) (9, 48, 85, 219). It also has been shown that achieving higher activity levels (2,100-2,700 kcal per week) after weight loss is necessary to prevent weight regain (48, 220). Basic logic states that both calorie restriction and increased exercise and LTPA are the most effective approaches to weight loss and weight loss maintenance. One important point to consider is that it is sometimes difficult for people who are overweight (especially those with BMIs greater than 40) to perform sufficient amounts of physical activity to lose weight. An early approach to weight loss for clients who are extremely obese is a medically supervised VLCD in combination with light-intensity, low-impact aerobic exercise and resistance training (42, 48).

To prevent significant weight gain, clients should strive for 150 to 250 minutes per week of moderate-intensity physical activity. This amount of exercise is likely to result in only modest weight loss. Moderate-intensity activity greater than 250 minutes per week is likely to be more effective for weight loss and preventing weight regain (4, 48, 220). Table 4.3 presents basic exercise guidelines for clients who are obese.

Exercise Modifications, Precautions, and Contraindications for Clients With Obesity

There are several precautions that the exercise professional needs to consider and be aware of when working with clients with obesity. Importantly, clients with obesity are likely to have one or more metabolic disorders such as hypertension, dyslipidemia, type 2 diabetes, or cardiovascular disease (CVD). Medical clearance is essential before starting an exercise program for most of these clients.

- Clients with obesity are prone to musculoskeletal injuries and diseases, particularly osteoarthritis and hip, low back, neck, and knee pain. Thus, a carefully graded progression is critical. Also it may be helpful to emphasize that joint pain usually improves, sometimes dramatically, following weight loss of as little as 5% to 10% of body weight. Low-impact aerobic exercise may be prudent, such as cycle ergometry or moderately paced walking.

- Both aerobic and resistance training may need to initially be performed intermittently in multiple bouts (5-15 minutes) per day.

- The exercise professional should focus on increasing duration and frequency before increasing intensity.

- Some machines may not be usable by clients who are obese and thus adaptive equipment such as a larger seat on a bicycle ergometer may be required.

- The exercise professional should be sensitive to the physical and emotional difficulties that

Table 4.3 General Exercise Guidelines for Clients Who Are Obese

Parameter	Guideline
Exercise intensity	40-85% heart rate reserve
Weekly exercise duration (to prevent weight gain)	150-300 min
Weekly exercise duration (to prevent regain)	300+ min per week
Weekly caloric expenditure for weight loss	1,200-2,000 kcal
Weekly caloric expenditure to prevent regain	2,000+ kcal
Exercise frequency	5 or more days per week, preferably 7 days per week
Minimum exercise duration per session	10 min (for very deconditioned clients)
Exercise duration goal per session	30 min (minimum)
Optimal exercise duration for weight loss	45-60 min per day
Optimal exercise duration to prevent regain	60-90 min per day
Modality	Aerobic activity is a priority, weight bearing preferred; resistance training should be incorporated to promote lean body mass preservation and contribute to health benefits and maintenance of resting metabolism; ideally, a combination is preferred.

References: (5, 48, 173, 220)

the client with obesity may experience when exercising in a facility or in a group.

- The exercise professional should encourage a client with obesity to increase daily NEPA and obtain a pedometer and initially determine his average daily steps. With this baseline measure, the client should increase daily steps by around 250 per day per week, with a goal of reaching 11,000 to 14,000 steps. This goal would include structured exercise and may take several months to achieve.

- The exercise professional should recognize that weight loss is most effectively induced with a low-calorie diet and increased physical activity. Thus the client with obesity should be encouraged to adhere to a low-calorie, high-fiber diet that is limited in saturated and trans fat and processed carbohydrate. It is important that clients with obesity become accustomed to exercise, as exercise minimizes the loss of fat-free mass and is a key predictor of long-term weight loss maintenance.

- Due to high risk for metabolic disorders, percent fat, weight, blood pressure, fasting blood glucose, and lipids should be assessed every three to six months.

- For safety and as a potential motivational tool, blood pressure should be periodically assessed before, during, and after exercise to ensure safe levels and to demonstrate the postexercise hypotension that commonly occurs after an exercise bout with enhanced conditioning and weight loss.

- The exercise professional must encourage adequate fluid intake in clients with obesity and also be attentive to maintaining a thermoneutral environment (66-72°F [19-22°C]), as persons with obesity are prone to hyperthermia.

Case Study

Preventing Weight Regain

Mr. A, a 66-year-old retired university professor, started a weight loss program with an initial body weight of 282 pounds (128 kg), BMI of 34.4, and 33.2% body fat. A medical history revealed prediabetes (fasting glucose of 109 mg/dl), prehypertension (resting blood pressure of 136/88 mmHg), and high triglyceride (191 mg/dl) and low high-density lipoprotein (HDL) (38 mg/dl) levels. He had no history of CVD. After medical clearance and a normal physician-supervised 12-lead clinical exercise stress test, a submaximal metabolic exercise test was administered. Flexibility and muscle strength were also assessed. Mr. A was advised to exercise aerobically every other day at a heart rate of 118 to 134 beats/min beginning with 10 to 15 minutes twice per day and progressing by 10% to 15% per week to 60 minutes per session.

A resistance training program beginning with multijoint exercise machines and specific single-joint exercises was implemented. The resistance training program was designed with an initial frequency of two or three days per week with one set and progressed over two months to three sets of 10 to 15 reps at 50% to 70% of estimated one repetition maximum (1RM). After two months, the resistance training program was advanced to three sets of 8 to 10 reps at 60% to 80% of 1RM two days per week plus a third day on which he would perform the previous program. After another two months, the program was changed to one day per week at 60% to 70% of 1RM for 10 to 15 reps per set, one day per week at 70% to 80% of 1RM for 8 to 10 reps per set, and one day per week at 80% to 90% of 1RM for 4 to 6 reps per set.

Mr. A was initially advised by his physician and referred to a registered dietician for counseling on how to adopt and adhere to a diet that was low in total fat, high in fiber, and calorie restricted to remove 500 kcal from his daily diet and target a 1.5-pound (0.7 kg) loss per week. After a year, laboratory measurements and all tests were repeated. The table shows the changes in body composition as a result of the weight loss program.

Test or measurement	Pre	Post	Change
Body weight	282 lb (128 kg)	219 lb (99 kg)	−63 lb (29 kg)
BMI	34.4	26.7	−7.7 units
% fat	33.2	21.2	−12
Fat-free weight	188.4 lb (85 kg)	174.8 lb (79 kg)	−13.6 lb (6 kg)
Fat weight	93.6 lb (42 kg)	44.2 lb (20 kg)	−49.4 lb (22 kg)
Maximal oxygen uptake (ml · kg^{-1} · min^{-1})	22.2	32.5	+10.3
Triglycerides (mg/dl)	191	89	−102
HDLs (high-density lipoproteins) (mg/dl)	38	53	+14
Fasting blood glucose (mg/dl)	109	89	−20

Recommended Readings

American College of Cardiology/American Heart Association Task Force on Practice Guidelines, Obesity Expert Panel, 2013. Expert Panel Report: guidelines (2013) for the management of overweight and obesity in adults. *Obesity* 22:S41-S410, 2014.

Flegal, KM, Kruszon-Moran, D, Carroll, MD, Fryar, CD, and Ogden, CL. Trends in obesity among adults in the United States, 2005 to 2014. *JAMA* 315:2284-2291, 2016.

Hill, JO. Understanding and addressing the epidemic of obesity: an energy balance perspective. *Endocrine Rev* 27:750-761, 2006.

Moore, GE, Durstine, JL, and Painter, PL, eds. *ACSM's Exercise Management for Persons with Chronic Diseases and Disabilities.* 4th ed. Human Kinetics: Champaign, IL, 2016.

U.S. Department of Health and Human Services and U.S. Department of Agriculture. Dietary Guidelines for Americans 2015–2020. Eighth Edition. December 2015. http://health.gov/dietaryguidelines/2015/guidelines. Accessed January 6, 2017.

TYPE 2 DIABETES MELLITUS

Type 2 diabetes is a disease of insulin resistance (36, 145). Normally in response to a mixed meal, blood glucose rises and pancreatic beta cells release insulin, a hormone that facilitates the uptake of glucose into muscle, fat, and other cells. Without adequate secretion and blood levels of insulin or with impaired insulin action or both, blood glucose increases to abnormal levels. Obesity is implicated because of the influence of the adipokines and their proinflammatory response, as well as the direct inhibitory effect of obesity on insulin receptors in muscle cells (117). As insulin resistance progresses, pancreatic insulin-producing cells produce less insulin, resulting in insulin deficiency and type 2 diabetes. Insulin resistance coupled with other metabolic dysfunction (45) also causes dyslipidemia in many persons with type 2 diabetes.

In summary, insulin resistance is initially present before type 2 diabetes. It can take up to 10 years for insulin resistance to progress to the diagnosis of type 2 diabetes. However, even though the clinical diagnosis of type 2 diabetes can be delayed long after the initial insulin resistance, the pathophysiology and the associated complications (endothelial dysfunction, kidney and eye problems, sensory difficulties associated with the disease, and so on) all can and do negatively affect tissues during this time (15, 24, 113). Over 75% of type 2 diabetes cases occur among obese, inactive adults (59). Persons with a BMI >35 have up to a 30-fold greater risk of developing type 2 diabetes than persons with a BMI of <23 (38). Table 4.4 presents the definitions and classification of normal, impaired, and diabetes levels of fasting and random or **postprandial** (after consuming a meal) blood glucose.

Epidemiology and Pathophysiology of Type 2 Diabetes

Approximately 29.1 million people in the United States have diabetes, and another 86 million are estimated to have prediabetes (28). There are four general classifications of diabetes:

1. Type 1, which is insulin dependent and thought to be the result of an autoimmune attack on the beta cells of the pancreas resulting in their destruction
2. Type 2, which is largely the result of insulin resistance
3. Gestational diabetes, which occurs during pregnancy
4. Diabetes due to other specific causes such as monogenic diabetes (i.e., neonatal diabetes mellitus and maturity-onset diabetes of the young), drug-induced diabetes (which may result after organ transplant or human immunodeficiency virus/acquired immune deficiency syndrome treatment), and exocrine pancreatic insufficiency (which may lead to cystic fibrosis–related diabetes)

Approximately 90% to 95% of all cases are type 2, which in the United States was estimated at 27.85 million in 2014 (28). The prevalence of type 2 diabetes is greatest among African Americans and Hispanic Americans. Among 12- to 19-year olds of all racial groups, Li and colleagues (119) reported

Table 4.4 Classification of Normal, Impaired, and Diabetic Fasting and Random Blood Glucose

Classification	Fasting blood glucose	Random (2 h after 75 g of glucose)
Normal	<100 mg/dl	<140 mg/dl
Prediabetes	100-125 mg/dl	140-199 mg/dl
Diabetes	>125 mg/dl[a]	>199 mg/dl[b]

[a]On two occasions after fasting 8 hours or more.

[b]On two occasions 2 hours after a 75-g glucose load or 2 hours after a mixed meal.

Reference: (8)

a prevalence of impaired fasting glucose, impaired glucose tolerance, and prediabetes of 13.1%, 3.4%, and 16.1%, respectively. Type 2 diabetes is directly and positively correlated with the mean increase in body weight over the past 2.5 decades (85), and this strong positive correlation has led to use of the term "diabesity" for type 2 diabetes (106).

Frequently, high levels of glucose are associated with several secondary complications such as these:

- Coronary artery disease–myocardial infarction: 70% of persons with diabetes die of heart disease (128)
- Congestive heart failure (a complication of heart disease) (128, 150)
- Cerebral vascular accident (stroke): Diabetes is a major risk factor for stroke (28)
- Hypertension: 71% of adults 18 years or older with diagnosed diabetes have a blood pressure greater than or equal to 140/90 mmHg or are on antihypertensive medications (28)
- Kidney disease: Diabetes was listed as the primary cause of end-stage renal disease in 44% of new cases in 2011 (28)
- High triglycerides and low HDLs are related to insulin action on adipose cells to increase storage and insulin resistance (63)
- Eye disease: Diabetes is a major cause of retinopathy and blindness (28)
- Neuropathies and autonomic dysfunction: decreased exercise capacity, decreased heart rate response and heart rate variability, and a slow recovery heart rate (28, 47, 193, 208)
- Peripheral artery disease (insufficient blood flow to limbs): 60% of nontraumatic amputations occur in persons with diabetes related to decreased blood flow and impaired healing (28)

Common Medications Given to Individuals With Type 2 Diabetes

Medications table 4.2 near the end of the chapter lists the common medications used for type 2 diabetes. Medical therapy for type 2 diabetes is targeted at improving insulin resistance, reducing liver secretion of glucose, and stimulating pancreatic beta cells to secrete insulin. Initial treatment should focus on lifestyle change therapy, which has been shown in multiple studies to possibly reverse type 2 diabetes (17, 171, 189). However, for multiple reasons, a large percentage of persons with type 2 diabetes are prescribed medications.

Effects of Exercise in Individuals With Type 2 Diabetes

Exercise has long been an essential component of the prevention and management of type 2 diabetes. Since type 2 diabetes is the result of acquired insulin resistance, the prevention and management of this disease can be conceptualized as a four-pronged strategy, depicted in figure 4.1.

Studies (36, 128, 180, 181) have shown that increased physical activity and structured exercise improve insulin-independent muscle glucose uptake independently of weight loss or a hypoglycemic diet. Aerobic exercise has been shown to enhance glucose delivery to exercising muscle, stimulate translocation of glucose transporter protein 4 to the cell surface, improve insulin receptor sensitivity, and increase phosphorylation and utilization of glucose intracellularly (155, 209). It has also been demonstrated that the effect of an acute exercise bout on glucose uptake persists into the recovery period (36, 128). As such, daily exercise provides an alternative mechanism (in the absence of insulin) for blood glucose disposal.

The benefits of sustained exercise are significantly enhanced when coupled with modest weight loss (5-7%) and a low-fat, high-fiber diet (109). In the Diabetes Prevention Program Outcomes Study (46), the lifestyle intervention was significantly better than metformin in reducing the risk of developing type 2 diabetes. In adults older than 55 years, lifestyle modification resulted in a 71% reduction in the risk for developing type 2 diabetes (46).

Key Point

Lifestyle intervention has been shown to be more effective than metformin in reducing the risk for developing type 2 diabetes.

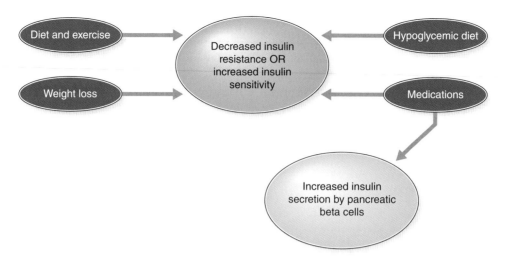

Figure 4.1 Model of lifestyle factors, medications, and effects on insulin and glucose management.

Resistance training has been shown (36, 41, 128, 180, 181) to be safe and essentially as effective as aerobic training in the prevention and management of type 2 diabetes. In women, muscle-strengthening and conditioning activities were found (77) to be associated with a 40% reduction in risk of type 2 diabetes. If women engaged in more than 150 minutes of aerobic exercise and more than 60 minutes of resistance training per week, risk of type 2 diabetes compared to that for inactive age-matched women was reduced by 67% (77). Long-term (at least six months) resistance training increases fat-free mass, resulting in increased insulin receptors and capacity for glucose uptake. Resistance training has also been shown to stimulate glucose uptake and lower glycosylated hemoglobin in a similar manner to aerobic exercise (36, 128, 180, 181, 223).

Recent studies have demonstrated the superior benefits on insulin resistance and glycemic control of combined resistance training and aerobic exercise in individuals with type 2 diabetes (12, 33, 41, 179). Several studies (36, 39, 128, 179) have demonstrated that glycated (or glycosylated) hemoglobin (HbA1c) levels—a long-term measure of blood glucose—improved significantly more in a combined resistance training and aerobic training group compared to resistance training–only and aerobic training–only groups, whereas improvements in blood pressure and lipids were similar among all groups. One potentially confounding factor was that the total exercise duration and caloric expenditure was greater in the combined group versus either the resistance training or aerobic training groups. It is also worth considering that accumulated bouts of aerobic exercise (e.g., three sessions of 10 minutes per day) may be as effective as one 30-minute continuous bout of exercise at improving insulin sensitivity (144).

Key Point

Several studies have demonstrated that HbA1c improves significantly more with a combined resistance training and aerobic training program compared to a resistance training–only or aerobic training–only program.

Exercise Recommendations for Clients With Type 2 Diabetes

Table 4.5 presents guidelines for exercise in persons with type 2 diabetes. Exercise professionals need to be aware of screening recommendations, contraindications, and precautions in clients with type 2 diabetes. All clients with type 2 diabetes should be advised to begin and sustain an individualized aerobic, resistance, and flexibility exercise program.

Table 4.5   General Exercise Guidelines for Clients With Type 2 Diabetes

Parameter	Guideline
Aerobic exercise frequency	Sedentary clients should start with two or three 10-min bouts of aerobic activity per day and progress to 30 min of continuous aerobic activity on 5 to 7 days per week
Aerobic exercise intensity	50-85% heart rate reserve; 12-16 rating of perceived exertion (RPE); talk test[a] is applicable for most clients
Aerobic exercise duration	Minimum of 10 min per session (even lower with peripheral neuropathy or peripheral vascular disease) with a minimum goal of 30 min per session; if weight loss needed, gradually progress to 60 min per session or per day; minimum goal is 150 min per week, up to 300 min or more if weight loss and prevention of weight regain needed
Aerobic exercise modes	Rhythmic, continuous; emphasize large muscle groups as with walking, biking, and swimming
Aerobic exercise caloric expenditure	Goal of 300+ per session and >2,000 per week
Resistance training frequency	2-3 days per week or, ideally, every other day or 48 h apart
Resistance training duration	30-60 min per session using 8-12 repetitions, 2-3 sets, 10-12 large-muscle multijoint exercises
Resistance training intensity	If just beginning a program, use 50-70% 1RM and gradually progress such that by 3-6 months the program consists of a nonlinear plan of 50-65% 1RM with high reps for one session, 65-80% 1RM with moderate reps for one session, and 80-95% 1RM for one session each week (occasionally may test the 1RM)
Resistance training exercise types	Large variety of possibilities depending upon the goals, interests, capabilities, and clinical status of the client (e.g., resistance bands; pneumatic, hydraulic, plate-loaded, or selectorized machines; free weights); goal is to primarily use free weights
Flexibility training[b]	Stretch all major muscle groups every other day, 1-2 static stretches per major muscle groups, hold stretches for 10-30 s each, 20-25 min total duration

[a]The talk test is a test of how comfortably a person can talk during exercise. The intensity at which a person can "just barely respond in conversation" is considered to be safe and appropriate for aerobic endurance improvement (165).

[b]Flexibility exercise is very important in persons with type 2 diabetes due to the association of poor range of motion with this disease.

References: (36, 128)

Exercise Modifications, Precautions, and Contraindications for Clients With Type 2 Diabetes

There are several guidelines that the exercise professional needs to consider and be aware of when working with clients who have type 2 diabetes (5, 36, 128):

- Individuals with type 2 diabetes need to be medically cleared before starting a vigorous exercise program and should undergo a thorough medical evaluation, particularly if they have any cardiovascular, kidney, nervous, renal, or visual complications or have ≥10% risk of a cardiac event over 10 years (5, 36).

- Individuals with type 2 diabetes who have a greater than 10% risk of a cardiac event over the next 10 years should undergo a medically supervised maximal clinical exercise test before starting an exercise program (5, 36).

- Individuals with type 2 diabetes are prone to **silent ischemia** (insufficient blood flow to the heart without clinical signs or symptoms). They may need to have a clinical exercise test with radionuclide injection that allows for detection of ischemic areas of the heart (78, 128).

- Hypoglycemia is the most common abnormal response to exercise. **Hypoglycemia** is clinically defined as a blood glucose of <70 mg/dl and is particularly common in individuals with type 2 diabetes on insulin or multiple oral hypoglycemic agents (36, 128).

Exercise should not occur when exogenous insulin action is peaking. Thus the exercise professional must be familiar with hypoglycemic oral agents and insulin preparations (see medications tables 4.2 and 4.3 near the end of the chapter).

- Blood glucose monitoring should be performed before and after an exercise session and when starting or progressing an exercise program (36).

- If preexercise blood glucose is <100 mg/dl, it is prudent to have the client ingest 20 to 30 g of carbohydrate before starting exercise (recheck glucose 10 minutes after ingestion).

- Avoid injecting insulin into exercising limbs; it is best to use an abdominal site if a type 2 diabetes client presents with a blood glucose above 200 mg/dl, and it is also prudent to check ketone bodies in urine (reagent sticks are available at most pharmacies). If no ketone bodies are present, light to moderate exercise is possible (30% to <60% $\dot{V}O_2$ or heart rate reserve), but vigorous exercise ($\geq$60%-90% $\dot{V}O_2$ or heart rate reserve) should be avoided.

- Be aware of possible dehydration, particularly if the client is hyperglycemic (207).

- For clients with retinopathy, avoid vigorous-intensity exercise and excessive elevations in blood pressure (36). Individuals with **autonomic neuropathy** (pathology of the autonomic nervous system) may have a blunted blood pressure and heart rate response to exercise. These clients should be referred to a medically supervised program.

- Individuals with type 2 diabetes who have kidney disease, peripheral artery disease, or peripheral neuropathy also should be referred to a medically supervised program.

- Be particularly cautious with vigorous exercise in all individuals with type 2 diabetes, as a high percentage of them have undiagnosed atherosclerosis of the coronary and peripheral arteries. Seventy-five percent of individuals with type 2 diabetes will die from CVD.

Case Study

Type 2 Diabetes

Mrs. D, a 58-year-old woman with obesity and type 2 diabetes, was referred to a clinical exercise physiologist by her primary physician for lifestyle management. She is 61 inches (155 cm) tall and weighs 178 pounds (81 kg). She has a history of stage 1 hypertension treated with Lisinopril and hydrochlorothiazide. She is a nonsmoker but has a history of abnormal lipids presently not medically treated. Her physician wanted to see if type 2 diabetes and lipids could be managed with lifestyle intervention. Mrs. D reported no significant musculoskeletal issues except for several two- to four-week bouts of low back pain. She completed a physician-supervised clinical exercise stress test, which was normal. A submaximal metabolic exercise test with body composition assessment was administered. Sit-and-reach, dorsiflexion, and shoulder extension range of motion tests were performed.

Mrs. D gradually progressed her aerobic exercise to 30 to 45 minutes per day, four days per week, at a target heart rate range of 115 to 135 beats/min. She was prescribed a general flexibility and combined aerobic and resistance training program to be done two or three days per week. The program included an 8-minute aerobic exercise warm-up, four resistance training exercises, 5 minutes of aerobic exercise, four resistance training exercises, 5 minutes of aerobic exercise, four resistance training exercises, and a 10-minute aerobic exercise cooldown incorporating flexibility exercises. She purchased a heart rate monitor and a pedometer and was advised to progress from a baseline of 5,500 steps per day to between 11,000 and 14,000 steps per day including her exercise routine. Mrs. D achieved all exercise goals. Labs and metabolic exercise test results were repeated. The table summarizes her progress and results.

Test or measurement	Pre	Post
Body weight	178 lb (81 kg)	152 lb (69 kg)
BMI	33.6	28.8
Fasting blood glucose (mg/dl)	138	102
Triglycerides (mg/dl)	250	140
High-density lipoproteins (mg/dl)	38	52
Low-density lipoproteins (mg/dl)	134	111
Sit-and-reach test	12 in. (30 cm)	16 in. (41 cm)
YMCA bench press test (reps with 35 lb [16 kg])	6	22
Estimated $\dot{V}O_2max$ (ml · kg^{-1} · min^{-1})	22.5	30.1
Ventilatory threshold heart rate (beats/min)	120	131

Recommended Readings

American Diabetes Association. Standards of medical care in diabetes—2016. *Diabetes Care* 39:S1-S112, 2016.

Centers for Disease Control and Prevention. *National Diabetes Statistics Report: Estimates of Diabetes and Its Burden in the United States.* Atlanta: U.S. Department of Health and Human Services, 2014.

Eberhardt, MS, Ogden, C, Engelgau, M, Cadwell, B, Hedley, AA, and Saydah, SH. Prevalence of overweight and obesity among adults with diagnosed diabetes—United States, 1988-1994 and 1999-2002. *MMWR* 53:1066-1068, 2004.

Philippides, G and Rocchini, A. Exercise training for type 2 diabetes mellitus and impact on cardiovascular risk: a scientific statement from the American Heart Association. *Circulation* 119:3244-3262, 2009.

Vinik, AI and Erbas, T. Neuropathy. In *Handbook of Exercise in Diabetes.* 2nd ed. Ruderman, N, ed. Alexandria, VA: American Diabetes Association, 463-496, 2002.

TYPE 1 DIABETES MELLITUS

Type 1 diabetes is an autoimmune disease that causes the body to attack pancreatic beta cells that produce and store insulin. As a result, exogenous insulin is needed to compensate for the lack of endogenous insulin production.

Even though type 1 diabetes was previously termed juvenile diabetes, type 1 diabetes can occur at any age. The onset of type 1 diabetes is typically by age 30, but the greatest occurrence is during puberty (19, 31, 40). The cause of the autoimmune condition is not fully known, but heredity and environmental factors are linked to a greater incidence (31).

Epidemiology and Pathophysiology of Type 1 Diabetes

Of the nearly 30 million people in the United States who have diabetes (28), only 5% to 10% who have diabetes are type 1 and therefore are insulin dependent (19, 28, 31, 40, 206). In 2008 and 2009, more than 18,000 youth were diagnosed with type 1 diabetes, and the trend is continuing (28). By 2012, about 208,000 people of the U.S.

population under 20 years of age were diagnosed with either type 1 or type 2 diabetes (28). Within this group, Caucasian children and adolescents are at the greatest risk of type 1 diabetes; worldwide, Chinese and South American people have a lower risk of developing type 1 diabetes (185).

Individuals with type 1 diabetes need exogenous insulin via injections or an infusion pump to regulate blood glucose levels. A lack of insulin results in hyperglycemia if not treated. High blood sugar levels have a cascading effect of increasing urine production and risk of dehydration and, if unchecked, **ketoacidosis** can occur. When the body cannot take in the glucose from the blood into the cells (the function of insulin), the body uses fat and protein for metabolism with, in the case of fat as fuel, ketones as an acidic by-product. Accumulation of ketones lowers the pH of the blood and results in ketoacidosis, with the following common symptoms:

- Dry mouth or excessive thirst
- Frequent urination
- Nausea and vomiting
- Abdominal pain
- Rapid breathing or shortness of breath
- "Fruity" breath
- Muscle weakness
- Mental confusion

Often, individuals who are unaware that they have type 1 diabetes see a physician or other health care professional for symptoms related to ketoacidosis and then are tested and diagnosed with the disease. Common tests include the HbA1c test or a random or fasting blood glucose test (133), with the result of a glucose test compared against normal values (see table 4.4). An HbA1c test reveals the average blood glucose level of the previous two to three months by measuring the percent of glucose that is attached to blood hemoglobin. An HbA1c level of ≥6.5% (7, 133) tested on two separate occasions indicates a diabetic condition, but not a distinction between type 1 and type 2 diabetes (191). If the individual is pregnant, however, an HbA1c test does not provide accurate results.

Key Point

An HbA1c test is a valuable test for type 1 diabetes because it reveals the individual's average blood glucose level for the previous two to three months rather than just the blood glucose level at the time of the test.

Common Medications Given to Individuals With Type 1 Diabetes

Insulin is commonly administered using a needle and syringe, a cartridge, or a prefilled pen usually to the lower abdomen; or, alternatively, it can be inhaled or delivered via an insulin pump. Note that insulin cannot be delivered in pill form (210). The particular type of insulin that is prescribed is based on the degree and rate the individual needs to affect her blood glucose levels (6, 211):

- Rapid-acting insulin reduces glucose levels within 15 minutes, but the effect lasts only for several hours.
- Short- (or regular-) acting insulin requires about 30 minutes before becoming effective but continues for 3 to 6 hours.
- Intermediate-acting insulin does not reduce blood glucose levels until 2 to 4 hours after administration, but it is effective for up to 18 hours.
- Long-acting insulin takes several hours to begin affecting glucose levels, and it keeps levels relatively even for 24 hours.

Inhaled insulin (Afrezza) is delivered as a fine powder using an air-propelled inhaler or nebulizer to the individual's lungs where it crosses the alveolar–capillary barrier to enter the bloodstream. At the time of this publication, Afrezza had received mixed responses from physicians and patients, however (22). An insulin pump continuously administers rapid- or short-acting versions of insulin through a catheter that is placed under the skin. If the wearer needs additional insulin, it can be administered manually (i.e., a bolus dose).

Medications table 4.3 near the end of the chapter lists the common medications used for type 1 diabetes.

Key Point

Insulin is categorized into four types (rapid-, short-, intermediate-, or long-acting) based on the length of the delay before the effects of the drug kick in and on the duration over which it regulates the individual's blood glucose level.

Effects of Exercise in Individuals With Type 1 Diabetes

Multiple studies have cited the positive effects of exercise on individuals with type 1 diabetes including reduced HbA1c levels (178, 221), improved body composition (26, 114, 152, 169), reduced high blood pressure and elevated blood lipid levels (26, 114, 152), and decreased mortality rates (112, 143). Despite its benefits, exercise can also cause hypoglycemia during (79, 84, 126, 168, 200, 201) or after the session or hours later during sleep (**nocturnal hypoglycemia**) (125, 126, 200).

Although these glucose-lowering effects of exercise are logical responses due to the pathophysiology of type 1 diabetes, not all exercise causes a hypoglycemic reaction. Several studies (194, 200) reported that only moderate-intensity exercise (40% to <60% $\dot{V}O_2$ or heart rate reserve) resulted in lower blood glucose levels during or after exercise while high-intensity interval training (HIIT) caused a postexercise increase in blood glucose or at least less of a decrease (13, 55, 79, 80, 90, 197). Further, HIIT has been shown to lower the incidence of nocturnal hypoglycemia (90, 195) but not in all studies (126).

Most of the studies that examined the effects of exercise on type 1 diabetes were based on the subjects performing aerobic exercise. The effects of resistance training on blood glucose levels are less certain (197), but research has shown that it can contribute to reducing the incidence of exercise-induced hypoglycemia (224).

Key Point

Exercise can cause hypoglycemia during or after a workout, or hours later when the individual is sleeping. The manifestation or the extent of low blood glucose can depend on the type and intensity of the exercise session.

Exercise Recommendations for Clients With Type 1 Diabetes

The guidelines for designing an exercise program for a client with type 2 diabetes who is taking insulin are also appropriate for a client with type 1 diabetes (37, 92). The goal is 150 minutes a week of moderate- to vigorous-intensity aerobic exercise attained via three or more weekly sessions, two or three nonconsecutive days a week of resistance training, and two or three days a week of flexibility and balance training (37). See table 4.6 for general exercise guidelines that are specific to type 1 diabetes.

Table 4.6 General Exercise Guidelines for Clients With Type 1 Diabetes

Component	Type	Frequency	Intensity	Volume
Aerobic exercise training	Large muscle groups and rhythmical movements (e.g., walking, jogging, biking, swimming, stair stepping)	3-7 days per week (with ≤2 days between training days)	Moderate (40% to <60% $\dot{V}O_2$ or heart rate reserve) to vigorous (≥60%-90% $\dot{V}O_2$ or heart rate reserve)	≥10 min (per session); goal is ≥150 min (per week)
Resistance training	All types of exercises qualify; an emphasis on larger muscle groups is ideal	2-3 nonconsecutive days per week	At least 8-10 exercises; 1-3 sets; 6-15 RM loads	20-30 min (depending on the number of exercises and sets)
Flexibility training	Static and dynamic stretching; yoga	2-3 days per week	To the point of tightness; repeat 2-4 times	Hold a static stretch for 10-30 s; repeat a dynamic stretch for 10-30 s
Balance training	Single-leg stands; tai chi; yoga	2-3 days per week	Light to moderate	Any duration

Reference: (37)

Exercise Modifications, Precautions, and Contraindications for Clients With Type 1 Diabetes

One of the goals regarding exercise and type 1 diabetes is to effectively balance the amount and timing of insulin administration with preexercise food (carbohydrate) intake and the type, duration, and intensity of the exercise session. During- or postexercise hypoglycemia can be avoided or mediated by increasing the time between the preexercise insulin administration and the beginning of the exercise session, reducing the amount of preexercise insulin, increasing the amount of carbohydrate consumed before exercising, lowering the amount of postexercise insulin, or a combination of these tactics (30, 72, 80, 92, 194).

The decision about how much (if any) carbohydrate to eat before exercise is based on preexercise blood glucose levels and the parameters of the upcoming session (37, 225):

- If preexercise glucose levels are under 100 mg/dl, consume 15 to 30 g of carbohydrate unless the duration of the session will be less than 30 minutes or at a very high intensity (no extra carbohydrate is needed) or if the session will be long (consume 0.5-1 g of carbohydrate per kilogram of body weight per hour).

- Preexercise glucose levels between 90 and 150 mg/dl commonly necessitate carbohydrate to be ingested from the beginning of the session and throughout the session at a rate of 0.5 to 1 g of carbohydrate per kilogram of body weight per hour.

- If preexercise glucose levels are between 90 and 150 mg/dl, delay consuming carbohydrate until levels fall under 150 mg/dl.

- Preexercise glucose levels between 250 and 350 mg/dl require a ketone test; if moderate to large amounts exist, exercise should not be performed. If ketones are low, light- to moderate-intensity exercise is acceptable, but wait until levels are under 250 mg/dl before performing high-intensity exercise.

- If preexercise glucose levels are over 350 mg/dl, measure ketones and delay the session if they are moderate to high. If ketones are negative or at trace levels, administer an appropriate insulin correction per the orders of the client's health care professional. If ketones are in an acceptable range, mild- to moderate-intensity exercise can begin, but the intensity should not be high until glucose levels are under 250 mg/dl.

In addition to checking blood glucose levels before exercise, it is also important to frequently check levels during the exercise session and consume carbohydrate and adjust insulin administration as needed. Further, if the client is taking certain medications in addition to insulin (see medications table 4.3 near the end of the chapter), it may be necessary to adjust the type, timing, and amount of insulin in light of an upcoming exercise session, as some of those medications can increase the incidence of exercise-induced hypoglycemia.

Key Point

A client who has type 1 diabetes should always check his blood glucose level before exercise to determine how to modify carbohydrate intake and insulin administration. It some instances, the individual may need to test for ketones, delay the start of the exercise session, or both.

Case Study

Type 1 Diabetes

Mr. M, 33 years old, has had type 1 diabetes since he was a child. He has a sedentary job and an inactive lifestyle, and as a result he has gained about 10 to 15 pounds (4.5-6.8 kg) every year since graduating from college (at that time, he weighed 180 pounds [81.6 kg]). He recently decided to hire an exercise professional to improve his body composition with the hope that, by losing weight and becoming more active, he could reduce the amount of insulin he has to take each day.

After Mr. M was cleared to exercise, the exercise professional performed an initial assessment battery consisting of the YMCA step test, 1RM bench press test, 1RM leg press test, and sit-and-reach test. The results revealed that Mr. M's cardiovascular endurance was "poor"; his upper and lower body strength was within the 20th percentile, and his low back and hip joint flexibility was "fair." After discussing the results with Mr. M, the exercise professional designed a beginning exercise program that included walking, resistance training, and flexibility exercises. The table shows the specific exercise guidelines for Mr. M.

Component	Aerobic exercise training	Resistance training	Flexibility training
Type*	Walking	• Bodyweight squat • Bodyweight lunge • Incline push-up • One-arm dumbbell row • Lateral shoulder raise • Hammer curl • Triceps pushdown • Abdominal crunch	• Spinal twist static stretch • Forward lunge static stretch • Side quadriceps static stretch • Sitting toe touch static stretch • Straight arms behind back static stretch • Cross arm in front of chest static stretch • Behind-neck static stretch
Frequency	3 days per week (Monday, Wednesday, Friday)	2 days per week (Tuesday and Saturday)	3 days per week (after walking)
Intensity	40% to <60% $\dot{V}O_2$max (or 40% to <60% heart rate reserve; will need to first measure resting heart rate)	2 sets of 12-15 repetitions	Stretch to the point of tightness; repeat each stretch twice
Volume	15 min	~20 min	Hold each static stretch for 10 s

*For a description of the exercises, consult NSCA's Essentials of Personal Training, 2nd ed., Coburn, JW, Malek, MH, eds. Champaign, IL: Human Kinetics, 2012, and Essentials of Strength Training and Conditioning, 4th ed., Haff, GG, and Triplett, NT, eds. Champaign, IL: Human Kinetics, 2016.

Recommended Readings

American Diabetes Association. Diagnosis and classification of diabetes mellitus. *Diabetes Care* 35:S64-S71, 2012.

Centers for Disease Control and Prevention. *National Diabetes Statistics Report: Estimates of Diabetes and Its Burden in the United States.* Atlanta: U.S. Department of Health and Human Services, 2014.

Colberg, SR, Sigal, RJ, Yardley, JE, Riddell, MC, Dunstan, DW, Dempsey, PC, Horton, ES, Castorino, K, and Tate, DF. Physical activity/exercise and diabetes: a position statement of the American Diabetes Association. *Diabetes Care* 39:2065-2079, 2016.

Mayo Clinic. Diseases and conditions: type 1 diabetes. www.mayoclinic.org/diseases-conditions/type-1-diabetes/basics/tests-diagnosis/con-20019573. Accessed December 21, 2016.

Tonoli, C, Heyman, E, Roelands, B, Buyse, L, Cheung, SS, Berthoin, S, and Meeusen, R. Effects of different types of acute and chronic (training) exercise on glycaemic control in type 1 diabetes mellitus. *Sports Med* 42:1059-1080, 2012.

DYSLIPIDEMIA

Dyslipidemia continues to be a growing health problem in the United States and around the world. Although genetics plays a role in the development of dyslipidemia, lifestyle factors such as diet, body weight and percent body fat, tobacco use, and exercise or physical activity levels affect the management and prevention of dyslipidemia.

Epidemiology and Pathophysiology of Dyslipidemia

Dyslipidemia refers to abnormal blood lipoprotein concentrations and is a major risk factor for atherosclerosis, heart attack, and stroke. Dyslipidemia exists when there is an elevated blood level of low-density lipoproteins, elevated serum triglyceride concentrations, or an abnormally low level of high-density lipoproteins. Excess cholesterol, particularly oxidized low-density lipoproteins (LDLs), becomes trapped within the **intima** (the inner lining of arteries) and eventually builds to the point that the lumen is narrowed and blood flow is impaired. The definitions of key blood lipids include the following:

- Total cholesterol (TC): This represents the total serum or plasma cholesterol.

- Triglycerides (TGs): These are lipids that are carried in the bloodstream to tissues. Most of the body's fat stores are in the form of TGs. Triglycerides are found also in muscle and are used for energy. High levels are independently associated with high risk for atherosclerosis.

- Chylomicrons (CMs): A chylomicron is a small fat globule composed of protein and lipid (fat). Chylomicrons are found in blood and lymphatic fluids where they serve to transport fat from the intestine to the liver and adipose tissue. High levels contribute to atherosclerosis.

- Very low density lipoproteins (VLDLs): These are lipoproteins produced in the liver and found in the bloodstream. They are the major carriers of TGs in the bloodstream.

High levels are associated with greater risk for atherosclerosis.

- Low-density lipoproteins (LDLs): These are manufactured by the catabolism of VLDLs in the bloodstream. Low-density lipoproteins are the primary carrier of cholesterol in the bloodstream (approximately 70% of all serum cholesterol). Intermediate-density lipoproteins or IDLs are a subfraction of LDLs. Low-density lipoproteins are commonly known as "bad cholesterol" because they are the major contributor to the development and progression of atherosclerosis. There are seven different fractions of LDL based on particle size, with the smaller, more dense LDLs being more **atherogenic** (facilitating the development of atherosclerosis and its progression).

- High-density lipoproteins (HDLs): These are composed of a high proportion of protein with little TG and cholesterol. High-density lipoproteins are involved in **reverse cholesterol transport**, which returns blood cholesterol to the liver and is protective against atherosclerosis. High-density lipoproteins are commonly referred to as "good cholesterol" and appear in two major subfractions: HDL2 and HDL3; HDL2 is a lipoprotein subfraction that is protective against atherosclerosis.

There are five primary blood lipid classifications as provided by the National Cholesterol Education Program; see table 4.7 for a summary.

In 2011-2012, 12.9% of U.S. citizens age 20 years and older had TC levels of >240 mg/dl, and 38.6% (non-Hispanic black men) to 48.1% (Mexican American men) of those over 20 years of age had a level of 200 to 240 mg/dl (27, 75). Among persons 20 years of age and older, 33.1% of white men and 12.4% of white women had HDLs less than 40 mg/dl (75). Among African Americans, 20.3% of men and 10.2% of women, and among Hispanic Americans, 34.2% of men and 15.1% of women, had HDLs below 40 mg/dl. Triglycerides have been shown (67, 74) to independently predict risk of CVD events. Over 10 years in the Framingham Heart Study (89), TGs decreased from a mean of 144.5 to 134.1 mg/dl in men and 122.3 to 112.4 mg/dl in women. Persons with the least increase in BMI had the most favorable improvements in HDLs and TGs.

Table 4.7   Lipid Guidelines Based on the National Cholesterol Education Program

Lipid component	Optimal (very low risk)	Near optimal, above optimal, desirable, or normal	Borderline high	High (high risk)	Very high
Total cholesterol (mg/dl)	<150	<200	200-239	240+	
LDLs (mg/dl)	<100	100-129	130-159	160-189	190+
HDLs (mg/dl)	≥60			<40	
Triglycerides (mg/dl)	<100	<150	150-199	200-499	500+

Reference: (146)

Of particular interest is the level of postprandial TGs in response to a high-fat Western-like meal (table 4.2 compares a Western with a prudent diet). Studies (16, 151) show that abnormal blood levels of postprandial lipids, particularly TGs, are a stronger predictor of atherosclerosis risk than fasting levels. (See Libby [120] for a description and discussion of development and progression of atherosclerosis.)

Common Medications Given to Individuals With Dyslipidemia

Medications table 4.4 near the end of the chapter lists common medications used in the management of abnormal lipids. Severe forms of dyslipidemia are usually caused by genetic defects such as familial hypercholesterolemia, which is due to a reduction in liver LDL receptors. Hypothyroidism can cause elevated LDLs, and insulin resistance or type 2 diabetes can cause high blood concentrations of TGs and low concentrations of HDLs.

Effects of Lifestyle Management and Exercise in Individuals With Dyslipidemia

Exercise, diet, and weight loss are powerful tools in the prevention and management of dyslipidemia. General nutrition tips for improving blood lipids include the following (202):

- Lose body fat (if needed) through a hypocaloric diet and exercise.
- Consume less than 7% of calories from saturated fat and little or no trans fat each day.
- Consume no more than 20% to 30% of daily calories from fat sources and limit mono- or polyunsaturated fat to 13% to 23% of daily calories.
- Consume no more than 200 mg of cholesterol per day (44, 93).
- Consume 0.25 cup (25 g) of berries (e.g., blueberries, strawberries) per day.
- Consume two or three fish meals (e.g., salmon, tuna, mackerel, sardines, trout) per week.
- Consume 25 g of soy protein per day.
- Consume 0.25 cup (31 g) of nuts (e.g., walnuts, almonds, pecans, pistachios) per day.
- Consume 0.5 to 1 cup (100-200 g) of cooked beans and legumes (e.g., black, pinto, garbanzo, lima, navy) four or more days per week.
- Consume 15 to 20 g of soluble fiber per day and 35 to 45 g of total fiber per day.
- Consume whole-grain products (e.g., oats, barley, brown rice, quinoa, bulgur, whole wheat).
- Limit sugars to no more than 5% of calories (or 20-40 g) per day.
- Limit all processed foods.
- Limit alcohol to one or two drinks per day for men and one drink per day for women.

Aerobic exercise, low saturated and trans fat, and a high-fiber diet coupled with body-fat loss have been documented to decrease TGs and LDLs and increase HDLs (186). For example, an acute bout of aerobic exercise at 60% to 85% of $\dot{V}O_2$max for 30 to 45 minutes lowers TGs and raises HDLs (186, 196). Further, cross-sectional studies have reported an inverse relationship between TGs and

LDLs and a positive relationship between HDLs and weekly volume of aerobic exercise (214, 215). Randomized studies have also shown that chronic aerobic exercise at a level of more than 1,200 kcal per week results in a sustained decrease of TGs and increase in HDL (183, 217). Paoli and colleagues (163) also found that high-intensity circuit training (three days per week for 50 minutes each session) that included resistance training was more effective in improving blood pressure, lipoproteins, and TGs than either lower-intensity circuit training or aerobic endurance training. In conjunction, the breakdown of TGs is increased during exercise and continues to be elevated in the recovery period. However, blood lipid responses among persons engaging in aerobic exercise is variable, suggesting a possible genetic influence (216).

Key Point

Lifestyle changes can improve dyslipidemia. This includes a low-fat diet, weight loss (if needed), and exercise (primarily aerobic exercise).

In any case, the effects of exercise on postprandial lipids appear to show that those who exercise regularly have a lessened increase of TGs in response to a high-fat meal (186, 196). In addition, randomized studies show that exercise training results in an improved postprandial lipid response to a high-fat meal (186, 196). Some studies found that accumulated bouts of exercise were effective in reducing postprandial lipids (3, 140). Trombold and colleagues (199) recently demonstrated that iso-energetic high-intensity aerobic exercise (alternating 2 minutes at 25% and 2 minutes at 90% $\dot{V}O_2$peak) was more effective than

moderate-intensity aerobic exercise (60 minutes at 50% $\dot{V}O_2$peak) for lowering postprandial lipids. A few studies support improved postprandial lipid levels in response to a systematic resistance training program (11, 186). The favorable effects of exercise training on postprandial lipids are most apparent when the exercise is performed 8 to 12 hours before consumption of a high-fat meal (226).

Exercise Recommendations for Clients With Dyslipidemia

The mechanism for the benefit of exercise is thought to be an increased activity of the catalytic enzyme, lipoprotein lipase, that peaks between 8 and 12 hours after a moderate to vigorous exercise bout (186, 196, 226). This finding illustrates a subacute beneficial effect of exercise and emphasizes the importance of daily physical activity. Other studies reported that the effects of accumulated (i.e., three 10-minute bouts interrupted by 20-minute recovery periods) versus continuous bouts (30 minutes, once per day) of exercise at equivalent intensities on postprandial lipids were similar (3, 144). Although the evidence is inconclusive, it appears that clients with dyslipidemia exercising at equal intensities and caloric expenditure may improve TGs and HDLs similarly following 4 to 12 weeks of either accumulated or continuous bouts. However, in these studies, subjects did 10-minute exercise bouts interrupted by 20 minutes of rest for three bouts versus 30 minutes continuously at 50% to 70% of $\dot{V}O_2$max. This is a total session time of 70 minutes, which is more time-consuming than a single 30-minute bout. Table 4.8 summarizes exercise guidelines for clients with dyslipidemia.

Table 4.8   General Exercise Guidelines for Clients With Dyslipidemia

Component	Type	Frequency	Intensity	Volume (per session)
Aerobic exercise training	Large muscle groups and rhythmical movements (e.g., walking, jogging, biking, swimming, stair stepping)	1-4 sessions per day; 4-7 days per week	40-85% heart rate reserve; 12-16 RPE	15-60 min
Resistance training	8-12 exercises preferably that train large muscle groups	2-3 days per week	50-85% 1RM	20-40 min
Flexibility training	12-16 static stretches that stretch all major muscle groups	3-7 days per week	Static stretch (to point of moderate tension), holding for 10-30 s; repeat 2-3 times	20-30 min

References: (56, 147, 166)

Exercise Modifications, Precautions, and Contraindications for Clients With Dyslipidemia

Clients with dyslipidemia may be on medications called **statins** such as Lipitor, Crestor, Zocor, Pravachol, Advicor, Mevacor, or Altacor (see medications table 4.4) that may cause muscle damage or muscle pain (**myalgias**) (70, 164). Ganga and colleagues (70) reported that in clinical practice, approximately 10% to 25% of clients treated with a statin experienced muscle problems. Krishman and Thompson (111) reported that muscle strength was diminished among persons being treated for dyslipidemia with a statin. It appears that resistance training or weight-bearing exercise while one is taking a statin may result in more myalgias and delayed-onset muscle soreness. A study of 37 subjects randomized to aerobic exercise only (19 subjects) or aerobic exercise plus 40 mg per day of simvastatin (18 subjects) showed that after 12 weeks of training, the addition of simvastatin reduced the increase in maximal oxygen uptake and skeletal muscle citrate synthase activity (138). Maximal oxygen uptake increased 10% in the exercise-only group but only 1.5% in the combination group (138). The exercise professional needs to be alert to any unusual lingering muscle soreness and consider referral to a physician or other health care professional. When starting an exercise program, it would be wise to begin at a low level of intensity (both aerobic and resistance training) and progress gradually to reduce risk of muscle damage or soreness.

Key Point

If a client is taking a statin, it is important to monitor for muscle soreness or pain. Exercise can worsen the muscle soreness or pain, which can be a side effect from statins.

Clients with dyslipidemia may have secondary conditions such as CVD, type 2 diabetes, or hypertension, and as a result will need medical clearance before exercise. It is important for the exercise professional to emphasize that comprehensive lifestyle change including weight loss, a healthy diet low in saturated and trans fat and high in fiber, and regular aerobic and resistance exercise is the most effective strategy to improve dyslipidemia.

Case Study

Dyslipidemia

Mr. B, who is 55 years old and has dyslipidemia, was referred to an exercise professional for lifestyle management. Mr. B had been on three cholesterol-lowering drugs and experienced significant myalgia of his shoulder and neck musculature and frequent headaches. The myalgia seemed to be aggravated when he attempted to increase his exercise volume or intensity, and he experienced considerable delayed-onset muscle soreness 36 to 48 hours after a vigorous exercise session. His physician placed him on Etia, a cholesterol-lowering medication that blocks cholesterol absorption. He does not have hypertension or type 2 diabetes and does not smoke.

The goal of his exercise program was to promote weight loss, as this would likely reduce his TC, LDL, and TG levels. A balance of aerobic exercise and resistance training would be performed, with an emphasis on the aerobic component.

After medical clearance was obtained, a metabolic exercise test was administered with a body composition analysis. Mr. B was prescribed to walk or jog every other day for 30 to 45 minutes at a target heart rate zone of 120 to 138 beats/min. Two or three days per week, he did a combined aerobic and resistance circuit for 45 to 50 minutes per session (20 minutes of aerobic exercise and 25 to 30 minutes of resistance training composed of 10 to 12 exercises at 60% to 80% of 1RM, one or two sets per exercise). His diet was low calorie, low fat, low in processed carbohydrate, and high

(continued)

Dyslipidemia *(continued)*

in fiber. After five to six months of training, Mr. B was jogging 3 or 4 miles (5-6 km) three days per week for 30 to 40 minutes per session.

He also progressed on the circuit, increasing loads by 40% to 50%. The table summarizes the improvements he made in several areas.

Test or measurement	Pre	Post
Maximal oxygen uptake (ml · kg^{-1} · min^{-1})	32.9	36.5
Body weight	219 lb (99 kg)	209 lb (95 kg)
Body fat (%)	26.8	23.2
Fat weight	58.6 lb (27 kg)	48.5 lb (22 kg)
Fat-free weight	160.4 lb (73 kg)	160.5 lb (73 kg)
Total cholesterol (mg/dl)	226	188
Triglycerides (mg/dl)	168	67
LDLs (mg/dl)	166	131
HDLs (mg/dl)	26	44

Recommended Readings

Carroll, MD, Kit, BK, Lacher, DA, and Sung, S. Total and high-density lipoprotein cholesterol in adults: NHANES, 2011-2012. NCHS Data Brief No. 132:1-8, 2013.

Ingelsson, E, Massaro, JM, Sutherland, P, Jacques, PF, Levy, D, D'Agostino, RB, Vasan, RS, and Robins, SJ. Contemporary trends in dyslipidemia in the Framingham Heart Study. *Arch Int Med* 169:279-286, 2009.

Mann, S, Beedie, C, and Jimenez, A. Differential effects of aerobic exercise, resistance training and combined exercise modalities on cholesterol and the lipid profile: review, synthesis and recommendations. *Sports Med* 44:211-221, 2014.

National Cholesterol Education Program. Third report of the National Cholesterol Education Program (NCEP) Expert Panel on Detection, Evaluation, and Treatment of High Blood Cholesterol in Adults (Adult Treatment Panel III) Final Report. *Circulation* 106:3143-3421, 2002.

Stone, NJ, Robinson, JG, Lichtenstein, AH, Merz, CNB, Blum, CB, Eckel, RH, Goldberg, AC, Gordon, D, Levy, D, Lloyd-Jones, DM, and McBride, P. 2013 ACC/AHA guideline on the treatment of blood cholesterol to reduce atherosclerotic cardiovascular risk in adults: a report of the American College of Cardiology/American Heart Association Task Force on Practice Guidelines. *J Am Coll Cardiol* 63:2889-2934, 2014.

HYPOTHYROIDISM AND HYPERTHYROIDISM

In hypothyroidism, or underactive thyroid, the thyroid gland does not make enough thyroid hormone to meet the body's needs. With hyperthyroidism, or overactive thyroid, the thyroid gland makes more than the body requires. Both conditions affect one's health in a number of ways. This, plus a number of medications that may be taken to treat the condition, needs to be considered when one is developing an exercise program.

Epidemiology and Pathophysiology of Hypothyroidism

Hypothyroidism is a condition in which the thyroid gland (located in the anterior neck region) does not produce enough of the hormone thyroxine. The signs and symptoms of an underactive thyroid include fatigue, cold intolerance, dry skin, unexplained weight gain, puffy face, hoarseness, muscle aches and weakness, elevated blood cholesterol, stiff and painful joints, loss of bone mineral density, hair loss, depression, slowed heart rate, and impaired memory (18). If hypothyroidism is untreated it can lead to **goiter** (enlarged thyroid gland) or **myxedema** (swelling of the skin and underlying tissues), which can be fatal.

Causes of hypothyroidism include iodine deficiency, autoimmune disease (Hashimoto's thyroiditis), and partial or total removal of the thyroid gland (29). Stress and a diet high in simple, processed carbohydrate and saturated and trans fat may contribute to hypothyroidism (107). The prevalence of hypothyroidism is estimated to be 3% of U.S. women, while subclinical hypothyroidism is thought to have a prevalence of 7% to 10% worldwide (108). Hypothyroidism is seven times more prevalent in women than in men (139). **Subclinical hypothyroidism** is characterized by low serum thyroid-stimulating hormone in the presence of normal levels of triiodothyronine and thyroxine (43). Subclinical hypothyroidism prevalence increases with age and is associated with an increased risk of cardiovascular complications such as atrial fibrillation and cardiovascular mortality (108).

Epidemiology and Pathophysiology of Hyperthyroidism

Hyperthyroidism, also called overactive thyroid, is a condition in which the thyroid gland produces and secretes excessive amounts of free (not bound to a protein) triiodothyronine or thyroxine (198). Graves' disease is the most common cause of hyperthyroidism.

Hyperthyroidism also can result from inflammation of the thyroid gland (thyroiditis) or from taking too much thyroid medication. In these cases, thyrotoxicosis can occur; even though the thyroid gland itself is not necessarily overactive, there is still too much thyroid hormone in the blood. The long-term effects of untreated thyrotoxicosis can lead to serious medical complications such as heart rhythm disturbances and osteoporosis (108).

Thyroid hormone is the main regulator of metabolism. If there is too much thyroid hormone, many functions of the body speed up with the resulting symptoms of nervousness, irritability, increased perspiration, tachycardia, tremors, anxiety, difficulty sleeping, heat intolerance, and muscular weakness (18). Further, weight loss often occurs in spite of a good appetite.

The National Health and Nutrition Examination Survey III assessed thyroid status in a randomly selected group in the United States (87) and reported that hyperthyroidism was prevalent in 1.2% of the selected group. Interestingly, 0.7% of this 1.2% were found to have subclinical hyperthyroidism with no clinical manifestation of the disease. Hyperthyroidism is approximately four to five times more prevalent among women than among men (115).

Cardiometabolic Effects of Hypo- and Hyperthyroidism

Thyroid hormone at **euthyroid** (normal thyroid) levels promotes decreased systemic vascular resistance, increased resting heart rate, greater left ventricular contractility, and increased blood volume. Thyroid hormone also activates **renin-angiotensin-aldosterone** (hormones produced in the kidneys, arteries, and adrenal glands), which results in increased sodium absorption (108). As a result of these and other effects of thyroid hormone, there is an increase in preload of the ventricles and increased cardiac contractility.

In hyperthyroidism, these effects are accentuated, and cardiac output can be 50% to 300% greater than normal (62). In hypothyroidism, the cardiovascular effects are diametrically opposite and cardiac output may decrease by 30% to

50% (108). Hyperthyroidism typically causes a decrease in diastolic blood pressure whereas hypothyroidism often causes an increase in diastolic blood pressure. One other important manifestation of untreated thyroid disease is that hyperthyroidism can cause a tachycardia whereas hypothyroidism may cause a bradycardia. Finally, of importance to exercise professionals is that hypothyroidism and hyperthyroidism can cause atrial fibrillation and chest pain and that hypothyroidism is frequently associated with an increase in premature ventricular contractions (108). The exercise professional must be alert to these abnormal cardiovascular effects, which can occur in individuals who have under- or overtreated hypothyroidism or hyperthyroidism.

Another sign of hypothyroidism is an elevation in TC and LDL levels (108). When hormones produced by the thyroid gland are low, the body does not break down and remove LDLs as efficiently as usual. As a result, an individual with hypothyroidism may be taking a cholesterol-lowering medication (see section on dyslipidemia). Both hypothyroidism and hyperthyroidism are associated with a reduced exercise capacity. Subclinical hypothyroidism also is associated with several cardiorespiratory and metabolic abnormalities that result in impaired exercise capacity (102, 103, 136). Table 4.9 summarizes some negative effects of hypothyroidism and hyperthyroidism on muscle metabolism and exercise capacity.

Common Medications and Treatment Given to Individuals With Hypo- and Hyperthyroidism

Treatment for hypothyroidism involves thyroid replacement therapy; the type of hormone administered is commonly a synthetic version of thyroxine such as levothyroxine. Because thyroxine affects almost all of the systems in the body, thyroid replacement therapy can cause a wide range of side effects on heart function, nervous system activity, muscle control, and overall metabolism (182). Therefore, thyroid replacement medication effects on submaximal and maximal exercise include tachycardia and elevated blood pressure (182).

The goal for treatment of hyperthyroidism is to relieve the effects of thyrotoxicosis (108). Antithyroid drugs such as propylthiouracil (PTU) and methimazole are effective because they inhibit thyroid hormone synthesis in the thyroid gland (182). Care must be taken, as antithyroid drugs can cause thyroxine levels to swing to hypothyroidism. Commonly, individuals start out with a higher dose and then adjust until euthyroidism is achieved.

Thyrotoxicosis causes an increase in the number of catecholamine receptors, so β-blockers are sometimes prescribed to reduce catecholamine response. The resulting effect on exercise is a decreased exercise heart rate and blood pressure that necessitates using rating of RPE rather than a target heart rate as an indicator of exercise intensity.

Medications tables 4.5 and 4.6 near the end of the chapter summarize medical therapy for both conditions.

Effects of Exercise in Individuals With Hypo- and Hyperthyroidism

For individuals with hypothyroidism, exercise can help promote weight loss, reduce cholesterol levels, increase metabolic rate, reduce stress, and improve mood state. For hyperthyroidism, potential benefits from exercise include reduced stiffness in the joints and muscles, a positive impact on bone mineral density, and increased muscle tissue. The common exercise benefits (e.g., increased aerobic capacity, increased muscular strength) are also achieved in individuals with thyroid disease.

Key Point

Exercise guidelines for hyperthyroidism and hypothyroidism essentially follow the guidelines for apparently healthy persons, provided that the hormone replacement results in a euthyroid state. The exercise professional needs to know the signs and symptoms of thyroid disease and adjust the exercise program accordingly.

Exercise Recommendations for Clients With Hypo- and Hyperthyroidism

The main goal of therapy for hypothyroidism and hyperthyroidism is to establish a euthyroid state (normal thyroid hormone levels). The exercise professional needs to be alert to the signs and symptoms of hypothyroidism and hyperthyroidism (see earlier discussions) and refer clients to medical professionals if needed. Once a euthyroid state is established, exercise guidelines for apparently healthy individuals can be applied.

Table 4.10 presents general guidelines for clients with hypothyroidism and hyperthyroidism who have been successfully treated to a euthyroid state.

Table 4.9   Negative Effects of Hypothyroidism and Hyperthyroidism on Exercise Capacity

Parameter	Hypothyroidism	Hyperthyroidism
Exercise intolerance	Decreased due to insufficient skeletal muscle blood flow and decreased availability of oxygen and bloodborne substrates such as glucose and free fatty acids compared to euthyroid; impaired vasodilation	Increased heart rate at submaximal exercise intensity, increased reliance on muscle glycogen, and reduced heart rate reserve compared to euthyroid
Heart rate response	Depressed with exercise compared to euthyroid	Elevated with exercise compared to euthyroid; slow response to increasing workloads
Systolic blood pressure	Depressed with exercise compared to euthyroid	Elevated with exercise compared to euthyroid
1-min heart rate recovery	Slower than euthyroid	Slower than euthyroid
Anaerobic threshold	Reduced compared to euthyroid	Reduced compared to euthyroid
Respiratory stress (breathing frequency × tidal volume)	Increased breathing frequency compared to euthyroid	Increased breathing frequency and tidal volume compared to euthyroid
Contractility of heart	Reduced, but restored when euthyroid achieved	Hypercontractility restored when euthyroid achieved

References: (102, 103, 108, 136)

Table 4.10   General Exercise Guidelines for Clients With Hypothyroidism and Hyperthyroidism

Parameter	Guideline
Aerobic exercise frequency	Sedentary individuals should start with two or three 5- to 15-min bouts of aerobic activity with the goal of achieving a minimum of 5-6 days per week; 7 days per week if weight loss is needed
Aerobic exercise intensity	40-85% heart rate reserve
Aerobic exercise duration (per session)	Sedentary individuals should start with two 5- to 15-min bouts of aerobic activity within the day and progress to 30-60 min of continuous aerobic activity
Aerobic exercise duration (per week)	A minimum of 150 min of moderate intensity (40% to <60% heart rate reserve) or 75 min of vigorous intensity (≥60%-90% heart rate reserve) or a combination of both; goal is 300 min for additional benefits and if weight loss is needed
Aerobic exercise caloric expenditure	1,200 minimum per week; >2,000 per week for additional benefits or if weight loss is needed
Resistance training	2-3 days per week; 8-12 large-muscle multijoint exercises; 60-80% 1RM planned in a periodized manner over a 4- to 6-month period
Flexibility training	5-7 days per week; 8-12 exercises addressing all major joints; static or dynamic stretching (if static, hold each stretch for 20-30 s and do 2-3 repetitions per stretch)

References: (21, 76)

Recommended Readings

Baskin, HJ, Cobin, RH, Duick, DS, Gharib, H, Guttler, RB, Kaplan, MM, and Segal, RL. American Association of Clinical Endocrinologists medical guidelines for clinical practice for the evaluation and treatment of hyperthyroidism and hypothyroidism. *Endocr Pract* 8:457-469, 2001.

Chakera, AJ, Pearce, S, and Vaidya, B. Treatment for primary hypothyroidism: current approaches and future possibilities. *Drug Des Devel Ther* 6:1-11, 2012.

Hollowell, JG, Staehling, NW, Flanders, WD, Hannon, WH, Gunter, EW, Spencer, CA, and Braverman, LE. Serum TSH, T(4), and thyroid antibodies in the United States population (1988 to 1994): National Health and Nutrition Examination Survey (NHANES III). *J Clin Endocrinol Metab* 87:489-498, 2002.

Klein, E and Danzi, S. Thyroid disease and the heart. *Circulation* 116:1725-1755, 2007.

Larsen, PR, Kronenberg, HM, Melmed, S, and Polonsky, KS. *Williams' Textbook of Endocrinology.* 10th ed. Philadelphia: Saunders, 374-421, 2002.

CHRONIC KIDNEY DISEASE

Chronic kidney disease is a progressive, long-term disease of the kidneys. Chronic kidney disease is divided into five stages based on kidney **glomerular filtration rate** (the rate at which the nephrons filter the body's fluids) and the presence and extent of kidney damage (149). The stages of chronic kidney disease range from stage 1, in which glomerular filtration rate is normal (but some kidney damage is present), to stage 5, in which there is severely impaired filtration and the kidneys function at less than 75% of normal. All stage 5 individuals require dialysis and become candidates for renal transplant (end-stage renal disease or ESRD). The majority of individuals with chronic kidney disease have either diabetes, hypertension, or both (175).

Epidemiology and Pathophysiology of Chronic Kidney Disease

The kidneys are the filtration system for the body. All of the blood in the body circulates through the kidneys. They are designed to filter toxins, waste products, and other materials for elimination through urine. They also function to return fluid and other constituents of blood back to circulation as part of the filtering process. Renal microstructure is composed of millions of microscopic nephrons, which are the anatomical filtering structures. At the center of each nephron is the glomerulus, where filtering occurs. Simply put, blood is circulated through nephrons, which absorb waste products and return fluid and non-waste material back to circulation. The waste products and retained fluid are then transported to the bladder in the form of urine. Normal urine is composed primarily of water and the waste products filtered out by the nephrons.

Damage to the nephrons via high levels of glucose, blood pressure, inflammation, and other mechanisms impairs their ability to filter waste products. In this state, blood returning to the circulation has increasing concentrations of waste products. These waste products damage organs and tissues in the system and produce progressive damage to nephrons, further hindering their ability to work normally. The end result of this disease process is progressive renal dysfunction and general end-organ (e.g., heart and liver) damage and dysfunction.

The pathophysiology of many chronic diseases predisposes a person to develop renal dysfunction and eventually ESRD. Causative factors that lead to chronic kidney disease and ESRD (and their underlying pathophysiology) are similar to those for many other chronic diseases. Chronic systemic inflammation, vascular dysfunction, and insulin resistance are part of the kidney dysfunction that leads to chronic kidney disease and ESRD (175).

Approximately 13% of adults in the United States have chronic kidney disease defined as a glomerular filtration rate of less than 60 ml per minute, and 44% of persons over 65 years of age meet this criterion (170).

Exercise testing may not be necessary in these individuals because they are limited by muscle fatigue, and a test is often a barrier to participation in an exercise program (5). Testing, if undertaken, and exercise training for those with chronic kidney disease should be administered by trained medical professionals in a medical environment (159, 184). Research (158, 159) has shown that functional capacity in individuals with ESRD is 60% to 70% of the functional capacity of age- and sex-matched peers without ESRD and, with training, can be increased by about 17%. A review and meta-analysis of studies assessing exercise tolerance in individuals on dialysis treated with erythropoiesis-stimulating agents found a 23.8% increase in $\dot{V}O_2$peak after treatment (98). Most individuals with chronic kidney disease can exercise, and those with ESRD often can exercise while receiving dialysis treatment (95, 96, 141, 162, 177). Moore and colleagues (142) found that most, but not all, individuals with ESRD who train with stationary cycling during dialysis improve their $\dot{V}O_2$peak. In this study, individuals who improved $\dot{V}O_2$peak had an increased tissue oxygen extraction rate, suggesting that oxygen delivery is not always the limiting factor in individuals with ESRD. Painter and colleagues (160) also reported that exercise training after renal transplantation resulted in higher levels of measured $\dot{V}O_2$peak and self-reported physical functioning. The most common issue with exercise in this population is that the progressive nature of ESRD leads to increasing physical inactivity and very low levels of physical functioning (97), thus emphasizing the need for structured and individualized exercise programs in this population (95, 158, 184).

Key Point

The progressive nature of ESRD leads to decreased physical activity and very low levels of physical functioning. This population benefits from a structured, individualized exercise program to stave off inactivity.

Common Medications Given to Individuals With Chronic Kidney Disease

There is a long and complex list of medications used in ESRD; consult the medications tables provided in the sections on type 2 diabetes, dyslipidemia, and hypertension (chapter 6), as the majority of individuals with ESRD are on several of these medications. The use of pharmaceutical therapy in these individuals is primarily aimed at treating the signs and symptoms of the disease, the associated comorbidities (e.g., coronary heart disease, type 2 diabetes, hypertension, and dyslipidemia), and other conditions associated with the onset and progression of ESRD (101, 170).

Most commonly, these individuals are on a diuretic to prevent edema and fluid accumulation, an antihypertensive (if hypertension is present), and hypoglycemic drugs if type 2 diabetes is present. Many individuals with chronic kidney disease are treated for anemia (148), often with an erythropoietin-stimulating agent. The exercise professional must be knowledgeable and informed about these medications.

Key Point

An erythropoietin-stimulating agent, a drug used to treat anemia, is often administered to individuals with chronic kidney disease.

Effects of Exercise in Individuals With Chronic Kidney Disease

The effects of exercise in people with ESRD are similar to those in apparently healthy people. Exercise training has been successfully used in individuals with ESRD during dialysis (158). These studies demonstrate that cardiovascular endurance exercise does improve functional capacity in individuals on dialysis (94-96, 141, 158, 162). The effects of both aerobic and resistance training in people with ESRD appear to be similar to those in persons without chronic kidney disease or ESRD but somewhat moderated through unknown mechanisms. Increased functional capacity as measured by a 6-minute

Recommended Readings

Johansen, KL and Painter, P. Exercise in Individuals with CKD. *Am J Kidney Dis* 59:128-134, 2012.

Johnson, CA, Levey, AS, Coresh, J, Levin, AA, Lau, J, and Eknoyan, G. Clinical practice guidelines for chronic kidney disease in adults: part I. Definition, disease stages, evaluation, treatment, and risk factors. *Am Fam Physician* 70:869-876, 2004.

National Kidney Foundation. K/DOQU clinical practice guidelines for chronic kidney disease: evaluation, classification, and stratification. *Am J Kidney Dis* 39:S1-S266, 2002.

Saran, R, Li, Y, Robinson, B, Abbott, KC, Agodoa, LY, Ayanian, J, Bragg-Gresham, J, Balkrishnan, R, Chen, JL, Cope, E, and Eggers, PW. U.S. renal data system 2015: annual data report: epidemiology of kidney disease in the United States. *Am J Kidney Dis* 67:A7, 2016.

Smart, NA, Williams, AD, Levinger, I, Selig, S, Howden, E, Coombes, JB, and Fassett, RG. Exercise and Sports Science Australia (ESSA) position statement on exercise and chronic kidney disease. *J Sci Med Sport* 16:406-411, 2013.

walk test or other valid assessments of functional capacity has been demonstrated in individuals with ESRD (158). An increased ability to carry out activities of daily living, as well as increased overall physical activity and functioning, has been reported (158). Studies of resistance training in individuals with ESRD have demonstrated increased muscle strength as well as other anabolic effects (94, 99, 100).

Aerobic and resistance exercise have been shown to reduce cardiovascular risk factors, and studies have reported a variety of beneficial effects including reductions in oxidative stress, inflammation, and blood pressure in clients with chronic kidney disease or ESRD (94, 95, 100, 158, 161, 177, 184).

Exercise Recommendations for Clients With Chronic Kidney Disease

The exercise recommendations for clients with chronic kidney disease or ESRD are similar to those for older adults and the management of comorbidities such as diabetes and hypertension (94, 96, 99, 158). It is advised that these recommendations be considered in light of each client's functional capacity. Medical clearance should be obtained before exercise programming. The exercise program should include aerobic and resistance training (184) and flexibility exercises.

Exercise guidelines for clients with chronic kidney disease or ESRD include performing aerobic endurance training most or all days of the week at a moderate intensity of 40% to <60% heart rate reserve or 12 to 13 RPE. Clients should aim for 20 to 60 minutes of activity, whether intermittent or continuous, with an overall goal of 150 minutes of aerobic endurance activity per week, depending on the level of physical functioning. Caution is recommended for vigorous intensity exercise (5). Resistance training can be done two or three days a week, with one set of 10 to 15 repetitions per exercise at 70% to 75% 1RM (5).

CONCLUSION

A key point of this chapter is that chronic metabolic disorders such as obesity, type 2 diabetes mellitus, type 1 diabetes mellitus, and dyslipidemia are largely preventable and that it has been consistently shown that inclusion of regular exercise and a healthy diet can significantly reduce the risk of contracting these diseases. The role of exercise in the management and treatment of these common metabolic disorders has been demonstrated to be safe and effective. Exercise professionals can play a key role in the support of individuals with metabolic diseases; however, a thorough understanding of the signs and symptoms, associated medications, and response to exercise for individuals with metabolic diseases is necessary.

Key Terms

adipokines
atherogenic
autonomic neuropathy
dyslipidemia
euthyroid
glomerular filtration rate
goiter
hyperthyroidism
hypoglycemia
hypothyroidism
intima
ketoacidosis

myalgias
myxedema
nocturnal hypoglycemia
obesity
overweight
postprandial
renin-angiotensin-aldosterone
reverse cholesterol transport
silent ischemia
statins
subclinical hypothyroidism

Study Questions

1. Which of the following is considered to be the most essential behavior to prevent weight regain?

   a. 60 to 90 minutes a day of physical activity

   b. regular assessment of leptin levels in the blood

   c. 3 days per week of a comprehensive resistance training program

   d. restriction of the level of carbohydrate in the diet, especially simple sugars

2. Which of these lipid-related blood elements is properly defined?

   a. chylomicrons: the primary form of fat in the body

   b. triglycerides: most likely contributor to atherosclerosis

   c. low-density lipoproteins: primary carriers of blood cholesterol

   d. very low density lipoproteins: remove cholesterol from the blood vessel walls

3. Which of the following exercise limitations or symptoms is likely to be present in a hyperthyroid client?

   a. reduced heart contractility

   b. faster heart rate recovery

   c. higher heart rate but slower response to increase of intensity

   d. lower blood pressure but higher rate of respiration during exercise

4. Which of the following exercise parameters falls outside the recommended exercise prescription for individuals with chronic kidney disease?

   a. An RPE between 14 and 16 is recommended.

   b. Exercise should be done only following medical clearance.

   c. Aerobic exercise should be performed most days of the week.

   d. Clients should accumulate at least 150 minutes of aerobic exercise per week.

Medications Table 4.1 Common Medications Used to Treat Obesity

Drug names	Mechanism of action	Most common side effects	Effects on exercise
orlistat (Xenical, Alli)	Lipase inhibitors, block absorption and digestion of fatty acids	Stomach pain, gas, diarrhea, leakage of oily stools	Unknown cardiovascular and metabolic effects; gastric symptoms are common and may affect exercise
Combination drug consisting of phentermine and topiramate (Qsymia)	Acts as a serotonin receptor agonist; phentermine is a sympathomimetic and anorectic (depresses appetite), and topiramate is an anticonvulsant with weight loss side effects	Paresthesia, dizziness, dysgeusia (rancid taste sensation), insomnia, constipation, dry mouth, insomnia, GI disorders, anxiety, depression	Unknown cardiovascular and metabolic effects; may decrease resting or exercise heart rate or both; may increase risk of hypoglycemia in persons with type 2 diabetes
lorcaserin (Belviq)	Exact mechanism of action not known; believed to decrease food consumption and promote satiety by selectively activating serotonin receptors in the brain (activation of these receptors may help a person eat less and feel full after eating smaller amounts of food)	Headache, dizziness, generalized GI symptoms including diarrhea and constipation; Caution: drug interactions include selective serotonin reuptake inhibitors (SSRIs), monoamine oxidase inhibitors (MAOIs), bupropion, and some botanical supplements	Unknown cardiovascular and metabolic effects; may decrease resting or exercise heart rate or both; may increase risk of hypoglycemia in persons with type 2 diabetes
Extended-release form of naltrexone and bupropion (Contrave)	Bupropion is an antidepressant medication that may decrease appetite; naltrexone may also curb hunger and food cravings	Suicidal thoughts, seizure risk, and added effects with alcohol; Caution: do not drink alcohol with Contrave	Increased resting heart rate and blood pressure (therefore may cause an abnormal heart rate and blood pressure response to exercise)

References: (23, 53, 132, 153)

Medications Table 4.2 Common Medications Used to Treat Type 2 Diabetes

Drug class and names	Mechanism of action	Most common side effects	Effects on exercise
insulin (Humulin, Novolin, Lantus); includes rapid-acting (Humalog, Humulin R, Novolin R), rapid- and intermediate-acting combination (Humalog 50/50, Humalog 70/30, Novolin 70/30), and long-acting (Humulin U, Lantus, Levemir) forms	Replaces the insulin normally produced by beta cells of the pancreas; both human and animal forms of the hormone are used	Pain, redness, swelling or itching at the injection site; hypoglycemia and resulting symptoms may occur; other less common side effects include allergic reactions and hypokalemia	Increases release of injected insulin if the injection is given in active skeletal muscle; increases uptake of glucose from arterial blood (which can cause hypoglycemia); Note: exercise decreases insulin resistance

Oral hypoglycemic drugs come in many different forms and have many different effects. The following is a sample of several classes.

Sulfonylureas

glipizide (Glucotrol) glimepiride (Amaryl), glyburide (Diabeta, Glynase)	Stimulate the beta cells to produce and release more insulin (many drugs are fast-acting)	Hypoglycemia, weight gain, nausea, skin rash	Increased risk of hypoglycemia; Note: need to monitor pre- and postexercise blood glucose levels until response to exercise is predictable

Dipeptidyl peptidase-4 (DPP-4) inhibitors

saxagliptin (Onglyza), sitagliptin (Januvia), alogliptin (Nesina), linagliptin (Tradjenta)	Stimulate the release of insulin by preventing breakdown of glucagon-like peptide 1 (GLP-1) and inhibit the release of glucose from the liver	Upper respiratory tract infection, sore throat, headache; inflammation of the pancreas (from sitagliptin)	Very little information on interactions with exercise; Caution: possible increased risk of hypoglycemia due to exercise

Biguanides

metformin (Fortamet, Glucophage, others)	Inhibit gluconeogenesis and the release of glucose from the liver, improve insulin sensitivity, may promote modest weight loss and modest decline in LDLs	Nausea, diarrhea, lactic acidosis (rarely)	May increase exercise heart rate response to submaximal exercise and interfere with the glucose-lowering action of the drug

Thiazolidinediones

rosiglitazone (Avandia), pioglitazone (Actos)	Improve insulin receptor sensitivity to insulin in muscle, liver, and adipocytes; inhibit the release of glucose from the liver; may slightly increase HDLs	Heart failure, heart attack, stroke, liver disease	May improve exercise capacity; Caution: possible increased risk of hypoglycemia due to exercise

Alpha-glucosidase inhibitors

acarbose (Precose), miglitol (Glyset)	Slow the absorption and breakdown of carbohydrate in GI tract	GI discomfort and other symptoms including gas and diarrhea	*Caution:* possible increased risk of hypoglycemia due to exercise

Combination drugs

kazano (alogliptin and metformin), oseni (alogliptin and pioglitazone)	Stimulate the release of insulin by preventing breakdown of GLP-1, inhibit the release of glucose from the liver, improve insulin sensitivity; may promote modest weight loss and modest decline in LDLs (from metformin) and improve insulin receptor sensitivity in muscle, liver, and adipocytes; may slightly increase HDLs (from pioglitazone)	Heart failure, heart attack, stroke, liver disease (from pioglitazone); upper respiratory tract infection, sore throat, headache, inflammation of the pancreas (from alogliptin); nausea, diarrhea, lactic acidosis (rarely) (from metformin)	Very little information on interactions with exercise; Caution: possible increased risk of hypoglycemia due to exercise (from alogliptin and pioglitazone); may increase exercise heart rate response to submaximal exercise; may interfere with glucose-lowering action (from metformin); may improve exercise capacity

References: (8, 50, 135)

Medications Table 4.3   Common Medications Used to Treat Type 1 Diabetes

Drug class and names	Mechanism of action	Most common side effects	Effects on exercise
Rapid-acting insulin: lispro (Humalog), aspart (Novolog), glulisine (Apidra) Short-acting insulin: regular Humulin (also called Humulin R), Velosulin (for insulin pump) Intermediate-acting insulin: Hypurin isophane (also called NPH) Long-acting insulin: insulin glargine (Basaglar, Lantus, Toujeo), insulin detemir (Levemir)	Replaces the insulin normally produced by beta cells of the pancreas	Pain, redness, swelling or itching at the injection site; hypoglycemia and resulting symptoms may occur	Increases release of injected insulin if the injection is given in active skeletal muscle; increases uptake of glucose from arterial blood (which can cause hypoglycemia)
pramlintide (Symlin)*	Blunts the increase in blood glucose levels after eating	Redness, swelling, bruising, or itching at the injection site, loss of appetite, stomach pain, excessive tiredness, dizziness, cough, sore throat, joint pain	Affects purposeful and desired blood glucose increase from preexercise snack and may result in decreased performance
Angiotensin-converting enzyme (ACE) inhibitors*	Reduce high blood pressure (if applicable)	Dry cough, dizziness, light-headedness, fainting, headaches, fatigue	May or may not decrease exercise submaximal and maximal heart rate, lower submaximal and maximal blood pressure
Statins*	Reduce risk (or levels, if already raised) of high blood lipids	GI discomfort, headaches, muscle aches, drowsiness, dizziness, myopathy, liver damage	May attenuate aerobic training benefits and increase myalgias when combined with exercise

*These medications do not directly affect blood glucose levels, but are taken by individuals who have type 1 diabetes to help manage their disease.

References: (8, 35, 49, 134, 203, 204)

Medications Table 4.4 Common Medications Used to Treat Abnormal Lipid Levels

Drug class and names	Most common side effects	Effects on exercise
Statins, HMG-CoA reductase inhibitors		
lovastatin (Mevacor), pravastatin (Pravachol), simvastatin (Zocor), atorvastatin (Lipitor), rosuvastatin (Crestor), ezetimibe and simvastatin combination (Vytorin, Zetia-Zocor)	GI discomfort, headaches, muscle aches, drowsiness, dizziness, myopathy, liver damage	May attenuate aerobic training benefits and increase myalgias when combined with exercise
Niacin		
niaspan (Niacor), Slo-niacin (over the counter)	Flushing of the face, neck, itching, dizziness, hypotension	No known effect on exercise responses unless hypotension occurs, then may increase heart rate responses
Fibrates, fibric acid		
gemfibrozil (Lopid), fenofibrate (Tricor), bezafibrate (Bezalip)	GI discomfort, aching muscles (more likely if also using a statin), rash, possible damage to gallbladder	May increase the risk of myalgias when combined with exercise
Bile acid binding resins		
cholestyramine (Questran), colesevelam (Welchol), colestipol (Colestid)	GI discomfort, heartburn, gas, constipation	No known effects on exercise responses
Cholesterol absorption blocker		
ezetimibe (Zetia)	GI discomfort	No known effects on exercise responses
Omega-3 fish oil		
Lovaza (as a prescription), over-the-counter supplements	No significant side effects	No known effects on exercise responses

References: (51, 130, 190)

Medications Table 4.5 Common Hormones Used in Thyroid Replacement Therapy

Hormone type	Drug names	Most common side effects	Effects on exercise
Synthetic	levothyroxine (Levothroid, Levoxyl, Synthroid, Unithroid)	Hyperthyroid symptoms from overdosing, tachycardia, palpitations, cardiomyopathy possible, tremors, anxiety, weight loss, nervousness, loss of sleep	Increased heart rate and blood pressure during submaximal and maximal exercise, tachycardia
Synthetic combination	levothyroxine (Synthroid) + liothyronine (Cytomel)	Essentially the same as for synthetic	Essentially the same as for synthetic
Natural (from animal glands)	thyroid (Armour thyroid)	Essentially the same as for synthetic	Essentially the same as for synthetic

References: (54, 182)

Medications Table 4.6 Common Therapies Used to Treat Hyperthyroidism

Therapy	Drug names	Most common side effects	Effects on exercise
Antithyroid drugs	methimazole (Tapazole), propylthiouracil	Can cause hypothyroidism	May increase exercise heart rate and blood pressure
β-blockers	propranolol (Inderal), metoprolol (Lopressor, Toprol XL)	Fatigue, decreased HDLs, increased triglycerides, increased cholesterol, impotence, increased blood glucose	Lower exercise heart rate and blood pressure
Iodine 131 (radioisotope therapy to ablate the thyroid)	Radioiodine	May cause complete destruction of thyroid requiring lifelong replacement therapy	No identified effects on exercise

References: (52, 131, 182)

5

Pulmonary Disorders and Conditions

Kenneth W. Rundell, PhD

James M. Smoliga, DVM, PhD, CSCS

Pnina Weiss, MD, FAAP

After completing this chapter, you will be able to

- understand the distinguishing physiological and physical characteristics of asthma, exercise-induced bronchoconstriction, pulmonary hypertension, chronic obstructive pulmonary disease, chronic restrictive pulmonary disease, and cystic fibrosis;

- recognize and identify the major signs or symptoms of asthma, exercise-induced bronchoconstriction, pulmonary hypertension, chronic obstructive pulmonary disease, chronic restrictive pulmonary disease, and cystic fibrosis;

- understand the major medication groups and their effects on individuals and the exercise response for those with asthma, exercise-induced bronchoconstriction, pulmonary hypertension, chronic obstructive pulmonary disease, chronic restrictive pulmonary disease, and cystic fibrosis;

- identify, program, and administer appropriate exercise for asthma, exercise-induced bronchoconstriction, pulmonary hypertension, chronic obstructive pulmonary disease, chronic restrictive pulmonary disease, and cystic fibrosis; and

- understand modifications, precautions, and the need to terminate exercise for asthma, exercise-induced bronchoconstriction, pulmonary hypertension, chronic obstructive pulmonary disease, chronic restrictive pulmonary disease, and cystic fibrosis.

The contributors would like to thank Sara Chelland for her assistance in the preparation of this chapter.

Regular physical activity promotes health and provides positive benefits to those suffering from chronic heart disease, diabetes, and other ailments; however, benefits of regular exercise for individuals with lung disease are less clear. Reduced corticosteroid use, improved quality of life scores, and decrease in severity of exercise-induced bronchoconstriction (EIB) have been associated with improved cardiopulmonary fitness from aerobic exercise (231, 309). Yet paradoxically, there is evidence that aerobic endurance exercise may contribute to asthma and EIB (280, 281). Likewise, air pollution has been associated with new-onset asthma and chronic obstructive pulmonary disease (COPD) (121, 151, 175, 248). This chapter explores the beneficial and detrimental effects of exercise as related to asthma, pulmonary hypertension, COPD, chronic restrictive pulmonary disease, and cystic fibrosis.

ASTHMA

Asthma is a chronic inflammatory lung disease that affects an estimated 25 million people in the United States, 6 million of whom are children (8, 54). In the United States, medical costs are estimated to be over $53 billion per year, and more than 10.5 million school days are lost annually because of asthma (7). Asthma results in approximately 3,500 deaths annually (9 per day) in the United States (53). Although roughly 90% of all individuals with asthma have a bronchoconstricting response to exercise and exercise can trigger a severe exacerbation, exercise-related asthma deaths are relatively uncommon with approximately nine per year in the United States (34); in these, mild intermittent or persistent asthma was identified.

Exercise-related exacerbations generally occur in approximately 10% of the population (248, 251); however, in some sports the prevalence is much higher. For example, with ice rink athletes, Nordic skiers, and swimmers, the prevalence of EIB is greater than 25% (210). Exercise-induced bronchoconstriction occurs in people with apparent asthma and those without apparent asthma. In either case, the mechanism is inflammatory; however, the precise trigger may differ from person to person (231, 309).

Key Point

Asthma is a chronic disease of the lungs characterized by airway inflammation, which leads to airway remodeling and hyperresponsiveness.

Pathology and Pathophysiology of Asthma

Asthma prevalence in the United States has increased dramatically in the last 30 years (53); however, this increase may in part be due to increased asthma awareness and overdiagnosis (190). Airborne pollutants from a variety of combustion sources (e.g., coal- and oil-burning furnaces, internal combustion engines and high automobile traffic, and gas cooking stoves) as well as high ozone levels can aggravate existing asthma and may be responsible for new-onset asthma in individuals who are genetically susceptible (162, 199). Changes in bacterial and viral infections, altered microflora, and diet may also contribute to allergic disease (278). Reduction in infection and contact with the microbial environment during prenatal and early life (i.e., the *hygiene hypothesis*) can affect the maturation of a normal immune response (155). Diminished microbial exposure during infancy may also affect sensitization to allergens (38, 158). Immune responses are primed in utero and reshaped during postnatal allergen exposure. The sensitivity to environmental antigens depends on the immunologic memory initiated during antigen encounters of early life (154).

Low socioeconomic status (SES) is associated with unfavorable conditions of high allergens such as dust mites, cigarette smoke, and cockroaches (318). Exposures have also been identified as a risk for the development of asthma (46). Asthma severity and related mortality are twice as common in persons with low SES; however, the prevalence of asthma is greater among those with high SES (301). This may be related to better health care and asthma diagnosis in the high-SES population.

A high prevalence of asthma has been reported for African Americans (109, 167). African Americans also suffer from a fourfold higher asthma mortality rate than Caucasians (202). Even after SES factors were accounted for, African Americans and Hispanics were shown to be at greater risk than Caucasians for both adult and childhood onset of asthma (188).

Several studies (47, 52, 302) suggest that asthma is a risk factor for obesity because of decreased exercise in this population, although recent studies (31) support obesity as a risk for asthma. Airway obstruction and peak flow variability are increased in obese populations while a decrease in fat mass and body mass index is related to improved airway function.

In asthma, mast cells, eosinophils, T lymphocytes, macrophages, neutrophils, and epithelial cells may all be actively involved in the inflammatory process and airway hyperresponsiveness (63, 309). Symptoms of asthma include recurrent episodes of wheezing, breathlessness, chest tightness, and coughing (especially during the morning and night, or in response to allergen exposure or exercise). Asthma episodes are associated with airflow obstruction that typically resolves spontaneously within 1 hour (309). An acute response is characterized by activation of airway inflammatory cells, whereas the subacute response involves persistent inflammation from resident inflammatory cells in the airway causing more persistent inflammation. Chronic inflammation, characteristic of moderate to severe asthma, is defined by resident inflammatory cells, airway remodeling, and persistent respiratory symptoms. Figure 5.1 reveals the structural changes in a person with asthma.

Degrees of Asthma Severity

A variety of factors or indices are used to classify asthma status; however, a key indicator of severity is the degree to which medication is needed to alleviate the symptoms (63). A classification system is shown in table 5.1.

Pathology and Pathophysiology of EIB

Exercise-induced bronchoconstriction is defined as a transient narrowing of the airways during or after the cessation of exercise (231). This response typically resolves spontaneously within an hour postexercise. According to most diagnostic criteria, EIB is defined as a 10% or greater decrease in

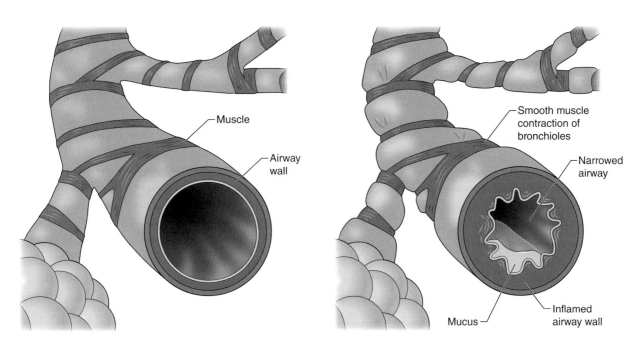

Figure 5.1 Schematic of a normal airway and a constricted airway of a person with asthma. Note the smooth muscle constriction, thickened mucosal layer, thickened basement membrane, denuded epithelium, and increased inflammatory cells of asthmatic airway.

Based on D. Doeing and J. Solway, 2013, "Airway smooth muscle in the pathophysiology and treatment of asthma," *Journal of Applied Physiology* 114:834-843.

Table 5.1   Components of Asthma Severity by Clinical Features Before Treatment

Severity	Days with symptoms	Nocturnal awakenings	Lung function	Interference with normal activity	Short-acting β_2-agonist use for symptom control
Intermittent	<2 days/week	<2 times/month	Normal FEV_1 between exacerbations; FEV_1 or PEF >80% predicted; FEV_1/FVC normal	None	<2 days/week
Mild persistent	>2 days/week but not daily	3 or 4 times/month	FEV_1 or PEF >80% predicted; FEV_1/FVC normal	Minor limitation	>2 days/week but not daily, and not more than 1 time on any day
Moderate persistent	Daily	>1 time/week but not nightly	FEV_1 or PEF 60% to 80% predicted; FEV_1/FVC reduced 5%	Some limitation	Daily
Severe persistent	Throughout the day	7 times/week	FEV_1 or PEF <60% predicted; FEV_1/FVC reduced >5%	Extreme limitation	Several times per day

FEV_1 = forced expiratory volume in the first second; FVC = forced vital capacity; PEF = peak expiratory flow.

Reprinted, by permission, from B. Carlin, 2013, Asthma. In *Clinical exercise physiology*, 3rd ed., edited by J.K. Ehrman, R.M. Gordon, P.S. Visch, and S.J. Keteyian (Champaign, IL: Human Kinetics), 342.

forced expiratory volume in the first second of a maximal exhalation (FEV_1). Exercise-induced bronchoconstriction can occur in those with apparent asthma and those without apparent asthma. Exercise is the most common instigator of an asthma attack. This hyperresponsive reaction to exercise occurs in approximately 90% of individuals who have asthma and, for those who have mild asthma, EIB may be the only apparent expression of the disease (14).

Key Point

Exercise-induced bronchoconstriction (EIB) is a condition in which there is a narrowing of the airways during or following exercise.

Exercise-induced bronchoconstriction prevalence has been estimated to be 4% to 20% in the general population (25, 231, 309, 313) and 11% to 55% in specific sport populations (183, 193, 252, 310, 313), with the highest prevalence found in winter sport athletes (310).

Exercise-induced bronchoconstriction is typically instigated by water loss from the airway surfaces consequential to the humidification of inspired air during exercise (15-17). Exercise-related inflammation and airway hyperresponsive-

ness can also be related to the allergen response or inhalation of airborne pollutants during exercise. Following the humidification process consequential to dry air inhalation, water loss from the airway surfaces increases osmolarity in airway cells; this is followed by an influx of water into the cells to restore osmolarity and trigger an inflammatory mediator release, which subsequently causes bronchial smooth muscle constriction (231, 309). The severity of the exercise-related response is determined by ventilation rate, ambient air water content and temperature during exercise, and the presence of an allergen (231).

Normally, water loss from the humidification process in the airways is continuously replenished via epithelial cells and submucosa (13, 60); however, evidence indicates that alterations in the subepithelial basement membrane may be in part responsible for an observed decrease in the ability to adequately respond to this airway surface evaporative water loss (169, 179). This may necessitate the recruitment of smaller airways into the humidification process, enhancing airway hyperreactivity (13).

Although the exercise environment may be the primary determinant of the EIB response in individuals with and without apparent asthma, it has been postulated that the mode of exercise may play a role, albeit minor, when ventilation is affected (252). For example, the prevalence and intensity of EIB are lessened when the mode of exercise is swimming and the environment is a pool, where the temperature is relatively warm and humidity is very high (51). However, to the contrary, high airway hyperresponsiveness and asthma have been identified in competitive swimmers; high trichloramine levels at the pool surface are thought to be the cause (51, 263). In stark contrast to an indoor swimming pool, the environmental conditions of an indoor ice arena include low temperatures and humidity in conjunction with high levels of particulates and pollutants (figure 5.2). The ultrafine particles emitted during ice resurfacing have been shown to exacerbate the asthmatic response, and chronic exposure can result in new-onset asthma (121, 193, 238, 249).

Therapy of Asthma and EIB

Although a cure is currently unknown, several pharmacotherapeutic agents are effective in the treatment of asthma and EIB. These treatments can support the removal or attenuation of airway inflammation and accompanying symptoms that allows the individual with asthma or EIB to lead a normal, physically active life. The key to a successful treatment, however, is the design of an individualized treatment strategy.

Medical intervention can control respiratory symptoms and offset lung function decline over time. Optimal treatment is the elimination of or reduction in airway inflammation and exacerbations, to minimize the use of rescue inhalers, and to reduce emergency department visits and hospitalizations. Successful treatment should strive to achieve optimal baseline pulmonary function and a reduction of symptoms.

Common Medications Given to Individuals With Asthma and EIB

Classic medications to treat asthma and EIB can be divided into two primary categories; however, a novel class of biologics called *monoclonal antibodies* has emerged that demonstrates efficacy in moderate to severe allergic asthma and high eosinophilic asthma (35, 146). Because asthma is

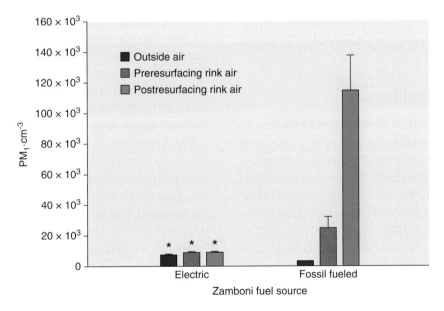

Figure 5.2 Particulate matter (<1.0 mm in diameter) measured in outside air and at ice level in seven ice rinks during prime usage hours (29 measurements). Note that the particulate matter concentration in the ice arena air is more than 20 times greater than that of the ambient air outside of the ice arena.

Data from K. Rundell, 2003, "High levels of airborne ultrafine and fine particulate matter in indoor ice arenas," *Inhalation Toxicology* 15: 237-250.

considered a disease of chronic airway inflammation, one group of medications, known as *controllers,* aims to provide long-term control by reducing inflammation. Medications in this category are taken on a daily basis and provide the foundation for asthma management (62). Other medications, known as *relievers,* are used to relieve acute obstruction, bronchoconstriction, or both. Drugs in this category are taken on an as-needed basis and are often used to supplement the controllers (41, 67, 231, 309).

Inhaled Corticosteroids

The National Institutes of Health defines anti-inflammatory medications as those that decrease inflammatory markers, resulting in reduced airway hyperresponsiveness (67). Inhaled corticosteroids (ICSs) are an effective, frequently used anti-inflammatory medication in the treatment of asthma (67, 314). Inhaled corticosteroids present significantly fewer adverse effects than oral corticosteroids (OCSs) and are generally well tolerated (35, 67). With long-term use, ICSs improve pulmonary function and reduce inflammation in individuals with asthma and also improve control of bronchial hyperresponsiveness (BHR). Despite that, ICS treatment plans longer than three weeks have shown diminished improvements in resting FEV_1 (296), peak expiratory flow (PEF) (28, 108, 136), frequency of symptoms (28, 108), and BHR (136, 231, 309).

Leukotriene Modifiers

Leukotriene modifiers demonstrate efficacy in providing **prophylaxis** (preventive treatment) for asthma and EIB; however, their effectiveness varies between individuals, with protection ranging from none to 100% (89, 116, 309). Additionally, leukotriene modifiers can allow a reduction in the dose of an ICS (89, 164). Thus, while it appears that leukotrienes are involved in the pathogenesis of asthma and EIB, evidence that leukotriene modifiers are not 100% effective (250, 309) supports the notion of multiple mediator involvement in airway inflammation and BHR. However, it should be noted that leukotrienes seem to play a primary role in eosinophilic asthma (138).

β_2-Adrenergic Agonists

β_2-adrenergic agonists are potent bronchodilators used in prophylaxis and rescue from acute asthma exacerbation and EIB and are one of the most effective preventive therapies for EIB (309) because they improve pulmonary function in nearly all individuals suffering from EIB (18).

The short-acting β_2-adrenergic agonists (SABAs) are functionally similar to long-acting β_2-agonists (LABAs); they relax airway smooth muscle, improve air flow, decrease vascular permeability, and moderately inhibit mediator release (67, 314). Long-acting β_2-agonists are effective only for a short duration, with a peak bronchodilatory effect within 60 minutes of administration (231, 309). Common recommendations include one inhaler per month as the maximal dosage; daily use implies a need for improved asthma control (i.e., via an ICS) (314). For example, it is recommended that if SABAs are used more than two or three times per week, an alternative treatment plan, such as the use of corticosteroids, should be examined and implemented (231). Moreover, SABAs were not found to prevent postexercise decreases in FEV_1 in elite speed skaters when compared to no medication (313) (figure 5.3).

Long-acting β_2-agonists function similarly to SABAs (i.e., prevent bronchoconstriction and improve expiratory flow), thereby reducing the frequency and intensity of asthma, EIB episodes, or both (33, 70). The effects of a LABA may last up to 12 hours, which can be particularly helpful for individuals with overnight asthma symptoms (219). Long-acting β_2-agonists have, however, been associated with increased mortality risk, so it is unclear whether daily use is safe. In conjunction with this, daily use of at least one LABA (salmeterol) has been shown to result in rapidly diminishing effectiveness of its long-duration effects in as little as one month (66). It should also be noted that LABAs are not recommended as standalone medications and should be used only in conjunction with an ICS.

A summary of medications given to individuals with asthma and EIB is found in medications tables 5.1 and 5.2 near the end of the chapter.

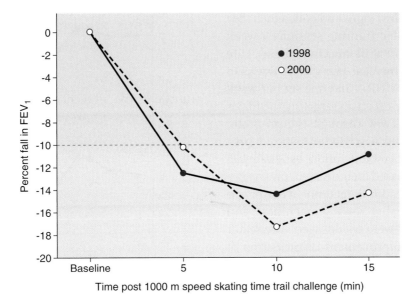

Figure 5.3 Postexercise decreases in FEV$_1$ before and following a SABA treatment in eight EIB-positive elite short track speed skaters. Values are for the greatest decrease in FEV$_1$ measured at 5, 10, or 15 minutes postexercise. No significant improvements from β_2-agonist intervention were noted for any pulmonary function measured. Initial testing was done during the 1998 season and follow-up testing was done during the 2000 season.

Data from R.L. Wilber, K.W. Rundell, and D.A. Judelson, 2001, Presented at the Thematic Poster Session, Science in Winter Sports, under the title "Mid expiratory flow rates of cold weather athletes with exercise induced asthma."

Effects of Exercise in Individuals With Asthma and EIB

As previously mentioned, a higher prevalence of asthma and EIB has been found in cross-country skiers, ice rink sport athletes, and swimmers (51, 248, 263), with respective causes likely from high minute ventilation breathing of cold dry air, air high in combustion emission pollutants, or air with high trichloramine levels found in indoor pool air. Exercise in high-ozone air has also been shown to cause acute decreases in lung function in both the asthmatic and nonasthmatic populations (248, 263). Most recently, long-term exposure to ozone while exercising has been related to the development of new-onset asthma in the child athlete (163). Studies on elite Nordic skiers (252, 313), ice rink athletes (193, 238, 251, 313), swimmers (110, 263), and youth soccer players (121) support the development of new-onset asthma and EIB from exercise-induced oxidative stress.

Key Point

While approximately 10% of the general population exhibits EIB, considerably greater prevalence is reported in sport participants such as cross-country skiers, ice rink athletes, and swimmers.

Most individuals with asthma are susceptible to EIB, yet their ability to exercise is often not limited (248). In cases in which resting lung function is impaired, exercise can be compromised (248). However, most individuals with asthma are able to exercise, compete in sports symptom-free, and improve their overall quality of life (80). Note that despite an extensive review paper by Del Giacco and colleagues (79) concluding that moderate-intensity (40% to <60% $\dot{V}O_2$ or heart rate reserve) aerobic exercise improves cardiovascular fitness in a person with asthma or EIB, there is not consensus that exercise creates an improvement in baseline lung function or BHR (50).

A 24-week study by Dogra and colleagues (84) included three aerobic training sessions a week at a minimum of 70% of maximal heart rate (MHR)—with a 5% increase every three weeks to a minimum of 85% MHR—and one set per week of resistance training exercises targeting the major muscle groups. Halfway through the program, participants followed a self-administered program that allowed personalization; for example, exercise mode was based on individual preference (outdoor jogging, treadmill, recumbent or upright cycling, and elliptical or rowing machines), and five weekly sessions were encouraged. The result was a significant improvement of measures of quality of life, asthma control, and aerobic fitness.

The EIB response typically occurs after exercise is stopped in the 6- to 8-minute-duration challenge test, but during longer bouts of exercise a gradual decline in lung function occurs and is followed by a larger fall in FEV_1 upon the cessation of exercise (32). Type of exercise (constant vs. interval), intensity, and duration determine whether bronchoconstriction occurs during or at cessation of exercise, or not at all (32).

Lung function in the EIB challenge test most often involves bronchodilation during the exercise bout followed by falls in expiratory flow rates 5 to 20 minutes after exercise (125, 277). The exercise bronchodilation is likely attributable to the larger tidal volumes during exercise causing airways to be stretched open, thus providing a mechanical protection against EIB (32).

After tidal volume decreases when exercise is stopped or intensity decreased, bronchoconstrictive influences dominate. Beck and colleagues (32) found that during 36 minutes of steady-state exercise, an initial bronchodilation occurs within the first few minutes, followed by a steady decline in lung function for the remaining period of exercise. Until this study, the decline in exercising lung function had gone unnoticed simply because challenge tests were of short duration. During interval exercise, lung function in the individual with asthma fluctuates with exercise intensity; it increases with high intensity and decreases during the rest interval. Beck and colleagues (32) also evaluated lung function during 36 minutes of interval exercise consisting of 6-minute alternating moderate- and light-intensity bouts. Lung function demonstrated a gradual fall during the 36-minute

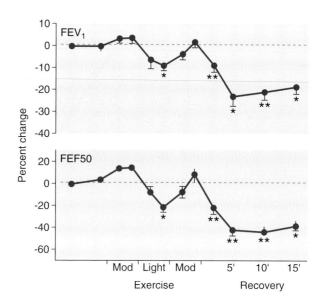

Figure 5.4 Change in FEV_1 and FEF50 during and after 36 minutes of interval-type exercise, alternating 6-minute periods of moderate- and light-intensity exercise. Note the dynamic nature of pulmonary function between exercise intensities but the overall decline over 36 minutes.

Based on K.C. Beck, K.P. Offord, and P.D. Scanlon, 1994, "Bronchoconstriction occurring during exercise in asthmatic subjects," *American Journal of Respiratory and Critical Care Medicine* 149: 352-357.

exercise period with a pattern of improvement during the moderate-intensity period and deterioration during the light-intensity period (figure 5.4).

Exercise Recommendations for Clients With Asthma and EIB

The prevalence of asthma and EIB in clients and athletes who compete in environments that are known to trigger asthma and EIB attacks (e.g., cold and dry) supports the fact that exercise is possible for clients with these conditions. Exercise prescription recommendations for clients with asthma and EIB should be based on the results of exercise testing and assessment, including a bronchial challenge test, so the exercise professional is aware of the client's threshold and response to exercise intensity, duration, mode, and, when possible, environmental stimuli.

It is important for clients with asthma and EIB to have adequate control of their symptoms and condition before initiating an exercise program. Commonly, aerobic exercise is paired with pharmaceutical therapy as a method to improve BHR, exercise capacity, and quality of life in clients with moderate or severe asthma (101, 114). The exercise professional should be aware that clients with asthma or EIB typically use a preexercise (15 minutes) medication such as a SABA, a mast cell stabilizing agent, or an inhaled anticholinergic agent (231). In conjunction, clients with asthma or EIB often take a daily controller medication that may include an ICS or leukotriene receptor antagonist (231). Although this comprehensive strategy greatly reduces the risk of the exercise session causing an adverse event (107), it is still recommended that the client and exercise professional, with input and approval from the client's physician or other health care professional, determine an individualized action plan before starting a program in case of an exacerbation of symptoms.

Exercise guidelines for clients with asthma or EIB include several specific recommendations. First, a 10- to 15-minute preworkout warm-up is highly recommended (176, 231, 276). An effective warm-up—especially using variable or interval high-intensity exercise, as opposed to continuous high- or light-intensity exercise (231, 276)—may produce a refractory period up to 2 hours (231) that reduces a client's propensity to develop EIB (203).

The intensity and duration of an aerobic workout need to begin at a lower level and gradually progress so as to not cause an exacerbation of symptoms. As a client's fitness level improves, the exercise professional should strive to assign an intensity of 40% to <60% $\dot{V}O_2$ or heart rate reserve for 20 to 60 minutes three to five times a week using an exercise mode that involves rhythmic and continuous movement of large muscle groups (19, 79, 213, 272). For example, a client with asthma or EIB can start with walking, then progress to a walk–jog program, then a run-only program. When clients are able to handle vigorous-intensity sessions of ≥60% to 90% $\dot{V}O_2$ or heart rate reserve without an exacerbation of symptoms, they can do interval training workouts of 10 to 30 seconds of high-intensity exercise followed by 30 to 90 seconds of rest (213).

For clients with asthma or EIB, the design of an initial resistance training program is similar to common guidelines for beginning, untrained individuals (two or three sessions a week of two to four sets using moderate loads) (19, 272).

Tables 5.2 and 5.3 show a summary of the aerobic and resistance training guidelines for clients with asthma and EIB.

Table 5.2 General Aerobic Exercise Guidelines for Clients With Asthma and EIB

Parameter	Guideline
Frequency	3-5 sessions per week
Intensity	40% to <60% $\dot{V}O_2$ or heart rate reserve
Mode	Large muscle mass activities (e.g., walking)
Duration	20-60 min of continuous activity

References: (19, 79, 213, 272)

Table 5.3 General Resistance Training Guidelines for Clients With Asthma and EIB

Parameter	Guideline
Frequency	2-3 sessions per week
Intensity	Moderate (60-80% 1RM)
Repetitions	6-12
Sets	2-4

References: (19, 272)

Asthma

Ms. S is a 26-year-old graduate student. She was never involved in organized sport but decided she needed to get physically fit and set a goal of completing a marathon. She began a running program but found that she was not making any progress. She reported, "I am wheezing and feeling a bit tight in the chest after about a block and half of running; when I slow to a walk, it seems to get worse and I get this cough." She added that she had these symptoms year-round but that they were worse during the allergy season. This persisted for approximately one month into her program. She was getting nowhere in terms of achieving her goal of completing a marathon.

Despite Ms. S's persistent attempt to train, her fitness was not improving. This led her to her family physician, who suggested that she might have EIB. He prescribed a β_2-agonist to be used before her workout sessions. She felt better and was able to run for about 30 minutes by the end of the first week. By the end of the second week of daily β_2-agonist use, that old feeling of wheezing, chest tightness, and cough returned and she was back to walking after the first or second block of running. She then made an appointment with an asthma specialist to be evaluated for her issues. After measurement of her resting lung function and the ability of a β_2-agonist to improve her function, it was decided that she would undergo a challenge test. Her resting FEV_1 was 110% of the age-, sex-, height-predicted value, and she did not improve her FEV_1 by at least 12% after β_2-agonist administration. However, this was likely because her daily use of the prescribed β_2-agonist for approximately one month now resulted in the development of a tolerance (**tachyphylaxis**). The high predicted FEV_1 suggested that there was minimal chronic inflammation, and the initial benefit provided by the preexercise use of the β_2-agonist is suggestive of EIB. Ms. S did test positive for grass allergy, which was currently in season, and dust mites and had mild to moderate nasal congestion, runny nose, and postnasal drip indicative of rhinoconjunctivitis. The challenge test was scheduled a week later, and Ms. S was given instructions to not use the β_2-agonist except as a necessary rescue during the week leading up to the test. The result from the challenge test showed a substantial posttest fall in FEV_1 of 77%, suggesting very hyperreactive airways (a fall of 10% is considered positive).

Recommended Readings

Bonini, M and Palange, P. Exercise-induced bronchoconstriction: new evidence in pathogenesis, diagnosis and treatment. *Asthma Res Pract* 1:2, 2015.

Del Giacco, SR, Firinu, D, Bjermer, L, and Carlsen, KH. Exercise and asthma: an overview. *Eur Clin Respir J* 2:27984, 2014.

Dogra, S, Kuk, J, Baker, J, and Jamnik, V. Exercise is associated with improved asthma control in adults. *Eur Respir J* 37:318-323, 2011.

Lucas, SR and Platts-Mills, TA. Physical activity and exercise in asthma: relevance to etiology and treatment. *J Allergy Clin Immunol* 115:928-934, 2005.

WebMD. Asthma health center. 2016. www.webmd.com/asthma/guide. Accessed October 28, 2016.

PULMONARY HYPERTENSION

Pulmonary hypertension (PH) is both a hemodynamic and pathophysiological condition in which mean pulmonary arterial pressure is greater than 25 mmHg at rest (118). Pulmonary hypertension may be further subdivided into six different categories representing a variety of pathophysiological mechanisms (118). Thus, management for an individual with a diagnosis of PH does not simply involve following a general protocol, but rather must consider the type of PH and underlying factors specific to each individual case.

Pulmonary arterial hypertension (PAH) is a specific clinical condition characterized by PAH in the absence of other causes of precapillary hypertension (118). Pulmonary arterial hypertension may have many underlying origins, including heredity and drug toxicity, or may be **idiopathic** (i.e., have an unknown cause). All causes of PAH produce similar pathophysiological changes in the cardiopulmonary system. However, PAH is rare, with an estimated incidence of 1 in 100,000 to 1,000,000 individuals (208). Nonetheless, the individual economic impact of PAH is substantial, with a 2015 systematic review reporting a range of approximately $2,500 to $12,000 per month of direct costs to each individual, plus unknown indirect costs (135).

The general condition of PH is not uncommon, with estimates of up to 1% of the global population, where it is often associated with other chronic cardiopulmonary or infectious diseases (150, 208, 229). The incidence and underlying cause of PH have considerable geographic variation, due to differences including population genetics, environment, infectious disease, and medical care. Further, differences in methodology between registries create barriers in accurately understanding the epidemiology of PH (201). Pulmonary hypertension is commonly associated with hypoxic cardiopulmonary diseases, including COPD and diffuse parenchymal lung diseases (229, 247).

Pathology and Pathophysiology of PH

The pulmonary circulatory system is a high-flow, low-pressure, low-resistance system relative to the rest of the circulation, with resting peak systolic pressure <25 mmHg and diastolic pressure <10 mmHg, such that normal mean **pulmonary arterial pressure** (PAP) is 14 ± 3 mmHg at rest. Right atrial and ventricular pressure during diastole is generally <5 mmHg, which is a pressure sufficient to allow a favorable pressure gradient for venous blood from systemic circulation to return to the right side of the heart. In accordance with the general principles of cardiovascular physiology, increases in blood pressure are rooted in an increase in cardiac output or an increase in vascular resistance. In PH, the latter is generally the causative mechanism, though the root of increased pulmonary vascular resistance is quite varied.

Previous classification systems of PH divided it into primary and secondary conditions, and though this schema is overly simplistic and has been abandoned (118), there remains value in understanding how various pathological conditions can lead to the development of PH. The pathogenesis of PH leads to decreased functional diameter of the lumen of pulmonary arteries and veins, depending on the category of PH. For instance, primary vasoconstriction, thromboembolic blockages, and parasitic infestations may all decrease blood vessel diameter and thus increase vascular resistance. Under hypoxic conditions, as in various chronic pulmonary diseases (229, 247) and sleep apnea (171), pulmonary arterial smooth muscle contracts to cause vasoconstriction. This mechanism normally promotes ventilation–perfusion matching, but in chronic hypoxic lung disease, the increased pulmonary vascular resistance resulting from hypoxic pulmonary vasoconstriction leads to the development of PH (106).

Pulmonary hypertension can lead to further systemic effects such as increased pulmonary vascular resistance, which necessitates greater pressures in the right ventricle for blood to be ejected into the pulmonary circulation. This causes overload in the right ventricle and subsequent dilation and, ultimately, right-sided heart failure. Blood pooling in the right side of the heart can lead to congestion in the vena cava and the hepatoportal circulation, which can cause liver dysfunction. Additionally, increased blood pressure can lead to pulmonary and systemic edema.

Animal model data also suggest that respiratory function is impaired in PH due to diaphragmatic muscle fiber weakness and atrophy (76), which contributes to **dyspnea** (labored breathing) and fatigue during exercise. Indeed, individuals with idiopathic PAH experience inspiratory and expiratory muscle weakness (207). This may be attributed to respiratory muscle overload (214). There is also evidence that this dysfunction extends beyond the diaphragm and affects skeletal muscles globally (228).

Given that PH negatively influences the heart, lungs, vascular system, and respiratory muscles, it follows that exercise capacity is limited in PAH and that this negatively influences quality of life (137). Interestingly, resting hemodynamic parameters were not found to be related to quality of life in individuals with PAH (137).

The signs and symptoms of PH are generally nonspecific, including dyspnea, fatigue, general signs of cardiovascular dysfunction (e.g., **syncope** [fainting], angina, various heart murmurs), and signs of pathologically elevated systemic blood pressure (e.g., ascites, edema, jugular distension). A detailed description of diagnostic and prognostic tests is beyond the scope of this chapter but is achieved through specialist referral and includes a variety of imaging procedures, blood tests, and direct measurement of right ventricular pressure via catheterization (118, 119).

Common Medications Given to Individuals With PH

It is important to recognize that pharmacotherapy targeted toward individuals with PAH is not necessarily the same as that for PH, due to differences in the pathophysiology. While pharmacotherapy that causes vasodilation to reduce pulmonary vascular resistance should be beneficial to individuals with PAH, these physiologic responses may impair gas exchange in individuals with hypoxic lung diseases (229). Thus, there is not a single standard pharmacotherapeutic regimen for treating PH; rather, the type of PH and associated comorbidities must be considered.

Pharmacotherapy in PH is dependent on the classification of the disease; thus there is not a specific drug profile that can be used for all individuals with PH. However, there are medications that are approved for managing PAH, and various pharmacotherapy algorithms are available with varying degrees of evidence (118, 119). Pharmacotherapy for PAH is targeted at improving function and delaying progression of the disease and more invasive procedures, such as lung transplantation. Various clinical outcome measures are used to assess the effectiveness of pharmacotherapy, but improved exercise performance can be expected in successfully managed individuals.

Vasoreactivity testing may be performed in individuals with PAH, and those who are vasoreactive may be treated with relatively high doses of calcium channel blockers. Vasoreactive individuals with baseline tachycardia are generally treated with diltiazem, and those with baseline bradycardia are generally treated with nifedipine. Generally, few individuals respond favorably to calcium channel blockers; those with idiopathic, heritable, and drug-induced PAH are most likely to respond (118, 119).

The three distinct targets of interest for specific pharmacological management of PAH are the endothelin, nitric oxide, and prostacyclin pathways, which counter vasoconstrictor pathways or activate vasodilator signaling pathways. For individuals with PAH who are not vasoreactive or respond poorly to calcium channel blockers, monotherapy targeting one of the relevant signaling pathways is indicated. Endothelin receptor antagonists, such as ambrisentan, bosentan, and macitentan, may be used to counter pulmonary vasoconstriction induced by elevated levels of endothelin-1. Phosphodiesterase inhibitors, such as sildenafil, tadalafil, and vardenafil, act through inhibiting degradation of cyclic guanosine monophosphate (cGMP), which improves nitric oxide bioavailability and thus promotes vasodilation. Vasodilation is also promoted through drugs that activate the prostacyclin pathway, including prostacyclin analogues (e.g., beraprost, epoprostenol, iloprost, and treprostinil) and selective prostacyclin receptor agonists (e.g., selexipag). There is good clinical evidence for each of these classes of drugs, but limited data regarding comparative efficacy preclude recommendation for a monotherapy of choice for most individuals with PAH. Combination therapy targeting two or more signaling pathways may be useful for managing PAH. Much of the evidence for combination therapy is centered on sequential combination therapy, such that one class of drugs is initiated and additional pharmacological management is added as needed to achieve targeted clinical outcomes. However, there is currently limited evidence for using combination therapy as a first line of pharmacological management (118, 119).

Drugs used in the management of PAH may be effective for some, but not all, of the other categories of PH. For instance, there is some evidence, though not strong, that individuals with PH due to left heart disease may benefit from PAH pharmacotherapy. Conversely, there is essentially no evidence for use of PAH drugs in individuals with PH due to lung disease or hypoxia, and vasodilators may impair gas exchange. Given the multifactorial nature of PAH and other types of PH, it is possible that individuals may also be managed with other types of drugs, such as anticoagulants, antiarrhythmics, diuretics, angiotensin-converting enzyme (ACE) inhibitors, and β-blockers, depending on underlying pathology. Yet the combination of PAH-specific drugs with antihypertensive agents may cause systemic hypotension.

A summary of medications given to individuals with PH is found in medications table 5.3 near the end of the chapter.

Effects of Exercise in Individuals With PH

Pulmonary arterial pressure normally rises during high-intensity exercise in healthy fit individuals due to increased cardiac output. The pulmonary circulation is normally a low-resistance system, with the pulmonary arteries having limited ability to dilate beyond that at rest (115). The lung is relatively fully perfused at rest; but during exercise, recruitment of additional blood vessels in less perfused regions helps accommodate some of the increase in cardiac output to offset changes in pulmonary arterial pressure. As cardiac output rises during high-intensity exercise, there is limited room to decrease pulmonary vascular resistance compared to that of the systemic circulation. Accordingly, PAP normally rises during high-intensity exercise (71). However, in some individuals the exercise-induced increase in PAP is actually pathological, and is referred to as **exercise pulmonary hypertension**.

The classification of exercise pulmonary hypertension is less straightforward than that for resting PH, since an increased mean PAP during exercise occurs in all healthy individuals. Exercise pulmonary hypertension is characterized by a high PAP accompanied by symptoms of PH, such as breathlessness, which are not present at rest. This condition may occur in individuals with mild left heart disease or pulmonary vascular dysfunction that is not severe enough to induce these effects under resting conditions (147). Previously, a mean PAP of >30 mmHg during exercise was considered diagnostic for exercise pulmonary hypertension, but it is possible for healthy, fit individuals to achieve this criterion during high-intensity exercise. Newer research indicates that a mean PAP of >30 mmHg, when combined with a total pulmonary resistance of >3 mmHg $\cdot$ min^{-1} $\cdot$ L^{-1}, has a high sensitivity and specificity for discriminating between healthy individuals and those with pulmonary vascular disease or right heart disease (147).

Because exercise can trigger PH before it manifests at rest, exercise testing may be useful in the identification of the early stages of PH by revealing subclinical impairments in right ventricle contractility in individuals with conditions associated with PH (61). For instance, in systemic sclerosis, pulmonary vascular resistance may be elevated and require increased right heart contractility at rest, which leads to irreversible right heart failure. However, individuals may be asymptomatic at rest in the early stages of the disease, but the observation of right ventricular impairment at rest can be useful in demonstrating the otherwise unnoticed presence of pulmonary vascular dysfunction so that it can be treated before it leads to irreversible right heart failure. Likewise, PAH is generally diagnosed late in the disease process (159), and therefore it is possible that exercise testing may be useful in detecting it earlier.

Exercise testing may be used to determine severity of PAH and provides valuable information regarding prognosis. Laboratory testing indicates that $\dot{V}O_2$ peak of less than 10.4 ml · kg^{-1} · min^{-1} is associated with poorer prognosis, as is inability to exceed a systolic blood pressure of >120 mmHg during peak exercise. Field tests of functional aerobic capacity are also useful in evaluating PH, and the 6-minute walk test is commonly used for this purpose. Interpretation of walk test scores must consider confounding factors that can influence test results, such as age and musculoskeletal function; therefore general recommendations, rather than specific targets, are most useful in understanding the functional capacity of individuals with PAH. A $\dot{V}O_2$ peak of more than 15 ml · kg^{-1} · min^{-1} and a 6-minute walk test result of >500 m (547 yd) are considered factors that contribute to a "stable and satisfactory" prognosis. In younger, more physically healthy individuals, >500-m (547-yd) walk distances may be achieved even by those with severe PAH, which makes this test less meaningful in this population.

Various measurements obtained during exercise have been demonstrated to be a better predictor of long-term survival than resting pulmonary hemodynamics (141). During exercise, a low $\dot{V}O_2$ peak, high PVR, and a small change in heart rate relative to rest are all associated with poorer prognosis in individuals with PAH (312). Additionally, **cardiac index** (cardiac output divided by body surface area) during exercise, but not rest, is related to aerobic function in PAH, and is one of the key predictors of survival in PAH (59, 141). Likewise, the relationship between mean PAP and cardiac output during exercise is linked to transplant-free survival of PH (141). Pulse oximetry values that drop more than 10% below resting levels are also associated with poorer prognosis.

Exercise Recommendations for Clients With PH

Pulmonary arterial hypertension is a chronic disease and does not have a cure, but treatments to diminish symptoms and slow the progression of the disease may be quite efficacious. Exercise was previously thought to be dangerous to clients with PH, as it was thought that increased stress on the cardiopulmonary system could accelerate heart failure. However, a significant body of evidence demonstrates that exercise is beneficial in improving symptoms, exercise capacity, and activities of daily living in clients with PAH and other forms of PH (21, 24, 118, 134, 206).

A systematic review and meta-analysis focused on clients with PAH and inoperable chronic thromboembolic PH revealed that exercise training increased the 6-minute walk distance and $\dot{V}O_2$ peak within three weeks of program initiation, which was generally maintained in studies of 12- to 15-week duration (319). Further, the meta-analysis (319) revealed improved quality of life and physical functioning following 15 weeks of training. The exercise protocols generally consisted of a combination of aerobic activity (i.e., treadmill walking, stationary cycling, or both) and resistance training. Some studies included specific respiratory muscle training and mental training. While Yuan and colleagues (319) demonstrated that exercise is beneficial for those with PH, the meta-analysis was limited to specific PH populations, which yielded only 12 studies (449 individuals).

Details of individual exercise protocols vary, but many share similar underlying structure. A commonly followed model of exercise programming in PH studies is three weeks of in-hospital training followed by 12 weeks at home. The initial three weeks allows clients to become familiar with correct exercise techniques, learn how to gauge proper intensity, and build confidence in their ability to perform the exercise. These initial three weeks may also include some educational components regarding the importance of adhering to the program and understanding the expected benefits. It may be beneficial to collect baseline and posttraining outcome data related to physical fitness (i.e., the 6-minute walk test) and quality of life following the initial few weeks of training to determine if the program is effective and to assist in convincing the client of the value of exercise.

The components of exercise protocols also share many similarities. Mereles and colleagues (206) performed the first major trial on the combination of exercise and respiratory training in severe PH. This protocol used interval training on a cycle ergometer, alternating between 30 seconds of lower-intensity and 60 seconds of higher-intensity exercise for 10 to 25 minutes per day in an in-patient setting. In that protocol, the higher-intensity training was 60% to 80% of heart rate achieved during initial maximal exercise test. Limitations for exercise intensity were based on the client's subjective physical exertion, a peak heart rate not more than 120 beats/min, and pulse oximetry values greater than 85%. Additionally, participants walked 60 minutes per day, performed 30 minutes of light resistance training, and did 30 minutes of specific respiratory muscle training five days per week. Upon discharge, individuals were asked to continue a similar routine, albeit for slightly decreased duration and frequency.

Subsequent exercise protocols for PH have used both interval and continuous training and have varied the approach to the aerobic exercise component. For instance, Chan and colleagues (57) and Weinstein and colleagues (311) had individuals walk for 30 to 45 minutes at 70% to 80% of heart rate reserve two or three times per week, while Grünig and colleagues (134) combined cycle ergometer interval training and walking similarly to Mereles (206). Fox and colleagues (113) took the approach of prescribing interval training for the first six weeks of rehabilitation, followed by continuous aerobic exercise in the second six weeks of rehabilitation, and included stair climbing in both components of the program. Such an approach may be useful for clients who are not able to initially engage in long periods of continuous activity. In addition, the general skeletal muscle dysfunction that has been associated with PAH (319) indicates that inclusion of resistance training in many published training protocols is justified (319).

Given the previously described respiratory muscle dysfunction in PAH (76, 207, 214), specific respiratory muscle training may be of particular benefit to clients with PH and has been included as a component of many of the training studies (319). Kabitz and colleagues (168) reported improved respiratory muscle strength and exercise capacity following 15 weeks of a combination of exercise and respiratory training in clients with PAH. Likewise, Saglam and colleagues (253) reported that six weeks of inspiratory muscle training improved pulmonary parameters, 6-minute walk distance, fatigue severity, and dyspneic symptoms.

Despite the evidence supporting the efficacy of exercise training for improving exercise capacity and activities of daily living for clients with PH, the number of randomized controlled trials remains small, with insufficient data to define optimal factors such as intensity, duration, and mode, and so there is no consensus on specific guidelines for exercise programming for clients with PH (119). In general, it is recommended that clients with PH should be physically active within the tolerance of their symptoms (118) and perform a combination of sustained light- to moderate-intensity workloads (20), specific respiratory muscle training, and resistance training. These programs are typically aimed at improving physical function and quality of life. It is also recommended that these clients undergo medically supervised testing to determine their symptom thresholds for exercise intensity and duration before initiating an exercise program. High-intensity aerobic or resistance training that exacerbates a client's symptoms or could elicit the Valsalva maneuver should be avoided (119). However, it must be noted that exercise programs may be specific to each subtype of PH. Further, exercise is often performed in combination with pharmacotherapy.

Key Point

Exercise training programs for clients with pulmonary hypertension commonly include the combination of light- to moderate-intensity training, specific respiratory muscle training, and resistance training. Importantly, clients should be tested in a medically supervised environment to determine their symptom thresholds before beginning an exercise program.

Case Study

Pulmonary Hypertension

A 63-year-old generally sedentary male with a body mass index (BMI) of 28 kg/m² initially presented to his general practitioner with a chief complaint of breathlessness while engaging in physically demanding activities, such as mowing the lawn and other infrequent laborious tasks. A physical exam revealed hypertension, but no other obvious signs of cardiovascular disease. Referral to a cardiologist to address the cause of dyspnea revealed mild left ventricular dysfunction and PH, based on diagnostic imaging findings. The client did not undergo catheterization or other invasive diagnostic procedures. Given that he was not dyspneic during lighter-intensity activity (e.g., walking the dog), he was considered to be in the relatively early stages of disease. He was prescribed an antihypertensive agent, encouraged to make dietary modifications, and encouraged to engage in a more physically active lifestyle to slow progression. He was referred to an outpatient clinic to undergo supervised exercise training, where he underwent exercise testing. He achieved 625 m (684 yd) in the 6-minute walk test, in which he achieved a heart rate of 108 beats/min and had a pulse oximetry reading of 92%. He did not undergo $\dot{V}O_2$ max testing. He was prescribed exercise at a target heart rate between 105 and 140 beats/min. He began walking for exercise, gradually progressing from 15 minutes to 30 minutes, four days per week. Additionally, he underwent supervised exercise training twice per week, during which he performed stationary cycling. The cycling was continuous intensity for the first two weeks, during which he averaged 105 to 112 beats/min for 20 minutes, with mild dyspnea at higher intensities. Interval training was then incorporated into his exercise routine, consisting of 2 minutes of higher intensity (115-125 beats/min) with 3 minutes of light pedaling as active recovery. Additionally, he performed three sets of deep breathing exercises at the end of each supervised training session. Over the course of six weeks, he progressed to 30 minutes of continuous cycling, averaging 115 beats/min without dyspnea. He reported that his symptoms of breathlessness during mowing the lawn and strenuous housework were reduced considerably, though not entirely absent.

Recommended Readings

Galiè, N, Humbert, M, Vachiery, JL, Gibbs, S, Lang, I, Torbicki, A, Simonneau, G, Peacock, A, Noordegraaf, AV, Beghetti, M, and Ghofrani, A. 2015 ESC/ERS Guidelines for the diagnosis and treatment of pulmonary hypertension. *Eur Heart J* 37:67-119, 2016.

Newman, J and Robbins, I. Exercise training in pulmonary hypertension. *Circulation* 14:1448-1449, 2006.

Pandey, A, Garg, S, Khunger, M, Garg, S, Kumbhani, DJ, Chin, KM, and Berry, JD. Efficacy and safety of exercise training in chronic pulmonary hypertension: systemic review and meta-analysis. *Circ Heart Fail* 8:1032-1043, 2015.

Pulmonary Hypertension Association. Recommendations for exercise in patients with PAH. 2016. www.phassociation.org/Patients/ExerciseConsensus. Accessed November 1, 2016.

Yuan, P, Yuan, XT, Sun, XY, Pudasaini, B, Liu, JM, and Hu, QH. Exercise training for pulmonary hypertension: a systematic review and meta-analysis. *Int J Cardiol* 178:142-146, 2015.

CHRONIC OBSTRUCTIVE PULMONARY DISEASE

Chronic obstructive pulmonary disease (COPD) is a progressive lung disease characterized by emphysema and chronic bronchitis, which decrease lung function. There is no known cure, and only heart disease and cancer kill more Americans than COPD. In the United States, more than 11 million people have been diagnosed with COPD while millions more are affected but undiagnosed (11). Worldwide, COPD mortality is rising (10), and the disease is responsible for over $36 billion in annual health care costs (9). Women are 37% more likely to have COPD than men, and about half of the deaths are in women (10). The number of individuals with COPD has increased by approximately 41% since 1982 (266).

Currently, smoking cessation is the only intervention that has conclusively been shown to slow the rate of lung function decline (286). Symptoms include chronic cough, sputum production, shortness of breath, exercise intolerance, muscle wasting, gas trapping, and frequent respiratory infections (266).

Treatment is typically SABAs, LABAs, anticholinergics, ICSs, or a combination of these drugs (217). Additionally, individuals should have an annual flu shot and the pneumococcal vaccine (217). Diagnosis of comorbid COPD and asthma occurs in 15% to 20% of individuals (189, 192, 200, 270). These individuals tend to experience more rapid disease progression than those with either disease alone (123, 170). Bronchial hyperresponsiveness and the diagnosis of asthma have been associated with greater decline in FEV_1 in both smokers and nonsmokers (181, 246, 284). The presence of BHR in individuals with COPD has been associated with an increase in exacerbations and mortality (157), and the coexistence of asthma and COPD is associated with increased health care utilization (271).

Key Point

Chronic obstructive pulmonary disease (COPD) is a progressive inflammatory lung disease that causes airflow obstruction due to thickened airway walls and inflammatory mucus due to the effects of emphysema and chronic bronchitis.

Pathology of COPD

Chronic obstructive pulmonary disease is characterized by progressive emphysema, chronic bronchitis, or both, and results in decreases in FEV_1 and FEV_1/FVC (**forced vital capacity**). These declines reflect both the reduction in exhalation force available and decline in lung capacity as a result of emphysema and obstruction to airflow in the smaller airways. Chronic obstructive pulmonary disease is characterized by airway wall thickening and by inflammatory cells in the airways. Neutrophils, T lymphocytes, and B lymphocytes are all present and contribute to lung function decline. However, airway wall thickening is strongly related to the progression of COPD (151). As COPD progresses, small airways become occluded by inflammatory mucus, which is a defining feature of chronic bronchitis. Obstruction of the small airways in COPD occurs by remodeling that is related to tissue repair and attenuated mucociliary clearance (151).

Pathophysiology of COPD

Eighty to ninety percent of COPD is related to smoking while the remainder is likely due to environmental exposure to toxic gases and particles (218). Despite the effects of smoking, Salvi and Barnes (257) presented data suggesting that the burden of nonsmoking COPD is much higher than previously believed; an estimated 25% to 45% of individuals with COPD have never smoked. Other factors that have been associated with COPD include exposure to air pollutants such as dust, cooking fumes, and internal combustion fumes; a history of repeated lower respiratory tract infections during childhood; pulmonary tuberculosis; chronic asthma; poor nourishment; poor SES; and an alpha-1 deficiency (12). Sood and colleagues (269) reported that exposure to wood smoke was associated with a 70% increased risk of COPD in both men and women in the United States, and that this association remained even after adjustment for age, tobacco smoking, and educational attainment. Likewise, biomass or coal cooking has been identified as high risk for COPD in low- and middle-income countries (126).

Airway inflammation also plays an important role in disease progression (82, 127, 128, 151, 235). The intensity of inflammation relates to the degree of airflow obstruction (82), and may result from oxidant-induced damage. About 3% of all COPD cases can be attributed to a genetic deficiency of alpha-1 antitrypsin, a condition that occurs in about 1 in 1,500 to 3,000 Americans of European descent. The main function of alpha-1 antitrypsin is to protect the lungs from inflammation caused by infection and inhaled irritants (130, 299).

Common Medications Given to Individuals With COPD

Inhaled SABAs are referred to as a "rescue" medication and used as needed. In some cases, however, inhaled SABAs are used daily. For example, albuterol and levalbuterol are often prescribed to be used as needed, while ipratropium, an anticholinergic drug, is used as a standalone drug or in combination with albuterol (Combivent).

Inhaled LABAs are used daily and should not be used as rescue medication for an acute exacerbation because they do not immediately open the airways. Long-acting β_2-agonists, such as salmeterol, formoterol, and arformoterol, are inhaled twice daily and provide 12 hours of bronchodilation. Indacaterol is also a LABA that provides 24-hour protection with a single dose, whereas tiotropium is a long-acting 24-hour anticholinergic bronchodilator.

Inhaled corticosteroids act as an anti-inflammatory medication and are often used in combination with a LABA and are taken twice daily. Examples include Advair (flovent and salmeterol), Dulera (mometasone and formoterol), Symbicort (budesonide and formoterol), and Breo (fluticasone and vilanterol). Daily ICS treatments are used to stabilize symptoms and reduce inflammation and mucus production, especially with individuals who have chronic bronchitis. A number of studies have shown ICSs to be less efficacious in COPD (29, 186, 225, 258), but an ICS combined with a LABA has beneficial airway anti-inflammatory effects not seen with ICSs alone (72). The combination of an ICS with a LABA bronchodilator improves lung function and decreases exacerbations as well as the frequency of rescue medication use (40, 140, 215, 222). Long-acting β_2-agonists and corticosteroids may interact to prevent downregulation of β_2-receptors in airway cells to prevent tachyphylaxis (265). The combination also facilitates translocation of glucocorticoid receptors into the nucleus of inflammatory cells, thereby amplifying the anti-inflammatory activity of the corticosteroid (265). Combination therapy of a LABA with an ICS improves symptom scores and reduces exacerbations by a third compared to a placebo (265).

Histone deacetylase-2 (HDAC-2) is significantly reduced in airway tissue from individuals with COPD compared with healthy nonsmokers (196). Histone deacetylase-2 has also been implicated in sensitivity to corticosteroids and plays a key role in suppressing inflammatory expression in the airways (282). Increasing HDAC-2 expression, activation, or both can be an approach to reversing corticosteroid resistance in COPD (165). Further, p38-kinase activity increases (42, 204) and interleukin production decreases (42, 58) in individuals with COPD. (Interleukin causes neutrophils to migrate, in this case, into the airways.) Another change includes a considerable increase in phosphatidylinositol-4,5-bisphosphate 3-kinase (PI3K) activity in individuals with COPD (156). The result is a loss of sensitivity to ICSs (42).

A summary of medications given to individuals with COPD is found in medications table 5.4 near the end of the chapter.

Effect of Exercise in Individuals With COPD

Exercise is considered an essential component of pulmonary rehabilitation in individuals with COPD (75, 120, 184, 220, 254). Decreased exercise capacity and loss of muscle strength disable an individual with COPD, increase time off work, increase social isolation, and contribute to mortality (78, 300). Exercise training by individuals with COPD can increase exercise capacity and improve quality of life, both socially and during daily activities (120). Additionally, an aerobic endurance exercise training program has been found to decrease systemic inflammation with a decrease in serum C-reactive protein and interleukin (303). The observed decreased dyspnea from an exercise training program in this population is not the result of improvement in lung function but rather from peripheral changes (303).

Exercise Recommendations for Clients With COPD

Although several studies have shown improvement in peripheral muscle strength, gas exchange, and aerobic endurance capacity with exercise interventions, there is no consensus on the optimal exercise program, as intensity and duration should be individualized to reflect the severity of symptoms (120) (see table 5.4). The addition of resistance training to aerobic training in clients with COPD (120) (see table 5.5) is associated with significantly greater increases in muscle strength and mass, but does not provide additional improvement in exercise capacity, dyspnea, or quality of life (37, 323). However, the addition of resistance training to an aerobic endurance program seems a reasonable strategy since muscle weakness is one of the extrapulmonary manifestations of COPD (323).

Resistance training, aerobic endurance training, and a combination resistance and aerobic endurance training program have similar efficacy for clients with COPD (160). As such, the program can be designed around the client's preference to maximize compliance. Improvements in exercise tolerance and an increase in muscle strength are indicative of a successful rehabilitation program.

Key Point

It is important that clients who have COPD follow both an aerobic training program and a resistance training program to improve their quality of life.

Table 5.4   General Aerobic Exercise Guidelines for Clients With COPD

Parameter	Guideline
Frequency	3-5 days per week
Intensity	30-80% of peak work rate*
Mode	Walking or cycling
Duration	20-60 min/session*

*Intensity and duration of exercise should be individualized to reflect the severity of symptoms.

Reference: (120)

Table 5.5   General Resistance Training Guidelines for Clients With COPD

Parameter	Guideline
Frequency	2-3 days per week
Intensity	Light to moderate; 40-80% 1RM
Repetitions	8-12
Sets	1-4
Rest periods between sets	2-3 min
Exercises	8-12 mostly large muscle groups and multijoint

Reference: (120)

Chronic Obstructive Pulmonary Disease

Mr. B is 60 years old and played ice hockey from a very young age through college. Thereafter, he exercised daily and competed in running and cross-country ski races through his 20s and 30s. He grew up in a house where both parents were smokers, and he remembers long rides in the car with the windows up and his parents smoking. When Mr. B began cross-country ski racing, it did not take too long before he was winning and training long hours. He began to develop a postrace hack and seemed to be sensitive to the volatilized fumes in the ski wax room, a place that he frequented on a daily basis. After 15 years of living in Vermont, heating with wood, and spending most winter nights in the wood-burning sauna, his family moved south.

Over time, Mr. B gradually stopped exercising due to work and family obligations. As a result, he gained about 40 pounds (18 kg), and he began to notice that it was more difficult going up stairs and that he was short of breath even with just light physical activity. He attributed this to old age and the extra body weight. He also noticed that he was constantly coughing, and he had contracted pneumonia three times in the last four years.

With encouragement from his wife, Mr. B scheduled an appointment with a pulmonologist. Findings demonstrated that his FEV_1 was 63% of predicted values with an FEV_1/FVC ratio of 68%. The reduced FEV_1 of 63% of predicted value coupled with the FEV_1/FVC ratio less than 0.70 suggests that Mr. B may have moderate COPD according to the Global Initiative for Chronic Obstructive Lung Disease criteria (table 5.6).

Table 5.6 Classification of COPD for Individuals With FEV_1/FVC Ratios Less Than 0.70

Classification	Post-bronchodilator FEV_1 reading (% of predicted)
Mild	≥80%
Moderate	50-79%
Severe	30-49%
Very severe	<30%

Adapted, by permission, from *Global Initiative for Chronic Obstructive Lung Disease*, 2016, Global strategy for the diagnosis, management, and prevention of chronic obstructive pulmonary disease.

Recommended Readings

Iepsen, UW, Jørgensen, KJ, Ringbaek, T, Hansen, H, Skrubbeltrang, C, and Lange, P. A systematic review of resistance training versus endurance training in COPD. *J Cardiopulm Rehabil Prev* 35:163-172, 2015.

National Heart, Lung, and Blood Institute. What Is COPD? 2014. www.nhlbi.nih.gov/health/health-topics/topics/copd/. Accessed January 27, 2017.

Pothirat, C, Chaiwong, W, Phetsuk, N, Liwsrisakun, C, Bumroongkit, C, Deesomchok, A, Theerakittikul, T, and Limsukon, A. Long-term efficacy of intensive cycle ergometer exercise training program for advanced COPD patients. *Int J Chron Obstruct Pulmon Dis.* 10:133-144, 2015.

Salvi, SS and Barnes, PJ. Chronic obstructive pulmonary disease in non-smokers. *Lancet* 374:733-743, 2009.

Spruit, MA, Singh, SJ, Garvey, C, ZuWallack, R, Nici, L, Rochester, C, Hill, K, Holland, AE, Lareau, SC, Man, WDC, and Pitta, F. An official American Thoracic Society/European Respiratory Society statement: key concepts and advances in pulmonary rehabilitation. *Am J Respir Crit Care Med* 188:e13-e64, 2013.

Wootton, SL, Ng, LC, McKeough, ZJ, Jenkins, S, Hill, K, Eastwood, PR, Hillman, DR, Cecins, N, Spencer, LM, Jenkins, C, and Alison, JA. Ground-based walking training improves quality of life and exercise capacity in COPD. *Eur Respir J* 44:885-894, 2014.

CHRONIC RESTRICTIVE PULMONARY DISEASE

Restrictive disease occurs from conditions that cause the restriction of lung expansion, loss of lung tissue, and a decrease in gas diffusion both in and out of the lungs. Dyspnea is compensated for by rapid breathing and shallow breaths. **Chronic restrictive pulmonary disease (CRPD)** is characterized by a decrease in total lung capacity (TLC), a modestly preserved FEV_1, airway resistance, and a decreased FVC that result in a FEV_1/FVC ratio greater than 80%. Restrictive lung disease is also characterized by a reduction in **functional residual capacity** (FRC, the volume of air in the lungs when respiratory muscles are fully relaxed).

Pathology and Pathophysiology of CRPD

Individuals with CRPD and disorders of the **pulmonary parenchyma** (the covering of the lungs) may experience increased effort of breathing and an exercise-related desaturation from a decreased gas transfer. In disorders of the pleura and thoracic cage, the abnormal compliance of the respiratory system results in a ventilation–perfusion mismatch and desaturation. Severe conditions of the spine, such as kyphosis, can result in respiratory failure and obesity and have been shown to dramatically reduce FRC (166).

Restrictive diseases are generally classified as intrinsic or extrinsic (table 5.7). Intrinsic restrictive disease is characterized by general fibrosis of lung parenchyma, while extrinsic resistive disease may involve the chest wall, pleura, respiratory muscles, or neuromuscular disorders. Dust, gases, fumes, fiberglass, and asbestos are occupational and environmental irritants that can cause CRPD. Additionally, radiation, medications, poisons, and autoimmune responses all have been linked to CRPD.

The prevalence and incidence of these conditions vary. While there is an overall prevalence of 3 to 6 cases per 100,000 for intrinsic lung diseases, the prevalence for idiopathic pulmonary fibrosis (IPF) is 27.9 to 63 cases per 100,000 (234). The prevalence for adults aged 35 to 44 is 2.7 per 100,000 and 175 cases per 100,000 for adults older than 75 years of age (273). In the United States, the prevalence of sarcoidosis is 10 to 40 per 100,000 and is 10 to 17 times higher in African Americans (273), with 1 in 10,000 persons having severe kyphosis (273).

Therapy of CRPD

Treatment strategies for CRPD are on an individual basis depending on disease severity, stability, and clinical history. Nonpharmacological treatments focus on avoiding airborne irritants (e.g., combustion exhaust and airborne trichloramines from indoor pools) and ceasing smoking and exposure to second-hand smoke, maintaining blood oxygen levels over 90% (as measured by pulse oximetry), participating in a structured exercise program (including breathing exercises, anxiety management, nutritional counseling, and health education), and considering flu and pneumonia vaccinations.

For individuals who have end-stage CRPD and have exhausted their treatment options with no attenuation of disease progression, a lung transplant is an option. The number of lung transplants performed each year in the United States is 1,400 with 2,000 on a waiting list at any given time (142). The 1-year survival rate after a lung transplant is about 90% with the 5-year survival rate of approximately 55%; only 33% survive 10 years (142). The median survival rate for adult recipients of a dual lung transplantation is 5.7 years, with bilateral transplants having a better survival rate of 7 years (320). The primary reason that individuals die from lung transplants is because of chronic rejection and subsequent deterioration of the transplanted lung. However, immunosuppression decreases the effectiveness of the immune system, leaving the individual vulnerable to infections.

Table 5.7 General Classifications of Intrinsic and Extrinsic Restrictive Pulmonary Diseases

INTRINSIC	
Disease or condition	**Cause or description**
Pneumoconiosis	Condition due to dust or environmental exposures (e.g., asbestosis, black lung, siderosis).
Radiation fibrosis	A complication of radiation treatment.
Hypersensitivity pneumonitis	Allergic reaction to inhaled particles.
Acute respiratory distress syndrome	Widespread inflammation triggered by another disease such as pneumonia or from trauma.
Infant respiratory distress syndrome	A developmental insufficiency of surfactant in the lungs. It is the leading cause of death in premature infants.
Tuberculosis	An infectious disease that is more common in individuals with HIV/AIDS and those who smoke. Approximately 5-10% of the U.S. population tests positive.
Idiopathic pulmonary fibrosis	No known cause. Involves the pulmonary interstitium and is associated with smoking.
Idiopathic interstitial pneumonia	Affects the pulmonary interstitium. May be related to pneumonia or drug toxicity.
Sarcoidosis	Can affect any organ and may be due to an abnormal immune response.
Eosinophilic pneumonia	High eosinophils; cause can be medication or an environmental trigger, parasitic infection, cancer, or immune response.
Lymphangioleiomyomatosis	Rare systemic disease that causes cystic lung destruction. Predominately in young women with tuberous sclerosis complex.
Langerhans cell histiocytosis	Rare disease that occurs almost exclusively in cigarette smokers. Abnormal proliferation of Langerhans cells that results in fibrosis.
Alveolar proteinosis	Rare disease characterized by accumulation of surfactant in alveoli, disrupting gas exchange. Trigger can be environmental exposure, malignancy, or lung infection.
EXTRINSIC	
Disease or condition	**Cause or description**
Kyphosis, pectus carinatum, pectus excavatum	Nonmuscular diseases of upper thorax. Lungs may not function optimally and gas exchange can be affected.
Obesity, diaphragmatic hernia, ascites	Obesity has been associated with asthma and affects tidal volume while breathing. Ascites is the accumulation of fluid in the peritoneal cavity usually caused by cirrhosis or liver disease.

Reference: (49)

Common Medications Given to Individuals With CRPD

The pharmacological treatment of CRPD includes corticosteroids, cyclophosphamide, nintedanib, pirfenidone, and supplemental oxygen therapy. Oral corticosteroids are used to suppress the immune system and decrease inflammation and are often supplemented with co-trimoxazole and macrolides for individuals with IPF who have a rapid progression of respiratory failure (226). Unfortunately, OCS use has been associated with increased risk of fracture and cataracts, adrenal suppression, and weight gain (4-6, 297). Further, Hanada and colleagues (139) found that long-term OCS treatment contributed to muscle weakness in individuals with interstitial lung disease. A combination of an ICS and a LABA has been shown to decrease frequency and severity of acute episodes and improve lung function in individuals with combined IPF and emphysema (86).

Cyclophosphamide suppresses inflammation and has been used to treat certain forms of pulmonary fibrosis. Cyclophosphamide treatments result in lung function stabilization in most individuals with fibrotic interstitial lung disease (260).

The drug is predominately taken orally but may also be administered intravenously. Nintedanib is an antifibrotic kinase inhibitor drug approved to treat IPF in the United States. In clinical trials, nintedanib has been shown to slow the decline in lung function in mild-to-moderate IPF (245). Pirfenidone is an antifibrotic and anti-inflammatory drug approved to treat IPF in the United States, Europe, Canada, and Asia. In clinical trials, pirfenidone has been shown to slow progression of mild-to-moderate IPF (262).

Supplemental oxygen therapy is also a treatment strategy for CRPD. Because scar tissue in the lungs diminishes movement of oxygen from the alveoli to the bloodstream and carbon dioxide from the blood to the alveoli, oxygen levels decrease in the blood in individuals with CRPD. Therefore, supplemental oxygen might be prescribed, but if oxygen levels are always low (<90%), then continuous supplemental oxygen may be required.

A summary of medications given to individuals with CRPD is found in medications table 5.5 near the end of the chapter.

Effects of Exercise in Individuals With CRPD

Pulmonary fibrosis is characterized by diminished exercise capacity due to progressive pulmonary restriction, decreased FVC, ventilatory inefficiency, impaired gas exchange, low oxygen saturation, and dyspnea (205, 241). A characteristic of IPF is lowered arterial oxygen pressure and saturation during exercise (152, 180). Exercise is typically recommended for individuals with lung disease although it may not improve fibrotic scarring. It will, however, improve the cardiovascular system and the ability of the muscles to use oxygen and decrease symptoms of dyspnea, thereby allowing a higher quality of life (88). Exercise is also helpful in preventing the deconditioning and weakness that occur when individuals with CRPD become less active due to dyspnea.

Exercise capacity is generally related to the severity of the disease. Vainshelboim and colleagues (292) identified a peak work rate of 62 watts (379 kgm/min), $\dot{V}O_2$peak of 13.8 ml $\cdot$ kg^{-1} $\cdot$ min^{-1}, tidal volume reserve of 0.48 L/breath, and a minute ventilation-to-carbon dioxide ratio at the anaerobic threshold of 34 as cutoff points associated with mortality in individuals with IPF. Leuchte and colleagues (185) found that comorbid PH significantly contributed to exercise limitations in individuals with severe lung fibrosis and suggested that treatment of PH may be beneficial in these individuals.

Cardiopulmonary exercise testing (CPET) for exercise tolerance evaluation should be done to aid in diagnosis and prognosis as well as for developing effective targeted treatments. Cardiopulmonary exercise testing can identify the presence of comorbidities in approximately 38% of individuals with IPF (291). Resting cardiopulmonary function can show moderate pulmonary restriction and impairments in diffusion capacity. Multifactorial limitations for a moderately diminished aerobic capacity can be revealed during CPET, although functional capacity can be normal. In a study by Vainshelboim and colleagues (291), aerobic capacity of 13.4 ml $\cdot$ kg^{-1} $\cdot$ min^{-1} (62% of predicted) was reduced with the presence of abnormalities in pulmonary gas exchange and desaturation, circulatory impairments, inefficient ventilation, and skeletal muscle dysfunction; however, functional capacity measured by the 6-minute walk test was normal (distance = 505 m [552 yd], 99% of predicted).

Key Point

People who have CRPD benefit from cardiopulmonary exercise testing because the results reveal an individual's tolerance for exercise, which is an important factor to consider when developing an effective exercise program.

In another study, Porteous and colleagues (237) suggested that right ventricular morphology, pulmonary vascular resistance, and FVC may improve exercise capacity in individuals with IPF. They found that right ventricular dilation was associated with a decrease of 50.9 m (56 yd) in the 6-minute walk test. For each 200-ml reduction in FVC, the walk distance decreased by 15 m (16 yd) (237).

Exercise Recommendations for Clients With CRPD

Current evidence indicates that exercise training in clients with CRPD is safe and beneficial at improving dyspnea and measures of quality of life (88, 290). Whole-body exercise training is a primary component of pulmonary rehabilitation for interstitial lung disease (ILD), and the standard exercise prescription for other chronic lung diseases is effective in ILD. The program often includes eight weeks of training with at least two supervised sessions per week and a minimum 30 minutes of aerobic training in each session. However, the unique presentation and underlying pathophysiology of ILD can require modifications in exercise prescription. Clients with connective tissue disorders may present with joint pain that requires alterations in exercise, which may involve a reduction in weight-bearing exercise. Clients with severe disease may present with severe dyspnea that can limit the intensity of exercise and training progression. Because exercise-induced hypoxemia is common in ILD and is more severe than seen in other chronic lung diseases, rehabilitation programs should include supplemental oxygen therapy. Pulmonary rehabilitation programs should also offer the opportunity to address the management of comorbidities, symptoms, and psychological factors (153).

It has been shown that a three-month rehabilitation program can significantly improve symptoms and physical activity levels in clients with IPF (122). This investigation also showed that while in the rehabilitation program, the rehabilitation group maintained higher levels of physical activity throughout the three-month program than the control group. Also, symptom scores improved by 9 ± 22 in the rehabilitation group and worsened in the control group (16 ± 12) (122). During a three-month follow-up in that study, self-reported physical activity levels (i.e., a metabolic equivalent of task-minutes) in the rehabilitation group were not different than those of the control group, demonstrating reversal of activity in the rehabilitation group; however, scores after the 6-minute walk tests did not change significantly.

A 12-week physical training program has been shown to improve or maintain exercise capacity in clients with IPF (despite disease progression) or fibrotic sarcoidosis (279). After completion of the 12-week program, exercise capacity (as measured by the 6-minute walk test) improved by 10% in 13 of 24 subjects (54.2%), 7 with IPF and 6 with sarcoidosis (279).

The 6-minute walk test has been shown to be a valid and responsive endpoint that can provide objective and clinically relevant information about the functional status and prognosis of clients with IPF. An analysis of 338 individuals with IPF showed that a baseline 6-minute walk test was significantly correlated with lung function measurements, patient-reported outcomes, and quality of life measures. Compared to the baseline, a change in the 6-minute walk test showed stronger correlations with change in lung function measurements and quality of life measures (216).

Improvements in dyspnea, 6-minute walk test, $\dot{V}O_2$, lactate threshold, and quality of life scores have been noted from pulmonary rehabilitation exercise programs in clients with IPF (77, 289, 293, 294). Pulmonary rehabilitation programs can also improve body composition and help the client maintain an appropriate body weight. Excess body weight can increase dyspnea during daily activities and affect the overall health of the client as discussed in other chapters. Clients with IPF and a BMI of >30 kg/m^2 who received a bilateral lung transplant were 1.71 times more likely to die within 90 days than bilateral lung transplant recipients with a BMI of 18.5 to 30 kg/m^2 (131). Rehabilitation programs can be inpatient, outpatient, or combined, or they can be community-based programs.

Given that CRPD refers to many diseases that are collectively grouped, research to determine exercise guidelines typically focuses on one of these conditions. This restricts the capacity to provide, or at least raises caution about providing, global exercise prescription recommendations for clients with CRPD. At a minimum, it is recommended that clients with CRPD be tested in a medically supervised setting to determine their symptom thresholds for exercise intensity and duration before initiating an exercise program, and that an individualized training plan based on these results be designed and implemented by a qualified exercise professional.

Chronic Restrictive Pulmonary Disease

Mr. J, a 69-year-old male with rheumatoid arthritis, presented at his annual checkup with a 10-month history of respiratory symptoms that included thoracic pain, chronic dry cough, and dyspnea upon exertion. His history included six years of working construction, where he had repeated exposure to fiberglass insulation and asbestos. Mr. J also grew up in a smoking household. He also had a smoking history of approximately eight years after college but managed to quit. At age 32, he began an exercise program, and after 20 years he stopped exercising because of work and life demands. At 64, he began exercising again and could not believe how hard it was to get back in good physical condition. He began with a walking program five days per week and after about six months began jogging, but he got very dyspneic. He thought it was probably the extra weight he had put on, but as he lost weight, the dyspnea did not improve and he gradually stopped exercising.

Pulmonary function tests revealed a modest decline of 10% below predicted FEV_1 with an FVC of 78% of predicted. On subsequent visits, Mr. J performed a 6-minute walk test (he covered 300 m [328 yd], with an exercise oxygen saturation of 84%), and a high-resolution computed tomography (CT) chest scan was performed (it revealed emphysema). Mr. J was diagnosed with combined pulmonary fibrosis and emphysema and desquamative interstitial pneumonia (DIP).

Treatment options were discussed and imple-mented. Treatment involved pharmacological interventions for mild-to-moderate IPF and an antidepressant. Mr. J was vaccinated for influenza and pneumococci and referred to an outpatient rehabilitation center.

Mr. J's exposure to tobacco smoke, fiberglass, and asbestos should not be ignored, especially considering his reported dyspnea during exercise and initial test results. His subsequent test results suggested IPF. His smoking and environmental exposure combined with dyspnea, chronic cough, and rheumatoid arthritis were suggestive of DIP, while the CT scan indicated emphysema.

The pulmonary rehabilitation program should include exercise training, nutritional counseling, energy-conserving techniques, breathing strategies, and psychological coun-seling. The exercise program should be based on pulmonary function test results, a physical exam, 6-minute walk test results, and perhaps exercising $\dot{V}O_2$, oxygen saturation, and disease stage. The program should include a plan to improve aerobic endurance and muscle strength to enable Mr. J to better carry out daily activities. The plan should include exercises for both arms and legs using a treadmill, stationary bike, or resistance training exercises. If long-duration exercise sessions are too difficult, the plan may involve short sessions repeated with rest breaks in between. While Mr. J is exercising, his blood oxygen levels may be monitored with a pulse oximeter attached to a finger.

Recommended Readings

Kagaya, H, Takahashi, H, Sugarwara, K, Kasai, C, Kiyokawa, N, and Shikoya, T. Effective home-based pulmonary rehabilitation in patients with restrictive lung diseases. *Tohoku J Exp Med* 218:215-219, 2009.

Markovitz, GH and Cooper, CB. Rehabilitation in non-COPD: mechanisms of exercise limitation and pulmonary rehabilitation for patients with pulmonary fibrosis/restrictive lung disease. *Chron Respir Dis* 7:47-60, 2010.

Troosters, R, Gosselink, R, Janssens, W, and Decramer, M. Exercise training and pulmonary rehabilitation: new insights and remaining challenges. *Eur Respir Rev* 19:24-29, 2010.

Vogiatzis, I, Zakynthinos, G, and Andrianopoulos, V. Mechanisms of physical activity limitation in chronic lung diseases. *Pulm Med* 2012:634761, 2012.

CYSTIC FIBROSIS

Cystic fibrosis (CF) is one of the most common life-limiting autosomal recessive diseases in the Caucasian population. As of 2015 there were 28,983 people living with CF in the United States (69). In the 1960s, the predicted median age of survival was 10 years; however, in 2015 it was 41.7 years (69). From 2000 to 2015, the percentage of individuals in whom CF could be detected at birth increased from 3.1% to 59.6% (69).

Pathology and Pathophysiology of CF

Cystic fibrosis is a multiorgan system disease caused by a mutation in a protein called the **cystic fibrosis transmembrane regulator (CFTR)**, which is located on the membrane of many cells and allows chloride and water to move out of cells into the lumen of many organs. Cystic fibrosis transmembrane regulator is located in cells that line the airway, sinuses, pancreas, intestine, bile duct, sweat gland, and vas deferens, which accounts for the clinical features. When the CFTR is defective, secretions outside the cell are not hydrated with water. Secretions become thick and viscous and may obstruct the organs. Local inflammation also occurs, which may injure and destroy the cells.

Almost all individuals with CF have significant sinusitis (74). In 85% of individuals, the pancreas is destroyed and the digestive exocrine enzymes cannot be produced (26, 242). Pancreatic insufficiency causes malnutrition, diarrhea, and fat-soluble vitamin deficiency. In the second to third decades of life, pancreatic endocrine function is often impaired and individuals develop diabetes (87, 315). In the gastrointestinal tract, obstruction from viscous secretions may result in intestinal obstruction, and rectal prolapse may

Key Point

Clients who have CF are at a greater risk than others to have diabetes, so an exercise professional, as directed by the client's physician or other health care professional, may need to modify the client's exercise program to account for any limitations.

occur (315). Cholestasis is also often present in individuals with CF and can cause cholelithiasis, liver injury, and cirrhosis (174). It is hypothesized that the obstruction of the vas deferens produces azoospermia and infertility (242, 298).

Pulmonary disease is the leading cause of mortality and morbidity in individuals with CF (36). Individuals born with CF have normal lungs, but thick secretions are inadequately cleared from the airways. The airways become inflamed and injured, which leads to bacterial colonization. Initially, infants are colonized with organisms such as staphylococcus aureus or haemophilus influenza (267). Later in life, individuals with CF are colonized with more virulent organisms such as pseudomonas aeruginosa (267), resulting in irreversible airway injury or **bronchiectasis** (a condition in which the walls of the bronchi are thickened from inflammation and infection), which leads to deterioration in lung function and potentially respiratory failure (242). The increased airway inflammation causes hemoptysis that erodes into bronchial veins or arteries and may cause acute failure.

Individuals with CF develop cough, wheezing, and bronchitis as their airways are hyperreactive and bronchoconstrict in response to irritants, exercise, and viral and bacterial infections. As the disease progresses, they develop worsening lower airway obstruction and frequent exacerbations characterized by an increased cough with productive sputum, dyspnea, hemoptysis, deterioration in lung function, and weight loss (111). Because of their COPD, illness, and malabsorption of vitamins and minerals, individuals with CF can develop postural abnormalities such as thoracic kyphosis, decreased bone mineral density, musculoskeletal pain, and arthritis (22, 45, 230).

Therapy and Common Medications Given to Individuals With CF

Therapy for CF is characterized as preventive and rescue. The primary therapy is geared toward improving mobilization of secretions, minimizing inflammation and lung injury, and decreasing bacterial colonization (195, 242). The cornerstone of CF therapy is chest physiotherapy (224). Chest physiotherapy may be performed individually by controlled, active breathing and coughing exercises. It may also be administered manually by a caregiver using percussion and postural drainage. Mucous clearance can be augmented by vests that give high-frequency chest compression (112). Handheld devices may also increase clearance by providing oscillation or positive expiratory pressure to the airways (112). Playing a wind instrument, singing, and jumping on trampolines have also been shown to be effective ways to promote mucous clearance (73).

A number of other agents are important in maintaining pulmonary function and decreasing exacerbations in individuals with CF. Inhaled hypertonic saline hydrates demonstrate efficacy in improving clearance of secretions (243, 283). Inhaled dornase alfa is used to reduce the viscosity of the purulent secretions to aid in clearance (132, 209). Oral ibuprofen and corticosteroids have also been used to decrease inflammation (27, 209).

Antibiotics are administered both preventively and for exacerbations. For example, nebulized antibiotics such as aminoglycosides are used to decrease bacterial colonization in individuals colonized with pseudomonas (100). Oral azithromycin, which has anti-inflammatory and antibiotic properties, may be given as a preventive measure (256). For individuals with pulmonary exacerbations, oral antibiotics are routinely given (44); however, if there is no clinical improvement, then intravenous antibiotics are typically prescribed (65). Finally, ivacaftor targets the defective CFTR and improves lung function in individuals with CF.

Nutritional support is of the utmost importance in individuals with CF who have pancreatic insufficiency associated with malabsorption of fats, vitamins, and minerals. Better lung function has been correlated to better nutritional status (268). Oral pancreatic enzymes are commonly administered, as well as fat-soluble vitamins (A, D, E, and K) to improve lipid digestion and absorption in pancreatic-insufficient individuals with CF (39, 83, 85, 99). In addition, high-calorie nutritional supplements are routinely given because of the generally low nutritional status in these individuals (1).

A summary of medications given to individuals with CF is found in medications table 5.6 near the end of the chapter.

Effects of Exercise in Individuals With CF

Unfortunately, individuals with CF participate in fewer hours of vigorous physical activity than their healthy counterparts (221). However, aerobic and anaerobic physical training have positive effects on their exercise capacity, strength, lung function, and health-related quality of life (212, 240). Physical training has also been used to improve sputum clearance and improve pulmonary function (244, 322) and it may be as effective as conventional percussion and postural drainage (55, 244, 321).

However, in individuals with CF, both the pulmonary disease and malnutrition may limit the ability to exercise (64, 232, 288). Progressive lung disease is associated with ventilatory limitation and dyspnea. Individuals with severe lung disease can develop arterial hypoxemia and carbon dioxide retention with exercise (30, 104, 129). Persons with CF are at risk for severe dehydration from exercise (177). They have elevated levels of sodium chloride in their sweat and can develop hyponatremic hypochloremic dehydration and are also at risk for pneumothorax and hemoptysis (103, 172). In addition, an individual with CF has a higher than normal loss of sodium chloride in the sweat, which can lead to a diminished thirst drive and possible voluntary dehydration (177).

Exercise Recommendations for Clients With CF

It is useful to have baseline cardiopulmonary exercise testing on clients with CF before beginning an exercise program in order to assess their current level of fitness and to enable effective exercise programming. Cardiopulmonary responses to exercise, including intensity and duration of exercise before the onset of coughing or other symptoms, a baseline maximal heart rate, and a goal rate of perceived exertion (for subsequent exercise prescription purposes), should be determined in this initial assessment (144).

The initial assessment should also include an evaluation of the client's posture, neuromuscular control of the muscles of the trunk (especially the abdominal muscles, obliques, lumbar extensors, and scapular retractors), and alignments of the spine, shoulder, scapulae, and rib cage. Clients with CF recruit abdominal muscles at lower workloads of exercise, earlier in the respiratory cycle, and to a higher recruitment level than clients without CF (56). Further, young adults with CF have compromised plate-like axial trabecular morphology that may increase fracture independent of normal bone mineral density (239).

A number of exercise programs for clients with CF have demonstrated an increase in both aerobic and anaerobic capacity, improvement in pulmonary function, and strengthened ventilatory muscles (23, 133, 145, 173, 261). Improved sputum clearance has also been related to exercise and is likely a mechanical airway clearance from the increased exercising ventilation (182). However, moderate-intensity exercise has been shown to block respiratory epithelial cell sodium channels, which could result in decreased mucus viscosity and enhanced expectoration (143). Moreover, a higher physical activity level and $\dot{V}O_2$ max are positively related to survival in CF (211, 236). Although most CF training studies have focused on aerobic training and have demonstrated improved lung function, $\dot{V}O_2$ max, dyspnea, and quality of life (259, 261, 287), anaerobic training may have different effects than aerobic training (43). Both aerobic and anaerobic training have been shown to improve muscle strength and muscle size, resulting in an increase in lean muscle mass (173, 227, 261). Therefore, the training program could include a variety of activities adapted to a client's needs and preferences to promote compliance and consistency for the long term.

Clients need to learn how to assess their own exertion level; this is often difficult due to ventilatory limitations and fluctuating health status (149), but it can be accomplished with heart rate monitoring, measures of dyspnea, or a Borg or OMNI scale of perceived exertion. The OMNI scale combines an exertion scale that is linked to a verbal and pictorial representation of increasing states of exertion ranging from not tired at all (0) to very tired (10) [(149)]. Children with CF appear capable of using the OMNI scale to regulate exercise intensity (149). Initially, vital signs such as respiratory rate, oxygen saturation, and rate of perceived exertion should also be monitored closely.

Key Point

Ventilatory limitations and fluctuating health status will affect the ability of a client who has CF to determine intensity during an exercise session. In conjunction with objective clinical monitoring, the client can use a Borg or OMNI scale to subjectively describe exercise intensity.

Aerobic exercise should optimally include three to five sessions per week and reach 70% of peak heart rate for 20 to 30 minutes (259, 261); however, exercise should be terminated if the Borg scale reaches 7 (on a 10-point scale). If necessary, the intensity should be modified to allow 30 minutes in the target heart rate range. Ideal exercises are walking and cycling. The client should have a cooldown period of light exercise for 10 minutes (68). See table 5.8 for a summary of the general aerobic exercise guidelines for clients with CF.

While some research evidence exists as to the efficacy of resistance training for clients with CF for improving various measures of strength and quality of life, there are currently insufficient data to provide guidelines for optimal resistance

Table 5.8 General Aerobic Exercise Guidelines for Clients With CF

Parameter	Guideline
Frequency	3-5 days per week
Intensity	40-70% of peak heart rate*
Mode	Walking, treadmill, cycling
Duration	20-30 min

Note: Maintaining adequate hydration pre-, during, and postexercise is very important.

*Intensity should be modified to allow 30 minutes in target heart rate range.

References: (259, 261)

training prescription (233, 264, 295). Studies have largely individualized prescribed programming based on initial testing results, and while the weight of available evidence is positive, systematic reviews highlight that this individualized approach limits the ability to provide specific guidelines. General guidelines include focusing on training the postural muscles (187, 197), making the loads progressive (227, 255, 295), and mobilizing tight joints and retraining the muscles that support them.

Once an exercise program is implemented, it is worthwhile to have a follow-up evaluation to reinforce the program and reassess tolerance in a client with CF. Also, after any pulmonary exacerbations, the client's exercise tolerance will need to be reassessed, and therefore a new program will need to be devised. If the client with CF develops a new oxygen requirement, formal cardiopulmonary exercise testing should also be repeated.

In addition, it is very important for clients with CF to maintain adequate hydration before, during, and after exercise. To aid with this, they should be encouraged to exercise during the cooler morning or evening hours or go to an air-conditioned facility.

Case Study

Cystic Fibrosis

Terrell, a 17-year-old male with CF, was referred for an exercise program. Lung function testing revealed that he had a mild decrease in FEV_1 of 2.96, which was 78% of his predicted normal value. He underwent cardiopulmonary testing using bicycle ergometry and reached 120 watts (734 kgm/min) with a maximal heart rate of 145 beats/min. His Borg score was 6 (on a 10-point scale) at maximum. His $\dot{V}O_2$ peak was 50 ml · kg^{-1} · min^{-1}, which was 77% of predicted. He was instructed to use the cycle ergometer for 30 minutes daily, keeping his targeted heart rate close to 110 beats/min and Borg score less than 5. He was monitored during his exercise for two weeks and intensities were adjusted as necessary. This would serve as one of his three daily recommended periods of chest physiotherapy.

Recommended Readings

Bradley, J and Moran, F. Physical training for cystic fibrosis. *Cochrane Database Syst Rev* 5:1-59, 2011.

Cropp, GJ, Pullano, TP, Cerny, FJ, and Nathanson, IT. Exercise tolerance and cardiorespiratory adjustments at peak work capacity in cystic fibrosis. *Am Rev Respir Dis* 126:211-216, 1982.

Dwyer, TJ, Alison, JA, McKeough, ZJ, Daviskas, E, and Bye, PT. Effects of exercise on respiratory flow and sputum properties in patients with cystic fibrosis. *Chest* 139:870-877, 2011.

Mogayzel, PJ, Naureckas, ET, Robinson, KA, Mueller, G, Hadjiliadis, D, Hoag, JB, Lubsch, L, Hazle, L, Sabadosa, K, Marshall, B, and the Pulmonary Clinical Practice Guidelines Committee. Cystic fibrosis pulmonary guidelines: chronic medications for maintenance of lung health. *Am J Respir Crit Care Med* 187:680-689, 2013.

O'Neill, PA, Dodds, M, Phillips, B, Poole, J, and Webb, AK. Regular exercise and reduction of breathlessness in patients with cystic fibrosis. *Br J Dis Chest* 81:62-69, 1987.

Radtke, T, Nolan, SJ, Hebestreit, H, and Kriemler, S. Physical exercise training for cystic fibrosis. *Paediatr Respir Rev* 19, 42-45, 2016.

Ratjen, F and Tullis, E. Cystic fibrosis. In *Clinical Respiratory Medicine: Expert Consult.* 4th ed. Spiro, SG, Silvestri, GA, and Agusti, A, eds. Philadelphia: Elsevier, 568-579, 2012.

Rowe, SM, Miller, S, and Sorscher, EJ. Cystic fibrosis. *N Engl J Med* 352:1992-2001, 2005.

Zach, M, Oberwaldner, B, and Hausler, F. Cystic fibrosis: physical exercise versus chest physiotherapy. *Arch Dis Child* 57:587-589, 1982.

CONCLUSION

This chapter examined and explained how regular physical activity can provide various positive benefits to persons with lung disease, including improvements in symptom expression, overall health, quality of life, reduced medication use, muscular and cardiovascular strength, and pulmonary performance. The effects of an exercise program also include a decrease in the severity of EIB if appropriate understanding of the pathophysiology of the condition and corresponding individualized attention are devoted to triggers, medication, and exercise stimuli. The exercise professional can have a profound positive impact on the quality of life, health, and fitness of clients with asthma, exercise-induced bronchoconstriction, pulmonary hypertension, chronic obstructive pulmonary disease, chronic restrictive pulmonary disease, and cystic fibrosis.

Key Terms

asthma
bronchiectasis
cardiac index
chronic obstructive pulmonary disease (COPD)
chronic restrictive pulmonary disease (CRPD)
cystic fibrosis (CF)
cystic fibrosis transmembrane regulator (CFTR)
dyspnea
exercise-induced bronchoconstriction (EIB)
exercise pulmonary hypertension

forced expiratory volume in the first second (FEV_1)
forced vital capacity
functional residual capacity
idiopathic
prophylaxis
pulmonary arterial hypertension (PAH)
pulmonary arterial pressure (PAP)
pulmonary hypertension (PH)
pulmonary parenchyma
syncope
tachyphylaxis

Study Questions

1. Which class of medications improves pulmonary function for nearly all clients who experience exercise-induced bronchoconstriction?

   a. leukotriene modifiers

   b. β_2-adrenergic agonists

   c. inhaled corticosteroids

   d. monoclonal antibodies

2. A decrease in FEV_1 is the primary diagnostic evidence for which of the following disorders?

   a. chronic obstructive pulmonary disease

   b. exercise-induced bronchoconstriction

   c. pulmonary hypertension

   d. asthma

3. Nutritional support for clients with cystic fibrosis might include which of the following?

   a. vitamin A, D, E, and K supplements

   b. high-fiber foods

   c. glycolytic enzymes

   d. calcium supplements

4. For clients with pulmonary hypertension, which of the following is true regarding exercise prescription?

  a. Interval training has been shown to be effective, but exercise testing should be done to determine severity of the disease.

  b. The Valsalva maneuver is actually encouraged, because it can improve respiratory muscle strength.

  c. Only light exercise is recommended, because moderate or higher intensity can increase pulmonary arterial blood pressure to harmful levels.

  d. Exercise is effective for clients with pulmonary arterial hypertension but not for clients for whom the cause of hypertension is unknown.

Medications Table 5.1 Common Anti-Inflammatory Controller Medications Used to Treat Asthma and EIB

Drug name	Chemical family
beclomethasone dipropionate	Corticosteroid
budesonide	Corticosteroid
flunisolide	Corticosteroid
fluticasone propionate	Corticosteroid
triamcinolone acetonide	Corticosteroid
montelukast	Leukotriene modifier
zafirlukast	Leukotriene modifier
zileuton	Leukotriene modifier
salmeterol	Long-acting β_2-agonist
theophylline	Methylxanthine

References: (95, 198)

Medications Table 5.2 Common Short-Acting Reliever Medications Used to Treat Asthma and EIB

Drug name	Chemical family
albuterol	Short-acting β_2-agonists
bitolterol	Short-acting β_2-agonists
metaproterenol	Short-acting β_2-agonists
pirbuterol	Short-acting β_2-agonists
terbutaline	Short-acting β_2-agonists
methylprednisolone	Oral corticosteroid
prednisolone	Oral corticosteroid
prednisone	Oral corticosteroid
ipratropium bromide	Anticholinergic

References: (95, 198)

Medications Table 5.3 Common Medications Used to Treat PH

Drug class and names	Mechanism of action	Most common side effects	Effects on exercise
Endothelin receptor antagonists			
ambrisentan (Letairis), bosentan (Tracleer), macitentan (Opsumit)	Block endothelin receptors of the smooth muscle of blood vessels, thus inhibiting pulmonary vasoconstriction	Peripheral edema, headache, flushing, throat irritation and respiratory tract infections, nausea, anemia, syncope	Improve exercise tolerance and delay time to worsening clinical symptoms
Phosphodiesterase inhibitors			
sildenafil (Revatio), tadalafil (Adcirca), vardenafil (Levitra, Staxyn)	Inhibition of cyclic GMP degradation thereby increasing nitric oxide bioavailability and subsequently increasing vasodilation	Headache, dyspepsia, nausea, flushing, visual disturbances, myalgia	No change in exercise capacity
Prostacyclin analogues			
epoprostenol (Flolan, Veletri), iloprost (Ventavis), treprostinil (Tyvaso)	Activate the prostacyclin pathway	Headache, hypotension, flushing, flulike symptoms, cough, throat irritation, nausea	Possible small improvement in exercise capacity or no change depending on symptom class level

References: (96, 117, 161, 191, 275)

Medications Table 5.4 Common Medications Used to Treat COPD

Drug class and names	Mechanism of action	Most common side effects	Effects on exercise
Short-acting (4-6 h) bronchodilators			
β_2-agonists: albuterol (Ventolin, Combivent), salbutamol (Airomir), levalbuterol (Xopenex HFA)	Cause bronchodilation by binding to airway β_2-adrenergic receptors resulting in smooth muscle relaxation of the airways	Headache, tachycardia, palpitations, muscle tremors, anxiety, nausea	Improve exercise tolerance by achieving relief of COPD symptoms
anticholinergics: ipratropium (Atrovent)	Causes bronchodilation (via smooth muscle relaxation) by nonselectively inhibiting muscarinic acetylcholine receptors, thereby reducing acetylcholine availability of the parasympathetic nerves that cause bronchoconstriction	Headache, cough, dry "cotton" mouth	No ergogenic effect
Long-acting (up to 12-24 h) bronchodilators			
β_2-agonists: salmeterol (Serevent), formoterol (Foradil Aerolizer), arformoterol (Brovana), indacaterol (Arcapta Neohaler)	Cause bronchodilation by binding to airway β_2-adrenergic receptors, resulting in smooth muscle relaxation of the airways	Headache, tachycardia, palpitations, muscle tremors, anxiety, nausea	May improve lung function during exercise, but research results inconsistent
anticholinergics: tiotropium (Spiriva), aclidinium bromide (Tudorza Pressair)	Cause bronchodilation (via smooth muscle relaxation) by nonselectively inhibiting muscarinic acetylcholine receptors, thereby reducing acetylcholine availability of the parasympathetic nerves that cause bronchoconstriction	Headache, cough, dry "cotton" mouth	May improve exercise tolerance
Oral corticosteroids			
prednisolone (Prelone)	Airway anti-inflammation and decrease mucus production	Short-term use: fluid retention, hypertension, hyperglycemia, mood changes, skeletal muscle atrophy; long-term use: weight gain, osteoporosis, easy bruising, myopathy and cataracts, increased risk of infections, stomach ulcers	No significant effect on exercise capacity
Inhaled corticosteroids			
budesonide (Pulmicort), fluticasone (Flovent), mometasone (Asmanex)	Glucocorticoids bind to airway receptors resulting in reduced lung inflammation and decreased mucus production	Sore mouth or throat, hoarse voice, yeast infections in throat or mouth	No significant effect on exercise capacity

References: (2, 102, 148, 223, 285, 305-308, 317)

Medications Table 5.5   Common Medications Used to Treat CRPD

Drug class and names	Mechanism of action	Most common side effects	Effects on exercise
Oral corticosteroids			
prednisone (Sterapred)	Immunosuppressant and anti-inflammatory agent	Increased risk of fracture and cataracts, risk of adrenal suppression, weight gain	May cause hypertension, myasthenia
Immunosuppressive cytotoxic agents			
azathioprine (Azasan, Imuran), cyclophosphamide (Cytoxan), methotrexate (Trexall, Rheumatrex)	Inhibit immune cell growth and proliferation thereby decreasing autoimmune activity; suppress inflammation	Blood in urine or stools, bleeding gums, chest pain, lower back or side pain, stomach pain, cough, shortness of breath	No known effect
Antifibrotic inhibitors			
nintedanib (Ofev), pirfenidone (Esbriet, Pirfenex, Pirespa)	Decrease lung fibrosis through inhibition or downregulation (or both) of various growth factor receptors; anti-inflammatory effects via reduced inflammatory mediators	Abdominal pain, diarrhea, nausea, vomiting, dizziness, dyspepsia, fatigue, skin rash, weight loss	May increase exercise tolerance

References: (3-6, 90, 92, 194, 274, 297, 316)

Medications Table 5.6   Common Medications Used to Treat CF

Drug class and names	Mechanism of action	Most common side effects	Effects on exercise
Inhaled hypertonic saline	Mucolytic	Cough, sore throat, chest tightness	No effect
Inhaled antibiotics			
tobramycin (Bethkis), aztreonam (Cayston)	Antibacterial	Cough, sore throat, chest tightness, fever, bloody, runny or stuffy nose	No effect
Recombinant deoxyribonuclease			
dornase alfa (Pulmozyme)	Mucolytic; acts by hydrolyzing excess DNA in pulmonary mucus	Change in or loss of voice, throat discomfort, skin rash	No known effect
Cystic fibrosis transmembrane regulator (CFTR) gene potentiator			
ivacaftor (Kalydeco)	Increases the likelihood the defective CFTR channel will remain open, allowing chloride ions to pass through and thus decreasing mucus viscosity	Dizziness, headache, body aches, abdominal or chest pain, cough, nasal congestion	No known effect
Pancreatic enzymes			
pancrelipase (Creon, Pancreaze)	Breakdown of carbohydrate, protein, fat due to pancreatic insufficiency	Headache, diarrhea, nausea, abdominal pain, constipation, mucus membrane irritation	No known effect

References: (81, 91, 93, 94, 97, 98, 105, 178, 304)

Cardiovascular Conditions and Disorders

Ann Marie Swank, PhD, CSCS

Carwyn Sharp, PhD, CSCS,*D

After completing this chapter, you will be able to

- describe the physiological effects of various cardiovascular conditions and disorders on an individual's health, fitness, and physical activity capacity;

- understand the effects of key medications associated with treatment of various cardiovascular conditions and disorders on physiological systems and the responses to exercise;

- design and implement a safe, effective, and efficient individualized exercise program for those affected by cardiovascular conditions and disorders; and

- understand the roles and responsibilities of the exercise professional as part of the team working with individuals affected by cardiovascular conditions and disorders to effectively and efficiently improve health, fitness, and physical capacity.

According to the Centers for Disease Control and Prevention, cardiovascular disease (CVD) is the leading cause of death in the United States for both men and women, even though a number of preventable risk factors for CVD have been identified. As such, significant interest exists in interventions, such as exercise, that prevent or reduce these risks, subsequently decreasing the associated mortality and morbidity. This chapter addresses the essentials of exercise training for individuals with the following cardiovascular conditions: hypertension, peripheral arterial disease, angina, chronic heart failure, myocardial infarction, conduction disturbances, atrial fibrillation, pacemakers, coronary artery bypass grafting (CABG), and other revascularization procedures.

The common underlying mechanism for these conditions is the process of **atherosclerosis**, defined as the development of plaque in arteries of the heart, periphery, brain, or more than one of these. Risk factors for the development of atherosclerosis include factors that cannot be modified, including age, sex, and family history, and those factors that can be modified, such as lipid profile, exercise history, smoking, diabetes, and sedentary behavior. The exercise professional needs to consider a comprehensive program when working with individuals with cardiovascular issues—one that includes risk factor management as well as exercise programming.

HYPERTENSION

Hypertension (HTN) is a considerable health concern in the United States with almost one out of three adults having the disease (39), which is also a positive risk factor for CVD, the number one cause of mortality for both men and women in the United States (45). While exercise has been shown to be effective in the treatment and prevention of HTN (45), prevalence and mortality continue to increase (5).

Hypertension is defined as a systolic blood pressure greater than or equal to 140 mmHg or a diastolic blood pressure greater than or equal to 90 mmHg (or both) confirmed on at least two separate occasions in adults (i.e., older than 18 years of age) (45). **Prehypertension** is defined as a systolic blood pressure between 120 and 139

mmHg and diastolic blood pressure between 80 and 89 mmHg (25). For nearly 95% of cases of HTN in the United States, the cause is not known (i.e., idiopathic) and the condition is referred to as primary hypertension (14). In contrast, secondary HTN is caused by some other medical condition such as renal dysfunction, drugs, or steroids (26). Hypertension is often called the "silent killer" due to the lack of symptoms until the disease process has significantly affected biological systems (16).

Pathophysiology of Hypertension

The two determinants of blood pressure are cardiac output and total peripheral resistance. **Cardiac output** is defined as the amount of blood expelled from the heart each minute, which is a function of blood volume. **Total peripheral resistance** is a measure of the tone or level of constriction of the blood vessels. Elevations in either or both of these variables contribute to HTN. Conditions that contribute to higher blood volume and ultimately HTN include excess salt intake, salt sensitivity, chronic kidney disease, and kidney dysfunction, among others (26). Factors contributing to increased tone of blood vessels include actions that increase sympathetic tone and the associated increase in catecholamine response, such as high stress levels, certain drugs, and exercise (20, 23). However, while various factors resulting in HTN (or more specifically, secondary hypertension) have been identified, it has been reported that 90% to 95% of cases are of unknown cause; these are referred to as primary or essential hypertension (14). When blood pressure has been elevated for an extended period of time, permanent damage to blood vessels, heart tissue, and other organ systems can occur as a result of the constant overload. This overload leads to coronary heart disease, stroke, renal failure, chronic heart failure, and peripheral vascular disease (25).

Common Medications Given to Individuals With Hypertension

The first treatment for HTN is to consider lifestyle changes including exercise, diet, and reduced salt intake for those individuals who may be salt sensitive or may be consuming excess salt (20, 48). However, since blood pressure is a function of both blood volume (cardiac output) and blood vessel tone (total peripheral resistance), medications that affect these two entities are very effective treatments for HTN (25). Diuretics (thiazides) decrease blood volume and therefore reduce blood pressure through this pathway. β-blockers, calcium channel blockers, angiotensin II receptor blockers, and angiotensin-converting enzyme (ACE) inhibitors all have the potential to reduce blood vessel tone and thus reduce blood pressure via this pathway. For some patients, combinations of medications are necessary to achieve effective control of blood pressure (26). The effects of these medications on exercise performance are listed in medications table 6.1 at the end of this chapter; however, of note, the medications to lower blood pressure may affect heat tolerance as well as reduce heart rate response (β-blockers) to a given level of exercise (45). Medications that affect blood vessel tone may also result in exertional hypotension associated with positional changes such as moving from a supine bench press to sitting or standing (52).

Effects of Exercise in Individuals With Hypertension

Normally during exercise, systolic blood pressure increases while the diastolic pressure either stays the same or is lowered (24, 57). During a single (acute) exercise session, the blood pressure response for an individual with HTN may be normal, diminished, or exaggerated depending, in part, on the baseline value presented before exercise and the effectiveness of the medications being taken. In addition to the expected benefits of exercise training, such as increased $\dot{V}O_2$max, increased efficiency (lower heart rate and blood pressure at fixed submaximal workloads), and weight loss, individuals with HTN often experience significant drops in both systolic and diastolic pressure. Meta-analyses have shown that following an eight-week aerobic exercise program, reductions of approximately 5 mmHg and 2 to 3 mmHg for systolic and diastolic blood

pressure, respectively, have been seen, as well as a decrease of 3 to 4 mmHg for both systolic and diastolic blood pressure with resistance training (16). This is related in part to reduced catecholamine activity and an increase in vasodilation capacity of blood vessels (16). Weight loss also contributes to the reduced resting and exercise blood pressure (9).

Exercise Recommendations for Clients With Hypertension

Exercise programming recommendations for clients with HTN should be based on the results of exercise testing and assessment such that the exercise professional is aware of the blood pressure response to exercise intensity and duration. In general, however, exercise recommendations for clients with HTN include the following:

- The mode for aerobic training should be large muscle group activities such as walking, jogging, or cycling with a frequency of most, if not all, days of the week and 30 minutes or more of either continuous or accumulated exercise throughout the day. Intensity should be moderate (i.e., 40% to <60% $\dot{V}O_2$ or heart rate reserve [16] or a rating of perceived exertion [RPE] of a 12 to 13 out of 20 on the Borg scale).

- Since postexercise is associated with reduced blood pressure for up to 4 hours, repeated bouts of exercise or performance of activities of daily living that include higher levels of energy expenditure should be encouraged throughout the day to enhance the positive exercise effects on blood pressure and fitness gains (45). These benefits include increased caloric expenditure, which may also be important because obesity is often a comorbidity for clients with HTN.

- Resistance training is recommended at a moderate level of 8 to 12 repetitions at 60% to 80% of one repetition maximum (1RM) using total body exercises for most clients (2, 16); however, some may benefit from lighter intensity (40% to 60% 1RM) and higher volume (up to 15 repetitions) (16). A circuit weight training format may be most appropriate and is time efficient.

Sample exercises to assist the exercise professional in developing a resistance training program for the client with HTN and a stepwise methodology for teaching clients have been developed (34).

The most important consideration for the exercise professional working with clients with HTN is to monitor blood pressure before, during, and after exercise (possible hypotensive response during recovery). A systolic pressure of 220 or a diastolic pressure of 105 may be considered exercise termination criteria (19). During resistance training, education regarding breathing patterns to avoid a Valsalva maneuver is important (19, 27). For the select patient who has been appropriately screened, high-intensity interval training (HIIT) may be appropriate, for example, a metabolic resistance training protocol (29). Tables 6.1 and 6.2 summarize guidelines for aerobic exercise and resistance training for clients with HTN.

Case Study

Hypertension

Mr. S presented to an exercise professional at his local health club with the primary goals of weight loss and increasing his "energy level." He is currently considered overweight with a BMI of 29. He is inactive and has a "desk job" selling insurance. He denies experiencing stress with his job or home life. His resting blood pressure is 118/76 controlled with an ACE inhibitor. He is 42 years old with a family history of HTN.

The exercise professional recommended a 10-week progressive walking to walk–jog program at an intensity starting at 40% of heart rate reserve and working up to 80% for five days per week. In conjunction, resistance training two days per week using a circuit weight training format was included. The exercise professional also recommended that Mr. S perform the exercise programming at the health club so his blood pressure and symptom response to exercise could be followed. Dietary counseling for his weight management was encouraged, and he was further reminded to be consistent with his blood pressure medication regimen.

Recommended Readings

Contractor, AS, Gordon, TL, and Gordon, NF. Hypertension. In *Clinical Exercise Physiology*. 3rd ed. Ehrman, JK, Gordon, PM, Visich, PS, and Keteyian, SJ, eds. Champaign, IL: Human Kinetics, 137-154, 2013.

Durstine, J, Moore, G, Painter, P, Macko, R, Gordon, B, and Kraus, W. Chronic conditions strongly associated with physical inactivity. In *ACSM's Exercise Management for Persons with Chronic Diseases and Disabilities*. 4th ed. Moore, G, Durstine, J, and Painter, P, eds. Champaign, IL: Human Kinetics, 71-94, 2016.

Pescatello, LS, Franklin, BA, Fagard, R, Farquhar, WB, Kelley, GA, and Ray, CA. American College of Sports Medicine position stand. Exercise and hypertension. *Med Sci Sports Exerc* 36:533-553, 2004.

Table 6.1   Aerobic Exercise Guidelines for Clients With Hypertension

Parameter	Guideline
Frequency	Preferably 5-7 days per week
Intensity	40 to <60% of $\dot{V}O_2$ or heart rate reserve; or 12-13 RPE (on Borg 6- to 20-point scale)
Mode	Activities that engage large muscle groups such as walking
Duration	Minimum of 30 min per day, may be 3-6 bouts of 10 min
Total weekly minutes	150 minimum to 250 or greater

Reference: (16)

Table 6.2   Resistance Training Guidelines for Clients With Hypertension

Parameter	Guideline
Frequency	2-3 days per week, preferably every other day
Intensity	(can start at 40%) 60-80% 1RM
Repetitions	8-12 (up to 15)
Sets	1-3
Rest periods between sets	30-60 s
Exercises	8-12 mostly large muscle groups and multijoint
Progression	2-5 lb for upper body, 5-10 for lower body

Reference: (16)

PERIPHERAL ARTERIAL DISEASE

Peripheral arterial disease (PAD) is defined as a narrowing of noncardiac arteries that may result in reduction of blood flow (18, 35); it affects approximately 8.5 million adults in the United States aged 40 years and older, with similar prevalence in males and females (39). An individual may have clinical PAD in that there is significant blockage of blood vessels in the periphery, but up to two-thirds of individuals 40 years or older who have PAD do not have symptoms (39). The classic symptom of PAD is called **intermittent claudication** (IC), an aching or cramping feeling in the legs, calf, or buttocks (or more than one of these) induced by exercise that is caused by insufficient blood flow to the muscles of the lower extremities and is relieved by rest. However, it is estimated that IC occurs in only 10% to 40% of cases of PAD (18, 35).

Pathophysiology of Peripheral Arterial Disease

The underlying disease process for PAD is atherosclerosis, defined as a condition in which the arteries become narrowed and hardened due to an excessive buildup of plaque along the wall of the affected artery (18). Atherosclerosis is the common underlying process for most cardiovascular conditions including angina, myocardial infarction, and stroke. The primary difference for each of these conditions is the location of the atherosclerosis, and for PAD the location is the noncoronary arteries such as those of the legs. The main risk factors for atherosclerosis of the periphery resulting in PAD are smoking, hyperlipidemia, and diabetes (18, 35).

Common Medications Given to Individuals With Peripheral Arterial Disease

Common medications for treating PAD include those for HTN (see medications table 6.1); antiplatelet–vasoactive agents such as cilostazol (Pletal); statins (for reducing cholesterol); and drugs that inhibit blood clotting such as pentoxifylline, Plavix, and aspirin (18). See medications table 6.2 near the end of the chapter. As is often the case with CVDs, PAD exists with comorbidities such as diabetes and past myocardial infarction, so the exercise professional needs to be aware of not just all medications and the potential interactions, but also the influence of exercise (28, 38). With the exception of the vasoactive agents, which may increase exercise capacity for the individual with PAD, all other medications just listed have a neutral impact on exercise capacity.

Effects of Exercise in Individuals With Peripheral Arterial Disease

Not all cases of PAD exhibit IC. If IC exists, then during an acute exercise session the individual's given level of external work is often limited by the onset of IC pain (18). The amount of work that can be performed by those with IC is likely to be low and depends in part on the severity of the lesion and the baseline fitness level of the individual. The expected benefits of exercise training, such as increased $\dot{V}O_2$max, increased cardiovascular efficiency (lower heart rate and blood pressure at a fixed submaximal level of work), and decreased weight are modest for individuals with PAD-induced IC because the associated onset of pain limits exercise intensity and duration. With chronic exercise training, individuals with IC associated with PAD demonstrate an increased amount of external work performed before the onset of IC pain occurs. The mechanism for this training effect is likely related to increased leg blood flow due to reduced tone of blood vessels, decreased blood viscosity, and a shift from reliance on anaerobic to aerobic metabolism (35).

Key Point

Consistent and chronic exercise training by individuals with intermittent claudication results in an ability to do more external work before the onset of pain.

Exercise Recommendations for Clients With Peripheral Arterial Disease

All clients with known CVDs, such as PAD, should obtain a medical clearance before commencing an exercise program. It is also highly recommended that clients with PAD, regardless of symptom severity, undergo exercise testing before initiating an exercise program so that the exercise professional can identify the level of exercise that results in symptoms (e.g., onset of pain and time to maximal pain), postexercise ankle pressure can be established, exercise prescription baseline information may be gathered (e.g., total walking distance before onset of pain), and, if not previously established, the presence of CVD may be determined (18).

Using the results of the exercise testing, it is recommended that exercise professionals design a program with the primary goals of decreasing cardiovascular risk factors and IC pain symptoms (18). Given the severe deconditioning of this population, the recommended mode of activity is weight-bearing large muscle group exercise such as walking, which has the added advantage of working the gastrocnemius (particularly affected by PVD), more so than cycling or swimming (18, 35). The recommended intensity is 40% to <60% heart rate reserve, or claudication pain of 3 out of 4 (18), for 30 to 60 minutes of accumulated activity, three to seven days per week (3, 18). These clients can benefit from intermittent training that entails exercising to a level of 3 out of 4 on a claudication pain scale (0 = no pain; 1 = onset of pain; 2 = moderate pain; 3 = intense pain; 4 = maximal pain), then resting until pain subsides and repeating the effort until 30 minutes without resting can be tolerated (3, 18). Resistance training can be performed three days per week with a moderate intensity of 10 to 12 repetitions for one or two sets of upper and lower body exercise (18). For clients with IC, their level of pain will determine the exercise intensity. For clients with PAD and no IC, RPE can also be used to determine exercise intensity (12 to 13 out of 20 is recommended).

It is also worthy to note that as clients with IC associated with PAD train and increase their fitness, comorbidities may become evident and will need to be addressed by the exercise professional (38). Tables 6.3 and 6.4 summarize guidelines for aerobic exercise and resistance training for clients with PAD.

Table 6.3 Aerobic Exercise Guidelines for Clients With Peripheral Arterial Disease

Parameter	Guideline
Frequency	Preferably 3-7 days per week
Intensity	40% to <60% heart rate reserve, but staying below level 3 out of 4 on the pain scale
Mode	Activities that engage large muscle groups such as walking
Duration	30-60 min per day, may be 3-6 bouts of 10 min each

References: (6, 35)

Table 6.4 Resistance Training Guidelines for Clients With Peripheral Arterial Disease

Parameter	Guideline
Frequency	2-3 days per week
Intensity	Moderate; 60-80% 1RM*
Repetitions	10-12
Sets	1-2 sets each for upper and lower body
Rest periods between sets	30-60 s
Exercises	8-12 mostly large muscle groups and multijoint
Progression	2-5 lb for upper body, 5-10 for lower body

*Intensity for those with intermittent claudication will be determined by pain.

Reference: (18)

Case Study

Peripheral Arterial Disease

Ms. J has a history of type 2 diabetes treated for 20 years with metformin (a blood glucose–lowering agent) and is morbidly obese with a BMI of 45. She has also been diagnosed with PAD and has difficulty walking short distances without profound cramping in her calf muscles indicating IC. She rates her pain with walking a level of 4 out of 4 on the IC pain scale. She sought the help of an exercise professional at a local fitness club for exercise programming.

Because of her obesity and low level of exercise tolerance, a unique exercise program was developed. Two chairs without handles were placed a short distance apart, and Ms. J walked between the chairs until her legs began to cramp. Then she sat down at the second chair until the pain of IC subsided. She continued this intermittent training for 10 weeks and demonstrated a 200% increase in the distance covered between the chairs. She was also able to walk to her

(continued)

Peripheral Arterial Disease *(continued)*

curbside mailbox at home to retrieve the mail for the first time in several years—an outcome that had significant impact on her self-esteem. She is continuing her chair exercise with her exercise professional and has been advised to work with a certified diabetes educator for diabetes control and nutrition. She is also beginning a modest-intensity lower body resistance training program under the direction of her exercise professional to build her muscle strength and endurance.

Recommended Readings

Cooper, C, Dolezal, B, Durstine, J, Gordon, B, Pinkstaff, S, Babu, A, and Phillips, S. Chronic conditions very strongly associated with tobacco. In *ACSM's Exercise Management for Persons With Chronic Diseases and Disabilities*. 4th ed. Moore, G, Durstine, J, and Painter, P, eds. Champaign, IL: Human Kinetics, 95-114, 2016.

Mays, RJ, Casserly, IP, and Regensteiner, JG. Peripheral artery disease. In *Clinical Exercise Physiology*. 3rd ed. Ehrman, JK, Gordon, PM, Visich, PS, and Keteyian, SJ, eds. Champaign, IL: Human Kinetics, 277-296, 2013.

ANGINA

The increasing prevalence of **angina**—chest pain that occurs in response to myocardial ischemia or reduced blood flow to the myocardium (18)—has been estimated at approximately 9 million Americans, more than 50% of them women (8). Symptoms reported by individuals to describe their angina include (a) pressure, tightness, or fullness in the chest or (b) back, jaw, and tooth pain, typically lasting 2 to 10 minutes; these symptoms may be different for men and women (18). Women are more likely to feel symptoms in the neck, jaw, throat, abdomen, or back. Angina can be characterized as stable or unstable. While these have similar symptoms or characteristics, **stable angina** is associated with the onset of a specific level of stress such as physical activity and is rapidly alleviated with rest or nitroglycerin, whereas **unstable angina** is far less predictable and often occurs at rest (18). There are a number of forms of unstable angina associated with acute coronary events. These individuals are typically not candidates for exercise programming until after the acute event has been stabilized. Thus this chapter focuses on recommendations related to stable (predictable) angina.

Pathophysiology of Angina

The underlying cause of angina is a narrowing of the coronary arteries due to atherosclerosis (18). For healthy individuals without significant atherosclerotic lesions present in their coronary arteries, as demand for oxygen increases, the heart is able to supply that demand with an increase in blood flow. For individuals with a narrowing in one or more arteries due to atherosclerosis, the supply of blood flow cannot keep up with demand, and angina is often the result as the cardiac tissue experiences varying levels of ischemia. The amount of external work, usually defined as the combination of heart rate, blood pressure, and wall tension of the heart that results in the development of angina, is very predictable and reproducible in these individuals (18).

Key Point

For individuals with angina, the blood pressure and heart rate resulting from physical activity (i.e., external work) that results in the development of angina is very predictable and reproducible. This means that an exercise professional is able to quickly determine the threshold below which such an individual can exercise without incurring angina and prescribe accordingly.

Key Point

The primary goal of exercise programming for a client with angina is to increase the amount of work that can be performed before the ischemic threshold is reached.

Common Medications Given to Individuals With Angina

Medications used to treat angina have the common action of reducing myocardial oxygen demand so that the narrowed artery can adequately supply the tissue with sufficient blood flow (7). See medications table 6.3 near the end of the chapter. The primary actions of drugs to treat angina include lowering the heart rate or blood pressure or dilating the artery, or both. Typical examples include nitrates–nitrites, calcium antagonists, and β-blockers (53) as well as newer medications such as Ranolazine and other novel agents that improve symptoms by nonhemodynamic mechanisms (7, 28). All of the medications just discussed have the potential to increase exercise capacity in individuals with angina. For individuals with angina who are taking only vasodilating agents, care should be taken with any postural changes as these can be associated with dizziness, syncope, or both.

Effects of Exercise in Individuals With Angina

The occurrence of chest pain is likely the limiting factor for exercise programming in this population. The heart rate and blood pressure (rate–pressure product) for individuals with angina is very predictable, and the amount of exercise necessary to induce angina symptoms is called the ischemic threshold (3). In addition to the expected benefits of exercise training such as increased $\dot{V}O_2max$, increased cardiovascular efficiency (lower heart rate and blood pressure at a fixed submaximal level of work), and decreased weight, the individual with angina will be able to perform an increased amount of work before reaching the ischemic threshold, which is a primary goal of exercise programming (18). The initial amount of exercise that can be tolerated is a function of both the size of the lesion(s) and the amount of collateral blood flow available to the tissue.

Exercise Recommendations for Clients With Angina

For those with angina a medically supervised graded exercise test should be undertaken, and a medical release to exercise independently must be obtained before an exercise program is initiated. Apart from safety reasons, the results of the graded exercise test may be used to assist the exercise professional in developing exercise programming recommendations.

- With knowledge of the intensity and duration of exercise that elicits symptoms of angina, the aerobic exercise recommendations include the use of large muscle group activities including walking, jogging, stepping, or cycling as the preferred mode of exercise (3, 18). Aerobic exercise can be performed four to seven days per week (preferably seven) for 20 to 60 minutes of continuous or accumulated activity at an intensity of 10 to 15 beats/min below the ischemic threshold, in addition to an increase in activities of daily living (3, 18).

- Light-intensity resistance training can be performed two or three days per week at 40% to 60% 1RM of 15 to 20 minutes per session to improve functional capacity (3, 18). As with all clients with cardiovascular conditions, a longer warm-up and cooldown may be necessary, and the medications may cause postural hypotension. Higher intensities and HIIT may be performed for those clients with higher exercise capacities and those who have been appropriately screened for this type of activity (31).

The most crucial consideration for the exercise professional when working with this population is to be aware of the symptoms that clients experience with their angina and what they need to do to relieve the pain. Usually slowing down or stopping exercise is all that is needed. If pain does not subside, then the client may need to take a nitroglycerine tablet that he has brought with him for any exercise he may perform. If nitroglycerine is not effective, then the client should be immediately transported to the emergency room for further treatment. The exercise professional and client should discuss this symptom mitigation plan before any exercise, including the location of all medicines. Tables 6.5 and 6.6 summarize guidelines for aerobic exercise and resistance training for clients with angina.

Table 6.5   Aerobic Exercise Guidelines for Clients With Angina

Parameter	Guideline
Frequency	4-7 days per week (preferably every day)
Intensity	10-15 beats · min^{-1} below ischemic threshold
Mode	Activities that engage large muscle groups such as walking, jogging, cycling
Duration	20-60 min per day of continuous or accumulated activity

References: (18)

Table 6.6   Resistance Training Guidelines for Clients With Angina

Parameter	Guideline
Frequency	2-3 days per week
Intensity	Light; 40-60% 1RM*
Repetitions	8-12
Sets	1-2 sets each for upper and lower body
Rest periods between sets	60 s or longer if needed
Exercises	Initially one per large muscle group and multijoint

*Intensity determined by angina symptoms if onset is less than 40% 1RM.
References: (18)

Case Study

Angina

Ms. R, 54 years old, has experienced some chest pain during her walks around her neighborhood, especially when walking up the hills. She consulted with her physician, and after a stress test and catheterization were performed she was found to have modest blockage in two vessels and chest pain at a metabolic equivalent (MET) level of 5. Her physician also recommended that she work with an exercise professional on the development of a strength program for her lower body to assist with walking the hills in her neighborhood and an aerobic program to improve her ischemic threshold.

Ms. R's exercise professional recommended that she continue walking at her current frequency and duration per week but ensure that she stays 10 to 15 beats/min below 5 METs, meaning that on hills she must slow down. The exercise professional also recommended that she wear a heart rate monitor and program an alarm if her heart rate gets to within 15 beats/min of her ischemic threshold. For resistance training, Ms. R meets with her exercise professional two days per week and starts with a circuit-style workout of one set of a single exercise per major muscle group at 40% to 50% 1RM. Before the start of all training sessions, her exercise professional also asks Ms. R if she has her nitroglycerine tablets in case she should experience angina symptoms.

Recommended Readings

Cooper, C, Dolezal, B, Durstine, J, Gordon, B, Pinkstaff, S, Babu, A, and Phillips, S. Chronic conditions very strongly associated with tobacco. In *ACSM's Exercise Management for Persons With Chronic Diseases and Disabilities.* 4th ed. Moore, G, Durstine, J, and Painter, P, eds. Champaign, IL: Human Kinetics, 95-114, 2016.

Thomas, S, Gokhale, R, Boden, WE, and Devereaux, PJ. A meta-analysis of randomized controlled trials comparing percutaneous coronary intervention with medical therapy in stable angina pectoris. *Can J Cardiol* 29:472-482, 2013.

CHRONIC HEART FAILURE

While the incidence of heart failure has remained stable in the United States in recent years, the risk of developing the disease after 40 years of age is approximately 20% and the prevalence, currently at 5.1 million, is increasing (59). The economic cost is also significant, with the 2012 global cost estimated at $108 billion (17, 40). **Chronic heart failure (CHF)**, sometimes called **congestive heart failure**, is defined as an inability of the heart muscle to pump blood at a rate consistent with the metabolic needs, resulting in fatigue or dyspnea (46). There are two forms of CHF: systolic and diastolic. **Systolic heart failure** is a condition in which the *contractility* of the left ventricle is impaired, resulting in an ejection fraction <35% of normal. **Diastolic heart failure**, on the other hand, reflects an inability of the left ventricle to *relax* normally and fill appropriately due to increased stiffness or thickness (12). Individuals with systolic heart failure have reduced ejection fraction (stroke volume / end-diastolic volume × 100) due to reduced pumping capacity of the heart, often related to previous myocardial infarction(s) (12). Diastolic dysfunction is associated with normal ejection fraction but reduced stroke volume due to stiffness of the ventricle and difficulty with filling (reduced end-diastolic volume).

Pathophysiology of Chronic Heart Failure

Chronic heart failure may be the result of ischemic (myocardial infarction with significant tissue loss) or nonischemic (chronic HTN) etiologies (46). With the reduction in cardiac output and stroke volume associated with a failing heart, both the sympathetic (54) and renin-angiotensin systems (55) are subsequently activated. Activation of the sympathetic system results in acute increases in heart rate and peripheral constriction of blood vessels (60). In conjunction, chronic increased activity of the renin-angiotensin system leads to pathological cardiac remodeling and further activation of the sympathetic nervous system. However, the chronic activation of both the sympathetic and renin-angiotensin systems and the concomitant reduction in blood flow lead to a shift to anaerobic metabolism with early onset of lactate accumulation. In combination, chronically reduced muscle function is experienced by these individuals. The hallmark symptom of CHF is severe exercise intolerance due in part to lactate accumulation at low exercise levels (12, 51).

Common Medications Given to Individuals With Chronic Heart Failure

The medications (30, 51) used to treat CHF have the overarching goal to interrupt the harmful effects of the chronic activation of the sympathetic and renin-angiotensin systems, effects that include increasing heart rate and constriction of blood vessels resulting in reduced blood flow to critical organ systems. These medications consist of antiarrhythmia drugs such as digoxin (increases myocardial contractility); β-blockers (block sympathetic nervous system, lower heart rate); diuretics (reduce blood volume overload); ACE inhibitors and calcium antagonists; and aldosterone receptor blockers (ARBs) (reduce blood pressure, dilate blood vessels) (59). See medications table 6.4 near the end of the chapter. Cardiac resynchronization therapy (CRT) (also known as biventricular pacing) is commonly used with CHF to increase heart function by restoring synchrony (59). Each of these medications as well as biventricular pacing has the ability to increase exercise capacity for individuals with CHF.

Effects of Exercise in Individuals With Chronic Heart Failure

Individuals with CHF typically have very low exercise capacities relative to other cases of CVD. Relative to their healthy counterparts, individuals with CHF experience fatigue and dyspnea at light workloads due in part to their reliance on anaerobic metabolism and impaired vasodilation capacity (12, 30, 51). These individuals also have reduced inotropic and chronotropic responses to exercise that are secondary to their condition as well as a function of the medications they are taking (59). While intense exercise was previously thought of as contraindicated for those with CHF, more recently it has been shown to be safe and efficacious in various ways (e.g., increased $\dot{V}O_2$max, cardiovascular efficiency, and various peripheral training responses such as increased muscle function) (1).

Exercise Recommendations for Clients With Chronic Heart Failure

Exercise programming recommendations for the client with CHF should be based on medically supervised maximal exercise testing and if possible oxygen consumption measurements, as identifying anaerobic threshold can be valuable for exercise prescription for this population.

- The recommended mode of exercise for aerobic conditioning is large muscle group activities including walking or cycling performed at an intensity of 40% to 70% $\dot{V}O_2$ or heart rate reserve, four to seven days per week, accumulating 20 to 60 minutes per day (12). Intensity can also be gauged by RPE of 12 to 14 out of 20.

- Resistance training has been shown to be safe and effective in this population using light-to-moderate loads (40-80% 1RM) in a circuit weight training format (3, 18).

- In conjunction, HIIT may be performed for those clients with higher exercise capacities and those who have been appropriately screened for this type of activity (29).

- As with other chronic CVD populations, performance of activities of daily living that include higher levels of energy expenditure should be encouraged throughout the day to aid in increasing caloric expenditure and fitness gains as well as enhancing the confidence level for clients with HF to perform these activities safely (28).

Special considerations for the exercise professional to take into account while working with clients who have CHF include extensive warm-up and cooldown and difficulty dealing with temperature extremes due in part to the medication regimen (12). Clients should be weighed daily, as significant weight gain in a short time could be indicative of water retention and decompensation (acute HF), a condition in need of emergency treatment. Tables 6.7 and 6.8 summarize guidelines for aerobic exercise and resistance training for clients with CHF.

Table 6.7   Aerobic Exercise Guidelines for Clients With Chronic Heart Failure

Parameter	Guideline
Frequency	4-7 days per week (preferably every day)
Intensity	40-70% $\dot{V}O_2$ or heart rate reserve; or 12-14 RPE (on Borg 6- to 20-point scale)
Mode	Activities that engage large muscle groups such as walking and cycling
Duration	20-60 min per day of continuous or accumulated activity

Reference: (18)

Table 6.8   Resistance Training Guidelines for Clients With Chronic Heart Failure

Parameter	Guideline
Frequency	2-3 days per week
Intensity	Light to moderate; 40-80% 1RM
Repetitions	10-15
Sets	1 set per exercise in circuit format
Rest periods between sets	≤30 s
Exercises	Initially one exercise per muscle group

Reference: (18)

Case Study

Chronic Heart Failure

Mr. B, age 53, has a history of two previous myocardial infarctions several years apart that have reduced his ejection fraction to 25%, resulting in a diagnosis of CHF. He has a job as a waiter in a restaurant and finds himself becoming more fatigued doing his job than previously. His current medications include a β-blocker, ARB, statin (for cholesterol lowering), and a daily aspirin, and in conjunction he has been active with the program recommended by his cardiac rehabilitation staff, showing gains in fitness as a result of this program.

He wanted to add resistance training to his regimen, and the exercise professional he is working with at the health club recommended a circuit weight training program starting at an intensity of 40% of his 1RM for four weeks.

The exercise professional prescribed 10 to 15 repetitions of each of the following exercises: leg press, chest press, seated hamstring curl, seated row, machine military press, biceps curl, triceps extension. Mr. B's exercise professional initially had him complete a single circuit of one set per exercise and added a second circuit when he was able to complete 15 repetitions per exercise with less than 30 seconds of rest between exercises. (Note that the fitness facility had set aside the machines in a fashion for circuit training.) After the initial four-week training phase, the exercise professional would reassess fitness and adjust the program accordingly. Mr. B may be a candidate for a HIIT program if his fitness level is high enough to tolerate such a program.

Recommended Readings

Brubaker, PH and Myers, JN. Chronic heart failure. In *ACSM's Exercise Management for Persons with Chronic Diseases and Disabilities*. 4th ed. Moore, G, Durstine, J, and Painter, P, eds. Champaign, IL: Human Kinetics, 135-142, 2009.

Keteyian, SJ. Chronic heart failure. In *Clinical Exercise Physiology*. 3rd ed. Ehrman, JK, Gordon, PM, Visich, PS, and Keteyian, SJ, eds. Champaign, IL: Human Kinetics, 259-276, 2013.

Swank, AM. Resistance training strategies for individuals with chronic heart failure. In *Resistance Training for Special Populations*. Swank, AM, and Hagerman, P, eds. New York: Delmar Cengage, 169-184, 2009.

MYOCARDIAL INFARCTION

An acute **myocardial infarction (MI)**—that is, a heart attack—is the result of the formation of a thrombus or clot associated with an atherosclerotic lesion that has formed in a branch or in branches of the coronary artery system (21, 49). Approximately 720,000 Americans have a heart attack each year (18), and 122,071 died of an acute MI in 2010 (i.e., over 334 per day) (40). The severity of the MI depends in part on the amount of tissue that is damaged and the extent of collateral blood flow. The severity of an MI can be reduced by prompt action on the part of the individual in recognizing the symptoms and proceeding to emergency care, reducing the amount of time cardiac tissue is ischemic. In an emergency room an intervention such as percutaneous transluminal coronary angioplasty (PTCA) can be performed quickly so that blood flow is restored. In order to preserve the integrity of the affected tissue, a 2-hour window from the onset of chest pain to the intervention is usually best for tissue salvage (37).

Pathophysiology of Myocardial Infarction

Clot formation that occludes blood vessels of the coronary circulation is usually initiated by a fissure or breakage of an unstable atherosclerotic lesion (47). The formation of an atherosclerotic lesion is related to risk factors including high blood pressure, hyperlipidemia, diabetes, and family history, among others (39). Chronic inflammation is also a key aspect to the development of lesions and the formation of a clot at a vulnerable part of the lesion. An example of a vulnerable location in the coronary circulation is any area of bifurcation (branching) of blood vessels, as blood flow in these areas can become more turbulent rather than laminar and contribute to plaque rupture (21, 49).

Common Medications Given to Individuals With Myocardial Infarction

Medications given to an individual following an MI have the underlying role of reducing workload on the heart and maximizing blood flow, as well as reducing the risk of formation of another clot (28). If there are associated comorbidities such as HF or angina, then additional medications may be necessary (38). Medications include β-blockers and vasodilators (reduce workload on the heart), ACE inhibitors (reduce afterload), aspirin, blood thinners that reduce the risk of clot formation, statins (reduce cholesterol), and calcium antagonists (reduce afterload). See medications table 6.5 near the end of the chapter. The medications that reduce the workload on the heart have the potential to increase exercise capacity for individuals recovering from an MI. The medications associated with clot prevention and cholesterol lowering are for assistance in risk factor modification and likely have no impact on exercise capacity. However, because these medications lower heart rate (β-blockers) and blood pressure (ACE, ARB, calcium), hypotension with exertion and body position changes may occur.

Effects of Exercise in Individuals With Myocardial Infarction

With an acute exercise session and an uncomplicated MI, fitness is reduced and the medications may reduce the hemodynamic response to exercise. If comorbidities are present, such as HF or angina, then the exercise professional has to be versed in the special considerations regarding these conditions (38). There is also the potential for life-threatening arrhythmias and conduction disturbances; thus initially exercise should take place in a monitored and supervised cardiac rehabilitation setting (33).

Key Point

Exercise training responses for the individual who has had an MI include a reduced potential for arrhythmias, reduced symptoms related to decreased blood vessel tone, and reduced catecholamine response to exercise (21, 49). Thus compliance with an exercise program has the capacity to reduce the risk of subsequent cardiac problems and symptoms, thereby enhancing quality of life.

With exercise training it can be expected that an individual with an MI will have the same responses as an otherwise healthy person, such as increased $\dot{V}O_2max$, increased cardiac efficiency (lower heart rate and blood pressure at a fixed submaximal workload), and reduced weight, although the response will be somewhat blunted depending on the amount of damage to the myocardial tissue.

Exercise Recommendations for Clients With Myocardial Infarction

For exercise prescription purposes, it is strongly advised that all clients who have experienced an MI consult their physician or other health care professional and undergo a medically supervised exercise test before engaging in an exercise program to assess, among other factors, the ability to safely engage in such activity and the duration and intensity at which the client can participate before the onset of symptoms of ischemia. In conjunction, to ensure safety, it is highly recommended that all such clients also engage in a supervised exercise program with appropriately qualified exercise professionals before participating in unsupervised exercise (21, 49).

- The recommended modes of aerobic exercise are large muscle group activities such as walking, cycling, or running (49). Intensity can be monitored by RPE (12 to 16 out of 20) or 40% to 80% of $\dot{V}O_2$ or heart rate reserve. The recommendation is at least three days per week for 20 to 60 minutes, continuous or accumulated (21).

- Resistance training may be performed at 40% to 80% of 1RM, and a circuit weight training format of 8 to 10 stations is appropriate (2, 34). For the appropriately screened client, HIIT may also be suitable and more efficient for producing fitness gains (36).

- In addition, engaging in activities of daily living may assist in reducing risk factors by increasing caloric expenditure and may improve overall fitness gains especially for those with low fitness levels (21).

Recommendations specific for the client with MI include a more extended warm-up and cooldown, especially the cooldown, as the time after exercise is the most vulnerable time for these clients especially with respect to development of arrhythmias. Tables 6.9 and 6.10 summarize guidelines for aerobic exercise and resistance training for clients with MI.

Table 6.9   Aerobic Exercise Guidelines for Clients With Prior Myocardial Infarction

Parameter	Guideline
Frequency	≥3 days per week
Intensity	40-80% $\dot{V}O_2$ or heart rate reserve; or 12-16 RPE (on Borg 6- to 20-point scale)
Mode	Activities that engage large muscle groups such as walking, jogging, or cycling
Duration	20-60 min per day of continuous or accumulated activity

References: (21, 49)

Table 6.10   Resistance Training Guidelines for Clients With Prior Myocardial Infarction

Parameter	Guideline
Frequency	2-3 days per week
Intensity	Light to moderate; 40-80% 1RM
Repetitions	10-15
Sets	1 set per exercise in circuit format
Rest periods between sets	≤30 s
Exercises	8-10

References: (2, 34)

Case Study

Myocardial Infarction

Mr. W is six months post-MI. He has participated in 36 sessions of cardiac rehabilitation and is now in a maintenance program at his local health club. He is 62 years old with only his age, sex, and hyperlipidemia (high cholesterol and high triglycerides) as significant risk factors. He is currently taking a β-blocker, an ACE inhibitor, and statin medication following his MI. He was very active before his MI and is interested in beginning a higher-intensity program than was provided at his cardiac rehabilitation facility.

After approval from his cardiologist, Mr. W's exercise professional suggested a HIIT program in the format of circuit resistance training, such as 10 to 15 repetitions of each of the following exercises: leg press, chest press, seated hamstring curl, seated row, machine military press, biceps curl, and triceps extension, at an initial resistance of 70% of his maximum. While supervised, Mr. W initially completed two circuits with less than 30 seconds rest between exercises. When Mr. W was able to complete three circuits of 15 exercises, the intensity was increased to 75% of maximum and repetitions were dropped to 10 per exercise.

Recommended Readings

Cooper, C, Dolezal, B, Durstine, J, Gordon, B, Pinkstaff, S, Babu, A, and Phillips, S. Chronic conditions very strongly associated with tobacco. In *ACSM's Exercise Management for Persons With Chronic Diseases and Disabilities*. 4th ed. Moore, G, Durstine, J, and Painter, P, eds. Champaign, IL: Human Kinetics, 95-114, 2016.

Squires, RW. Acute coronary syndromes: unstable angina and acute myocardial infarction. In *Clinical Exercise Physiology*. 3rd ed. Ehrman, JK, Gordon, PM, Visich, PS, and Keteyian, S, eds. Champaign, IL: Human Kinetics, 215-234, 2013.

ATRIAL FIBRILLATION

Chronic **atrial fibrillation** is a conduction defect of the atria (the two top chambers of the heart) associated with chaotic and very rapid atrial depolarizations that result in irregular and sometimes rapid ventricular response (41). Atrial fibrillation is one of the most common arrhythmias, along with premature ventricular contractions (58). While precise incidence and prevalence of this condition have been difficult to determine, it was recently estimated, using modeling techniques for health insurance claims, that the incidence would increase from approximately 1.2 to 2.6 million cases from 2010 to 2030 (15). The most critical aspects of treatment are the prevention of clots that may form in the atria due to lack of coordinated contraction and controlling the rapid ventricular response.

Pathophysiology of Atrial Fibrillation

While the specific underlying mechanism for atrial fibrillation is not well understood, it is known that reentry or "circus" movements of electrical impulses in the atrial tissue cause the atria to fire at rates greater than 300 beats/min, eliminating effective atrial contraction (41). These impulses bombard the atrial-ventricular (AV) node; however, not all impulses reach the ventricle as the AV node is refractory to most of the impulses. Thus the refractory nature of the AV node protects the ventricle from the high rates exhibited by the atria. Atrial fibrillation is present in a number of conditions including HTN, HF, coronary heart disease, and valvular heart disease (38). The frequency of fibrillation is highly variable between individuals, and the exercise professional should consult with the individual's physician or other health care professional to understand frequency and duration of fibrillation episodes. An episode of atrial fibrillation may last less than 24 hours or longer than seven days, and in some individuals may be classified as permanent (i.e., longer than one year).

Common Medications Given to Individuals With Atrial Fibrillation

The most important considerations for medications for atrial fibrillation are to prevent clot formation due to inactive atrial tissue and control the ventricular response to increased rate of atrial stimulation (28, 41). Medications for preventing clot formation include Coumadin (warfarin) and Plavix. Coumadin requires careful monitoring of clot times to ensure that the dose is appropriate. Medications that slow conduction through the AV node and decrease the ventricular response include digitalis, calcium antagonists, and β-blockers. The medications just discussed that control the ventricular response to exercise would likely have the impact of increasing exercise capacity for the individual with atrial fibrillation. In conjunction, many of these individuals may have undergone some type of surgical procedure for an accompanying or causative condition such as catheter ablation or maze procedure. The exercise professional should be aware and knowledgeable of these conditions and surgical procedures in conjunction with current medications. See medications table 6.6 near the end of the chapter.

Effects of Exercise in Individuals With Atrial Fibrillation

Exercise programming for atrial fibrillation is most affected by the associated underlying condition (38). The reader is referred to each of these potential conditions as discussed in this chapter for specifics of the acute and chronic exercise responses. Atrial fibrillation has the potential to reduce exercise capacity due to the reduction of atrial contribution to the stroke volume and car-

diac output (about 20%) (41). This loss of cardiac output may contribute to early onset of fatigue. There is also the potential that exercise would induce a greater than normal ventricular heart rate response.

Exercise Recommendations for Clients With Atrial Fibrillation

Those with atrial fibrillation have a reduced exercise tolerance; however, the extent of this reduction is highly variable and largely reflective of any coexisting heart disease (41). Due to this variability and for safety reasons, it is recommended that clients seek a medically supervised graded exercise test to provide information for exercise prescription based on the ventricular and perceived exertion responses to exercise.

- Aerobic exercise prescription recommendations for clients with atrial fibrillation should consist of large muscle group activities such as walking, cycling, or running at an intensity assessed by RPE of 13 to 16 out of 20, corresponding to workloads of 50% to 85% of peak $\dot{V}O_2$ (41). Exercise can be performed four to seven days per week with either continuous or accumulated durations of 30 to 60 minutes per day.

- Resistance training can be performed at a moderate intensity and with a circuit weight training format of 8 to 10 exercises performed between 40% and 80% 1RM (2, 34). As with other cardiovascular conditions, performance of activities of daily living for the client with atrial fibrillation should be encouraged throughout the day.

- For the appropriately screened client, HIIT may be suitable and valuable for increasing training outcomes (29).

For the exercise professional, there are three important issues that need attention in working with clients with atrial fibrillation. The most important aspect is the variable ventricular response that makes heart rate unreliable as a measure of exercise intensity. Rating of perceived exertion may be the best measure, and clients need to be educated about appropriate use of this scale to monitor intensity. The final consideration is awareness of the comorbidities such as HF or HTN that may be present and how they interact with the specific considerations related to atrial fibrillation (38). Tables 6.11 and 6.12 summarize guidelines for aerobic exercise and resistance training for clients with atrial fibrillation.

Table 6.11 Aerobic Exercise Guidelines for Clients With Atrial Fibrillation

Parameter	Guideline
Frequency	4-7 days per week
Intensity	50-85% $\dot{V}O_2$peak; or 13-16 RPE (on Borg 6- to 20-point scale)
Mode	Activities that engage large muscle groups such as walking, jogging, or cycling
Duration	30-60 min per day of continuous or accumulated activity

Reference: (41)

Table 6.12 Resistance Training Guidelines for Clients With Atrial Fibrillation

Parameter	Guideline
Frequency	2-3 days per week
Intensity	Light to moderate; 40-80% 1RM
Repetitions	10-15
Sets	1 set per exercise in circuit format
Rest periods between sets	≤30 s
Exercises	8-10

References: (2, 34)

Case Study

Atrial Fibrillation

Mrs. M has a history of past MI that has resulted in an ejection fraction of 20% and thus CHF. Her underlying heart rhythm is atrial fibrillation. She has recently been experiencing an increase in fatigue during her activities of daily living, including grocery shopping, vacuuming, and doing the laundry. She met with her cardiologist and received a recommendation to pursue light- to moderate-level exercise training (both aerobic and resistance) to support her need to be able to perform activities of daily living without undue fatigue. Her exercise professional recommended a circuit weight training program two or three times per week of 8 to 10 large muscle group exercises such as leg press, chest press, and cable pulldown, at an intensity of 40% 1RM, to increase her lower and upper body muscular strength and fitness. Mrs. M's exercise professional also prescribed aerobic conditioning using a stationary bicycle and treadmill–walking at an initially light to moderate intensity (i.e., RPE of 9-13), building her volume from three 10-minute bouts, three or four days per week, depending on her tolerance.

Recommended Readings

Myers, J and Atwood, J. Atrial fibrillation. In *ACSM's Exercise Management for Persons with Chronic Diseases and Disabilities*. 4th ed. Durstine, JL, Moore, GE, Painter, PL, and Roberts, SO, eds. Champaign, IL: Human Kinetics, 143-148, 2016.

PACEMAKERS AND IMPLANTABLE CARDIOVERTER DEFIBRILLATORS

Cardiac conduction defects or disorders that may require a pacemaker or an implantable cardioverter defibrillator (ICD) can be defined as a block at any level of the conduction system of the heart that results in either a very low, very high, or chaotic heart rate causing symptoms such as light-headedness or syncope (11, 50). Pacemakers are available in a variety of forms, including rate-responsive, biventricular pacers (for bundle branch blocks), AV pacers (for restoring conduction between atria and ventricles), and those combined with ICDs. Regardless of the underlying design of the pacing system, the purpose is to correct abnormal conduction activity in the heart and restore normal rhythm. Optimizing normal rhythm ensures maximal heart rate, stroke volume, and cardiac output responses to exercise.

Pathophysiology of Pacemakers and ICDs

There are a variety of conditions that may affect the integrity of the conduction system of the heart and therefore result in a need for a pacemaker or ICD. These conditions include, but are not limited to, coronary artery disease; HF with bundle branch block; status as a survivor of sudden cardiac death syndrome and MI that interrupts blood flow to the conduction system; and **sick sinus syndrome**, defined as aging-associated degeneration of the sinoatrial node (11). These conditions can lead to the development of a cardiac arrhythmia such as bradyarrhythmia (an abnormally slow heart rate) or heart block (an interruption or delay in the heart's electrical conduction system). This may be subsequent to impaired blood flow to the cardiac tissue as with coronary artery disease or formation of scar tissue that physically affects cardiac signal conduction.

Common Medications Given to Individuals With Pacemakers or ICDs

The pacemaker itself could be considered the "medication" for the particular condition that resulted in the need. Details regarding the vast array of pacemaker technology available are beyond the scope of this chapter, and the reader is referred to additional resources as outlined in the recommended readings. For the exercise professional, the comorbidity (38) that created the need for pacing will have the associated medications (and many of these comorbidities have been discussed in previous sections of this chapter). If the pacemaker is effective at restoring normal conduction for the heart, then exercise capacity should be enhanced.

Effects of Exercise in Individuals With Pacemakers or ICDs

In regard to exercise programming for individuals with a pacemaker or ICD, the response to training is most affected by the effectiveness of the pacemaker and the associated comorbidities (11, 38, 50). If the pacemaker is effective at restoring normal or near-normal electrical activity, then exercise capacity will be increased. The increase in quality of life for individuals with pacemakers will be proportional to their ability to adequately perform activities of daily living and symptom relief of dyspnea, hypotension, light-headedness, and syncope. If the pacemaker is effective, the response to exercise training will be consistent with the expectations associated with the underlying comorbidities (38).

Exercise Recommendations for Clients With Pacemakers or ICDs

Various conditions may lead to the treatment of a client with a pacemaker or ICD. As such, exercise programming recommendations for these clients should be consistent with recommendations for the associated comorbidity. Due to the presence of these comorbidities, it is recommended that an initial medically supervised exercise test be conducted to determine exercise tolerance and thresholds, and also to evaluate the pacemaker response under the perturbation of exercise. A subsequent medical release to exercise should be requested and obtained by the exercise professional before initiating an exercise program.

- For several weeks after the pacemaker is implanted it is recommended that aerobic and resistance training be limited to lower body large muscle group activities and be modest in order to allow for the preservation of lead integrity (2, 11, 50). The exercise intensity can range from workloads corresponding to 40% to 80% of $\dot{V}O_2$ peak on four to seven days per week and duration of continuous or accumulated activity of 20 to 60 minutes (11, 50). Note that it is likely that clients with pacemakers will benefit from supervision of their initial exercise program, perhaps as part of cardiac rehabilitation.

- Resistance training can also be undertaken with an emphasis on lower body exercises performed in a circuit training format at 40% to 60% 1RM (2, 11, 34).

- As a comprehensive part of exercise programming for the client with a pacemaker or ICD, incorporating activities of daily living throughout the day should also be encouraged.

Important specific considerations for the exercise professional with clients with pacemakers or ICDs include the following. For clients with ICDs, their target heart rates for exercise training need to be at least 10% to 15% below the rate that will trigger an incorrect firing of the device (11). The client as well as the exercise professional also needs to be aware of symptoms associated with pacemaker malfunction that may include undue fatigue. While variable, symptoms may include syncope, dyspnea, dizziness, palpitations, or tachy- or bradycardia. It is further recommended that exercise professionals become familiar with the type of pacemaker for each client they are working with. Tables 6.13 and 6.14 summarize guidelines for aerobic exercise and resistance training for clients with a pacemaker or ICD.

Table 6.13   Aerobic Exercise Guidelines for Clients With a Pacemaker or ICD

Parameter	Guideline
Frequency	4-7 days per week
Intensity	40-80% $\dot{V}O_2$ peak
Mode	Activities that engage large muscle groups such as walking, jogging, or cycling
Duration	20-60 min per day of continuous or accumulated activity

References: (11, 50)

Table 6.14 Resistance Training Guidelines for Clients With a Pacemaker or ICD

Parameter	Guideline
Frequency	2-3 days per week
Intensity	Light; 40-60% 1RM
Repetitions	10-15
Sets	1-3 sets per exercise in circuit format
Rest periods between sets	≤30 s
Exercises	8-10; emphasis on lower body

References: (2, 11, 34)

Case Study

Pacemakers and ICDs

Ms. A is a participant in her company's wellness program. She is 75 years old with no history of heart disease and no significant risk factors. As part of that program she received a medically supervised graded exercise test and exercise prescription before beginning her exercise program. The baseline 12-lead electrocardiogram performed in a supine position indicated a second-degree heart block Mobitz type II with a ventricular response of 40 beats/min. This type of heart block is at the level of the AV node and is somewhat rare and usually associated with aging. What is surprising was that Ms. A was able to function with such a low heart rate. Needless to say, her exercise test was canceled for the day and she was taken to the emergency room. After consultation with her cardiologist, Ms. A underwent surgery to install a rate-responsive dual-chambered pacemaker. She indicated after the surgery how much better she felt to have a heart rate of 72 beats/min rather than 40.

She returned avidly to her walking program with her family. It was also recommended that she consider a modest resistance training program, so she joined her daughter for exercise counseling with an exercise professional on a beginning program. Ms. A's exercise professional prescribed a circuit-style resistance training program with an initial intensity of 40% 1RM, one set of 10 repetitions per exercise, and an emphasis on her lower body to facilitate her walking program: leg press, chest press, leg extension, seated row, seated hamstring curl, seated military press, calf raise, back extension.

Recommended Readings

Brawner, C and Lewis, B. Pacemakers and implantable cardioverter defibrillators. In *ACSM's Exercise Management for Persons with Chronic Diseases and Disabilities*. 4th ed. Durstine, JL, Moore, GE, Painter, PL, and Roberts, SO, eds. Champaign, IL: Human Kinetics, 149-154, 2016.

Stewart, K and Spragg, DD. Cardiac electrical pathophysiology. In *Clinical Exercise Physiology*. 3rd ed. Ehrman, JK, Gordon, PM, Visich, PS, and Keteyian, SJ, eds. Champaign, IL: Human Kinetics, 297-313, 2013.

VALVULAR DISORDERS

Valvular heart disease (VHD) may be defined as damage to one of the valves that normally allows passive blood flow from the atria to the ventricles and from the ventricles to the aorta, pulmonary artery, or both (43). The symptoms experienced by individuals with VHD depend on the degree of damage as well as the valve affected and may include dyspnea, fatigue, pain, and palpitations. Causes include rheumatic fever, congenital issues, infection, and aging. **Rheumatic fever** is an inflammatory disease that affects the integrity of heart valves first, before affecting other body systems, and is still a major concern in developing countries (43). While VHD results in less than 1% of all CVD-related deaths, it has been estimated that 5 million American adults are diagnosed with moderate to severe VHD each year (43).

Pathophysiology of Valvular Disorders

Valves affected by VHD manifest in two ways. The valves can become stenotic (narrowed) due to fibrosis or calcification (e.g., aortic or pulmonary stenosis) (56), or valves can be "incompetent," meaning that they do not close completely, and regurgitation of blood back into a heart chamber is the result. The long-term impact of VHD regardless of location is an increase in pressure and size (hypertrophy) in all chambers of the heart (56).

Common Medications Given to Individuals With Valvular Disorders

Atrial fibrillation and coronary heart disease are common comorbidities with VHD, and the exercise professional needs to be familiar with the medications associated with each of these conditions (38). Medications that may be used for individuals with VHD include ACE inhibitors (medications table 6.5), antiarrhythmics (medications table 6.4), antibiotics (no effects on exercise), diuretics (medications table 6.1), inotropes (digitalis) (medications table 6.6), β-blockers (medications table 6.3), and anticoagulants (medications table 6.2); the impact of these medications on the associated comorbidity has been discussed previously in this chapter (28). The type and amount of medication depend on the severity and location of the valve affected (generally aortic and pulmonary VHD are more serious) and the presence of comorbidities. For the most part, the medications just listed should have a positive impact on exercise capacity, with the most impact on the more severe disease. Ultimately, valve replacement surgery may be necessary to alleviate significant symptoms not helped by medications.

Effects of Exercise in Individuals With Valvular Disorders

The exercise response for acute exercise varies and depends on the valve affected and the severity of the disease present (43). When VHD is modest with minimal symptoms, then the response to exercise is near normal, and so too are the cardiovascular and body composition benefits (43). Individuals with modest VHD will show the training responses associated with their most significant comorbidity, and the reader is referred to other sections of this chapter for details on those comorbidities. For severe VHD, in which symptoms are present at rest, exercise training may be contraindicated until other effective treatment can be performed (43).

Exercise Recommendations for Clients with Valvular Disorders

Exercise programming recommendations have a wide range and are reflective of the varied location and severity of VHD experienced between clients. In order to best understand and recognize the individual nature of the response to exercise for those with VHD, supervised exercise testing is recommended before exercise training.

- In general, the mode for aerobic exercise should be large muscle group activities such as walking, cycling, or jogging, and the intensity can range from workloads equivalent to 40% to 80% of peak $\dot{V}O_2$ monitored by both heart rate and RPE (12-16 out of 20) (43). Recommended duration is continuous or accumulated activity of 20 to 60 minutes per day, which may consist of multiple bouts of as little as 10 minutes, at a frequency of four or more days per week (43), in conjunction with engagement in activities of daily living.

- Resistance training can be performed at a very light level of 30% to 50% 1RM for clients with VHD and symptoms (2, 18, 34).

Specific recommendations for the exercise professional include using a longer warm-up and cooldown (10-15 minutes), being cognizant of the special considerations for any present comorbidities, and potentially avoiding all resistance training for clients with symptomatic aortic or pulmonary stenosis. Tables 6.15 and 6.16 summarize guidelines for aerobic exercise and resistance training for clients with valvular disorders.

Table 6.15 Aerobic Exercise Guidelines for Clients with Valvular Disorders

Parameter	Guideline
Frequency	≥4 days per week
Intensity	40-80% $\dot{V}O_2$peak; or 12-16 RPE (on Borg 6- to 20-point scale)
Mode	Activities that engage large muscle groups such as walking, jogging, or cycling
Duration	20-60 min per day of continuous or accumulated activity in bouts of ≥10 min

Reference: (43)

Table 6.16 Resistance Training Guidelines for Clients With Valvular Disorders

Parameter	Guideline
Frequency	1-2 days per week
Intensity	Very light; 30-50% 1RM
Repetitions	10-15
Sets	1-3 sets per exercise in circuit format
Rest periods between sets	≤30 s
Exercises	8-10; emphasis on lower body

References: (2, 11, 34)

Case Study

Valvular Disorders

Mr. T is 23 years old with a history of mitral valve prolapse. He denies significant symptoms from this condition and indicates that his "valve problem has never limited his activity." He has no other significant health problems and wants to run the half marathon in his city with help from an exercise professional. Since he is asymptomatic and his physician has cleared him to train for this event, the exercise professional developed a 12-week progressive program that started with brisk walking, progressed to walk-jogging, and then finally to jogging. Mr. T completed the half in less than 2.5 hours.

Recommended Readings

Parker, M. Valvular heart disease. In *ACSM's Exercise Management for Persons With Chronic Diseases and Disabilities*. 4th ed. Moore, G, Durstine, J, and Painter, P, eds. Champaign, IL: Human Kinetics, 155-162, 2016.

CARDIOVASCULAR SURGICAL PROCEDURES: CORONARY ARTERY BYPASS GRAFT AND PERCUTANEOUS TRANSLUMINAL CORONARY ANGIOPLASTY

Coronary artery bypass grafting (CABG) may be defined as open heart surgery in which the rib cage is opened and a section of a blood vessel is grafted from the aorta to the coronary artery to bypass the blocked section of the coronary artery and improve the blood supply to the heart (22, 44). There are also less invasive procedures available to perform the bypass. Coronary artery bypass grafting provides the surgical "bypass" of the lesion using either the saphenous vein or the internal mammary or gastroepiploic arteries. This procedure becomes necessary as a result of atherosclerotic lesions in blood vessels of the heart. Lesions are usually considered clinically significant at 50% blockage as identified by cardiac catheterization. Bypassing the blockage is achieved by harvesting an appropriate blood vessel, such as the saphenous vein from the leg, radial artery, or other viable donor vessel, and grafting around the coronary artery obstruction. Coronary artery bypass grafting is usually the final choice for treatment of atherosclerotic heart disease after medical management or catheter-based techniques such as percutaneous transluminal coronary angioplasty have not been effective in alleviating symptoms.

Percutaneous transluminal coronary angioplasty (PTCA) and percutaneous coronary intervention (PCI) are catheter-driven treatments for coronary atherosclerosis in which a balloon-tipped catheter is guided to the site of the lesion and expanded with the purpose of reducing the plaque and restoring blood flow (22, 44). A variety of catheter-driven techniques are available including stent placement, rotational atherectomy, and laser. More than 700,000 individuals undergo PTCA each year (22).

Pathophysiology of CABG and PTCA

When atherosclerosis, defined as the accumulation of plaque on a wall of the artery, becomes significant (>50%) or advanced, leading to an appreciable occlusion of the coronary arteries, this blockage is the underlying pathology associated with a need for catheter-driven procedures such as PTCA or PCI or surgical treatment such as CABG (22). Risk factors associated with the development of atherosclerotic lesions include HTN, hyperlipidemia, diabetes, and family history, among others (39).

Common Medications Given to Individuals With CABG or PTCA

Common medications for individuals who have undergone CABG or PTCA are prescribed for the primary purpose of risk factor reduction and decreased work on the heart, as well as reducing mortality and morbidity, and include lipid-lowering medications (statins) (medications tables 6.2 and 6.5), calcium channel blockers (medications table 6.1), β-blockers (medications tables 6.1, 6.3, 6.4, 6.5, and 6.6), anticoagulants (medications tables 6.2, 6.5, and 6.6), and antiarrhythmics (medications table 6.4) (28). The medications associated with reduced workload on the heart (calcium antagonists and β-blockers) have the ability to increase exercise capacity, although the surgery itself has a substantial impact on exercise tolerance.

Effects of Exercise in Individuals With CABG or PTCA

If the surgery and intervention are successful, both acute and chronic responses to exercise are near normal (22). The chronic aerobic training responses most relevant to this population include an increase in the arrhythmia threshold as well as other more commonly expected improvements in cardiovascular and muscular functioning from such training (e.g., increased $\dot{V}O_2$ max, lower heart rate and blood pressure at fixed submaximal workloads, decreased weight) (22). Other training outcomes related specifically to individuals with CABG or PTCA include restoration of normal contractility, increased chronotropic response, and reduced symptoms of angina.

Anecdotally, CABG and PTCA clients may express feeling so much better after their surgery or intervention that they think they are "cured" such that exercise and other lifestyle changes are not necessary. The exercise professional will need to provide education regarding the lifetime of surgical grafts (5-7 years for saphenous; 20-25 for arterial) and the importance of lifestyle changes in maximizing that lifetime. The surgery or intervention is not a cure but rather a treatment for a symptom.

Exercise Recommendations for Clients With CABG or PTCA

As previously discussed in this chapter regarding those with cardiovascular pathology requiring CABG or PTCA, medically supervised graded exercise testing should be undertaken to determine the safety of exercise training as well as the thresholds needed for exercise programming. The initial exercise programming for CABG should be done as part of cardiac rehabilitation. In the early stages after PTCA, patients do better than with CABG and can likely exercise in a health club setting with qualified personnel.

- The mode for aerobic exercise is usually large muscle group activities such as walking, jogging, or cycling; brisk walking in particular has been shown to be highly efficacious (22). The intensity can be at workloads corresponding to 40% to 80% of $\dot{V}O_2$ or heart rate reserve (22, 44).

Rating of perceived exertion can also be used to determine intensity (12-16 out of 20) for the client who has been educated regarding use of the RPE scale. Exercise training can be performed four to seven days per week for 20 to 60 minutes of continuous or accumulated activity.

- In conjunction, performance of activities of daily living that include higher levels of energy expenditure should be encouraged to enhance fitness gains and caloric expenditure, as well as encourage the client after revascularization to have confidence in performing these activities.

- Resistance training can be performed in a circuit weight training format using 8 to 10 exercise stations, beginning with a light-intensity program (40-60% 1RM) and progressing to 80% 1RM as tolerated (2, 34).

Specific considerations in exercise training for clients following CABG or PTCA include the following. If symptoms related to angina return, this may be an indicator of vessel occlusion and requires immediate attention; the client needs to be made aware of this concern. For clients who have undergone invasive CABG, the chest wall needs to be observed and healed before upper body exercises are added to the exercise programming. This recovery usually takes about two to four weeks, and the medical supervisor can confirm when upper body exercises can be added to the program. Flexibility and range of motion are critical considerations for post-CABG care if the surgery was invasive. For selected clients, HIIT may be tolerated as their program progresses (29). Tables 6.17 and 6.18 summarize guidelines for aerobic exercise and resistance training for clients with CABG or PTCA.

Table 6.17 Aerobic Exercise Guidelines for Clients With CABG or PTCA

Parameter	Guideline
Frequency	4-7 days per week
Intensity	40-80% $\dot{V}O_2$peak; or 12-16 RPE (on Borg 6- to 20-point scale)
Mode	Activities that engage large muscle groups such as brisk walking, jogging, or cycling
Duration	20-60 min per day of continuous or accumulated activity

References: (22, 44)

Table 6.18 Resistance Training Guidelines for Clients With CABG or PTCA

Parameter	Guideline
Frequency	2-3 days per week
Intensity	40-80% 1RM
Repetitions	10-15
Sets	1-3 sets per exercise in circuit format
Rest periods between sets	≤30 s
Exercises	8-10

References: (2, 34)

Case Study

CABG and PTCA

Mr. D was brought into the emergency room at a local hospital with chest pain, profuse sweating, nausea, and dyspnea. After it was determined that he was having an MI, he was sent to the catheterization lab for emergency PTCA to alleviate the blockage in his coronary arteries and restore blood flow. Unfortunately, the PTCA resulted in a tearing of the affected coronary artery, and Mr. D was rushed into emergency CABG. After successful quadruple bypass surgery, Mr. D was referred to cardiac rehabilitation for exercise training and risk factor education. He successfully finished 36 sessions of rehabilitation and was referred to his exercise professional at a local fitness club for the development of a subsequent program.

Mr. D's exercise professional prescribed an integrated aerobic and resistance training program of brisk walking four days per week and two sessions of resistance training on nonconsecutive days. Mr. D was trained in the use of RPE during rehabilitation, so for his aerobic conditioning he was initially prescribed 20 to 25 minutes of continuous brisk walking at an RPE of 12 to 16, based on information from his progression during rehabilitation. For resistance training, he was prescribed two sets of a circuit—seated leg press, leg extension, seated hamstring curl, calf raise, seated machine alternating chest press, lat pulldown, seated shoulder press, biceps curl, and triceps extension—at 60% 1RM, with 10 repetitions for each exercise and 30 seconds recovery between each.

Recommended Readings

Cooper, C, Dolezal, B, Durstine, J, Gordon, B, Pinkstaff, S, Babu, A, and Phillips, S. Chronic conditions very strongly associated with tobacco. In *ACSM's Exercise Management for Persons With Chronic Diseases and Disabilities*. 4th ed. Moore, G, Durstine, J, and Painter, P, eds. Champaign, IL: Human Kinetics, 95-114, 2016.

Patterson, MA. Revascularization of the heart. In *Clinical Exercise Physiology*. 3rd ed. Ehrman, JK, Gordon, PM, Visich, PS, and Keteyian, SJ, eds. Champaign, IL: Human Kinetics, 239-258, 2013.

CONCLUSION

The important overarching theme of this chapter for the exercise professional is that many of the conditions covered exist as comorbidities; that is, it is quite rare to find these cardiovascular conditions in isolation. For example, the individual with CHF likely has a history of a past MI. Thus the exercise professional must be aware of the issues associated with each condition and how they may interact to influence the exercise response. Exercise programming that results in an increase in fitness for individuals with comorbidities may tease out the true limiting factor for the exercise professional to focus on as she designs and modifies the exercise training. Within the limits of safety for each client, exercise professionals are limited only by their creativity for designing safe and effective exercise programming.

Key Terms

angina
atherosclerosis
atrial fibrillation
cardiac conduction defect
cardiac output
chronic heart failure (CHF)
congestive heart failure
coronary artery bypass grafting (CABG)
diastolic heart failure
hypertension
intermittent claudication
myocardial infarction (MI)

percutaneous transluminal coronary
   angioplasty (PTCA)
peripheral arterial disease (PAD)
prehypertension
rheumatic fever
sick sinus syndrome
stable angina
systolic heart failure
total peripheral resistance
unstable angina
valvular heart disease (VHD)

Study Questions

1. When exercising with individuals who have hypertension, what precaution might be necessary for individuals taking β-blockers?

    a. watching out for signs of increased blood volume

    b. use of an alternate index of intensity, besides heart rate

    c. care in changing postural positions to avoid transient hypertension

    d. ensure that the individual has eaten recently, as blood sugar may be depressed

2. Which of the following is true of exercise with individuals with stable angina?

    a. The ability to exercise will differ each day, since symptoms can appear at rest.

    b. It is possible to know at what intensity the angina will appear and to design an exercise regimen accordingly.

    c. A supervised exercise test is not necessary before training, given the predictable nature of this particular disorder.

    d. During aerobic exercise, heart rate should be around 3 to 5 beats/min below the threshold where symptoms appear.

3. What is one underlying cause of low exercise tolerance in individuals with chronic heart failure?
   a. ischemia or tissue death in the left ventricle
   b. low total fluid volume in the cardiovascular system
   c. leg pain appearing during normal activities such as walking
   d. increased muscle lactate accumulation at low-intensity exercise

4. What is the most common long-term physiological result of valvular disorders?
   a. cardiac arrhythmias
   b. lifetime reliance on diuretics
   c. myocardial hypertrophy and increased cardiac pressure
   d. regular chest pain with onset during low-intensity exercise

Medications Table 6.1   Common Medications Used to Treat Hypertension

Drug class and names	Most common side effects	Effects on exercise
Diuretics (thiazides)		
chlorothiazide (Diuril), hydrochlorothiazide (HydroDIURIL), furosemide (Lasix), indapamide (Lozol), spironolactone (Aldactone)	Weakness, confusion, potassium depletion, fatigue, thirst, gout	No effect on exercise responses unless dehydrated
β-blockers		
atenolol (Tenormin), bisoprolol (Zebeta), metoprolol (Toprol XL), carvedilol (Coreg), acebutolol (Sectral)	Dizziness, wheezing, fatigue, depression, impotence, decreased high-density lipoprotein (HDL)	Decreased submaximal and maximal blood pressure and heart rate, decreased maximal oxygen uptake in hypertension
Calcium channel blockers		
amlodipine (Norvasc), isradipine (Dynacirc), diltiazem (Cardizem), verapamil (Calan), nifedipine (Procardia)	Headache, dizziness, edema, heartburn, constipation, palpitations	May or may not decrease exercise submaximal and maximal heart rate, lower submaximal and maximal blood pressure
Angiotensin II receptor blockers		
losartan (Cozaar), valsartan (Diovan), olmesartan (Benicar), irbesartan (Avapro)	Muscle cramps, dizziness, hypotension, orthostatic intolerance	May or may not decrease exercise submaximal and maximal heart rate, lower submaximal and maximal blood pressure
Angiotensin-converting enzyme (ACE) inhibitors		
lisinopril (Zestril, Prinivil), benazepril (Lotensin), ramipril (Altace), quinapril (Accupril)	Cough, rash, fluid retention, hypotension, orthostatic intolerance	May decrease exercise submaximal and maximal heart rate, lower submaximal and maximal blood pressure

Reference: (4)

Medications Table 6.2 Common Medications Used to Treat Peripheral Arterial Disease

Drug class and names	Most common side effects	Effects on exercise
Antiplatelet–vasoactive agents		
cilostazol (Pletal), pentoxifylline (Trental)	Headache, diarrhea, palpitations, dizziness	Increased time or distance to onset of symptoms
Statins		
atorvastatin (Lipitor), fluvastatin (Lescol), lovastatin (Mevacor), pravastatin (Pravachol), rosuvastatin calcium (Crestor), simvastatin (Zocor)	GI discomfort, headaches, muscle aches, drowsiness, dizziness, myopathy, liver damage	May attenuate aerobic training benefits and increase myalgias when combined with exercise
Anticoagulants		
pentoxifylline (Trental), clopidogrel (Plavix; commonly paired with aspirin)	Bloating, dizziness, indigestion	May cause excessive bleeding in response to injury

Reference: (6, 32)

Medications Table 6.3 Common Medications Used to Treat Angina

Drug class and names	Most common side effects	Effects on exercise
Nitrates		
nitroglycerin (Nitrolingual)	Dizziness, headache, nausea, flushing, blurred vision	Increased time to symptoms
Calcium channel antagonists		
amlodipine (Norvasc), diltiazem (Cardizem), nifedipine (Procardia)	Constipation, headache, dizziness, nausea, tachycardia, fatigue, swelling of feet or lower legs	Typically no significant effects on exercise; may decrease blood flow to working muscles; may decrease lactate threshold; may reduce maximal heart rate
β-blockers		
atenolol (Tenormin), bisoprolol (Zebeta), Metoprolol (Toprol XL), carvedilol (Coreg), acebutolol (Sectral)	Dizziness, wheezing, fatigue, depression, impotence, decreased HDL	Decreased submaximal and maximal blood pressure and heart rate, decreased maximal oxygen uptake in hypertension
Antiischemic nonhemodynamic agents		
ranolazine (Ranexa)	Dizziness, nausea, vomiting, dry mouth, headache, constipation	No significant effect on exercising heart rate or blood pressure

References: (7, 53)

Medications Table 6.4 Common Medications Used to Treat Chronic Heart Failure

Drug class and names	Most common side effects	Effects on exercise
Antiarrhythmics		
digoxin (Lanoxin)	Dizziness, syncope, tachycardia, bradycardia, arrhythmia	No effects
β-blockers		
atenolol (Tenormin), bisoprolol (Zebeta), metoprolol (Toprol XL), carvedilol (Coreg), acebutolol (Sectral)	Dizziness, wheezing, fatigue, depression, impotence, decreased HDL	Decreased submaximal and maximal blood pressure and heart rate, decreased maximal oxygen uptake in hypertension
Diuretics (thiazides)		
chlorothiazide (Diuril), hydrochlorothiazide (HydroDIURIL), furosemide (Lasix), indapamide (Lozol), spironolactone (Aldactone)	Weakness, confusion, potassium depletion, fatigue, thirst, gout	No effect on exercise responses unless dehydrated
Angiotensin-converting enzyme (ACE) inhibitors		
lisinopril (Zestril, Prinivil), benazepril (Lotensin), ramipril (Altace), quinapril (Accupril)	Cough, rash, fluid retention, hypotension, orthostatic intolerance	May decrease exercise submaximal and maximal heart rate, lower submaximal and maximal blood pressure
Calcium channel antagonists		
amlodipine (Norvasc), diltiazem (Cardizem), nifedipine (Procardia)	Constipation, headache, dizziness, nausea, tachycardia, fatigue, swelling of feet or lower legs	Typically no significant effects on exercise; may decrease blood flow to working muscles; may decrease lactate threshold; may reduce maximal heart rate
Aldosterone receptor blockers		
eplerenone (Inspra), spironolactone (Aldactone)	Nausea, vomiting, stomach cramps, diarrhea, hyperkalemia	No significant adverse effects on exercise responses

References: (59)

Medications Table 6.5   Common Medications Used to Treat Myocardial Infarction

Drug class and names	Most common side effects	Effects on exercise
β-blockers		
atenolol (Tenormin), bisoprolol (Zebeta), metoprolol (Toprol XL), carvedilol (Coreg), acebutolol (Sectral)	Dizziness, wheezing, fatigue, depression, impotence, decreased HDL	Decreased submaximal and maximal blood pressure and heart rate, decreased maximal oxygen uptake in hypertension
Vasodilators		
hydralazine (Apresoline), minoxidil (Loniten)	Headaches, tachycardia, joint pain, fluid retention	Postural hypotension
Angiotensin-converting enzyme (ACE) inhibitors		
lisinopril (Zestril, Prinvil), benazepril (Lotensin), ramipril (Altace), quinapril (Accupril)	Cough, rash, fluid retention, hypotension, orthostatic intolerance	May decrease exercise submaximal and maximal heart rate, lower submaximal and maximal blood pressure
Anticoagulants		
pentoxifylline (Trental), clopidogrel (Plavix; commonly paired with aspirin)	Bloating, dizziness, indigestion	May cause excessive bleeding in response to injury
Statins		
atorvastatin (Lipitor), fluvastatin (Lescol), lovastatin (Mevacor), pravastatin (Pravachol), rosuvastatin calcium (Crestor), simvastatin (Zocor)	GI discomfort, headaches, muscle aches, drowsiness, dizziness, myopathy, liver damage	May attenuate aerobic training benefits and increase myalgias when combined with exercise
Calcium channel antagonists		
amlodipine (Norvasc), diltiazem (Cardizem), nifedipine (Procardia)	Constipation, headache, dizziness, nausea, tachycardia, fatigue, swelling of feet or lower legs	Typically no significant effects on exercise; may decrease blood flow to working muscles; may decrease lactate threshold; may reduce maximal heart rate

Reference: (10)

Medications Table 6.6 Common Medications Used to Treat Atrial Fibrillation

Drug class and names	Most common side effects	Effects on exercise
Anticoagulants		
pentoxifylline (Trental), clopidogrel (Plavix; commonly paired with aspirin)	Bloating, dizziness, indigestion	May cause excessive bleeding in response to injury
Inotropes		
digitalis (Crystodigin)	Diarrhea, drowsiness, muscle weakness, fatigue, headache, blurry vision, tachycardia, bradycardia	May decrease heart rate
Calcium channel antagonists		
amlodipine (Norvasc), diltiazem (Cardizem), nifedipine (Procardia)	Constipation, headache, dizziness, nausea, tachycardia, fatigue, swelling of feet or lower legs	Typically no significant effects on exercise; may decrease blood flow to working muscles; may decrease lactate threshold; may reduce maximal heart rate
β-blockers		
atenolol (Tenormin), bisoprolol (Zebeta), metoprolol (Toprol XL), carvedilol (Coreg), acebutolol (Sectral)	Dizziness, wheezing, fatigue, depression, impotence, decreased HDL	Decreased sub-maximal and maximal blood pressure and heart rate, decreased maximal oxygen uptake in hypertension

References: (13, 42)

Immunologic and Hematologic Disorders

Don Melrose, PhD, CSCS,*D

Jay Dawes, PhD, CSCS,*D, NSCA-CPT,*D, FNSCA

Misty Kesterson, EdD, CSCS

Benjamin Reuter, PhD, ATC, CSCS,*D

After completing this chapter, you will be able to

- describe the immunologic and hematologic disorders and the characteristics associated with the various diseases,

- understand the short-term and long-term effects of the diseases,

- describe the pathophysiology of each disease,

- discuss the common medications used in the treatment of each disease,

- discuss the benefits and contraindications of exercise for each disease, and

- develop an exercise program for an individual with each disease.

The immune system consists of molecules, cells, tissues, and organs that function to defend the body against infection by foreign substances, such as bacteria, viruses, parasites, and other infectious organisms that might cause disease or illness (66). **Systemic autoimmune diseases** represent a broad range of related diseases characterized by altered immune system function that results in the immune cells attacking healthy tissue (186). Consequently, these conditions often result in an inappropriate inflammatory response and widespread tissue damage to multiple bodily systems. Common autoimmune disorders include rheumatoid arthritis, lupus, chronic fatigue syndrome, and fibromyalgia.

The etiology of the hematologic disorders is known, but the exact etiology of most autoimmune disorders is unclear. Immunologic and hematologic disorders may stem from a combination of genetics, history of infection, environmental factors, and endocrine function (186). For most autoimmune and hematologic disorders, the main focus of an intervention relates to minimizing symptomatology and further damage, developing effective management and coping strategies, improving functional abilities, and improving quality of life rather than curing the condition.

The most common hematologic disorders include human immune deficiency (HIV) or acquired immune deficiency syndrome (AIDS), sickle cell anemia, and hemophilia. The latter two conditions affect the tissues and systemic structures by different means. Sickle cell anemia alters the red blood cells and transportation of the blood to the tissues, causing damage to the structures and organs (50). Hemophilia, on the other hand, results in repetitive and often life-threatening bleeding. If left untreated, it can lead to other clinical manifestations and poor quality of life (162).

RHEUMATOID ARTHRITIS

Rheumatoid arthritis (RA) is an autoimmune disease that causes chronic inflammation of the joints of the body (59, 199). The risk for developing the disease is less than 5% for either sex, although it is higher for women than for men

(56). It typically affects people over the age of 40, but can occur earlier. The long-term effects of the disease are atrophy of muscles (190), joint deformity, and disability (22). This disability results in a gradual decline in physical mobility and quality of life and in premature death (110). As an autoimmune disease, RA has been found to be linked to other serious conditions, such as cardiovascular disease, anemia, lupus, interstitial lung disease, Sjogren's syndrome or dry eyes and mouth, vasculitis, osteoporosis, and reduced kidney function (45, 93, 97, 201). Individuals with RA are also at a great risk for falls and osteoporosis. There are many psychosocial issues associated with RA as well, such as depression, decrease in quality of life, work disability (204), decreased self-efficacy, and changes in lifestyle and environment (86).

History and Demographics of Rheumatoid Arthritis

Rheumatoid arthritis is the most common autoimmune disease (206). It typically occurs in individuals with ancestors from Asia or Europe (103). The condition manifests more often in women (70% of the time) (110) and in smokers (211) and affects 1% of the world's population (171). Family history has also been identified as a risk factor for RA (4). Interestingly, pregnancy may cause remission of the disease, and there is a decreased risk of disease development in women who breast-feed their babies (120). Zhang and colleagues (223) suggest that there is a relationship between low socioeconomic status, lower education levels, and pain perception in those with RA. Many individuals with RA are inactive (101).

Pathophysiology of Rheumatoid Arthritis

Inflammation is typically a normal protective response against foreign substances. But in the case of RA, the immune system releases antibodies that cause an inflammation to attack the cartilage and synovial lining of the joints (synovitis). The synovia provides a protective layer for the joint and tendon. As the inflammation progresses it causes a thickening of the lining of the joint and the joint becomes filled with synovial fluid. Most frequently, it begins with the wrists, fingers, and hands; individuals with RA initially complain of pain, stiffness, and localized swelling. The swelling and inflammation can cause lumps beneath the skin or rheumatoid nodules and deformity of the joint. Joint damage and disabilities increase gradually over a period of 10 to 20 years characteristically (171). As the disease progresses, the inflammation spreads to other systems, damaging other tissue, such as the lining of the heart (myocarditis) and lungs (interstitial lung disease) and vessels associated with other organs, such as the kidneys (97). RA is often characterized by high blood pressure, fever, inability to maintain body mass, and fatigue or unexplained tiredness (211).

In 2010, the American College of Rheumatology in collaboration with the European League Against Rheumatism developed an updated system to classify RA. The main purpose of the new system was to encourage identification of RA before symptoms such as nodules or joint damage become apparent. Criteria include the number of joints affected and size of the joints, the presence of rheumatoid antibodies, acute response, and duration of symptoms. Classification for RA requires a score >6 out of a possible 10 (14).

At this time there is no cure. The predominant treatment and management goal should be to control the inflammation caused by the disease. Through control of inflammation, the pain commonly associated with RA can be minimized (84). This has the effect of allowing individuals to maintain activity levels and health (59) and reducing the long-term complications associated with the disease.

Common Medications Given to Individuals With Rheumatoid Arthritis

Individuals suffering from RA typically use medications aimed at reducing the inflammatory process associated with this disorder. According to Wasserman (211), these medications may include **nonsteroidal anti-inflammatory drugs (NSAIDs)** that block the inflammatory responses and affect the function of the white blood cells. Nonsteroidal anti-inflammatory drugs are typically used for the short-term management of RA (211).

Disease-modifying antirheumatic drugs (DMARDs) reduce the progression of joint damage and disability. Disease-modifying antirheumatic drugs are classified as synthetic DMARDs, **biological response modifiers**, and glucocorticoids. The DMARDs are taken alone or in conjunction with other DMARDs, with NSAIDs, or with corticosteroids or biologics; this is commonly referred to as combination therapy. The DMARDs suppress the immune system, putting individuals at risk of infections and cancer. Synthetic DMARDs are slow to act, usually taking weeks to months to show benefits. They are often given early in the diagnosis of RA to minimize the joint damage. Their side effects are minimal (71).

The biologics act as an inhibitor that blocks the body's immune response. Biologic response modifiers are genetically engineered agents that act to stimulate the body's response to infection (19). Intra-articular **corticosteroid** injections reduce joint inflammation and thus pain and have also been found to improve range of motion (147). Corticosteroids mimic the hormone cortisol and help to control inflammation. However, the effect lasts for only a few weeks or months. There are many forms of corticosteroids, allowing individuals many choices of application. See medications table 7.1 near the end of the chapter.

Effects of Exercise in Individuals With Rheumatoid Arthritis

Individuals with RA should meet the minimum requirements for exercise prescribed for healthy populations (2). Without regular exercise, individuals with RA will suffer the same effects of a sedentary lifestyle seen in healthy individuals (52). Consistent cardiovascular training can be helpful to reduce the health risks of cardiovascular disease (160), obesity, and diabetes. It has been found that moderate intensity aerobic exercise (65% to <75%

of calculated maximal heart rate [MHR]) can be beneficial for individuals with RA, providing many protective cardiovascular, strength, and functional benefits (63, 173), and possibly even altering the pathophysiology of the disease (199).

Resistance training can reduce RA-associated muscle atrophy and subsequent strength loss (190) that can lead to osteoporosis and frequent falls. Regular resistance training can be beneficial for most individuals, including those with RA. A number of studies have examined resistance training in individuals with RA and reported positive results (30, 131, 190). Strasser and colleagues (190) found positive physiological effects with a resistance training program that progressed to three or four sets of 10 to 15 reps at about 70% 1RM (one repetition maximum) for all major muscle groups.

The training programs for individuals with RA examined by Strasser and colleagues (190) and Breedland and colleagues (30) were programs that used both resistance training and cardiovascular training. Both training interventions were relatively short (eight weeks and six months, respectively). Cycle ergometry was initiated at 60% heart rate reserve for 40 minutes twice a week. The Breedland and colleagues (30) study or "FIT program" incorporated an educational component in addition to the physical training, teaching self-management techniques to assist individuals in managing their disease. Research has also reported positive effects on balance and range of motion from other types of training such as yoga (75) and tai chi (98).

When prescribing exercise, it is important that the exercise professional consider how clients perceive the benefits of exercise and their limitations, the environment, and barriers to

Key Point

Exercise professionals should be very aware of how clients respond to training and be willing to adjust frequency, intensity, and time as needed. For clients with RA, these adjustments may be based on pain.

exercise (207), as well as home exercise programs versus supervised exercise programs. There are also social benefits of participating in supervised group exercise programs.

Exercise Recommendations for Clients With Rheumatoid Arthritis

Program design guidelines for clients with RA are summarized in table 7.1. Exercise professionals should consider the client's interests, fitness levels, classification of RA, current and acute pain levels, and goals when prescribing exercise. A warm-up should consist of dynamic activity, performed at light to moderate intensity. For those with a high rheumatism classification or those experiencing inflammation or pain, no-impact to low-impact large-muscle activities should be encouraged, such as walking, swimming, biking, elliptical or rowing machines, or water activities (e.g., water aerobics and water walking or running). Persons with RA should start at a light to moderate level of exercise but progress to moderate- to high-intensity aerobic activities. Running and sport (if tolerated) should be conducted two to five days per week with a goal of most, if not all, days per week, at an intensity of 55% to 85% maximum predicted heart rate (30, 203, 224). Clients should be encouraged to do resistance training to strengthen all major muscle groups at 40% to 80% 1RM two or three days per week, progressing from one or two sets initially to three or four sets of 10 to 15 reps. A combination of intermittent aerobic activities and resistance training at an intensity that is tolerated can be recommended. Exercise professionals should consider the primary joints affected by the RA and modify activities accordingly. Balance and range of motion from other types of training such as yoga, tai chi, and stretching should be encouraged as well. It's important to monitor the client's pain levels and adjust exercise accordingly. The cooldown should consist of 5 to 10 minutes of light-intensity aerobic activity and static stretching.

Table 7.1 Program Design Guidelines for Clients With Rheumatoid Arthritis

Type of exercise	Frequency	Intensity
Resistance training		

Multijoint movements
  a. Bodyweight resistance
  b. May use resistance bands, suspension training, and manual resistance
  c. Basic weight training such as resistance machines and free weights
Mode of resistance training can vary based on how well exercise is tolerated.
	Frequency will vary based on postexertion symptomatology.
	Strive for two or three sessions per week.
		Avoid exercises with impact unless tolerated.
		Choose 8-10 exercises using a full-body approach.
		Slowly progress over time to 2-3 sets of 10-15 repetitions.
		Use light to moderate intensity, 40-80% 1RM.
		If doing multiple sets, consider 1-2 min between sets to start; be prepared to adjust as needed.

Aerobic training		
Aerobic exercise mode should be low impact and well tolerated. Water aerobics, water walking or running, swimming, and biking are good suggestions. Mode of aerobic training can vary based on how well exercise is tolerated. Consider combination of intermittent aerobic activities and resistance training.	Begin conservatively, working up to two to five sessions per week. If tolerated, sessions can be increased slowly over time. Sessions can be performed most, if not all, days of the week.	Using 55-85% MHR, begin with 3- to 10-min bouts as tolerated, progressing to 2- to 15-min bouts. Strive for 20-60 min of continuous exercise. Tolerance may vary widely between clients.
Flexibility training		
Full-body flexibility exercises, starting with static stretching Also consider range of motion, functional activities, yoga, tai chi, and stretching.	1-3 days per week	8-10 static stretches, held 5-10 s initially, progressing to 20 s as tolerated

Note: MHR, maximal heart rate.

References: (30, 203, 224)

Case Study

Rheumatoid Arthritis

Sex: Female

Age: 58

Height: 5 feet, 8 inches (1.73 m)

Weight: 150 pounds (68 kg)

Body fat: 23%

Body mass index: 22.8

Resting heart rate: 75 beats/min

Blood pressure: 122/82 mmHg

Estimated $\dot{V}O_2$: No test was performed due to limited mobility

History

Ms. K, who is 58, was diagnosed with RA 20 years ago. Since her diagnosis, she has had numerous foot surgeries, as well as three wrist surgeries due to RA damage. For the past 18 months, she has been performing tai chi twice a week. Due to compromised ankle motion and arthritic changes in her knees from RA, she is unable to perform any weight-bearing aerobic exercise. Ms. K is eager to increase her strength and to understand how resistance training can

(continued)

be performed within the limitations of her RA. Having met with her primary physician, she was encouraged to seek the advice of a certified exercise professional for further advice on exercise.

Intake

Ms. K met with an exercise professional at her local fitness club. The exercise professional took a full medical history and did basic range of motion testing for all joints, took an estimate of cardiopulmonary capacity, and conducted an isometric strength battery. Ms. K was also encouraged to seek the advice of a registered dietician to aid in this process.

Goals

Ms. K and her exercise professional agreed on the following goals:

1. Increase aerobic capacity
2. Increase overall strength
3. Increase flexibility and joint mobility

Initial Training

The exercise professional encouraged Ms. K to incorporate nonimpact aerobic activity for a change of pace, such as water walking two or three days per week. Ms. K seemed to enjoy the socialization of the group water classes that incorporated a combination of nonimpact aerobic activity, strengthening associated with the resistance of the water, and stretching into a 1-hour session. The exercise professional guided Ms. K to progress slowly so as to avoid excessive fatigue and a possible flare.

Exercise Progression

After eight weeks, Ms. K met with the exercise professional to reevaluate her progress. She was doing so well that they decided to incorporate some resistance training for all the major muscle groups into her program as tolerated, with a goal of one or two times a week, 8 to 10 exercises for two or three sets of 10 repetitions at 70% 1RM, with her aerobic class schedule. She started at two times a week and has been able to increase to three times a week. The exercise professional recommended that Ms. K progress slowly so as to avoid excessive fatigue and a possible flare.

Outcomes

Ms. K did not experience any flares during the time period and is enjoying her improved aerobic capacity, joint mobility, and strength.

Training Recommendations and Contraindications for Clients With RA

1. Make exercise a regular part of the daily routine.
2. Choose aerobic exercises at a tolerated intensity such as biking, walking or jogging, swimming, water walking, water aerobics, tai chi, or yoga.
3. Avoid ballistic motions when training. Use smooth, controlled movements that will reduce the chance of injury and allow proper control of movement.
4. Vary the modes of aerobic and resistance training to avoid repetitive-motion injuries.
5. Allow extra time for adaptation when beginning any new form of training. Reduce intensity of the following workout until fatigue and soreness subside.
6. Sometimes joint pain is reflective of muscle stiffness. Gentle flexibility exercise may help alleviate joint pain.
7. Work within the physical and mental limitations of RA. Remember, moving regularly makes the difference.

LUPUS

Lupus erythematosus (lupus) is a multisystem idiopathic disease characterized by both acute and chronic inflammatory destruction of the skin, joints, blood elements, kidneys, serosa, nervous system, and other tissues (112). This autoimmune disease encompasses a broad range of cutaneous pathology (170). For individuals with lupus, autoantibodies in the bloodstream may target healthy tissues rather than fight foreign infectious agents that cause defects in both humoral and cellular immune responses (124, 216).

At one end of the lupus disease spectrum is a condition referred to as **discoid lupus erythematosus** (DLE), which primarily affects the skin without internal disease. On the opposite end of the spectrum, **systemic lupus erythematosus** (SLE) is much more serious. Systemic lupus erythematosus may be classified as either nonorgan threatening or organ threatening (216).

History and Demographics of Lupus

According to the Lupus Foundation of America (135), it is estimated that 1.5 million Americans, and up to 5 million people worldwide, have some form of lupus. Incidence rates of the most common type of lupus, SLE, are dependent on sex and race (41, 193). Similar to most autoimmune disorders, lupus appears to disproportionately affect females (10:1 female-to-male ratio), with the onset of symptoms typically occurring between the ages of 15 and 45 (216). For this reason, lupus is described as predominantly a young woman's disease that shortens life expectancy, and it is associated with significant health issues and reduced quality of life (124). With regard to the occurrence of SLE and race, the highest rates are seen among Afro-Caribbean people, followed by Asians, and then Caucasians (105). Some of the signs and symptoms associated with lupus are fatigue, sleep disturbances, low levels of physical fitness, depression, cognitive impairment, malar and discoid rash, photosensitivity, oral ulcers, arthritis, renal disorder, neurologic disorder, hematologic disorder, and antinuclear antibodies (23, 69, 99, 163).

Pathophysiology of Lupus

The exact cause or causes of lupus are uncertain. Although lupus is an autoimmune disorder, at this time it appears that the activation of this disease is likely the culmination of several predisposing features, such as genetics, environmental factors, and various hormonal factors (172). The primary physiological factors associated with SLE are cytokine dysregulation, polyclonal B-cell activation, autoantibody production, and increased immune complex formation involving hyperactive B and T cells (150). Assuming the proper predisposition to develop lupus, a variety of environmental "triggers" have been identified that may activate this illness or produce a flare of symptomatology. Such triggers include ultraviolet rays from the sun; ultraviolet rays from fluorescent bulbs; sulfa drugs that produce photosensitivity; penicillin or other antibiotic drugs; an infection, cold, or other viral illness; exhaustion; injuries; and emotional stress or stressful traumas to the body (135).

Presently, there is no known cure for lupus. The majority of treatment options for this condition focus on the prevention of symptom "flare-ups" as well as minimizing tissue damage and health complications associated with this disorder (216). Treatment regimens for lupus involve a variety of strategies including anti-inflammatory medications, exercise, nutritional supplementation, corticosteroids, and in some cases chemotherapy (216).

Common Medications Given to Individuals With Lupus

Many of the medications used by persons with lupus are also used by those with RA. See medications table 7.2 near the end of the chapter. Most are selected to reduce the inflammatory process. They include NSAIDs, corticosteroids, antimalarial medications, immunosuppressive medications, and dehydroepiandrosterone (DHEA) (158, 195). Nonsteroidal anti-inflammatory drugs are not known to have negative impacts on exercise performance; to the contrary, they have been shown to reduce exercise-induced fatigue (58, 133). Some evidence suggests that NSAIDs like ibuprofen may inhibit certain prostaglandins responsible for signaling translational responses to resistance exercise (143). This could over time attenuate the exercise recovery process. Most who take antimalarial drugs experience no side effects; however, should they occur, they are usually minor and persist for only a short time. Side effects that may interfere with exercise could include skin rashes, loss of appetite, abdominal bloating and cramps, and possibly muscle weakness (195). Corticosteroids can affect longer-term exercise responses in multiple ways, most of which are negative. Negative effects may include weight gain, redistribution of fat, hypertension, and increased cholesterol (195). Collectively, the most commonly used immunosuppressant medications do not appear to inhibit exercise response or capacity, but may have side effects that make exercising difficult or uncomfortable. For example, these drugs are known to increase susceptibility to colds and infections, suppression of fever symptoms, nausea, vomiting, diarrhea, abdominal pain, headache, dizziness, and sensitivity to sunlight (195). DHEA is an unapproved medication for those with lupus. It is not known to have negative effects on exercise performance or responses, and DHEA has been shown to be beneficial to people who are elderly as it may enhance muscle mass and strength as a result of heavy resistance training (208). Possible side effects of DHEA include acne, facial hair growth, oily skin, excessive sweating, lowered high-density lipoprotein in women, and increased estrogen levels in postmenopausal women.

Effects of Exercise in Individuals With Lupus

While there is not an extensive body of literature regarding the physiological effects of exercise on individuals with lupus, there is a growing body of work on the effects of exercise on attenuation of lupus-related symptoms. Much of the research in this area specifically used individuals with SLE. Most recently, the effects of a one-year high-intensity aerobic training program using women with mild to moderate SLE found improvements in $\dot{V}O_2$ max and no change in health-related quality of life. It was noted that individuals with lupus tolerated this training very well as the organs showed no sign of further damage (29). Other investigations have reflected this observation (47, 152). With regard to managing the symptomatology of lupus, other investigations using aerobic exercise have shown

improvements in fatigue and improved exercise tolerance, aerobic capacity, quality of life, and anxiety and depression (62, 107, 194). The utilization of resistance training in research protocols is much less common. One investigation comparing the efficacy of light-intensity cardiovascular training versus moderate resistance training in individuals with lupus found that both forms of training improved quality of life, but cardiovascular training was more effective (6). Another investigation used a similar design to compare the same two types of training and found that both forms of training were safe and did not worsen SLE disease activity. This investigation showed improvements in fatigue, functional status, cardiovascular fitness, and muscular strength (174). The benefits of exercise to the individuals with lupus notwithstanding, it should be noted that excessive levels of physical activity or exercise may intensify fatigue and result in excessive pain in the joints following a training session. This can result in the cessation of physical activity for several days in order to recover (216). For some clients, exercise programming may focus on symptom management and improving or maintaining one's ability to perform basic activities of daily living and not pushing physical limits (216).

Exercise Recommendations for Clients With Lupus

Program design guidelines for clients with lupus are summarized in table 7.2. Due to the nature of lupus and the variability of symptoms, initial exercise programming for this population should be both individualized and conservative. As with otherwise well populations, signs and symptoms of poor adaptation to training should be observed. Such indicators may include but are not limited to excessive or prolonged soreness, joint pain, and fatigue well beyond lupus symptoms and lack of exercise tolerance or lack of progress. Routinely communicating with the client is necessary to ensure progress.

Many clients with lupus suffer from significant reductions in cardiorespiratory health and capacity (23). Thus it is not uncommon for these clients to experience a higher incidence of comorbidity, such as obesity, hyperlipidemia, high blood pressure, and metabolic syndrome, than the general population (23). Therefore, a great deal of emphasis has been placed on improving the aerobic fitness levels of those with lupus (23). Additionally, it is prudent that they not exceed a 10 to 12 rating on Borg's perceived exertion scale. It is recommended that clients initially begin with three 10-minute bouts or two 15-minute bouts, three or four days per week as symptoms allow. Clients should progress to one 30-minute bout of continuous cardiovascular exercise three or four days per week as tolerance and symptoms allow. However, it should be noted that this is a conservative approach. Because lupus symptoms and tolerance levels vary dramatically, clients may progress at widely differing levels.

Resistance training has been proposed as a potential method to support, protect, and strengthen joints that may be negatively affected by lupus (216). Furthermore, strength training may also help improve the ability to successfully complete basic activities of daily living (ADL), improve physical parameters, aid in the reduction of postexertional fatigue, and enhance the chances of maintaining independent living.

With a novice client, it is recommended that resistance training programs include 8 to 10 exercises focusing on the large muscle groups, performed two or three days per week depending on the client's current training status and symptomatology. Initially, clients should aim for two or three sets of 10 to 12

Key Point

Clients with lupus should allow extra time for adaptation when beginning any new form of training. Reduce intensity during the following workout until fatigue and soreness subside. Moving regularly makes the difference.

repetitions (40-60% 1RM) per exercise at light- to moderate-intensity levels. Rest periods of 1 to 2 minutes are recommended; however, client symptoms may necessitate longer rest. Should severe or prolonged muscle soreness or fatigue ensue following training, the intensity of the next training session should be modified and the total volume of training reduced to improve exercise tolerance and prevent further symptom flare-ups.

Stretching may aid in improving or maintaining flexibility and joint range of motion by lengthening tight and shortened muscle fibers related to musculoskeletal pain caused by lupus (216). It is recommended that the client initially attempt to hold each stretch at the point of mild discomfort for approximately 5 to 10 seconds and progressively increase the duration of each stretch up to 10 to 20 seconds.

Table 7.2   Program Design Guidelines for Clients With Lupus

Type of exercise	Frequency	Intensity
Resistance training		
Multijoint movements a. Bodyweight resistance b. May use resistance bands, suspension training, and manual resistance c. Basic weight training such as resistance machines and free weights Mode of resistance training can vary based on how well exercise is tolerated.	Frequency will vary based on postexertion symptomatology. Strive for two or three sessions per week.	Choose 8-10 exercises, using a full-body approach. Slowly progress over time to 2-3 sets of 10-12 repetitions. Use light to moderate intensity, 40-60% 1RM; can progress to 65-75% 1RM. If doing multiple sets, consider 1-2 min between sets to start; be prepared to adjust as needed.
Aerobic training		
Aerobic exercise mode should be low impact and well tolerated. No mode-specific contraindications are implicated. Mode of aerobic training can vary based on how well exercise is tolerated.	Begin conservatively, working up to three or four sessions per week. If tolerated, sessions can be increased slowly over time. Sessions can be performed most, if not all, days of the week.	Using 60% $\dot{V}O_2$peak or 70-80% MHR, begin with three 10-min bouts as tolerated, progressing to two 15-min bouts. Strive for 30 min of continuous exercise. Tolerance may vary widely between clients.
Flexibility training		
Full-body flexibility exercises, starting with static stretching	Daily or as tolerated	8-10 static stretches, held 5-10 s initially, progressing to 20 s as tolerated

References: (6, 62, 107, 174, 194, 216)

Lupus

Sex: Female

Race: African American

Age: 32

Height: 5 feet, 5 inches (1.65 m)

Weight: 185 pounds (84 kg)

Body fat: 32%

Body mass index: 30.8

Resting heart rate: 77 beats/min

Blood pressure: 142/94 mmHg

Temperature: Normal

History

Mrs. D is a parts manager at an auto dealership. Her job entails standing for long periods of time and retrieving sometimes heavy auto parts for customers. She was diagnosed with SLE eight years ago and currently has untreated hypertension. She experiences acute inflammatory arthritis in her joints and persistent muscle pain. Over the past several months she has experienced generalized weakness, reduced mobility, and overall fatigue. She currently takes NSAID medication to help with arthritis pain. Due to her symptoms, she has avoided regular physical activity. Additionally, she has taken a leave of absence from work as it has become too painful to stand for long periods of time.

Goals

Mrs. D would like to work toward the following goals:

1. Strengthen her body and improve her physical capacity
2. Return to work and daily activities with less pain and fatigue
3. Reduce blood pressure
4. Improve body composition

Initial Intake

Before beginning an exercise intervention, Mrs. D's primary physician gave her clearance to begin a modest but progressive exercise regimen. Mrs. D met with an exercise professional at her local fitness club. The exercise professional took a full medical history, took an estimate of cardiopulmonary capacity (e.g., the University of Houston Non-Exercise Test), and performed an isometric strength battery. Body composition was assessed using bioelectric impedance. The exercise professional recommended a progressive resistance training program, flexibility training, and a regimen of cardiopulmonary exercise. It was also recommended that Mrs. D seek nutritional counseling to help promote general health, aid with weight loss, and help to address her hypertension.

Training sessions began with three 5-minute aerobic intervals consisting of walking, twice per week. Heart rate changes were monitored during aerobic training. Following aerobic training, gentle static stretching was performed for all major muscle groups. All stretches were held for 10 seconds and repeated a second time as tolerated. Resistance training consisted of basic multijoint, bodyweight movements. Five or six movements that were reasonably well tolerated by the client were initially performed for one set of up to 10 to 12 repetitions. Two-minute rest periods were used. All resistance training movements were executed in a slow, controlled manner. Movements were terminated below the level of volitional fatigue and within the client's pain-free range of motion.

Exercise Progression

Aerobic interval time was gradually increased by 1 to 2 minutes each week until several weeks later; a single 30-minute effort was tolerated at each training session. Resistance training was then to progress from bodyweight movements to elastic bands to most other forms of resistance training. Resistance training was to progress until two or three sets of 8 to 10 movements could be performed; it could turn out to be necessary to use a split program in which different body parts are worked on different days. Static flexibility training could be performed separately or incorporated between resistance training sets. Training schedules were to be flexible to reduce the instances of flare-ups and pain. Progress could be slower to accommodate reduced recovery.

Outcomes

With consistent effort over several months, Mrs. D was able to reach most of her goals. She was eventually able to return to full capacity at work. The pain in her joints, muscle weakness, and fatigue were significantly reduced, but not to normal levels. With dietary modification, moderate weight loss, and increased physical activity, blood pressure was reduced.

Training Recommendations and Contraindications for Clients With Lupus

1. Making exercise a regular part of the daily routine can lessen the chances of flare-ups.
2. Choose low-impact aerobic exercises such as biking, walking, swimming, tai chi, or yoga.
3. Avoid ballistic motions when training. Use smooth, controlled movements that will reduce the chance of injury and allow proper control of movement.
4. Vary the modes of aerobic and resistance training to avoid repetitive-motion injuries.
5. Allow extra time for adaptation when beginning any new form of training. Reduce intensity of the following workout until fatigue and soreness subside.
6. Sometimes joint pain is reflective of muscle stiffness. Gentle flexibility exercise may help alleviate joint pain.
7. Work within the physical and mental limitations of lupus. Remember, moving regularly makes the difference.

CHRONIC FATIGUE SYNDROME

Chronic fatigue syndrome (CFS) is an autoimmune disorder of unknown origin that is characterized by persistent, medically unexplained fatigue lasting for at least six months and is unrelieved by bed rest (9, 24). Although symptoms and fatigue levels vary considerably among individuals with CFS, most people experience significant reductions in health, physical activity, and overall quality of life (53).

History and Demographics of Chronic Fatigue Syndrome

Although awareness of CFS has increased mainly over the last few decades, cases of individuals with CFS-like symptoms were recorded in the medical literature as early as the late 1800s. Historically, CFS has been known as Iceland disease, Royal Free disease, and chronic Epstein-Barr syndrome (53). In the 1980s and 1990s, CFS was nicknamed the "yuppie flu" as it was thought to be more prevalent among well-educated, upper middle class persons and professionals (10). However, studies reveal that CFS incidence rates actually appear to be highest among minority groups with lower levels of education and occupational status (10, 113). The prevalence rate of CFS in the general population is unclear; however, the literature indicates that approximately 0.007% to 2.8% of adults may suffer from this condition (10, 74). While CFS is not considered sex specific, women constitute approximately 83% of all diagnosed cases (222). The onset of the condition generally occurs sometime between the ages of 20 and 50 (53).

Other than debilitating fatigue, the myriad other symptoms associated with CFS include sore throat, nausea, dizziness, painful lymph nodes, headaches, low-grade fever, nonrestorative sleep, sleep disturbances, cognitive impairment, and depression (74, 148, 220). In addition, CFS is often present in conjunction with a variety of other conditions, such as irritable bowel syndrome, multiple chemical sensitivities, and temporomandibular joint (TMJ) disorder (10). Furthermore, many individuals with CFS experience chronic musculoskeletal impairments such as myalgia. Approximately 35% to 75% also meet the diagnostic criteria for fibromyalgia (148). This has led some to conclude that fibromyalgia should be considered an important subclass of CFS (148, 192). Most recently, a new set of diagnostic criteria has been proposed. These proposed diagnostic criteria include the presence of **postexertional malaise** (35). With respect to exercise, this would present as enhanced CFS symptomatology following vigorous exercise.

Pathophysiology of Chronic Fatigue Syndrome

Currently, the exact cause or causes of CFS are unclear, even though numerous researchers have investigated the possible infectious and immunologic, neuroendocrine, sleep, and psychiatric mechanisms that may lead to the onset of this peculiar disorder (21, 167). The etiology of CFS is complex (220). It is unclear if there is one factor or multiple subsets of poorly understood illnesses that interact. At this time there are no known diagnostic markers for this condition; thus the primary diagnostic criteria for CFS are based on self-reported symptoms and the exclusion of other potential medical and psychiatric conditions such as HIV/AIDS, lupus, sleep apnea, alcoholism, disordered eating, and psychotic disorders (10, 74). Currently, research on CFS focuses on immune, adrenal, genetic, and biopsychosocial models, sleep, and nutrition (220).

It has been hypothesized that viral infection, immunologic dysfunction, abnormalities in the hypothalamic–pituitary–adrenal axis, serotonin pathways, neurological-mediated hypertension, central nervous system dysfunction, nutritional deficiencies, or some traumatic event may potentially trigger the onset of this condition (10, 21, 24, 32, 49). Others speculate that due to the high levels of psychiatric comorbidity associated with CFS, it is nothing more than a somatic expression of depression or anxiety disorder (10, 148). Afari

and Buchwald (10) suggest that since a unifying pathophysiology for CFS has yet to emerge, this condition may be a heterogeneous condition with different pathophysiological disturbances that manifest with the same or similar symptoms.

At the time of this writing, no known cure for CFS exists. As a result, the majority of treatment options focus on managing the condition and minimizing the debilitating associated side effects (220). Commonly used management strategies include pharmacological intervention, stress management, counseling, proper nutrition, nutritional supplementation, educational interventions, group therapy, energy conservation, and regular physical activity (21, 74). Thus, it appears that using a combination of management strategies is an effective way to treat and manage the symptoms associated with CFS.

Common Medications Given to Individuals With Chronic Fatigue Syndrome

According to the University of Maryland Medical Center (200), no medications are specifically approved to treat CFS. Medications for CFS are aimed predominantly at symptom management. Due to the diversity of symptoms associated with this condition, numerous types of medications may be used (24). See medications table 7.3 near the end of the chapter. The number of possible medications for CFS management is extensive and varies greatly based on individual symptoms. Consequently, medications and other treatments regarded as common for CFS often vary greatly between resources. A number of pharmacological and nonpharmacological treatments are applied to individuals with CFS (26). Common medications include sleep medications, pain relievers, antidepressants, and stimulants. Less common medications may include antivirals and immune modulators. Alternative interventions include substances such as vitamins, minerals, essential fatty acids, CoQ10, and specific amino acids.

Antidepressant and immunosuppressant medications are not known to negatively affect exercise or exercise response; however, potential side effects of the drugs may make exercising uncomfortable. While stimulants may have some negative side effects that are not compatible with optimal exercise performance, they can also have effects that are beneficial to exercise. For example, it is well established that acute caffeine ingestion can enhance muscular endurance and improve muscle performance during short-duration maximal dynamic contractions (70, 92). Westover and colleagues (212) did note that prevalent use of stimulant medications was associated with a significant decrease in peak heart rate and an increased risk of chronotropic incompetence.

Effects of Exercise in Individuals With Chronic Fatigue Syndrome

While research indicates that there are numerous benefits to engaging in regular physical activity (e.g., improved health and psyche, ability to perform functional activities, improved energy, and reductions in fatigue levels), individuals with CFS often complain of exercise intolerance. The most common complaint about exercise is severe postexertional fatigue or malaise (10, 61). According to Komaroff and Buchwald (126), as many as 75% of individuals with CFS complain of postexertional malaise immediately following strenuous physical activity. For this reason, many individuals with CFS avoid physical exertion. This aversion to physical activity can perpetuate fatigue and lead to significant reductions in overall health, fitness, functional ability, and quality of life (108). Needless to say, this can have a profound impact on all aspects of life and cause significant levels of distress and social and occupational impairment. In fact, some individuals become so deconditioned they have difficulty performing basic ADL, such as light cleaning or driving a car. In extreme cases, individuals are unable to maintain employment due to poor health and symptomatology.

To date, there is some evidence for the use of resistance training. Enhancing muscular fitness can profoundly affect quality of life for those with CFS. Strengthening of major muscle groups may significantly reduce fatigue by improving mechanical efficiency during performance of physical activity and many ADL (205). However, it is not recommended that these individuals perform resistance training exercises to the point of volitional fatigue, as this may exacerbate symptomatology and potentially lead to **kinesiophobia**, or a fear of movement (205). Adolescents have been shown to be responsive to limited resistance training, producing significant improvements in physical exercise capacity (90, 91). However, other forms of exercise have been found to be effective at either reducing CFS symptoms or at the very least not exacerbating symptoms. Learnmonth and colleagues (130) found that 15 minutes of moderate-intensity aerobic cycling exercise had no significant adverse effects on pain or function within a 24-hour period. Other interventions have shown effectiveness at reducing symptoms and improving function by using a combination of graded exercise therapy accompanied by cognitive behavioral therapy (42, 202, 214). Alternative modes of exercise such as yoga and qigong have also been shown to be efficacious and feasible for relieving CFS-related fatigue and sleep disturbances (43, 169).

Exercise Recommendations for Clients With Chronic Fatigue Syndrome

Program design guidelines for clients with CFS are summarized in table 7.3. Setting forth general exercise programming guidelines for clients with CFS can be very difficult due to the wide array of symptoms experienced by these clients, as well as the severity of symptoms (24). Since exercise has a propensity to aggravate symptoms associated with CFS and initially may worsen a client's condition, it is prudent for the client to begin with exercises that are known to be tolerated well, such as light walking or water aerobics in a heated pool. The client can slowly and progressively increase the intensity as tolerance allows (24). This approach would be indicative of a symptom-contingent approach to exercise prescription. Another common approach is time-contingent based on the availability of the client's energy stores (202, 214). Similar to the situation with other autoimmune disorders, the primary goal of exercise programming for these clients should not be pushing the limits of their functional capacity. Instead, the focus should be on breaking the chronic fatigue and pain cycle by improving physical fitness and functional capacity without perpetuating fatigue.

When training persons with CFS, the exercise professional must be able to manipulate a variety of acute training variables based on the severity of symptoms and level of fatigue on a daily basis (60). On days when a client is experiencing profound fatigue or symptom flare-ups, exercise intensity and duration should be reduced accordingly. Furthermore, on "good" days, the temptation to increase exercise intensity and duration in order to "make up for lost time" should be avoided as it may lead to enhanced muscle microtrauma, pain, and postexertional fatigue (24). Excessive physical exertion often leads to increased pain and fatigue, which decreases the likelihood of the client maintaining good exercise adherence. For this reason, emphasis on the importance of energy conservation, to allow for maximal recovery and reduction of symptomatology due to overexertion,

is vital. As a general rule with regard to avoiding excessive fatigue and promoting adherence, at the end of each training session clients should always feel as if they could have done more.

Initially persons with CFS should focus on performing multijoint exercises using partial to full weight-bearing bodyweight activities. In this situation, using gravity as external resistance before adding additional loads is advised. Once the client is able to perform approximately 10 to 15 repetitions with proper form and without significant fatigue, the use of other modalities of training, such as manual resistance, free weights, resistance training machines, and tubing, can be progressively introduced. A recommendation for selecting an appropriate resistance training intensity is to select an intensity at which the client feels he could perform for at least two or three additional repetitions at the end of each

Table 7.3 Program Design Guidelines for Clients With Chronic Fatigue Syndrome

Type of exercise	Frequency	Intensity
Resistance training		
Multijoint movements 　a. Bodyweight resistance at first 　b. May progress to resistance bands, suspension training, and manual resistance 　c. Basic weight training such as resistance machines and free weights Mode of resistance training can vary based on how well exercise is tolerated. Graded exercise therapy is also widely used with CFS.	Frequency will vary based on postexertion symptomatology. Begin with 1-2 times per week, likely not to exceed 2-3 times per week.	Choose 8-10 exercises, using a full-body approach. Start with 1 set of 10-15 repetitions. Slowly progress over time to 2-3 sets of 10-15 repetitions. Set intensity should fall short of volitional fatigue. Increases in intensity beyond this point should be based on postexercise symptomatology. If doing multiple sets, consider 1-2 min between sets to start; be prepared to adjust as needed.
Aerobic training		
Aerobic exercise mode should be low impact and well tolerated. No mode-specific contraindications are implicated. 　a. Water aerobics 　b. Walking 　c. Cycling 　d. Rowing Mode of aerobic training can vary based on how well exercise is tolerated.	Begin conservatively, using one or two sessions per week. If tolerated, sessions can be increased slowly over time. Sessions can be performed most, if not all, days of the week. Multiple light sessions in a day can be used.	Begin with 5- to 10-min sessions; progress with frequency and duration before intensity. Use light to moderate RPE levels for training.
Flexibility training		
Full-body flexibility exercises 　a. Dynamic drills 　b. Static stretches	Daily or as tolerated	8-10 dynamic exercise drills occurring over 5-10 m, should be light intensity, low amplitude, focusing on proximal-to-distal mobility and stability. Postural control is important for all movements. 8-10 static stretches, held 15-60 s as tolerated

Note: RPE, rating of perceived exertion.

References: (10, 24, 60, 61, 95, 148, 202, 205, 214)

set. This conservative approach to loading may improve muscular fitness and reduce postexertional fatigue (61).

When clients with CFS are introduced to a resistance training program, performing one set of each exercise for each of the major muscle groups may be sufficient to improve general fitness levels, as well as provide the exercise professional with greater insight as to how the training program should be manipulated to improve exercise tolerance and reduce postexertional fatigue. As fitness and confidence levels improve, the client's overall volume of training may be slowly and progressively increased. Dawes and Stephenson (61) recommend that the client be able to perform approximately two or three sets of 10 to 15 repetitions per exercise before significantly increasing the training intensity in order to minimize the deleterious effects of exercise frequently experienced in this population. Exercise selection should be centered on movements that reflect ADL of the individual client. In addition, consider the use of movement-based training, such as very low level power, agility, and dynamic balance types of exercises that emphasize concentric force production rather than eccentric loading (61).

Cardiorespiratory training has been shown both to improve health-related fitness and to reduce the severity of many symptoms associated with this condition, especially fatigue (10, 24, 148). Cardiorespiratory training may also be beneficial when one is seeking to attain or maintain ideal body weight and body composition. Effectively managing one's weight may reduce additional stress on the musculoskeletal system via excess body fat. Initially, cardiorespiratory or aerobic forms of activity should emphasize low-impact modalities that engage large muscle groups, such as pool therapy, walking, and cycling (24, 61). Light- to moderate-intensity aerobic exercise performed on all or most days of the week is recommended and well tolerated (61). Therefore, the intensity of these activities should generally correlate with a light to moderate rating on an RPE scale (205). When progressing a cardiorespiratory training program, it may be effective to increase the frequency and duration of the activity before significantly increasing the intensity (61). Furthermore, initially employing shorter, more frequent bouts (e.g., 5-10 minutes) of light

to moderate aerobic exercise on all or most days of the week may help improve exercise tolerance and adherence by reducing the effects of postexertional fatigue and muscle soreness.

Flexibility and mobility are often relatively poor in this population (95). For this reason, performing some form of dynamic and static stretching on a daily basis is recommended (61). Dynamic flexibility training should be performed before more vigorous activity and after a 5- to 10-minute generalized warm-up. Dynamic flexibility drills for this population should focus on light-intensity and low-amplitude movements at a speed that allows the client to maintain good postural control. For people who are severely deconditioned, these mobility-type drills may even constitute the majority of the workout based on daily symptomatology and fitness level. Drill progression should first emphasize proximal-to-distal mobility and stability. This may be accomplished via performing exercises that focus on stabilizing the trunk, such as bridges and planks, then progressing to exercises that emphasize moving the extremities at the glenohumeral and hip joints. This should be followed by exercises that progressively increase the load placed on the cardiorespiratory system, such as treadmill walking, cycling, or rowing. Finally, specific dynamic mobility exercises should be incorporated to prepare the client for the main training session. Ironically, for many clients who are severely deconditioned, the warm-up alone may initially provide a sufficient stimulus to improve their overall fitness level without the incorporation of additional training.

When performing static stretching exercises, the client should focus on performing at least one stretch for each of the major muscle groups, holding each stretch for approximately 10 to 15 seconds. As tolerance improves, the duration of each stretch may be increased to 20 to 30 seconds, additional sets may be added, or both (61).

Key Point

Engaging in regular physical activity has the potential to be very beneficial to people with CFS. However, when even slightly overdone, exercise can trigger post-exertional malaise (fatigue). An individualized, daily approach to exercise prescription is necessary when training people with CFS.

Chronic Fatigue Syndrome

Sex: Male

Race: Caucasian

Age: 45

Height: 5 feet, 9 inches (1.75 m)

Weight: 176 pounds (80 kg)

Body fat: 27%

Body mass index: 26.0

Resting heart rate: 72 beats/min

Blood pressure: 128/84 mmHg

Temperature: Normal

History

Mr. J is a physician assistant. His job entails obtaining patient histories, doing physical examinations, ordering lab results, and assisting with surgical operations. He gradually began experiencing symptoms consistent with CFS shortly after turning 40. His initial symptoms, which he attributed to aging, were tiredness and fatigue. New symptoms began to appear with time. Newer symptoms included frequent headaches, night sweats, and irritable bowel. In addition to NSAID medications, he takes Modafinil for tiredness and Tramadol for pain. Since becoming symptomatic, Mr. J has avoided any unnecessary physical exertion. In addition, performing well at work has become more difficult.

Goals

Mr. J would like to work on the following goals:

1. Strengthen his body and improve his physical capacity
2. Avoid exacerbating CFS symptoms
3. Reduce reliance on pain medications
4. Complete work and daily activities with less pain, fatigue, and tiredness

Intake

Before the start of an exercise intervention, Mr. J's primary physician gave him clearance to commence an exercise regimen. Mr. J met with an exercise professional at his corporate fitness center. The exercise professional took a full medical history, but pain and fatigue made it impractical to test for even submaximal cardiopulmonary or muscular fitness. Body composition was assessed using skinfold calipers. The exercise professional recommended a progressive resistance training program and flexibility training, as well as a regimen of cardiopulmonary exercise. Mr. J was also referred for nutritional counseling to help promote general health and improve body composition.

Initial Exercise

The primary goal of training clients with CFS is to avoid postexertional malaise; therefore training should not be carried out to the point of volitional fatigue. Additionally, training should not cause significant postexertional symptoms in the 12 to 48 hours postexercise. Any activities should be light and low impact. Due to very low tolerance for physical activity, Mr. J's initial form of training consisted of graded exercise therapy (GET). Graded exercise therapy programming began with a single 5-minute session of dynamic stretching followed by simple muscular contractions and extensions, two times per week. Five to 10 total exercises were used depending on tolerance. Programmatic flexibility was required. A full-body approach to this type of training was used. Physical limits were set by trial and error. The endpoint of GET training was set by number of repetitions or a clock. Rest is an important element of this type of training.

Exercise Progression

Upon the client achieving a favorable tolerance to GET, standard forms of training were gradually incorporated into the training regimen. Five- to 10-minute moderate-intensity walking intervals were introduced, performed one or two times per week. Over the course of several weeks, interval lengths and frequency were increased as long as there was no postexertional malaise. Gradually, dynamic stretching exercises were supplemented with resistance band and standard resistance training modes, one or two times per week. Up to 8 to 10 resistance exercises were eventually used for two or three sets of 12 to 15 repetitions. To accommodate client needs, the rest period remained flexible during training.

Outcomes

With consistent effort over the period of a year, Mr. J was able to reach most of his goals. He was able improve his physical capacity enough to get through his workday without undue fatigue and pain. While symptoms were reduced, they were not completely alleviated. He still uses medications but is not as reliant on them as he once was.

Training Recommendations and Contraindications for Clients With Chronic Fatigue Syndrome

1. Graded exercise therapy involves a gradual start that progresses slowly over time and should be applied to those with CFS. Be prepared for progression to take much longer than in apparently healthy clients.

2. Exercise professionals should be very aware of how clients respond to training and should be willing to adjust frequency, intensity, and time as needed. Work that is overdone can trigger postexertional malaise (fatigue).

3. All training should be light and low impact.

4. Resistance training should start with bodyweight activities, progressing to lower-level modes of resistance such as tubes and bands. Machines and free weights may also be used.

5. Avoid ballistic motions when training. Use smooth, controlled movements that will reduce the chance of injury and allow proper control of movement.

6. Consider time-based work intervals. Consider varying types of activity from session to session.

FIBROMYALGIA

Fibromyalgia (FM), or fibromyalgia syndrome, is a condition similar to CFS; the primary characteristic of FM is chronic widespread musculoskeletal pain, with a secondary emphasis on fatigue (53, 148). Due to their relationship, it is often difficult to separate these illnesses. In fact, 20% to 70% of individuals diagnosed with FM also suffer from CFS, and 35% to 70% of those diagnosed with CFS meet the diagnostic criteria for FM (88). A recent Canadian study found that almost one in four people (23%) with CFS also reported having FM and that approximately one in five people (21.2%) with FM also reported having CFS (181). For the aforementioned reasons, some researchers have suggested that FM should be considered a subclassification of CFS (192).

History and Demographics of Fibromyalgia

The American College of Rheumatology (55) reports that FM affects 2% to 4% of people and that 90% of all cases occur in women. The typical onset of FM occurs between the ages of 20 and 40 (213). Interestingly, prevalence rates of FM vary based on the different classification criteria. Jones and colleagues (116) found that FM prevalence is higher in men when the modified 2010 criteria are used as compared to the criteria that require input from a physician or other health care professional. The specific criteria used appear to have important implications for use in research and the clinical setting (116). However, Reifenberger and Amundson (175) have also observed this condition in both adolescents and persons who are elderly. Jiao and colleagues (115) found that young and middle-aged patients experienced worse FM symptoms as compared to older patients. In addition, they found that females with FM had lower quality of life in all age groups. This included both lower physical and mental health.

In addition to pronounced tenderness to palpation and profound fatigue, common symptoms associated with this disorder include generalized stiffness, anxiety, depression, nonrestorative sleep, heightened pain perception, gastrointestinal distress, headaches, sensitivity to light, joint swelling, mood swings, cognitive impairments (a.k.a. "fibro fog"), irritable bowel and bladder syndrome, and Raynaud's phenomenon, a condition that involves the narrowing of blood vessels when a person is cold or feeling strong emotions (183). Similar to CFS, diagnosis is based on self-reported symptoms rather than laboratory or diagnostic criteria (183). The American College of Rheumatology cites three specific criteria needed to diagnose FM. These include the following:

1. Pain and symptoms experienced over the past week, based on the total of the painful areas of the body, the severity of fatigue, waking unrefreshed, and cognitive problems, plus the number of other general physical symptoms

2. Symptoms lasting at least three months at a similar level

3. No other health problem that would explain the pain and other symptoms

Based on these criteria, a history of widespread pain in the axial skeleton occurring for greater than three months, in combination with bilateral tender points in at least 11 of 18 specified anatomical sites, is required (54, 183).

Pathophysiology of Fibromyalgia

To date, the exact etiology of FM is unknown. Some researchers speculate that this condition may be triggered by minor upper body injury, viral illness, or chronic stressors (179). Jay and Barkin (114) describe a pathophysiology that includes central-sensitivity syndrome, in which there are problems with central pain processing.

As a result, individuals with FM have a lower threshold for responding to pain as well as other stimuli such as heat, noise, and even strong odors. Jones, Clark, and Bennett (119) suggest that in order to better understand FM's pathophysiology, a greater understanding of several factors, such as altered pain processing, neuroendocrine abnormalities, neurotransmitter changes, and sleep disturbances, is imperative. For instance, individuals with FM have been shown to exhibit significantly greater levels of substance P, a neurotransmitter that aids in the regulation of pain sensitization, than the general population (24).

As with CFS, there is no cure for FM. Management strategies for this condition typically include antidepressive medications, counseling, group therapy, massage, acupuncture, biofeedback, dietary modifications, therapeutic exercise, trigger point injections, joint manipulation, and myofascial release techniques (48, 54, 180, 183). However, at this time it appears that a combination of these therapies is the most efficacious strategy when managing the symptoms associated with FM (183).

Common Medications Given to Individuals With Fibromyalgia

People with FM generally take a wide variety of medications to ameliorate the myriad side effects characterizing this condition. See medications table 7.4 near the end of the chapter. Most often these medications are used to reduce pain, improve sleep quality, and improve psychological well-being (depression and anxiety). Muscle relaxants may also be prescribed in this population as a method of pain management (165). Currently, only three medications are approved for use in the treatment of FM by the U.S. Food and Drug Administration: pregabalin (Lyrica), duloxetine (Cymbalta), and milnacipran (Savella). None are approved by the European Medicines Agency, and only two are approved by Health Canada: pregabalin and duloxetine (20, 33).

Nonsteroidal anti-inflammatory drugs are not known to have negative impacts on exercise performance; to the contrary, NSAIDs have been shown to reduce exercise-induced fatigue (58, 133).

Some evidence suggests that NSAIDs like ibuprofen may inhibit certain prostaglandins responsible for signaling translational responses to resistance exercise (143). This may attenuate recovery from exercise. Antidepressants and muscle relaxants are not known to negatively affect exercise or exercise response; however, side effects of the drugs may potentially make exercising uncomfortable. Sleep aids in general are not known to interfere with exercise or exercise response but may make it difficult especially if one is training in the morning.

Effects of Exercise in Individuals With Fibromyalgia

According to findings by Wilson and colleagues (217), about half of those who are newly diagnosed with FM received recommendations for initiating an exercise program. There is an abundance of evidence to support the use of exercise as a cornerstone in the management of FM (31, 109, 141, 144, 146, 168, 182, 217). This research shows that both aerobic exercise and strength training can reduce the severity of many symptoms associated with FM, including pain levels, fatigue, depression, and sleep disturbances (28). As obesity and overweight are common in persons with FM, weight control has also been found to be an effective tool in reduction of symptoms (180). People with FM often have a very narrow therapeutic window for physical activity due to the high levels of pain and stiffness associated with this disorder. In addition, exercise is frequently a symptom aggravator. For this reason, many people with FM avoid physical activity, fearing that their symptoms will be intensified. As a result, the majority of individuals with FM remain aerobically unfit with poor muscle strength and limited flexibility (118). Thus, training programs for this population should emphasize increasing functional activity levels without causing postexertional pain and fatigue. Gradually accumulating at least 5,000 steps per day may result in clinically significant reductions in pain intensity (121). Kibar and colleagues (123) found that balance training for persons with FM had a positive effect on static balance. Furthermore, it was noted that balance deficit contributed to the depression associated with risk of falling.

Jones and colleagues (119) found that stretching alone or in conjunction with strength training could elicit improvements in overall FM disease activity. Alternative forms of treatment have also been shown to reduce symptoms, such as mindfulness meditation, aquatic exercise, and qigong (27, 36, 134, 184).

Exercise Recommendations for Clients With Fibromyalgia

Program design guidelines for clients with FM are summarized in table 7.4. Postexertional complaints are typically seen in strength and conditioning programs that use higher-intensity, higher-impact movements and fail to allow clients to self-adjust their exercise intensity (117). Thus, light- to moderate-intensity exercise performed on all or most days of the week is recommended. In addition, because symptom severity may vary dramatically on a daily basis, the exercise professional must be able to manipulate exercise volume, intensity, and duration based on pain tolerance and acute bouts of fatigue. It would be advisable to assess the client's severity of symptoms before exercise activity.

Resistance training may be beneficial to those with FM by helping improve isometric and dynamic muscle strength, as well as power (96). By improving strength and power, clients with FM may be able to perform ADL with greater ease, thus conserving energy and minimizing the effects of fatigue. It is recommended that the exercise professional initially select at least one exercise for each of the major muscle groups in order to promote overall muscular development (85). If musculoskeletal aggravation occurs during the use of any of the selected exercises or on the days following training, the exercises used can be modified or substituted with others that may be better endured. Initially beginning with two training sessions per week with at least three days between sessions is a conservative frequency of training. As clients' functional abilities and tolerance improve, they may progress to three training sessions per week with at least 48 hours between sessions. Some clients with FM may actually better tolerate a four-day per week split routine in which different muscle groups are trained on

Table 7.4 Program Design Guidelines for Clients With Fibromyalgia

Type of exercise	Frequency	Intensity
Resistance training		

Multijoint movement considerations
  a. Bodyweight resistance
  b. Resistance bands, suspension training, and manual resistance
  c. Basic weight training such as resistance machines and free weights
Mode of resistance training can vary based on how well exercise is tolerated. If tolerated well, basic weight training can be used.
	Frequency will vary based on postexertion symptomatology.
	Begin with 1-2 times per week, likely not to exceed 3-4 times per week. Once acclimated, consider a split program in which different body parts are exercised by day to achieve greater frequency.
		Avoid movements involving significant impact.
		Choose 8-10 exercises, using a full-body approach.
		Start with one set of 10-15 repetitions with 40-60% 1RM.
		Slowly progress over time to 3 sets of 10-15 repetitions.
		Set intensity should fall short of volitional fatigue.
		Increases in intensity beyond this point should be based on postexercise symptomatology.
		If doing multiple sets, consider 1-2 min between sets to start; be prepared to adjust as needed.

Aerobic training		

Aerobic exercise mode should be low impact and well tolerated. No mode-specific contraindications are implicated.
  a. Water aerobics
  b. Walking
  c. Cycling
  d. Rowing
Mode of aerobic training can vary based on how well exercise is tolerated.
	Begin conservatively, using one or two sessions per week, possibly more than once per day with interval training. If tolerated, sessions can be increased slowly over time. Sessions can be performed 3-4 days per week.	Begin with 5- to 10-min sessions, 1-2 times per day, at light to moderate intensity (30% to <60% $\dot{V}O_2$ or heart rate reserve or 55% to <75% MHR, not exceeding 9-13 on the 6- to 20-point Borg scale).
		Progress to 10- to 15-min sessions, 1-2 times per day, at light to moderate intensity until ultimately reaching 30-40 min per day.

Flexibility training		
Full-body, passive, static, flexibility exercises	As part of other training sessions, between sets or intervals Can also exist as a regular training program if other forms of exercise are not well tolerated	Do 8-10 dynamic, low-amplitude stretches held 10-15 s at first, then progressing up to 20-30 s. Stretching intensity should not reach the point of pain but rather until the muscle is taut.

References: (27, 36, 60, 85, 96, 117-119, 121, 123, 127, 184)

different days. This reduces the intensity of each individual workout by dispersing the training load and volume typically performed on two days of training over four days. It may also be beneficial to intermittently incorporate cardiovascular and flexibility exercises between sets in order to provide clients with an opportunity to rest between resistance training exercises, thus enhancing exercise tolerance while still effectively using their time (60).

Selecting the appropriate intensity level for those with FM is often a trial-and-error process that requires the exercise professional to select an appropriate training load to elicit a positive adaptation without creating significant increases in pain or discomfort. LaFontaine (127) recommends that clients with FM use a light resistance, approximately 40% to 60% of their estimated 1RM (176). Clients should start by performing at least one set of 10 to 15 repetitions and gradually increase the volume of training as tolerance improves and fitness levels increase. Once the client is able to perform 12 to 15 repetitions with proper form and without undue pain and fatigue, the amount of resistance can progressively be increased with initial reductions in the volume. Thus, the number of repetitions performed should initially decrease as the training load increases in order help to prevent excessive muscular microtrauma.

Daily cardiorespiratory exercise should be encouraged. Typically, low-impact, light-intensity aerobic exercises such as walking, bicycling, or water aerobics in a heated pool are generally well tolerated by the FM population (118). Furthermore, because repetitive motion has a propensity to aggravate the symptoms of FM, some people may tolerate shorter 5- to 10-minute training intervals throughout the day instead of one long exercise session. LaFontaine (127) recommends beginning at a light intensity for 10 to 15 minutes twice per day and increasing the duration of the activity to 30 to 40 minutes three or four days a week as tolerated. In an investigation of vigorous-versus light-intensity aerobic training, Häuser and colleagues (102) found that vigorous-intensity aerobic work only moderately improved physical fitness and general well-being.

Performing passive and slow static stretching intermittently throughout training sessions may also enhance the client's tolerance to training by allowing an opportunity for the clients to rest between exercises. Stretching at regular intervals throughout the day may also be beneficial for reducing pain and stiffness and improving mobility, and may aid in the prevention of muscle pain and stiffness after remaining in one position for an extended period of time. Initially the client should attempt to hold each stretch for approximately 10 to 15 seconds or as tolerance allows. As tolerance improves, the duration of each stretch may be

Key Point

For clients with FM, progression in all health-related fitness areas takes much longer than in apparently healthy clients. Clients with FM will require exercise accommodations and interventions similar to those with chronic fatigue syndrome. Carefully implemented aerobic, resistance, and flexibility programs can reduce the severity of symptoms associated with FM. Training programs for this population should focus on increasing functional activity levels without post-exertional pain and fatigue. Alternative treatments such as meditation and aquatics are also useful.

progressively increased up to 20 to 30 seconds. While each stretch can be held for a greater duration, stretching longer than 30 seconds may be too intense and increase discomfort. Thus, it may be beneficial to stretch more frequently rather than for longer durations. Additionally, stretching on a daily basis may help manage the muscle pain and stiffness often experienced by these clients. Stretch intensity should remain relatively low with an emphasis on stretching only to the point at which the muscles feel taut, never to the threshold of pain or tenderness. This is an important consideration as overstretching may increase the likelihood of microtrauma in muscle tissues in conjunction with increased pain and stiffness.

Case Study

Fibromyalgia

Sex: Female

Race: Caucasian

Age: 43

Height: 5 feet, 3 inches (1.60 m)

Weight: 145 pounds (66 kg)

Body fat: 32%

Body mass index: 25.7

Resting heart rate: 72 beats/min

Blood pressure: 142/94 mmHg

Temperature: Normal

History

Mrs. P is a receptionist in a dental office. Her job entails sitting for long periods of time, entering information into a computer, and retrieving dental records. For several years she has noticed diffuse muscle discomfort throughout her upper body and thighs. She has made several modifications to her workstation to help alleviate her issues, but this has been unsuccessful. Her physical discomfort has made working quite difficult as well as straining her relationships at home. Following a serious car accident, she noticed

(continued)

a marked increase in her symptoms and great difficulty sleeping. After minimal success with physical therapy, she was diagnosed with FM by her primary physician. The physician prescribed NSAIDs, antidepressants, and a sleep aid. Having attempted alternative forms of treatment, Mrs. P sought the help of an exercise professional who was knowledgeable about FM.

Goals

Mrs. P hopes to work with her exercise professional to reach the following goals:

1. Alleviate consistent muscular pain
2. Improve quality of work and home life
3. Establish exercise programming as a regular part of treatment
4. Improve overall fitness

Initial Training

Having received clearance from her primary physician, Mrs. P met with a certified exercise specialist at a facility near her home. The exercise professional took a full medical history. Traditional submaximal aerobic and muscular exercise testing was attempted, but results were not accurate due to Mrs. P's low physical capacity. As an alternative, the exercise specialist performed the University of Houston Non-Exercise Test to assess her aerobic capacity and a dynamometer battery consisting of handgrip strength and back and leg strength. Body composition was measured using bioelectric impedance. The exercise professional recommended a slow but progressive approach to achieving a regular exercise program for Mrs. P and recommended a progressive resistance training program, flexibility training, and regimen of cardiopulmonary exercise. Ultimately, the exercise program will need to become a regular part of Mrs. P's treatment plan. It was also recommended that she seek the counsel of a registered dietician to help promote better general health.

Exercise Progression

Resistance training began with a combination of 8 to 10 movements consisting of both body-weight and resistance band exercises, two days per week. One set of 10 to 15 repetitions was performed for each exercise. While 1- to 2-minute rest periods were appropriate, early training rest periods were variable. Each session was completed with light full-body static stretching. Each stretch was held for 10 to 15 seconds. Aerobic sessions were scheduled on days in which resistance training was not done. Because of Mrs. P's preference, aerobic training was conducted twice per week in a swimming pool. Her group instructor aided her in completion of one or two 5- or 10-minute intervals of activity. All early training was kept below the point of volitional fatigue.

Resistance training frequency was increased to three or four times per week. While repetitions remained in the 10 to 15 range, the number of sets was increased to two or three. To accommodate this change, different muscle groups were trained on different days. Aerobic training progressed from intervals to single sessions of 20 to 30 minutes, three or four days per week. The client also began to explore other aerobic modes. Her training schedule remained flexible and was adjusted as needed depending on her symptoms.

Outcomes

Following some minor setbacks as she learned her exercise tolerances, Mrs. P was able to establish a routine that fit within the structure of her life. Her physical condition improved, as did her quality of life. The combination of her therapies and dietary modifications has been effective. Although she still deals with pain, it is dramatically less than before. The strain on her home and work relationships is better.

> ## Training Recommendations and Contraindications for Clients With Fibromyalgia
>
> 1. Be prepared for progressions in all health-related fitness areas to take much longer than in apparently healthy clients.
> 2. Exercise professionals should be very aware of how clients respond to training and be willing to adjust frequency, intensity, and time as needed. Avoiding painful movement is vital to this process.
> 3. Aerobic training should be light and low impact in the beginning.
> 4. Resistance training can include many different modes, but should begin sparingly until tolerance can be determined. Consider bodyweight activities, lower-level modes of resistance such as tubes and bands, and machine- and free-weight movements.
> 5. Avoid ballistic motions when training. Use smooth, controlled movements that will reduce the chance of injury and allow proper control of movement.
> 6. Consider aerobic modes initially that are predictable modes of exercise so the client can more effectively exercise in a steady state.
> 7. Consider interspersing low-level static stretching between resistance training sets or aerobic intervals.
> 8. Alternative modes of training are also useful. Consider aqua exercise, qigong, or mindfulness meditation.
> 9. As celiac disease is common to those with FM, consider testing for gluten sensitivity.

HIV/AIDS

Human immunodeficiency virus (HIV) is a retrovirus that causes **acquired immune deficiency syndrome (AIDS)**, a condition that gradually destroys the immune system, making it difficult to effectively fight off opportunistic infections and making people more prone to unusual cancers and other abnormalities (3, 166, 215).

History and Demographics of HIV/AIDS

The first case of AIDS was reported to the Centers for Disease Control and Prevention (CDC) in 1981 (76). Since this first documented case, AIDS has become a worldwide epidemic (185). According to Merson (151), approximately 25 years later, more than 65 million individuals had been infected with HIV and over 34 million had died of AIDS (219). It has been estimated that in the United States alone over 1 million individuals are living with HIV/AIDS, with approximately a quarter of these individuals remaining unaware that they are infected (77). Furthermore, it has been estimated that as many as 50,000 new HIV infections occur every year (38). Of the new infections, 44% are in the African American population with the Hispanic and Latino population making up 21%, the Caucasian population 31%, and the Asian population 2% (39). It is estimated that new HIV infections fell by 35% in the years between 2000 and 2015 (219).

Pathophysiology of HIV/AIDS

Serological tests are used to detect the presence or absence of two serotypes of HIV currently recognized as HIV-1 and HIV-2, with the predominant virus worldwide being HIV-1 (3, 76). Human immunodeficiency virus-1 was identified in 1984 as the primary causative viral agent for AIDS (76). In 1986, HIV-2 was discovered in AIDS patients in West Africa (37).

Both HIV-1 and HIV-2 are spread via a host transmitting the virus through a portal of exit into another host or reservoir. This often occurs through the transmission of bodily fluids, such as blood, semen, and vaginal secretions (5). Thus, engaging in behaviors that put people in direct contact with these secretions, such as unprotected sexual intercourse and sharing contaminated intravenous needles, increases an individual's risk of contracting the virus—as does receiving contaminated blood via transfusion, blood products, and organ transplants (76). The CDC reported in 2010 that 63% of new HIV transmissions were men who had had sexual intercourse with men compared to 25% of individuals infected through heterosexual sex and 8% by injection (39). In addition, this virus may also be transmitted from nursing mothers who are infected with HIV/AIDS via breast milk to their children (5). When compared to HIV-1, the HIV-2 immunodeficiency appears to develop more slowly with milder symptoms, and is initially less infectious in the early stages but becomes more so as the disease progresses.

Human immunodeficiency virus attacks white blood cells of the immune system, CD4 helper T cells, which are critical to immune function. The destruction of these cells leads to a progressive deterioration of the immune system, making individuals more susceptible to opportunistic infections, unusual cancers, and other abnormalities (3, 166) such as nephropathy and renal failure (153).

There are three stages associated with HIV (3, 136, 166). Symptoms vary based on the stage of infection (219). In stage I acute HIV infection, individuals are able to transmit HIV but remain asymptomatic and relatively healthy, though they may experience influenza-type symptoms. Individuals may remain in stage 1 for months to years. Stage 2, often referred to as AIDS-related complex (ARC), is characterized by asymptomatic HIV infection (8) with a moderate reduction in CD4 cells and the development of more pronounced signs and symptoms, such as weight loss,

muscle wasting, weakness, fatigue, diarrhea, rare cancers, and swollen or enlarged lymph nodes. Stage 3 is the most severe stage of HIV, acquired immunodeficiency disease, and is associated with a significant depletion of CD4 cells, in the presence of malignancy and opportunistic infection and cancers. This stage can take 2 to 15 years to develop (219).

Common Medications Given to Individuals With HIV/AIDS

There is no cure for AIDS or HIV; however, with the advent of new antiviral agents, many individuals infected with HIV are living much healthier and higher-quality lives than those diagnosed several decades ago (125). Thus treatment and management options focus on suppressing the symptoms associated with this disorder for as long as possible. See medications table 7.5 near the end of the chapter. The pharmacological intervention of HIV medicines is called antiretroviral therapy (ART). Commonly used HIV medication classes include nucleoside reverse transcriptase inhibitors (NRTIs), also known as analogues or "nukes," non-nucleoside reverse transcriptase inhibitors (NNRTIs), protease inhibitors, fusion inhibitors, entry inhibitors, integrase inhibitors, and pharmacokinetic enhancers. The HIV regimen requires a combination of these medications from different drug classes (11).

Highly active antiretroviral therapy (HAART) is a method used to reduce the number of HIV particles in the blood as measured by viral load, thus improving T-cell count and immune function (3). However, Malita and colleagues (139) reported that individuals using HAART for an extended period of time may be at increased risk of developing cardiovascular and metabolic complications (79). Highly active antiretroviral therapy has been associated with the development of lipodystrophy syndrome, indicative of increased central adiposity (lipohypertrophy), and peripheral lipoatrophy, peripheral insulin resistance, chronic kidney disease (44, 153), diabetes, dyslipidemia (128), hypertriglyceridemia, osteoporosis, and osteopenia.

Many of the drugs, especially NRTIs and NNRTIs, bind and alter (or block) the reverse transcriptase enzyme that the HIV virus uses to make copies of itself. A risk of myocardial infarction and lactic acidosis is associated with NRTIs; therefore, caution should be used with exercise. NRTIs have been found to impair mitochondrial function and reduce insulin sensitivity, making individuals more susceptible to type 2 diabetes mellitus (80).

Pharmokinetic enhancers are used to increase the effectiveness of other drugs used in the HIV regimen, by reducing the breakdown of those drugs. Anti-infectives and antineoplastics are prescribed to help stave off opportunistic infections. Protease inhibitors (PIs) block the enzyme protease, which spreads HIV to other cells. Protease inhibitors have greatly reduced the risk of morbidity and mortality for those suffering from HIV/AIDS (3).

While these drugs are effective in the treatment of HIV and AIDS, they have side effects, as well as interactions with other drugs. Over an extended period of time, individuals can develop resistance to the drugs. Secondary complications associated with ART are metabolic, causing an increase in risk factors for cardiovascular disease (CVD) such as dyslipidemia, insulin resistance, and changes in adiposity (198). Additionally, the endothelial dysfunction related to HIV replication is a determinant for arterial inflammation and thrombosis (128). Risks for CVD are exponentially heightened due to age, genetic predisposition (family history of CVD), or choices related to lifestyle (smoking) (83). Statins and other medications are taken to counteract the effects of ART. Other complications due to medications include peripheral neuropathy (34).

Exercise is beneficial in helping with decreasing central fat distribution but can increase peripheral fat wasting. Persons with HIV/AIDS are at an increased risk for hyperlipidemia and hypertriglyceridemia; of course, exercise can be beneficial in helping to increase high-density lipoprotein cholesterol while decreasing triglycerides (34).

Effects of Exercise in Individuals With HIV/AIDS

Exercise participation has been associated with improvements in immune function and long-term survival in HIV (189). However, with disease progression, factors such as fatigue, muscle wasting, muscle weakness, chronic diarrhea leading to dehydration, and opportunistic infection may significantly reduce exercise capacity (166). For this reason, while exercise is encouraged in all stages of HIV, it is particularly recommended that individuals engage in strength and conditioning activities in the early stages of this disease as this may help forestall or reverse disease progression (78).

Aerobic training is commonly used to help improve cardiovascular fitness, improve fatigue levels, and reduce central body fatness (139, 155, 191). In addition, nutritional intervention and supplementation, androgen supplementation, growth hormone administration, and resistance training are commonly used to counteract the negative effects associated with muscle wasting (68). Of these treatments, resistance exercise may be a preferred option because of affordability, its relatively few side effects, and its availability. Furthermore, because muscular strength is positively affected by resistance training, both functional ability and quality of life can be greatly improved (164).

Exercise Recommendations for Clients With HIV/AIDS

Program design guidelines for clients with HIV/AIDS are summarized in table 7.5. Designing an exercise program for clients with HIV infection is largely dependent on the stage of immunodeficiency. Clients in stage 1 are typically asymptomatic, with relatively few training restrictions. However, with disease progression, exercise capacity may steadily diminish and physical exhaustion and muscular fatigue may become a greater concern.

Cardiorespiratory training is commonly recommended for clients with HIV as a method of improving aerobic capacity and reducing the likelihood of cardiovascular-related issues, such as atherosclerosis, myocardial infarction, hypertension, congestive heart failure, and sudden cardiac death (177, 189). Either moderate (40% to <60% $\dot{V}O_2$ or heart rate reserve) or vigorous training (≥60%-90% $\dot{V}O_2$ or heart rate reserve) can be recommended based on the client's preference (191). However, disease status, symptoms, and current fitness level should be considered.

Table 7.5 Program Design Guidelines for Clients With HIV/AIDS

Type of exercise	Frequency	Intensity
Resistance training		

Multijoint movements
  a. Bodyweight resistance
  b. May use resistance bands, suspension training, and manual resistance
  c. Basic weight training such as resistance machines and free weights
Mode of resistance training can vary based upon how well exercise is tolerated
	Frequency will vary based on postexertion symptomatology
	Strive for two or three sessions per week
		Choose 8-10 exercises using a full-body approach.
		Slowly progress over time to 2-3 sets of 8-12 repetitions.
		Use light to moderate intensity, 40-80% 1RM.
		If doing multiple sets, consider 1-2 min between sets to start; be prepared to adjust as needed.

Aerobic training		
Aerobic exercise mode should be low to moderate impact. Mode of aerobic training can vary based on how well exercise is tolerated.	Begin conservatively, working up to three or four sessions per week. If tolerated, sessions can be increased slowly over time. Sessions can be performed most, if not all, days of the week.	Intensity (moderate or vigorous) is subject to the client's preference, disease status, symptoms, and current fitness level; strive for 30 min of continuous exercise. Tolerance may vary widely between clients.
Flexibility training		
Full-body flexibility exercises, starting with static stretching		8-10 static stretches, held 5-10 s initially, progressing to 20 s as tolerated

References: (89, 155, 177, 191)

Resistance training is also a commonly prescribed exercise modality as it has the potential to significantly influence muscle performance via increases in lean body mass and strength. However, appropriate resistance training protocols and guidelines are difficult to find for this population. Resistance training at high intensities (>80% 1RM) for relatively short periods has a positive influence on the accrual of lean body mass in persons with HIV without compromising immune function and is independent of the side effects associated with hormone therapies (68).

It is recommended that resistance training programs for persons with HIV concentrate on multijoint exercises emphasizing large muscle groups. Training intensity should generally be at a moderate level (60-80% 1RM), which should allow for comfortable performance of 8 to 12 repetitions per set. Alternatively, lighter-intensity muscular endurance training (40-60% 1RM) can be performed with 15 to 25 repetitions per set. Initial training should use one set per exercise, with training volume increased very gradually as tolerated by the client but not to exceed two

Key Point

For clients with HIV/AIDS, implement resistive exercises and other therapeutic exercises as tolerated to maintain muscle strength and function and prevent muscle wasting. Assess exercise tolerance frequently.

sets per exercise for the higher-volume muscular endurance training (89).

Finally, strength and conditioning activities are considered low risk for the transmission of HIV because there is little exposure to bodily fluids. However, cuts, scrapes, bloody noses, and open wounds increase exposure to bodily fluids and may increase the risk of HIV transmission. Thus, any time blood or body fluids, excluding sweat, are present, standard precautions should be followed to minimize risk of disease transmission. For this reason, it is recommended that the exercise professional be familiar with the universal and standard precautions as recommended by the CDC (1, 187).

HIV/AIDS

Sex: Female

Age: 32

Height: 5 feet, 5 inches (1.65 m)

Weight: 140 pounds (64 kg)

Body fat: 27%

Body mass index: 23.3

Resting heart rate: 70 beats/min

Blood pressure: 130/76 mmHg

Estimated $\dot{V}O_2$: 19.6 ml · kg^{-1} · min^{-1} (from the 1.5-mile [2.4 km] walk/run test)

History

The client, Mrs. N, has been infected with HIV for over 10 years. Before her infection, she played softball and ran the 400-m hurdles in college. Post-HIV diagnosis, she became more sedentary due to fear of aggravating or triggering symptoms of the disease. She was also reluctant to join a gym because she had been told by a previous health club that the patrons and staff were fearful of handling equipment after she had used it. She would like to begin an exercise program again. However, she has not been physically active, other than walking, for the last three years. She walks for 20 to 30 minutes three times per week. Recently she participated in a research study investigating the effects of a HAART on T-cell activation during asymptomatic HIV infection. During the study she complained of fatiguing very easily and experienced mild nausea and diarrhea. However, after she completed the study her symptoms subsided and she is currently asymptomatic.

Goals

Mrs. N would like to work on the following goals:

1. Strengthen her body and improve her physical capacity

2. Remain asymptomatic

3. Improve health and maintain current immune function

Intake

Before Mrs. N began her exercise program, her physician had encouraged her to seek the advice of a knowledgeable exercise professional. Other than diminished capacity, she has no physical limitations. She performed a 3-minute step test for aerobic capacity, push-up test for upper body endurance–strength, and the leg press test for lower body strength. Test results confirmed a low capacity for her age and sex. The exercise professional recommended a progressive resistance training program, cardiopulmonary exercise, and flexibility exercise. It was also recommended that she seek dietary advice from a registered dietician to help promote health.

Initial Training

Training sessions began with low-impact aerobic training three times per week. Mrs. N's choice of activity was stationary cycling and she began at 40% of her heart rate reserve for 20 minutes. Aerobic training was followed by resistance training and basic static stretching. A full-body approach to resistance exercise was used, as was basic dynamic stretching. Eight to 10 exercises were performed for 30 seconds, 8 to 10 exercises for one set. The repetition range was 12 to 15. A combination of bodyweight and dumbbell exercises was chosen.

Exercise Progression

Over a period of two months, the exercise professional progressed Mrs. N's aerobic training to four days per week with alternating modes of riding a stationary cycle and walking on a track. Mrs. N's intensity increased to

(continued)

60% heart rate reserve and each session was lengthened to 30 minutes. Also, Mrs. N's exercise professional recommended a split resistance training routine; over the four days, she completes two full-body workouts and instead of one set per body part, Mrs. N did two or three sets.

Outcomes

After eight weeks of training, a retest of muscular endurance and strength demonstrated significant increases in upper and lower body strength as well as $\dot{V}O_2$ max. Mrs. N's health has remained good despite side effects from the medications.

Training Recommendations and Contraindications for Clients With HIV/AIDS

1. Implement resistive exercises and other exercises as tolerated to maintain muscle strength and function and prevent muscle wasting.
2. Use extreme caution during aerobic exercise and other forms of exercise.
3. Monitor exercise tolerance frequently for excessive fatigue and weakness.
4. Use Universal Precautions for Prevention of Transmission of HIV and Other Bloodborne Infections established by the Centers for Disease Control and Prevention.

SICKLE CELL DISEASE

Sickle cell disease is a group of inherited blood disorders that is characterized by a genetic mutation of hemoglobin. This abnormality can cause an alteration of the shape of the red blood cell into a lengthened sickle profile (15). Sickle cell *anemia,* the most common and most severe of all of the forms of sickle cell disease, occurs when there are two abnormal sickle genes for hemoglobin; sickle cell *trait* has one normal and one sickle hemoglobin gene.

History and Demographics of Sickle Cell Disease

The sickle cell mutation was first recognized in Africa (51). The condition is most common in individuals of African descent (64) but also affects individuals of Arab, Indian, and Hispanic nationalities (15, 159). It is least common in Caucasian individuals. It is estimated that the number of babies born with sickle cell disease between 2010 and 2050 will be over 14 million, and the disease has been declared a global health problem by the World Health Organization (64). It has been suggested that those with low socioeconomic conditions are at a higher risk of experiencing sickle cell disease, but this has been refuted in other studies suggesting it is more of a lack of education and participation in research studies (17). The life expectancy for someone with sickle cell disease is now 40 to 60 years of age (compared to only 14 years in 1973) in the United States due to improvements in health care (159). Between 80,000 and 100,000 people in the United States have sickle cell disease (129). The National Collegiate Athletic Association mandates sickle cell trait screening in all athletes due to the risks involved with sport participation.

Pathophysiology of Sickle Cell Disease

Sickle cell disease can be diagnosed from birth. Signs and symptoms associated with the disease are swelling of the hands and feet, fatigue and jaundice, acute crises associated with certain triggers, and chronic pain. When the red blood cell of someone with sickle cell anemia becomes deoxygenated, the response is to change into an elongated sickle or crescent shape. Cells of this shape have a shorter life span than normal cells. Additionally, the altered shape and lack of flexibility make it more difficult for blood to flow through the microvasculature (51). Individuals with sickle cell disease suffer from pain (also called crises) due to the decrease in blood flow to tissue. This decrease in blood flow is associated with vascular occlusion and arterial and venous thromboembolism (67) due to inflammation, endothelial dysfunctions, and hypercoagulation of the red blood cells (156). Those with sickle cell disease are at a higher risk for early mortality due to multiorgan damage. The malformed sickle cells and hypercoagulation cause the red blood cells to stick to one another, causing thrombosis to form and to affect many organ functions. The loss of blood flow to tissues can lead to infection, acute chest syndrome (damage to the lungs due to reduced blood flow), stroke, and pulmonary hypertension (137). The spleen is responsible for acting as a filter for the blood and getting rid of infection. In the case of the spleen, the sickle cells reduce the blood flow from the spleen, causing anemia, infection, and septicemia (7, 111, 159). Anemia can range from mild to moderate and even severe depending on the individual. Other major tissues can be affected as well, such as the eyes, kidneys, liver, bones, and joints.

Quality of life conditions associated with sickle cell disease, such as low cognitive function and impaired attention, result from the pain and sleep disorders corresponding with insufficient peripheral capillary oxygen saturation (SPO$_2$) (106). Supplementary oxygen can be beneficial in helping to improve sleep and raise low SPO$_2$ levels.

Common Medications Given to Individuals With Sickle Cell Disease

According to the CDC (40), treatment for sickle cell disease is largely based on symptomatology. See medications table 7.6 near the end of the chapter. Treatment options can range from over-the-counter medications, such as aspirins and ibuprofen, to prescription medications such as hydroxyurea for pain, antiplatelet therapy or blood thinners, antioxidants, and anti-inflammatory medications. Nonsteroidal anti-inflammatory medications (ibuprofen) are typically given for acute and chronic pain, while morphine is commonly prescribed to combat pain associated with acute chest syndrome and other acute and chronic pain. Many of these medications may be associated with numerous side effects, including nausea, vomiting, gastrointestinal distress, and constipation. Due to splenic dysfunction, individuals with sickle cell disease are at a high risk for life-threatening bacterial infections (pneumonia, influenza, salmonella, staphylococcus, and chlamydia) that affect the blood, lungs, bones, brain, and brain stem (159). Therefore, penicillin is commonly prescribed prophylactically (138), and medical records are checked to make sure people are up to date on their vaccinations. Hydroxyurea is used to help reduce pain associated with sickle cell disease but can reduce the effectiveness of the immune system. Other therapies associated with sickle cell disease are red blood cell transfusion and hematopoietic stem cell transplantation. To date, hematopoietic stem cell transplantation is considered the only cure for sickle cell disease (65).

Effects of Exercise in Individuals With Sickle Cell Disease

Connes and colleagues (51) report limited research on the effects of aerobic exercise in individuals with sickle cell anemia. Exercise capacity is lower in children and young adults with this disease (132) due to adaptations in the vascular structure, low hemoglobin concentrations, and reduced blood flow to the tissue (12). Those with

Key Point

For clients with sickle cell disease, obtain medical permission for physical training depending on the level of severity. Monitor exercise capacity closely.

sickle cell anemia are at an increased risk of lung and cardiac dysfunction. According to Alvarado and colleagues (16), children with sickle cell anemia have a tendency to demonstrate impaired heart rate recovery following maximal exercise. This is associated with an autonomic nervous system dysfunction, specifically, vagal function. Low oxygen saturation and high ventilation rate with exercise often lead to hypoxia, which can precipitate variability in the heart rate. Also noted are lower $\dot{V}O_2$ max and anaerobic thresholds (12). Anemic situations such as hypoxia, cardiopulmonary disease, and inflammation can result in reduced exercise capacity. The 6-minute walk test is often used to indirectly measure exercise capacity in children.

As reported by Eichner (72) in the realm of sport, exertional sickling is the number one leading killer of athletes in National Collegiate Athletic Association Division I football. These deaths all occurred during the conditioning phase and consisted of sudden cardiac arrest, asthma, and exertional heatstroke. Eichner recommends that athletes be screened before participation. There is discussion as to whether these athletes should be allowed to play at all. However, so as to not exclude them from exercise that is beneficial, these athletes are encouraged not to go all out but to set their own pace, resting periodically. Those with sickle cell disease are not recommended to participate in maximal testing. Athletes should be educated on the warning signals and learn to heed the warnings and seek medical help. Exercise professionals and coaches should monitor environmental conditions and adjust athletes' workloads and intensities accordingly.

Exertional rhabdomyolysis or sickling has been identified in active duty soldiers. Exertional sickling and exertional heat illness pose a risk for sudden death for military personnel just as it does with athletes (73). The intense nature of the conditioning of the soldier shares many of the dangers associated with conditioning for sports. Therefore, recommendations are similar.

A recent study (210) compared the effects of incremental cycle ergometer exercise in individuals with sickle cell anemia and healthy individuals. The exercise was a single bout of incremental exercise to ventilatory threshold. Monitoring postexercise showed no significant hematologic changes in either sickle cell anemia or healthy subjects. This study indicates that light- to moderate-intensity aerobic exercise may be beneficial and safe in individuals with sickle cell anemia. However, as emphasized by the investigators, further research is needed to help quantify the exact amount and intensity of exercise that can safely be prescribed.

Exercise Recommendations for Clients With Sickle Cell Disease

Two studies have reported positive effects of exercise in clients with sickle cell anemia. Strength and aerobic exercise in children of less than 30 minutes allowed a decrease in the use of analgesics as well as improving range of motion in some areas of the body (13). More recently, Tinti and colleagues (197) published a case study on the positive effects of aquatic exercise consisting of aerobic exercise and stretching for 45 minutes twice a week. Results showed a reduction in pain, small strength increases, and improved life quality. Clearly, more research is needed to address the lack of solid exercise prescription recommendations for clients with sickle cell anemia. Connes and colleagues (51) recommend that clients with sickle cell disease begin slowly and progress based upon how well exercise is tolerated, avoid extreme temperature exposure and hydrate frequently, and incorporate frequent rest breaks with exercise bouts up to 20 minutes. There are no consistencies in exercise recommendations. Recommendations need to be based on the client's exertional capacity and symptomatology. It is advised that clients with a known enlarged spleen avoid contact sports (209).

Sickle Cell Disease

Sex: Male

Race: African American

Age: 25

Height: 6 feet, 5 inches (1.96 m)

Weight: 240 pounds (109 kg)

Body fat: 32%

Body mass index: 28.5

Resting heart rate: 60 beats/min

Blood pressure: 120/70 mmHg

History

Mr. T, a young man diagnosed with sickle cell disease at birth, wants to begin an exercise program. He has not been physically active, other than walking, for the last five years. Before that he had participated in a high-intensity program. While doing pull-ups and sit-ups he began to experience severe leg and back pain. He continued to exercise, and during a 2-mile (3.2 km) run he began to have severe leg cramps that continued hours after exercising, along with symptoms similar to those for the flu. His symptoms continued to intensify to the point that he went to the emergency room. There he was diagnosed with exertional rhabdomyolysis.

Goals

Mr. T would like to work on the following goals:

1. Lose weight and fat mass
2. Improve aerobic and physical capacity without sickling

Intake

Before Mr. T began his exercise program, his physician had encouraged him to seek the advice of a knowledgeable exercise professional. Other than diminished capacity, he has no physical limitations. He performed a 6-minute walk test for aerobic capacity, push-up test for upper body endurance–strength, and the leg press test for lower body strength. Test results confirmed a low capacity for his age and sex. The exercise professional recommended a progressive resistance training program, cardiopulmonary exercise, and flexibility exercise. It was also recommended that he seek dietary advice from a registered dietician to help promote health.

Initial Training

Training sessions began with low-impact cardiovascular training three times per week. Mr. T's choice of activity was water walking or jogging and swimming due to its low impact. He tolerates the water walking and jogging fairly well at a light intensity for 20 minutes. He has enjoyed some resistance training along with basic static stretching. A full-body approach to resistance exercise was used at a light intensity, with 10 to 12 repetitions increasing to a moderate intensity, and one set of a combination of bodyweight and dumbbell exercises was chosen.

Exercise Progression

Over a period of two months Mr. T continued to do his water walking and jogging and gradually increased his ability to swim to four days per week. Cardiovascular training was conducted four days per week for 30 minutes. He began to alternate training sessions between the pool, the treadmill and elliptical, and the weights. He was able to increase to a full-body workout of two or three sets at a moderate to high intensity, making sure to breathe properly.

Outcomes

In three months' time, with his workout program Mr. T has noted some weight and fat loss with a repeated body composition and now weighs 230 pounds (104 kg) at 28% body fat. His weights and aerobic work have been beneficial in improving his aerobic capacity as well.

Training Recommendations and Contraindications for Clients With Sickle Cell Disease

1. Obtain medical permission for physical training depending on the level of severity.
2. Physical capacity should be evaluated before starting exercise programming.
3. Physical activity should be limited to less than 20 minutes with frequent breaks.
4. Exercise professionals should be very aware of how clients respond to training and be willing to adjust frequency, intensity, and time as needed. Avoiding activities that prove too taxing on the cardiovascular system is vital to this process.
5. All training should be light intensity and should be progressed as needed based on tolerance to activity.
6. Resistance training can include many different modes. Monitor intensity levels accordingly, ensuring that the client is breathing properly.
7. Alternative modes of training are also useful. Consider aqua exercise as a possible form of aerobic exercise.
8. Consider avoiding contact sports, especially in persons with an enlarged spleen.
9. Hydration is important.
10. Use caution in extreme weather conditions.

HEMOPHILIA

Hemophilia is a genetic disease that occurs due to a lack of specific blood protein factors that allow clotting (221). Depending on the severity of the disease, a person with hemophilia may have mild symptoms (e.g., slower clotting than normal) or more severe symptoms such as severe bleeding that requires medical intervention. It is important to remember that hemophilia has a "range of severity," depending on the level of deficiency in one of the protein factors (221). Severe hemophilia usually appears within the first 18 months of life (122). The severity of hemophilia A or B is commensurate with the percentage of circulating clotting factor activity. Individuals with levels less than or equal to 1% activity are categorized as having severe disease, those with 2% to 5% as having moderate disease, and those with 6% to 40% as having mild hemophilia (178).

History and Demographics of Hemophilia

Hemophilia is hereditary and is carried recessively on the X chromosome (188). This means that it is more common in males than females. Since the disease is recessive and on the X chromosome, females with the disease would have both parents as carriers; but males, who have a single X chromosome, would need only a single parent as a carrier for the disease (221). Hemophilia A occurs in 1 in 5,000 male live births, hemophilia B in 1 in 30,000 (142). Diagnosis of the disease usually occurs by 6 years of age, and often earlier when the disease is severe (221). Most individuals with hemophilia are deficient in clotting factor VIII (218).

A study of U.S. demographics, comorbidities, and health status found that those living with hemophilia experience a wide variety of comorbidities (57). In this study of 141 participants with hemophilia A and B, 47.5% had liver disease. The rate of liver disease in the U.S. population is 1.1%. The rate of HIV infection in this population was 14.2%, as compared to 0.25% in the U.S. population. The same investigation found that almost 50% of persons with hemophilia were overweight or obese. As compared to the older participants, those at the younger end of the age spectrum were more obese than overweight (57). The average occurrence of hemophilic joint arthritis in this population was

33.3%. This average was higher in the older end of this population spectrum (44%). In comparison, the arthritis rate among U.S. males aged 18 to 44 is 6.8% (57). Forsyth and colleagues (82) found that spontaneous joint bleeding was reported in 76% of persons with hemophilia. Joint bleeding typically progresses from early synovitis to ultimate end-stage, irreversible joint damage (140).

Pathophysiology of Hemophilia

Severe hemophilia is typically identified in infancy, often due to knowledge of family history or unusual bleeding (221). According to the Mayo Clinic (145), **hemophilia A** is the most common type of hemophilia, characterized by insufficient clotting factor VIII. **Hemophilia B** is the second most common type, caused by insufficient clotting factor IX. **Hemophilia C** is the mildest form, caused by insufficient clotting factor XI. Since there is no cure for hemophilia, the key is to control the disease. This is typically accomplished by using clotting factors. Before clotting factors VIII and IX were isolated, the life span for an individual with hemophilia was quite short. Before the 1940s, the average life span of a person with hemophilia was 27 years; with technological improvements it increased to 60 years by the 1980s (218). A survey of the 2007 Healthcare Cost and Utilization Project–Nationwide Inpatient Sample (NIS) found that the mortality rates of hemophilia patients (2.2%) were comparable to the all-cause in-hospital mortality rates (1.9%) (87). The overall median age of death for hemophilia-related hospitalizations was 68.3 years as opposed to 72.3 years for all hospitalizations. With the development of recombinant factor production, the risk of AIDS and hepatitis transmission with clotting factor administration has been minimized (218).

Common Medications Given to Individuals With Hemophilia

According to the National Hemophilia Foundation, the preferred treatment for hemophilia is factor replacement therapy with factors made from human plasma. This treatment includes injecting the missing protein (clotting factor) into the person's vein. Clotting factor VIII is used for hemophilia A, while clotting factor IX is used for hemophilia B (159). This process allows for immediate use of the protein to facilitate clotting. Treatments are determined based on bleeding patterns and severity of the disorder. Regular treatment is referred to as **prophylaxis**, and treatment that is provided on an as-needed basis is referred to as "on-demand" (157). According to the National Institutes of Health (159), other types of treatment are also possible. Desmopressin is a man-made hormone used to treat people who have mild hemophilia A. This hormone stimulates the release of clotting factor VIII. Desmopressin is not known to interfere with exercise response or adaptations. Antifibrinolytic medicines are used in conjunction with gene replacement therapy to help keep blood clots from breaking down. These medications are not known to interfere with exercise response or adaptations, but may have side effects that make exercise unpleasant. See medications table 7.7 near the end of the chapter.

Effects of Exercise in Individuals With Hemophilia

Anderson and Forsyth (18) note that people with bleeding disorders vary widely in how they respond to taking part in sport and exercise. Unfortunately, inactivity among people with hemophilia is all too common. Despite concerns, there is little doubt as to the positive benefits of exercise for persons with hemophilia. As with healthy populations, regular exercise can significantly improve quality of life (154). Individuals with hemophilia are at risk for joint bleeding and may have preexisting joint damage from previous bleeds (81). This means that exercise programming should be conservative. Although the literature is relatively limited, it appears that individuals with hemophilia respond positively to aerobic, resistance, and aquatic training (25, 188).

People with hemophilia who engage in resistance training programming will benefit from muscular strength increases as the muscles around affected joints are strengthened (104). The benefits of resistance training for this population are multifold. Tiktinsky and colleagues (196) researched the effect of resistance training on people with severe hemophilia and found that in addition to muscular strength increases, bleeding frequency decreased from two or three times per week to one or two times per week. This investigation also documented two people with hemophilia who had engaged in long-term resistance training (more than 11 years); they reported a marked decrease in bleeding frequency and severity. Another study that used resistance training as part of a training regimen reported no exercise-induced pain or bleeding as a result of exercise (154). This investigation noted improvements in joint motion, muscular strength, and distance walked in 6 minutes. The greatest gains were seen in those with the most severe joint damage and comorbidities.

Aerobic exercise has also been found to be beneficial. In response to an acute high-intensity aerobic exercise session to volitional fatigue, Groen and colleagues (94) found significant increases in clotting factor VIII in persons with mild and moderate hemophilia A. Moderate aerobic exercise was found to be more effective than mild at improving markers of bone metabolism and handgrip strength in individuals with moderate hemophilia A. Improvements in clotting factors also occurred in persons with moderate hemophilia as a result of moderate-intensity aquatic exercise (25). Regular aquatic exercise has also been found to improve muscular strength around affected joints. Not much has been published regarding flexibility programming and hemophilia. However, Anderson and Forsyth (18) state that stretching is one of the most important parts of a conditioning program. Mulvany and colleagues (154) used a stretching program as part of a conditioning program. In this investigation, significant improvements in range of motion were found in all joints. As with healthy populations, regular exercise can significantly improve quality of life among people with hemophilia (154).

Exercise Recommendations for Clients With Hemophilia

Program design guidelines for clients with hemophilia are summarized in table 7.6. Exercise for clients with hemophilia is recommended in conjunction with medical treatment (188). Forsyth and colleagues (81) recommend a regular physical activity program including strength, aerobic, balance, and range of motion activities to help reduce the risks of osteoporosis, falls, and hemophilia-related joint changes. It is advisable that the person programming exercise for clients with hemophilia be familiar with the disease. Forsyth and colleagues (81) recommend that this person be someone associated with a hemophilia treatment center. With any type of exercise, it is important that people with hemophilia be given exercise options based on their capabilities. For instance, joint pain and limited range of motion may necessitate the use of alternative forms of exercise. Given the rather sparse and varied nature of investigations of exercise and hemophilia, providing solid guidelines is difficult. However, what has been done has been progressive over time and shown to be safe and effective. With regard to resistance training, research suggests that training can occur between two and five times per week. Starting at the lower end of this frequency spectrum, as well as those of other intensity indicators, is advisable upon initiating a program. Investigations have used a full-body approach, fewer multijoint exercises, and more isolated muscle group approaches. Intensity ranges are suggested to be between one and three sets, 10 to 20 repetitions (40-70% 1RM), 1 to 2 minutes of rest. Modes of resistance training can vary from resistance bands to machine weights, isometric exercises, and free weights.

Typically clients with hemophilia have low cardiopulmonary fitness. Initially, light- to moderate-level aerobic exercise is preferable. Mulvany and colleagues (154) used the estimated MHR formula (i.e., 220 – age) to develop individualized exercise training programming with a progression

Key Point

Advances in prophylaxis have made it easier and safer for people with hemophilia to exercise; however, bleeding due to injury is still possible. Always consider the timing of treatment in relation to physical activity.

Table 7.6   Program Design Guidelines for Clients With Hemophilia

Type of exercise	Frequency	Intensity
Resistance training		

Multijoint movement considerations
  a. Bodyweight resistance
  b. Resistance bands, suspension training, and manual resistance
  c. Basic weight training such as resistance machines and free weights
Mode of resistance training can vary based on how well exercise is tolerated. If tolerated well, basic weight training can be used.
	Frequency will vary based on postexertion symptomatology.
	Begin with two sessions per week, depending on total volume. Once acclimated, consider a split program in which different body parts are exercised by day to achieve greater frequency up to 5 times per week.
		Avoid movements involving significant impact.
		Choose 8-10 exercises, using a full-body approach.
		Start with 1 set of 10-20 repetitions at 40-70% 1RM.
		1-3 sets can be used depending on training level.
		Set intensity should fall short of volitional fatigue at first and may progress.
		Increases in intensity beyond this point should be based on postexercise symptomatology.
		If doing multiple sets, consider 1-2 min between sets to start; be prepared to adjust as needed.

Aerobic training		

Aerobic exercise mode should be low impact and well tolerated. No mode-specific contraindications are implicated.
  a. Water aerobics
  b. Walking
  c. Cycling
  d. Rowing
Mode of aerobic training can vary based on how well exercise is tolerated.
	Begin conservatively, using two or three sessions per week, possibly more than once per day with use of interval training. If tolerated, sessions can be increased slowly over time. Sessions can be performed 3-4 days per week.	Begin with 15- to 20-min sessions with a progression from 50% to 70% MHR. Progress to 30-min sessions most days of the week.

Flexibility training		
Full-body, passive, static, flexibility exercises	Can also exist as a regular training program if other forms of exercise are not well tolerated.	8-10 dynamic, low-amplitude stretches held for 30 s at first, then progressing up to 60 s. Stretching intensity should not reach the point of pain but rather muscle tautness.

References: (18, 25, 81, 94, 104, 154, 188, 196)

from 50% to 70% estimated maximal heart rate. While some success has been shown with an acute high-intensity bout, not much is known about how such exercise will be tolerated over time. Exercise sessions should start out at 15 to 20 minutes of continuous exercise two or three times per week. Aquatic exercise may also be used to achieve a desired aerobic effect. The National Hemophilia Foundation (18) recommends that adults gradually increase aerobic exercise until 30 minutes of moderate-intensity activity is achieved on most days of the week. Flexibility training should include a full-body approach. Static stretches should be slow and gentle and held for at least 30 seconds. Over time, the number and duration of stretches can be increased. Should bleeding occur, stretches should cease until bleeding is under control.

Hemophilia

Sex: Male

Race: Hispanic

Age: 19

Height: 5 feet, 8 inches (1.73 m)

Weight: 220 pounds (100 kg)

Body fat: 29%

Body mass index: 33.5

Resting heart rate: 72 beats/min

Blood pressure: 142/94 mmHg

Temperature: Normal

History

Mr. R is a 19-year-old college student with factor IX deficiency (hemophilia B). His disease severity is classified as moderate. He was diagnosed with this disease at 5 years old following episodes of intense bruising and bleeding. He has experienced joint tenderness, pain with movement, and decreased range of motion. Due to his symptoms, he has avoided physical activity for many years. As a result he has gained a significant amount of weight during his teenage years. In turn, his joint problems have gotten worse. He routinely receives factor IX for acute bleeds and recombinant factor IX for replacement therapy from a hemophilia care center. His physician has also prescribed NSAIDs for his joint pain. Working during college is important to Mr. R; however, maintaining a job has been difficult. Mr. R has come to the realization that his condition is not improving and that he needs to make a change for the better. He consulted his physician for further advice and was advised to exercise.

Goals

Mr. R would like to work on the following goals:

1. Reduce the amount of pain he experiences on a daily basis
2. Improve quality of life
3. Reduce body weight to take stress off joints
4. Make physical exercise a regular part of his treatment program

Intake

Having consulted with his hemophilia treatment center, Mr. R has located a certified exercise professional who knows about his condition. The exercise professional took a full medical history. Due to limited range of motion as well as joint pain, exercise testing was not possible. As an alternative, the exercise professional performed a walk test for time to assess Mr. R's aerobic capabilities and a dynamometer battery for strength. Bioelectric impedance was used to measure body composition. The exercise professional made a referral to a registered dietician who was knowledgeable about hemophilia.

Initial Training

Due to the client's condition, slow progression was necessary. In addition, alternative forms of training were required to accommodate limited ranges of motion. The primary training emphasis of the program was to help increase cardiopulmonary capacity, overall muscular strength especially around the affected joints, and muscular flexibility. Frequency of resistance training was variable until any joint swelling or other symptomatology subsided. Mr. R's initial strengthening program was based on his available range of motion at each joint and history of pain. The most fragile joints were targeted for this early phase of training. This generally consisted of exercises performed at 40% to 50% of the client's tested isometric maximum voluntary contraction (MVC), which was used as a guide. All exercises were performed for one set of 10 repetitions within the pain-free range of motion, below the point of volitional fatigue. Exercise options could include resistance bands, bodyweight exercises, dumbbell exercises, or other functional strengthening activities. Cardiovascular training was performed twice weekly and was low impact. Exercises chosen consisted of aquatic exercise, treadmill, or cross-country skiing. Typical intensity began at 50% MHR. The goal was to reach 10 to 20 minutes of consistent activity. If this goal was not reached in one interval, 5- and 10-minute intervals were used to reach it. Flexibility training followed cardiovascular training, as the fibrous joints of persons with hemophilia are more responsive to the warming of active exercise. To begin, stretches were held for 20 to 30 seconds within the pain-free range of motion.

Exercise Progression

With adequate adaptation, resistance training intensity increased by 5% to 10% per week up to a maximum of 70% of the client's MVC. Training frequency was increased to three or four times per week. With the strengthening of the most affected joints, a full-body approach could now be used. Full-body training was divided into two training sessions. Set volume increased from one to three sets per body part. Repetitions progressed to the 10 to 20 range. Aerobic training progressed to three or four 30-minute sessions per week at 70% of the client's MHR. Low-impact movements were still used. The same full-body approach to flexibility was maintained; however, the length of static stretches gradually increased up to 60 seconds.

Outcomes

Mr. R's progression took longer than anticipated, but he was eventually able to adopt a regular program. With persistence, he was able to increase muscular strength around his most affected joints. This made a definite difference in his physical capabilities and in his daily life.

Training Recommendations and Contraindications for Clients With Hemophilia

1. Obtain medical permission for physical training depending on the level of severity.
2. Physical capacity should be evaluated before starting exercise programming.
3. Evaluate joint range of motion limitations before exercise selection.
4. Coagulation medication should be available for potential light to moderate bleeds.
5. Use estimated MHR to help determine aerobic exercise intensity.
6. Flexibility exercise should be performed after active warm-up.
7. Be prepared for progressions in all health-related fitness areas to take much longer than in apparently healthy clients.
8. Exercise professionals should be very aware of how clients respond to training and be willing to adjust frequency, intensity, and time as needed. Avoiding painful movement is vital to this process.
9. All training should be light and low impact.
10. Resistance training can include many different modes but should begin sparingly until tolerance can be determined. Consider bodyweight activities, lower-level modes of resistance such as tubes and bands, and machine- and free-weight movements.
11. Avoid ballistic motions when training. Use smooth, controlled movements that will reduce the chance of injury and allow proper control of movement.
12. Consider aerobic modes initially that are predictable modes of exercise so the client can more effectively exercise in a steady state.
13. Alternative modes of training are also useful. Consider aqua exercise as a possible form of aerobic exercise.

Recommended Readings

Cheatham, SW. Fibromyalgia: current concepts for the strength and conditioning professional. *Strength Cond J* 35(4):11-18, 2013.

Coelho, JD and Cameron, KL. Hemophilia and resistance training: implications for the strength and conditioning professional. *Strength Cond J* 21(5):30-33, 1999.

Dawes, J and Stephenson, MD. ONE-ON-ONE: training those with chronic fatigue. *Strength Cond J* 30(6):55-57, 2008.

Ferreira, MP and Norwood, JM. Strength training for the athlete with HIV/AIDS: practical implications for the performance team. *Strengh Cond J* 19(6):50-57, 1997.

Williams, C and Dawes, J. Guidelines for training individuals with lupus. *Strength Cond J* 29(2):56-58, 2007.

CONCLUSION

Immunologic and hematologic disorders are serious life-altering diseases. It is important for the exercise professional to recognize signs and symptoms of these diseases. It may be that an individual has a previous undiagnosed illness, and recognition by the exercise professional will allow proper diagnosis by appropriate medical professionals.

When working with clients who have previously diagnosed immunologic and hematologic disorders, the exercise professional should monitor the client to ensure that the exercise prescription is beneficial and not harmful. The guidelines provided in this chapter are general, and it is critical to remember that each client is an individual. Furthermore, in some instances, clients with the disorders discussed in this chapter respond to exercise differently from healthy clients. Even if a client is asymptomatic, the exercise professional should always remember the existence of the chronic disorder. The benefits of exercise for both improved health and quality of life cannot be underestimated. The qualified exercise professional can have a positive impact on individuals with immunologic and hematologic disorders by recognizing limitations and designing exercise programming that adapts to meet the needs and abilities of the client.

Key Terms

acquired immune deficiency syndrome (AIDS)
biological response modifiers
chronic fatigue syndrome
corticosteroid
discoid lupus erythematosus
disease-modifying antirheumatic drugs (DMARDs)
fibromyalgia
hemophilia
hemophilia A
hemophilia B
hemophilia C

highly active antiretroviral therapy (HAART)
human immunodeficiency virus (HIV)
inflammation
kinesiophobia
lupus erythematosus
nonsteroidal anti-inflammatory drugs (NSAIDs)
postexertional malaise
prophylaxis
rheumatoid arthritis
sickle cell disease
systemic autoimmune diseases
systemic lupus erythematosus

Study Questions

1. Which of these is a characteristic of rheumatoid arthritis?
   a. occurs more frequently in men
   b. usually affects neck and back first
   c. is curable with regular exercise and medication
   d. originates with immune system attack on joint synovial lining

2. What is the difference between discoid lupus erythematosus (DLE) and systemic lupus erythematosus (SLE)?
   a. SLE affects only T-cells.
   b. DLE is not an autoimmune disease.
   c. SLE does not shorten life expectancy.
   d. DLE does not usually affect internal organs, only the skin.

3. A colleague presents the following initial exercise plan for a sedentary new client with lupus.

   Walking on a treadmill at 60% $\dot{V}O_2$peak for 30 minutes a day, twice a week to start, progressing to four times per week. Resistance training beginning with eight bodyweight exercises covering all major muscle groups, 1 set each at 50% estimated 1RM at a frequency dictated by symptoms. Full-body flexibility exercises held for 5 seconds, daily after treadmill exercise completed.

   Given this scenario, what recommendation should the exercise professional make?
   a. Reduce treadmill intensity to 30% $\dot{V}O_2$peak.
   b. Increase resistance training to 4 days per week.
   c. Split treadmill exercise into three 10-minute bouts.
   d. Eliminate flexibility exercises until treadmill intensity progresses to 70% $\dot{V}O_2$peak.

4. The most important consideration for clients with hemophilia when one is designing an exercise program is
   a. infection control
   b. postexertional malaise
   c. side effects from DMARDs and related medications
   d. the potential for joint damage and limits on range of motion

Medications Table 7.1   Common Medications Used to Treat Rheumatoid Arthritis

Drug class and names	Mechanism of action	Most common side effects	Effects on exercise
NSAIDs (nonsteroidal anti-inflammatory drugs)			
celecoxib (Celebrex), diflunisal (Dolobid), etodolac (Lodine), ibuprofen (Advil, Motrin, Rufen), meloxicam (Mobic), nabumetone (Relafen), naproxen (Naprosyn, Aleve), oxaprozin (Daypro, Duraprox), piroxicam (Feldene), salsalate (Disalcid), sulindac (Clinoril), tolmetin (Tolectin), ketoprofen (Orudis, Oruvail)	NSAIDs block formation of COX-1 and COX-2 enzymes that control the formation of prostaglandins. COX-1 enzymes control the formation of prostaglandins involved in normal organ function, and COX-2 enzymes control the formation of prostaglandins involved in the body's inflammatory response. By blocking the prostaglandins, the individual experiences less swelling and pain.	Upset stomach, headache, easy bruising, hypertension, fluid retention, dyspepsia, gastritis, increased risk of heart attack or stroke, reduced blood clotting, reduced kidney function in those with hypertension or preexisting kidney problems, elevated liver enzymes, worsened asthma or inflammatory bowel disease, severe headache and neck stiffness, possible skin rashes	NSAIDs are not known to have negative effects on exercise performance; however, some delay in exercise-induced fatigue has been associated with NSAID intake. Some evidence suggests that NSAIDs may attenuate exercise recovery.
Corticosteroids			
prednisone, prednisolone, hydrocortisone, methylprednisolone (Medrol); dexamethasone (Decadron); triamcinolone (Aristospan); methylprednisolone (Solu-Medrol); topical steroids	Corticosteroids slow and stop the processes in the body that make molecules involved in the inflammatory response. In addition, these drugs also reduce the activity of the immune system by affecting the function of the white blood cells.	Acne, Cushing's syndrome, weight gain, redistribution of fat, increased skin fragility, hair growth on the face, irritability, agitation, psychosis, mood swings, insomnia, increased susceptibility to infections, stomach irritations or ulcers, irregular menses, potassium deficiency, increased cholesterol and triglycerides, suppressed growth in children, necrosis of bone, osteoporosis, cataracts, glaucoma, muscle weakness, premature atherosclerosis, pregnancy complications	Corticosteroids are not known to interfere with exercise performance or exercise responses. Long-term health adaptations can be negated as increases in cholesterol, weight, and blood pressure are possible.
Conventional synthetic disease-modifying antirheumatic drugs (csDMARDs)			
methotrexate, hydroxychloroquine, sulfasalazine, leflunomide, cyclophosphamide, azathioprine	Reduce the progression of joint damage; often taken in combination with biologics	Weight gain, nausea and vomiting, severe infection, stomach pain, diarrhea, cancer, kidney damage, liver problems, increased risk of infection, skin rash	The reduction of inflammation should cause an improvement in physical function. Monitor for any unusual weakness and fatigue. Assess functional ability and disability associated with DMARDs. Assess for dizziness that might affect gait, balance, and other functional activities. Monitor pulmonary function during exercise.

Drug class and names	Mechanism of action	Most common side effects	Effects on exercise
Biologics			
abatacept, adalimumab, anakinra, certolizumab pegol, etanercept, infliximab, golimumab, rituximab	Each medication stops the inflammatory response differently; slows, modifies, or stops the disease	Serious infections, tuberculosis, lymphoma, congestive heart failure	Be alert for seizures or increased seizure activity. Assess for joint pain. Monitor for dizziness or trembling that might affect gait, balance, or other functional activities.
JAK (a subcategory of DMARDs)			
tofacitinib	Is an inhibitor, blocks certain pathways involved in the body's immune response	Bronchitis, headache, high cholesterol, low blood counts, increased liver enzymes; nasal, inflammation, gastrointestinal issues	Possibly beneficial for skeletal muscle adaptation.

References: (46, 100, 147, 161, 211)

Medications Table 7.2   Common Medications Used to Treat Lupus

Drug class and names	Mechanism of action	Most common side effects	Effects on exercise
NSAIDs (nonsteroidal anti-inflammatory drugs)			
celecoxib (Celebrex), diflunisal (Dolobid), etodolac (Lodine), ibuprofen (Advil, Motrin, Rufen), meloxicam (Mobic), nabumetone (Relafen), naproxen (Naprosyn, Aleve), oxaprozin (Daypro, Duraprox), piroxicam (Feldene), salsalate (Disalcid), sulindac (Clinoril), tolmetin (Tolectin), ketoprofen (Orudis, Oruvail)	NSAIDs block formation of COX-1 and COX-2 enzymes that control the formation of prostaglandins. (COX-1 enzymes control the formation of prostaglandins involved in normal organ function, and COX-2 enzymes control the formation of prostaglandins involved in the body's inflammatory response. By blocking the prostaglandins, the individual experiences less swelling and pain.)	Upset stomach, headache, easy bruising, hypertension, fluid retention, dyspepsia, gastritis, increased risk of heart attack or stroke, reduced blood clotting, reduced kidney function in those with hypertension or preexisting kidney problems, elevated liver enzymes, worsened asthma or inflammatory bowel disease, severe headache and neck stiffness, possible skin rashes	NSAIDs are not known to have negative effects on exercise performance; however, some delay in exercise-induced fatigue has been associated with NSAID intake. Some evidence suggests that NSAIDs may attenuate exercise recovery.
Corticosteroids			
prednisone, prednisolone, hydrocortisone, methylprednisolone (Medrol); dexamethasone (Decadron); triamcinolone (Aristospan); methylprednisolone (Solu-Medrol); topical steroids	Corticosteroids slow and stop the processes in the body that make molecules involved in the inflammatory response. In addition, these drugs also reduce the activity of the immune system by affecting the function of the white blood cells.	Acne, Cushing's syndrome, weight gain, redistribution of fat, increased skin fragility, hair growth on the face, irritability, agitation, psychosis, mood swings, insomnia, increased susceptibility to infections, stomach irritations or ulcers, irregular menses, potassium deficiency, increased cholesterol and triglycerides, suppressed growth in children, necrosis of bone, osteoporosis, cataracts, glaucoma, muscle weakness, premature atherosclerosis, pregnancy complications	Corticosteroids are not known to interfere with exercise performance or exercise responses. However, long-term health adaptations can be negated as increases in cholesterol, weight, and blood pressure are possible.
Antimalarial medications			
hydroxychloroquine (Plaquenil), chloroquine (Aralen), quinacrine (Atabrine)	Antimalarial drugs help control lupus by modulating the immune system without predisposing the individual to infection, protecting against UV light, and improving skin lesions that don't respond to topical treatment therapy.	Potential side effects can include skin rashes and pigment change, dry skin, loss of appetite, abdominal bloating, stomach cramps, and retinal damage; less common side effects include headaches, muscle aches, weakness, nervousness, irritability, dizziness, neurological side effects, and exacerbation of psoriasis.	Antimalarial medications are not known to interfere with exercise performance, responses, or adaptations. Secondary side effects could make exercising uncomfortable.

Drug class and names	Mechanism of action	Most common side effects	Effects on exercise
Immunosuppressive medications			
azathioprine (Imuran), mycophenolate mofetil (Cellcept), cyclosporine (Neoral, Sandimmune, Gengraf), methotrexate (Rheumatrex), leflunomide (Arava), cyclophosphamide (Cytoxan), chlorambucil (Leukeran), nitrogen mustard (Mustargen)	Immunosuppressive medications suppress the attack by interfering with the synthesis of DNA to keep the cells of the immune system from dividing.	Increased risk of infection, suppressed signs of illness, increased cancer risk, nausea, vomiting, stomach pain, diarrhea, liver test abnormalities, hepatitis, pancreatitis, allergic reaction, headache, dizziness, tremors, skin rashes, possible anemia, uric acid production	Immunosuppressive medications are not known to interfere with exercise performance or exercise responses. Secondary side effects could make exercising regularly difficult due to enhanced susceptibility to infections.
DHEA (dehydroepiandrosterone)			
	DHEA is a mild male hormone that has not been approved by the FDA for the treatment of lupus. Although DHEA levels are commonly low in individuals with inflammatory diseases like lupus, the exact mechanism by which it works remains controversial.	Acne, facial hair growth, oily skin, excessive sweating, lowered high-density lipoprotein in some women, increased estrogen levels in postmenopausal women	DHEA is not known to interfere with exercise capacity, response, or adaptations.

References: (58, 143, 158, 195, 208)

Medications Table 7.3 Common Medications Used to Treat Chronic Fatigue Syndrome

Drug class and names	Mechanism of action	Most common side effects	Effects on exercise
NSAIDs (nonsteroidal anti-inflammatory drugs)			
celecoxib (Celebrex), diflunisal (Dolobid), etodolac (Lodine), ibuprofen (Advil, Motrin, Rufen), meloxicam (Mobic), nabumetone (Relafen), naproxen (Naprosyn, Aleve), oxaprozin (Daypro, Duraprox), piroxicam (Feldene), salsalate (Disalcid), sulindac (Clinoril), tolmetin (Tolectin), ketoprofen (Orudis, Oruvail)	NSAIDs block formation of COX-1 and COX-2 enzymes that control the formation of prostaglandins. (COX-1 enzymes control the formation of prostaglandins involved in normal organ function, and COX-2 enzymes control the formation of prostaglandins involved in the body's inflammatory response. By blocking the prostaglandins, the individual experiences less swelling and pain.)	Upset stomach, headache, easy bruising, hypertension, fluid retention, dyspepsia, gastritis, increased risk of heart attack or stroke, reduced blood clotting, reduced kidney function in those with hypertension or preexisting kidney problems, elevated liver enzymes, worsened asthma or inflammatory bowel disease, severe headache and neck stiffness, possible skin rashes	NSAIDs are not known to have negative effects on exercise performance; however, some delay in exercise-induced fatigue has been associated with NSAID intake. Some evidence suggests that NSAIDs may attenuate exercise recovery.
Antidepressants			
amitriptyline (Elavil), doxepin (Sinequan), desipramine (Norpramin), nortriptyline (Pamelor), clomipramine (Anafranil), imipramine (Tofranil, Janimine), bupropion (Wellbutrin), nefazodone (Serzone), mirtazapine (Remeron), fluoxetine (Prozac), sertraline (Zoloft), paroxetine (Paxil), cymbalta (Duloxetine)	There are multiple classes of antidepressant drugs. Based on the class of antidepressant, these drugs work through different mechanisms. Tricyclic antidepressants affect brain chemicals involved in pain management. Other antidepressants affect different neurotransmitters. Serotonin reuptake inhibitors (SSRIs) interfere with the natural reuptake of neurotransmitters.	Headache, agitation, nausea, vomiting, constipation, dry mouth, reduced sexual drive, restlessness, slightly increased heart rate, interactions with other drugs	Potential side effects may make the process of exercise uncomfortable. A physician or other health care professional should be consulted if symptoms become too severe.
Immunosuppressive medications			
azathioprine (Imuran), mycophenolate mofetil (Cellcept), cyclosporine (Neoral, Sandimmune, Gengraf), methotrexate (Rheumatrex), leflunomide (Arava), cyclophosphamide (Cytoxan), chlorambucil (Leukeran), nitrogen mustard (Mustargen)	Immunosuppressant medications suppress the attack by interfering with the synthesis of DNA. This keeps the cells of the immune system from dividing.	Increased risk of infection, suppressed signs of illness, increased cancer risk, nausea, vomiting, stomach pain, diarrhea, liver test abnormalities, hepatitis, pancreatitis, allergic reaction, headache, dizziness, tremors, skin rashes, possible anemia, uric acid production	Immunosuppressive medications are not known to interfere with exercise performance or exercise responses. Secondary side effects could make regularly exercising difficult due to enhanced susceptibility to infections.
Stimulants			
caffeine, dexamphetamine, methylphenidate, modafinil	Stimulants work by increasing dopamine levels in the brain. Therapeutic stimulants increase dopamine in a slow and steady manner similar to the way it is produced naturally in the brain.	Appetite suppression, headache, upset stomach, increased blood pressure, dizziness, dry mouth, nervousness, sleeplessness or insomnia, weight loss	Possible greater power output, enhanced aerobic endurance, and resistance to fatigue. Prevalent use of stimulant medications may interfere with heart rate response during exercise.

Drug class and names	Mechanism of action	Most common side effects	Effects on exercise
Sleep aids			
zolpidem tartrate (Ambien), eszopiclone (Lunesta), zaleplon (Sonata), rozerem (Ramelteon), lorazepam (Ativan), triazolam (Halcion), temazepam (Restoril), diazepam (Valium), alprazolam (Xanax), diphenhydramine	Sleep aids work through a variety of mechanisms. Many prescription sleep aids work on select gamma-amino butyric acid (GABA) receptors in the brain that control levels of alertness or relaxation.	Dry mouth, daytime drowsiness, blurred vision, constipation, difficulty urinating, muscle relaxation, euphoria, poor memory	Potential side effects may make the process of exercise uncomfortable.

References: (24, 26, 58, 133, 143)

Medications Table 7.4   Common Medications Used to Treat Fibromyalgia

Drug class and names	Mechanism of action	Most common side effects	Effects on exercise
Drugs used as pain relievers			
pregabalin (Lyrica): Licensed as an antiepileptic, used to treat chronic pain	Pregabalin binds to the alpha 2 delta subunit of voltage-gated Ca$^+$ channels in the central nervous system.	Blurred vision, drowsiness, fluid retention in peripheral areas, lack of coordination, weight gain, loss of ability to focus, dizziness, dry mouth	Potential side effects may make the process of exercise uncomfortable. A physician or other health care professional should be consulted if symptoms become too severe.
Antidepressants			
amitriptyline (Elavil), doxepin (Sinequan), desipramine (Norpramin), nortriptyline (Pamelor), clomipramine (Anafranil), imipramine (Tofranil, Janimine), bupropion (Wellbutrin), nefazodone (Serzone), mirtazapine (Remeron), fluoxetine (Prozac), sertraline (Zoloft), paroxetine (Paxil), cymbalta (Duloxetine)	There are multiple classes of antidepressant drugs. Based on the class of antidepressant, these drugs work through different mechanisms. Tricyclic antidepressants affect brain chemicals involved in pain management. Other antidepressants affect different neurotransmitters. Serotonin reuptake inhibitors (SSRIs) interfere with the natural reuptake of neurotransmitters.	Headache, agitation, nausea, vomiting, constipation, dry mouth, reduced sexual drive, restlessness, slightly increased heart rate, interactions with other drugs	Potential side effects may make the process of exercise uncomfortable. A physician or other health care professional should be consulted if symptoms become too severe.
Analgesics—pain killers			
acetaminophen (Tylenol), tramadol (ConZip, Rybix, ODT, Ultram)	These generally are centrally acting in that they decrease the perception of pain by reducing the flow of pain signals from the brain.	Analgesics can cause allergic symptoms like hoarseness, swelling, difficulty breathing, hives, itching, itching rash, upset stomach, constipation, diarrhea, dizziness, and headache.	Potential side effects may make the process of exercise uncomfortable. A physician or other health care professional should be consulted if symptoms become too severe.
NSAIDs (nonsteroidal anti-inflammatory drugs)			
celecoxib (Celebrex), diflunisal (Dolobid), etodolac (Lodine), ibuprofen (Advil, Motrin, Rufen), meloxicam (Mobic), nabumetone (Relafen), naproxen (Naprosyn, Aleve), oxaprozin (Daypro, Duraprox), piroxicam (Feldene), salsalate (Disalcid), sulindac (Clinoril), tolmetin (Tolectin), ketoprofen (Orudis, Oruvail)	NSAIDs block formation of COX-1 and COX-2 enzymes that control the formation of prostaglandins. (COX-1 enzymes control the formation of prostaglandins involved in normal organ function, and COX-2 enzymes control the formation of prostaglandins involved in the body's inflammatory response. By blocking the prostaglandins, the individual experiences less swelling and pain.)	Upset stomach, headache, easy bruising, hypertension, fluid retention, dyspepsia, gastritis, increased risk of heart attack or stroke, reduced blood clotting, reduced kidney function in those with hypertension or preexisting kidney problems, elevated liver enzymes, worsened asthma or inflammatory bowel disease, severe headache and neck stiffness, possible skin rashes	NSAIDs are not known to have negative effects on exercise performance; however, some delay in exercise-induced fatigue has been associated with NSAID intake. Some evidence suggests that NSAIDs may attenuate exercise recovery.

Drug class and names	Mechanism of action	Most common side effects	Effects on exercise
Sleep aids			
zolpidem tartrate (Ambien), eszopiclone (Lunesta), zaleplon (Sonata), rozerem (Ramelteon), lorazepam (Ativan), triazolam (Halcion), temazepam (Restoril), diazepam (Valium), alprazolam (Xanax), diphenhydramine	Sleep aids work through a variety of mechanisms. Many prescription sleep aids work on select gamma-amino butyric acid (GABA) receptors in the brain that control levels of alertness or relaxation.	Dry mouth, daytime drowsiness, blurred vision, constipation, difficulty urinating, muscle relaxation, euphoria, poor memory, and morning tiredness	Potential side effects may make the process of exercise uncomfortable.
Muscle relaxants			
cyclobenzaprine (Amrix, Fexmid, Flexeril)	Act primarily within the central nervous system at the brain stem to reduce tonic somatic motor activity influencing both gamma and alpha motor system.	Blurred vision, dizziness, light-headedness, drowsiness, dryness of mouth	Potential side effects may make the process of exercise uncomfortable.

References: (33, 58, 133, 143, 165)

Medications Table 7.5   Common Medications Used to Treat HIV/AIDS

Drug class and names	Mechanism of action	Most common side effects	Effects on exercise
Nucleoside reverse transcriptase inhibitors (NRTIs)			
abacavir (Ziagen), didanosine, emtricitabine, lamivudine, stavudine, tenofovir disoproxil, zidovudine, azidothymidine (AZT)	Inhibit reverse transcriptase, cause DNA chain termination	Nausea, vomiting, hypersensitivity, lethargy, fatigue, cough, myalgia, arthralgia, malaise, chills, lactic acidosis, mitochondrial toxicity, dilated cardiomyopathy, neuropathy	Risk of myocardial infarction and lactic acidosis
Non-nucleoside reverse transcriptase inhibitors (NNRTIs)			
delavirdine, efavirenz, etravirine, rilpivirine	NNRTIs bind to and alter the enzyme HIV needs to make copies of itself (reverse transcriptase). Inhibit viral synthesis. Increase CD4 cell count. Slow progression of HIV infection and decrease severity.	Fatigue, headache, diarrhea, increased amylase, increased liver enzyme, nausea, vomiting, decreases in bone mineral density, dyslipidemia, hepatotoxicity, hypersensitivity reaction, fat redistribution, insomnia, severe rash with or without fever	Sudden and severe change in muscle strength or energy level
Protease inhibitors (PIs)			
atazanavir, darunavir, fosamprenavir, indinavir, nelfinavir, ritonavir, saquinavir, tripranavir	Block protease, an enzyme that HIV needs to make copies of itself. Prevent maturation of virus. Increase CD4 cell counts and decrease viral load with slowed progression of HIV.	Headache, depression, insomnia, heart block, nausea, abdominal pain, hyperglycemia, fat redistribution, myalgia, fever, spontaneous bleeding, hemophilia, intracranial hemorrhage, decrease in bone mineral density, myocardial infarction, cholelithiasis, kidney stone, insulin resistance, GI intolerance, hepatitis, jaundice, trunk fat increase, chronic kidney disease increase, renal atrophy	Arrhythmias, palpitations, chest discomfort, shortness of breath, fainting, fatigue or weakness all possible. May affect blood glucose levels. May affect gait and balance. Use caution with aerobic exercise and assess exercise tolerance frequently.
Fusion inhibitor			
enfuvirtide	Blocks HIV from entering CD4 cells of the immune system. Prevents entry of HIV 1 into cells by interfering with the fusion of the virus with cellular membranes. Improves CD4 cell count.	Fatigue, conjunctivitis, cough, pneumonia, sinusitis, diarrhea, nausea, abdominal pain, anorexia, dry mouth, pancreatitis, weight loss, injection site reaction, myalgia, limb pain, hypersensitivity reactions, herpes simplex	Monitor for excessive fatigue and weakness.
Entry inhibitor			
maraviroc	Blocks proteins on the CD4 cells that HIV needs in order to enter the cells	Hepatotoxicity, dizziness, cough, upper respiratory tract infection, abdominal pain, appetite disorder, rash, musculoskeletal pain, allergic reaction, fever, immune reconstitution syndrome, increased risk of infection	Musculoskeletal pain, muscle tenderness, or weakness is possible. May affect gait, balance, and other functional activities.

Drug class and names	Mechanism of action	Most common side effects	Effects on exercise
Integrase inhibitors			
dolutegravir, elvitegravir, raltegravir	Block HIV integrase, an enzyme HIV needs to make copies of itself; decreased viral replication and resistance to other agents	Dizziness, fatigue, myocardial infarction, abdominal pain, gastritis, hepatitis, vomiting, renal failure, decrease in bone mineral density, dyslipidemia, nausea, diarrhea, lipohypertrophy, rhabdomyolysis, weakness, increase in creatine phosphokinase levels, insomnia, depression, rash, headache	Monitor for symptoms of myocardial infarction. Dizziness or weakness might affect gait, balance, or functional activities. May cause an increase in blood pressure, muscle cramps, and twitching, edema, and weight gain from water retention. May cause anemia, which causes unusual fatigue, shortness of breath with exertion
Pharmokinetic enhancers			
cobicistat	Used in HIV treatment to increase the effectiveness of an HIV medicine in an HIV regimen		

References: (34, 46, 80)

Medications Table 7.6   Common Medications Used to Treat Sickle Cell Disease

Drug class and names	Mechanism of action	Most common side effects	Effects on exercise
NSAIDs (nonsteroidal anti-inflammatory drugs)			
celecoxib (Celebrex), diflunisal (Dolobid), etodolac (Lodine), ibuprofen (Advil, Motrin, Rufen), meloxicam (Mobic), nabumetrone (Relafen), naproxen (Naprosyn, Aleve), oxaprozin (Daypro, Duraprox), piroxicam (Feldene), salsalate (Disalcid), sulindac (Clinoril), tolmetin (Tolectin), ketoprofen (Orudis, Oruvail)	NSAIDs block formation of COX-1 and COX-2 enzymes that control the formation of prostaglandins. (COX-1 enzymes control the formation of prostaglandins involved in normal organ function, and COX-2 enzymes control the formation of prostaglandins involved in the body's inflammatory response. By blocking the prostaglandins, the individual experiences less swelling and pain.)	Upset stomach, headache, easy bruising, hypertension, fluid retention, dyspepsia, gastritis, increased risk of heart attack or stroke, reduced blood clotting, reduced kidney function in those with hypertension or preexisting kidney problems, elevated liver enzymes, worsened asthma or inflammatory bowel disease, severe headache and neck stiffness, possible skin rashes	NSAIDs are not known to have negative effects on exercise performance; however, some delay in exercise-induced fatigue has been associated with NSAID intake. Some evidence suggests that NSAIDs may attenuate exercise recovery.
Penicillin			
	Binds to bacterial cellular wall, resulting in cell death	Seizures, diarrhea, epigastric distress, nausea, vomiting, pseudomembranous colitis, interstitial nephritis, rash, urticaria, leukopenia, allergic reaction (anaphylaxis), superinfection	Watch for seizures. Monitor for allergic reactions and anaphylaxis. Assess muscle aches and joint pain (arthralgia). Monitor for signs of fatigue, weakness, myalgia, or leukopenia (fever, sore throat, signs of infection). Monitor injection site for pain, swelling, and irritation.
Hydroxyrea			
	Interferes with DNA synthesis; may alter characteristics of red blood cells; death of rapidly replicating cells; decreased frequency of painful crises and decreased need for transfusions in sickle cell anemia	Drowsiness, anorexia, diarrhea, nausea, vomiting, constipation, hepatitis, stomatitis, dysuria, infertility, renal tubular dysfunction, alopecia, erythema, pruritus, rashes, leukopenia, anemia, thrombocytopenia, hyperuricemia, chills, fever, malaise	Be alert for signs of leukopenia (fever, sore throat, signs of infection), thrombocytopenia (bruising, nose bleeds, bleeding gums), or unusual weakness and fatigue due to anemia. Assess drowsiness that might affect gait, balance, and other functional activities. Implement resistance exercises and aerobic training to maintain muscle strength and aerobic capacity. Use caution with aerobic exercise. Assess tolerance frequently (blood pressure, heart rate, fatigue levels).

References: (46, 149)

Medications Table 7.7 Common Medications Used to Treat Hemophilia

Drug class and names	Mechanism of action	Most common side effects	Effects on exercise
Antidiuretic, antihemorrhagic drugs			
desmopressin acetate (DDAVP)	Desmopressin releases clotting factor VIII from where it is stored in the body tissues.	Headache, nausea, upset stomach or stomach pain, diarrhea, flushing of the face, water retention	Side effects may make exercise unpleasant, but are not known to interfere with exercise response or adaptations.
Antifibrinolytic agents			
epsilon aminocaproic acid (Amicar)	Amicar acts by stopping the activity of the enzyme plasmin, which dissolves clots	Upset stomach, pain in the stomach, tiredness, dizziness, diarrhea	Side effects may make exercise unpleasant, but are not known to interfere with exercise response or adaptations.
tranexamic acid (Cyklokapron)	Blocks the breakdown of clots, thereby preventing bleeding	Pale skin, trouble breathing with exertion, unusual bleeding or bruising, tiredness or weakness, dizziness, diarrhea	Side effects may make exercise unpleasant, but are not known to interfere with exercise response or adaptations.
Blood product			
cryoprecipitate	Cryoprecipitate is a source of clotting factor VIII, fibrinogen, fibronectin, clotting factor IX.	This is a replacement therapy and is not known to have side effects.	There are no known side effects that would affect exercise response or adaptation.

References: (157, 159)

8

Neuromuscular Conditions and Disorders

Patrick L. Jacobs, PhD, CSCS,*D, FNSCA

Stephanie M. Svoboda, MS, DPT, CSCS

Anna Lepeley, PhD, CSCS

After completing this chapter, you will be able to

- describe the physiological characteristics of the various neurological disorders;

- discuss the health-related consequences for each of the special populations with neurological disorders;

- explain how different neurological disorders affect the ability to exercise, acute exercise responses, and chronic adaptation to exercise training;

- explain the benefits of appropriate exercise conditioning in persons with various neurological disorders; and

- design appropriate exercise programming specific to the needs of individuals with particular neurological disorders.

The nervous system is a complex, highly specialized organized network of nerve cells responsible for the coordination of all volitional and involuntary actions and functions of the human body. The nervous system anatomically consists of the central nervous system (CNS), made up of the brain and spinal cord, and the peripheral nervous system (PNS), which includes nerves that connect the CNS with the rest of the body, including skeletal muscle and organs. Functionally, the PNS is divided into the somatic system, which mediates volitional movement; the autonomic system, which is responsible for control of internal organs; and the enteric system, which regulates the gastrointestinal system. The PNS is also composed of ascending (afferent or sensory) and descending (efferent or motor) neural tracts.

Neuromuscular disorders are medical conditions that result in a decline in functioning of the body's various nervous systems or the muscular system. These medical conditions may arise from biological causes or from genetic defects. Neurological disorders may also be caused by injuries to the brain or spinal cord or in some cases by degenerative diseases. The location and severity of the tissue damage determine the short-term outcomes of the injury or disease process, as well as the long-term potential for recovery. Direct trauma to the brain may result in cerebral palsy if the injury occurs during pregnancy, during childbirth, or within the first three years of life. Injury to the adult brain produces traumatic brain injury, while interruption of blood flow to the brain may result in a stroke. Multiple sclerosis and Parkinson's disease are neurological disease processes that affect the peripheral nerves and the brain tissue in different populations.

Neuromuscular disorders can be classified as either progressive or nonprogressive. Progressive neurological disorders are conditions that involve a continuing and progressive deterioration of functioning. These disorders include multiple sclerosis, Parkinson's disease, and muscular dystrophy. These progressive neuromuscular conditions vary in rate of development and commonly have periods of relapse and periods of remission. Progressive neuromuscular disorders are generally caused by disease processes or genetic factors.

Nonprogressive neurological disorders are conditions that do not continue to exhibit declining neurological functioning following an initial episode of disease or mechanical injury. There are significant reductions in function with an initial episode with no further primary declines thereafter. These nonprogressive conditions include cerebral palsy, stroke, head injury, and spinal cord injury. Nonprogressive disorders are generally a result of traumatic injury to the CNS, either the brain or spinal cord.

Key Point

Common progressive neuromuscular disorders include multiple sclerosis, Parkinson's disease, and muscular dystrophy. Cerebral palsy, traumatic brain injury, stroke, and spinal cord injury are nonprogressive neurological disorders.

MULTIPLE SCLEROSIS

Both voluntary and involuntary actions of the human body are controlled and coordinated by the nervous system. The functional units of the nervous system, neurons, possess the unique ability to generate electrochemical signals that are transmitted along the neural axon. Some neurons are surrounded by a myelin sheath. **Myelin** is a fatty white substance that establishes an electrically insulating layer, or sheath, around the neuron that is essential for proper functioning of the nervous system. The myelin sheath increases electrical resistance across the neuron membrane, thereby preventing leakage of electrical impulses.

Demyelination, the loss of the myelin sheath, is the primary characteristic of some neurodegenerative autoimmune diseases in which the deterioration of the myelin layer dramatically weakens the electrochemical signals. Significant loss of myelin slows or blocks all electrochemical signals from the brain to the body.

The most common of these diseases is multiple sclerosis, which affects either or both of the CNS (brain and spinal cord) and the PNS. Other neurodegenerative autoimmune diseases that involve loss of myelin include transverse myelitis, Guillain-Barre syndrome, leukodystrophy, and Charcot-Marie-Tooth disease. Common characteristics of these diseases include muscular weakness, tingling or numbness, visual limitations, heat sensitivity, reduced coordination and balance, fatigue, and disturbance of cognitive processes including speech, memory, or both.

Pathology of Multiple Sclerosis

Multiple sclerosis (MS) is a progressive autoimmune disorder characterized by deterioration of the myelin sheath. The myelin sheath covers billions of nerve cells in the body, and its purpose is to aid in the speed and transmission of CNS signals. In individuals with MS, the myelin sheath and the underlying neurons undergo demyelination that leads to a breakdown in signal transmission.

Individuals afflicted with the disease experience a wide array of symptoms that vary between individuals (36, 84). These symptoms are due to the breakdown in nerve signal transmission and depend on where exactly the demyelization occurs. Individuals most commonly experience fatigue, numbness, walking problems, balance impairments, coordination impairments, bladder dysfunction, bowel dysfunction, vision problems, dizziness, vertigo, sexual dysfunction, cognitive dysfunction, pain, emotional changes, spasticity, and depression (12, 24, 36, 42, 84, 112, 195). In addition, other less common symptoms may be seen, such as speech disorders, swallowing problems, headache, hearing loss, seizures, tremors, breathing problems, and itching (11, 60, 178). Despite these symptoms, people with the disease experience a normal life span. It is often difficult to diagnose MS, as these symptoms can appear similar to symptoms of other diseases.

Individuals affected by MS also experience a wide range of disease courses and outcomes. There are four types of MS: *relapsing–remitting, secondary progressive, primary progressive,* and *progressive–relapsing.* Eighty-five percent of cases are initially diagnosed as relapsing–remitting MS (26). In these cases, patients experience clearly defined **exacerbations** or **flare-ups**. These are times when the CNS experiences inflammation and in turn, previously seen symptoms rapidly worsen or new symptoms arise. Exacerbations vary among individuals and can last anywhere between days and months. Exacerbations are interrupted by **remission** periods, or times in which patients' neurological functions stabilize and do not worsen. During remission, people may return to their preexacerbation condition with no symptoms, or they may experience some small ongoing symptoms (166).

Fifteen percent of MS cases are diagnosed as primary progressive, which is a type of MS in which neurological function deteriorates from disease onset without any significant remissions, although the symptoms may briefly plateau or possibly even appear to be temporarily improved. Otherwise, these patients experience slowly deteriorating neurological function (166).

Of the 85% of relapsing–remitting MS cases, 50% will be considered as secondary progressive within the first 10 years of diagnosis and 90% within 25 years (240). These individuals will experience less recovery following attacks and disability progressing over time with deteriorating neurological function (166).

Pathophysiology of Multiple Sclerosis

Multiple sclerosis is most commonly seen in Caucasian women (224). Women are two to three times more likely to develop the disease than men, and Caucasians are twice as likely to develop the disease as any other race (181). The disease is most often diagnosed between the ages of 20 and 40 and is the most prevalent neuromuscular disease seen in young adults (72, 202). The National Multiple Sclerosis Society estimates that 2.3 million people are affected worldwide (138, 166). Although MS is most commonly seen in adults, estimates suggest that 8,000 to 10,000 individuals under 18 years old suffer from this disease (164).

The definitive cause of MS is unknown; however, scientists offer four possible explanations for its origin: immunologic, environmental, infectious, and genetic (228). Some speculate that individuals with MS experience an abnormal immune-mediated response in which myelin and nerve fibers are attacked by the body (202). Specifically, the myelin sheath is attacked by a white blood cell group called T cells. In turn, this causes tissue damage and inflammation, leading to scar tissue (sclerosis) and blockage in signal transmission. This blockage in signal transmission causes messages to become lost or distorted, leading to the symptoms of MS.

Secondly, scientists hypothesize that MS may be caused by environmental factors (9). This theory originated from epidemiological data showing that persons are more susceptible to MS the farther they live from the equator (219). Along the same lines, it was also theorized that these individuals get less sunlight, leading to less vitamin D, and therefore do not receive the positive impact that vitamin D has on immune function (9). In addition, a pattern of children being born in an environment with a low risk for developing MS and moving to a high-risk environment before puberty increased their chances of developing the disease (5, 10).

Scientists have also shown that demyelination and inflammation can be caused by viruses; therefore they are looking at several different viruses or bacteria as a possible cause for MS: measles, canine distemper, human herpes virus-6, Epstein-Barr, and Chlamydia pneumoniae (9, 100).

Finally, the role of a person's genetics in relation to developing MS is being explored (79). Individuals may be genetically susceptible to but may not directly inherit MS; however, there may be certain gene markers making a person more susceptible to developing MS if exposed to the necessary stimuli. For example, if a person has a first-degree relative with the disease, the chances increase from 1 in 750 to 1 or 2 out of 40 that he or she will also develop the disease (165).

Common Medications Given to Individuals With Multiple Sclerosis

Multiple sclerosis is a disease process without a cure. The progression of MS and the associated symptoms vary appreciably with a variety of medical treatments for those symptoms. See medications table 8.1 near the end of the chapter for listings of common medications for persons with MS, the mechanism of action, and the most common side effects of those drugs as well as common effects of these medications on the ability to engage in exercise training.

Individuals with MS are commonly prescribed medications in three primary categories. First, after they have been diagnosed with MS, a physician is likely to prescribe a disease-modifying drug in an attempt to reduce the frequency and severity of attacks, reduce the damage to the CNS, and slow the progression of the disease (193). Some of these medications, such as interferon, have the potential for reducing the capacity to exercise as well as the capacity to recover between training sessions.

Secondly, if a person with MS is experiencing a significant exacerbation interfering with her ability to function or her safety, a physician may administer a large dose of corticosteroid to reduce the time of the flare-up (130). Corticosteroid medications such as prednisone and methylprednisolone reduce inflammation of the CNS but carry with them a risk of reducing exercise capacity.

Finally, individuals with MS may also take medications to help manage the following symptoms: bladder and bowel dysfunction, depression, erectile dysfunction, dizziness and vertigo, fatigue, nausea and vomiting, pain, itching, spasticity, and tremor (70, 73, 211). Medications may alleviate these symptoms, which may allow an increased ability to engage in purposeful exercise training. Conversely, side effects of these medications include drowsiness, dizziness, blurred vision, fatigue, and weakness, which may reduce exercise capacity and balance.

Effects of Exercise in Individuals With Multiple Sclerosis

The efficacy for exercise, specifically resistance training, in persons with MS has been widely established (116). The goals of an exercise program for persons with MS are to improve and maintain important functions such as activities of daily living. Participating in exercise will not cure or slow the disease progression (48), but it will allow people to experience a higher quality of life (152). Progressive resistance training (PRT) has been shown to positively affect strength. For example, Dodd and colleagues (55) assigned individuals with relapsing–remitting MS to either a PRT group or a control group for 10 weeks. After training two times per week for 10 weeks, the PRT group improved their strength, muscular endurance, fatigue level, and quality of life more than the control group.

Another research team examined the effects of an eight-week PRT program in subjects with MS. These subjects improved their isometric strength, muscular endurance, maximal power, muscular hypertrophy, and walking speed following the intervention (48). A third research group also demonstrated the efficacy of PRT in people with MS; subjects in this study were assigned to either a PRT group or a control group. Individuals in the intervention group trained their lower extremity muscles two times per week for 12 weeks. At the conclusion of 12 weeks, the PRT group improved their muscle strength and functional mobility (38). Filipi and colleagues (65) examined the effects of PRT on balance and gait parameters as well as muscular strength in patients with MS. These individuals exercised two times per week for six months. They demonstrated improvements in balance, gait, and muscle forces generated during gait.

Exercise Recommendations for Clients With Multiple Sclerosis

Clients with MS can benefit from both resistance and aerobic training (38, 39). Program design guidelines for clients with MS are summarized in table 8.1. Persons with MS may benefit from using seated resistance machines as opposed to upright free weight activities if their balance is compromised. Resistance training should be initiated with resistance levels at the 15RM (repetition maximum) level for one to three sets each of four to eight exercises using a total body program. Training criteria can potentially be increased progressively but slowly, over weeks, to three or four sets per exercise at 8RM to 15RM intensity for two or three sessions per week.

The modes of aerobic training suitable for persons with MS include indoor recumbent cycling, arm–leg ergometry, aquatic exercise, and treadmill walking. Aerobic training recommendations call for two or three weekly sessions at a light to moderate intensity beginning with 10- to 40-minute sessions. These clients will also benefit from a general static stretching program of low-duration stretching, as opposed to dynamic stretching, since persons with MS are quite prone to spasticity and many have balance limitations (167).

Aquatic exercise, either swimming laps or participating in cardiovascular or resistance training in the pool, is a popular and efficient way for this population to exercise (197). The water temperature should be kept cool, less than 85°F (29°C), to avoid overheating (108).

Table 8.1 Program Design Guidelines for Clients With Multiple Sclerosis

Type of exercise	Frequency	Intensity	Volume
Resistance training			
Modes of training a. Weight training machines and free weights b. Bodyweight resistance c. Elastic tubing	Begin with one or two sessions per week. Increase to two or three weekly sessions as tolerated.	Begin with four to eight exercises with resistance of 15RM emphasizing multijoint approach. Increase intensity slowly and progressively to 8- to 10RM. Recovery periods of 2-4 min.	Start with 1-3 sets per exercise of 10-12 reps. Potentially increase to 3-4 sets per exercise. If multiple sets, then 1-2 min between sets.
Aerobic training			
Modes of training a. Treadmill walking b. Cycling c. Arm and leg cycling d. Rowing e. Aquatic exercise	Begin with one session per week. Progress to 2-3 days per week.	Begin with light to moderate intensity of 30% to <60% $\dot{V}O_2$ or heart rate reserve, 55% to <75% MHR, or RPE of 9-13 on Borg 6- to 20-point scale. Increase intensity gradually.	Begin with 10- to 20-min sessions. Gradually increase to 30- to 40-min sessions.

References: (38, 39)

Exercise Modifications, Precautions, and Contraindications for Clients With Multiple Sclerosis

Fatigue is a common symptom seen in clients with MS (121). This may limit a person's ability to exercise on a given day. To avoid further increasing fatigue, exercise should not be performed maximally or to volitional fatigue or failure. In addition, all exercises need to be progressed slowly.

Clients with MS are very sensitive to external and internal increases in heat (45). An increase in internal body temperature of as little as half a degree can further complicate a demyelinated nerve's ability to conduct an impulse (199). Due to this sensitivity, exercise should be performed in a cool (72-76°F [22-24°C]) indoor air-conditioned facility; exercise in the sun or any humid environment is not recommended. Sensitivity to the heat may be further compromised by a decreased sweating response seen in some clients with MS (45). Pre- and postexercise cooling is a good strategy for helping with the natural increase in temperature with exercise. In addition, the client

Key Point

Persons with MS should always perform exercise training in well-ventilated areas with relatively cool temperatures. Even slight increases in internal body temperature may acutely limit nerve conduction in demyelinated nerves and over time may hasten further demyelination.

should remain well hydrated in order to further combat heat stresses.

Another concern arises when a client is experiencing an exacerbation, or flare-up. Exercise should be discontinued until the attack has completely subsided. When it is deemed safe to return to exercise, it may be necessary to adjust the exercise prescription to match the person's new level of ability. It is possible for people to regain all preattack functions, but they may now also have some new symptoms.

Also, clients with MS often use wheelchairs, canes, and walkers. Persons administering exercise programs to this population should be familiar with proper use of this equipment and proper ways of aiding transfers.

Case Study

Multiple Sclerosis

Mrs. F is a 46-year-old woman who was diagnosed with relapsing–remitting MS four years ago. She works at home on the computer. She has difficulty getting around the community and recently started walking with a rolling walker that has a folding seat. She gets fatigued easily. She wanted to do more activities outside of her home, so she enrolled at a fitness center. Her daughter hired an exercise professional to work with Mrs. F three days per week for an hour at a time.

Mrs. F's neurologist cleared her to exercise with instructions not to exercise if she is having an exacerbation of symptoms or if she is overly fatigued on a particular day. Mrs. F is taking disease-modifying drugs, has a body mass index (BMI) of 32, and has prehypertension. She self-reported that she has not exercised in years.

The exercise professional started Mrs. F's exercise sessions in a cool-water pool. The sessions began with shallow-end water walking and deep-end water "jogging" for cardiovascular conditioning. Mrs. F was also instructed in resistance exercises with aqua-dumbbells and flexibility activities.

After one month of water activities, Mrs. F started exercising in the gym for half of her sessions. She started her sessions with a cardiovascular warm-up of either recumbent cycling or recumbent arm–leg ergometry. She performed strengthening exercises using the seated machines in the gym. Next, she performed balance and posture activities. All sessions concluded with static stretching.

After three months of training, Mrs. F self-reported that she felt better than she had in years and had more energy. She started working outside of her home three half-days per week. In the three-month period, she canceled two sessions due to feeling fatigued and did not experience any exacerbations. She improved her muscular strength and endurance, flexibility, aerobic endurance, and ability to get around the community. She also reduced her blood pressure slightly and improved her BMI to 30.

Recommended Readings

Dalgas, UE, Stenager, E, and Ingemann-Hansen, T. Multiple sclerosis and physical exercise: recommendations for the application of resistance-, endurance- and combined training. *Mult Scler* 14:35-53, 2008.

Kjølhede, TK, Vissing, K, and Dalgas, U. Multiple sclerosis and progressive resistance training: a systematic review. *Mult Scler* 18(9):1215-1228, 2012.

Latimer-Cheung, A, Pilutti, L, Hicks, A, Martin Ginis, K, Fenuta, A, MacKibbon, K, and Motl, R. Effects of exercise training on fitness, mobility, fatigue, and health-related quality of life among adults with multiple sclerosis: a systematic review to inform guideline development. *Arch Phys Med Rehabil* 94:1800-1828, 2013.

Motl, R and Pilutti, L. The benefits of exercise training in multiple sclerosis. *Nat Rev Neurol* 8:487-497, 2012.

White, L and Dressendorfer, R. Exercise and multiple sclerosis. *Sports Med* 34(15):1077-1100, 2004.

PARKINSON'S DISEASE

Parkinson's disease (PD) is a progressive neurological disorder that influences volitional movement. This disease develops slowly and is most prevalent in older persons. The most common symptom of PD is muscular tremors. However, this disease commonly results in muscular stiffness and slow movements. Other symptoms include a lack of facial expression, lack of arm swing during walking, and slurred speech. While there is no cure for PD at this time, medications may reduce the symptoms.

Pathology of Parkinson's Disease

Parkinson's disease is the second most common neurodegenerative disease. It is a progressive brain disorder caused by the death or impairment of neurons in the substantia nigra region of the brain. These neurons are responsible for the production of dopamine, a chemical that sends messages to the area of the brain that is responsible for smooth and coordinated body movements. The hallmark signs of PD include tremor of a limb, **bradykinesia** (slowness of movement), rigidity, and poor balance (97). In addition, individuals may demonstrate small, cramped handwriting, stiff facial expressions, a shuffled walk or a festinating gait pattern, muffled speech, difficulty swallowing, and depression (97, 127). Diagnosis of PD is difficult and may be done only after a thorough examination by a neurologist. Additional blood work and magnetic resonance imaging tests may be ordered to rule out other diseases that also show parkinsonism symptoms, but there is no one test that can identify PD (30). Each case is unique in that the progression and level of disability vary greatly between individuals (187).

Pathophysiology of Parkinson's Disease

The cause of PD is currently unknown. Speculation exists that there might be a genetic or environmental link to PD (4). Approximately 15% to 25% of people with PD report having a relative with PD (185). Scientists are studying gene mutations that affect dopamine cell function, but no definitive result has been obtained yet (223). Being exposed to environmental toxins such as manganese, carbon monoxide, and certain peptides may increase the risk of developing PD (114).

Common Medications Given to Individuals With Parkinson's Disease

There are currently no medications to slow or stop the progression of PD, but there are many medications used to treat the associated symptoms. Most PD symptoms are due to a lack of dopamine; therefore, increasing dopamine can help a person to experience more natural body movements and less stiffness (232).

The most commonly prescribed medication used in the treatment of PD is levodopa (22), which is altered by brain enzymes to produce dopamine; this in turn minimizes the slowness, stiffness, and tremor commonly seen in PD. Common side effects of levodopa include nausea and loss of appetite as well as light-headedness, confusion, hallucinations, and reduced blood pressure (78, 249). These side effects could potentially limit exercise capacity and efficiency or place the individual at increased risk of injury. Levodopa was first used 30 years ago, and since then another class of drugs, dopamine agonists, has been developed. The different dopamine agonists vary in chemical structure, duration of action, and side effects but may also reduce the capacity for exercise training and balance.

In addition to levodopa and dopamine agonists, other medications are available to improve body coordination that work by mechanisms other than via dopamine receptors. These medications are classified as anticholinergic, monoamine oxidase B (MAO-B) inhibitors, catechol-O-methyl transferase (COMT) inhibitors, and others, each of which has several brand names (98, 265).

Anticholinergic medications are used to reduce spasm activity in persons with PD but

carry increased risk of blurred vision, drowsiness, and confusion with limitations in memory (207, 230). The COMT inhibitors are used to prolong the duration of activity of levodopa (103). Common side effects of COMT inhibitors include drowsiness and dyskinesia (involuntary muscle movements) (6). Medications table 8.2 near the end of the chapter provides an outline of the side effects of each of these drug classes and the limitations (e.g., reduced exercise capacity and balance) that these medications may place on the capacity of the person to engage in regular training sessions.

If medications are not successful in treating the symptoms of PD, the individual may be a candidate for brain surgery (253). A deep brain stimulator is implanted into the brain with the goal of minimizing symptoms.

Effects of Exercise in Individuals With Parkinson's Disease

It was previously thought that people with PD should not participate in resistance training programs for fear of increasing rigidity (206); however, studies have found that resistance training in individuals with PD improves numerous outcome measures. Resistance training has been shown to increase muscle strength, mobility and walking capacity, muscular endurance, balance, and fat-free mass in people with PD (21).

People with PD have been shown to experience strength gains similar to those in age-matched peers without PD following an eight-week resistance training program, in which participants trained the lower body two times per week (210). In addition to documenting increased strength, this study also found that people with PD increased their stride length, walking velocity, and postural angles following resistance training.

Another research group examined the effects of two different training interventions on balance outcome measures in individuals with PD (89). In this study, subjects with PD were assigned to either a balance training intervention or a program with balance training and high-intensity resistance training. Both groups trained three times per week for 10 weeks. Both training groups increased their performance during a balance test, but this increase was more profound in the group that included resistance training. In addition, both groups improved their strength; however, the strength gains were much higher in the combined group.

Dibble and colleagues (53) examined the safety and feasibility of high-force eccentric resistance training for individuals with PD. Participants engaged in 12 weeks of eccentric ergometer training three times per week. It was found that creatine kinase levels did not exceed the threshold for muscle damage, subjective reports of muscle soreness were low, participants were compliant, and total work and isometric force increased over time. In another study, the same research group contrasted the effects of a 12-week eccentric resistance training ergometer intervention with an evidence-based exercise program (52). Both groups trained three days per week for 10 weeks. The eccentric training group displayed significantly greater improvements in all outcome measures including gait speed, timed up and go, quality of life measures, and muscle force.

In 2007, Hass and colleagues not only added to the body of literature with evidence for the efficacy of resistance training in individuals with PD but also demonstrated the efficacy of creatine monohydrate in people with PD (82). Subjects were assigned to either a creatine or a placebo group; all subjects in the study participated in two sessions per week of resistance training for 12 weeks. Muscle endurance and fat-free mass increased in both groups; both groups improved their one repetition maximum (1RM) strength (more in the creatine group), and the creatine group also significantly improved the three-repetition sit-to-stand time.

The effects of a moderate-volume, high-load resistance training program in individuals with PD have also been examined. In one study, sub-jects with PD were assigned to either a standard care group or a resistance training group that underwent eight weeks of lower extremity exercise two days per week. The training group increased leg press strength more than the control group after the eight-week training period (213).

Exercise Recommendations for Clients With Parkinson's Disease

Persons with PD may benefit from participation in appropriate programs of exercise. However, the research on the application of exercise training in persons with PD has not established specific recommendations for this group. Therefore, recommendations for exercise with PD are typically based on the general recommendations for older adults. Program design guidelines for clients with PD are summarized in table 8.2. Resistance training may be performed initially with one set each of several exercise movements, emphasizing multijoint exercises. Training should begin with light to moderate resistance levels of 40% to 80% 1RM for 10 to 12 repetitions per set. Frequency of training may begin with one or two sessions per week and increase to three or four weekly sessions as tolerated.

In addition to a sound aerobic and resistance training program, these clients will likely benefit from balance training. Clients with PD have a difficult time moving their center of mass outside their base of support, and also have poor reaction times, which can result in falls. They should be instructed in basic reaching and balance activities; however, it may not be appropriate to exercise on unstable surfaces (foam, BOSU, BAPs board, and so on).

Clients with PD also tend to become rigid and develop contractures over time. These clients can benefit from stretching, flexibility, and mobility programs for all major muscle groups and joints. Specifically, clients with PD tend to develop a kyphotic posture, so more time should be spent on stretching their anterior trunk muscles

Table 8.2 Program Design Guidelines for Clients With Parkinson's Disease

Type of exercise	Frequency	Intensity	Volume
Resistance training			
Modes of training a. Weight training machines and free weights b. Bodyweight resistance c. Elastic tubing	Begin with one or two sessions per week. Potentially progress to 4 days per week, split routine.	Begin with 8-10 exercises with resistance of 40-60% 1RM (and progress to 60-80% 1RM), emphasizing multijoint approach.	Start with 1 set per exercise of 10-12 reps. Increase to 2-3 sets per exercise as tolerated. If multiple sets, then 1-2 min between sets.
Aerobic training			
Modes of training a. Walking b. Cycling c. Rowing d. Reciprocal press–pull exercise	Begin with one session per week. Progress to 4 or more days per week as tolerated.	Begin with light to moderate intensity of 30% to <60% $\dot{V}O_2$ or heart rate reserve, or 55% to <75% MHR, or RPE of 9-13 on Borg 6- to 20-point scale. Increase intensity gradually.	Begin with 15- to 20-min sessions. Gradually increase to 30-min sessions.

Reference: (61)

(abdominal muscles) rather than performing trunk flexion exercises like crunches.

Exercise Modifications, Precautions, and Contraindications for Clients With Parkinson's Disease

Safety is the most important consideration when working with a person with PD. As previously mentioned, these clients experience changes in their movement patterns, such as a slower walking speed, decreased ability to pick up their feet, decreased speed of movement, and poor balance. These clients find it difficult adapting to a dynamic environment; therefore, the exercise professional should take care to train at times when the facility is not too busy or provide a quiet room to exercise in. In addition, the floor should be clear of anything the client could trip over (exercise equipment, area rugs, cords, and so on).

Depending on the person, the client may be a candidate to participate in group classes or may need closer supervision. The exercise professional should be near the client at all times in case of a loss of balance. Also, because of tremor and poor coordination, upright or free weight exercise might not be safe in this population. These clients should not use a treadmill and instead can benefit from walking over ground or using a stationary bicycle with foot straps. Along the same lines, these clients should typically use resistance training machines rather than free weights.

In addition to safety, clients with PD should ask their physician when is the best time to exercise given their medication schedule. There is a window after taking medication during which symptoms are most controlled, and this would likely be the best time for a client to exercise. Clients should also be reminded that it is very important not to skip taking their medications unless instructed to do so by their physician.

The exercise professional must be cognizant that heart rate, blood pressure, and thermoregulation might have to be monitored more closely in clients with PD due to autonomic nervous system dysfunction (269). These clients are at risk for orthostatic hypotension and should be reminded to avoid the Valsalva maneuver. Finally, they are more susceptible to fatigue and should be instructed to work at submaximal levels.

Parkinson's Disease

Mr. B is a 72-year-old man who was diagnosed with PD by a neurologist one year before joining the fitness center. He has a mild resting tremor and a decrease in walking speed; he fell one time at home last year but was not injured. Mr. B completed two months of physical therapy after the fall but had not been exercising since being discharged from physical therapy. When he joined the fitness center, he reported that he was too nervous to exercise alone and would like to work with an exercise professional three times per week; he reported that he could afford 30-minute sessions. After meeting Mr. B for a consultation, the exercise professional learned that he would like to become active again and is afraid of falling.

The neurologist cleared Mr. B for exercise but did not give any specific instructions or precautions. Mr. B was taking levodopa, his BMI was 27, and his blood pressure was 123/75 mmHg. He had no other significant past medical or surgical history or cardiovascular contraindications to exercise.

Mr. B's exercise sessions consisted of recumbent cycling, supervised overground walking, strength training using machines, balance training, and flexibility training. Mr. B began his first sessions with cycling to warm up. As he became more confident, he began arriving to his appointments early and performing his cycling before his sessions with the exercise professional. After Mr. B felt comfortable cycling on his own, he spent the beginning of his sessions walking while supervised. During walking he was coached to stand upright, swing his arms, and take long steps. The coach stayed close to Mr. B during this activity in the event of loss of balance.

After the cardiovascular warm-up, Mr. B performed resistance training for all major muscle groups. He used the following machines most often: leg press, leg curl, leg extension, chest press, shoulder press, seated row, triceps extension, and biceps curl. Exercises were performed for three sets of 10 repetitions with a 45-second break in between sets.

After resistance training, Mr. B was instructed in double- and single-leg balance activities on even surfaces. All sessions concluded with flexibility activities focusing on all major muscles with an emphasis on trunk extension and knee extension.

After three months, Mr. B feels more confident in the weight room and trains on Saturdays without his coach. He reports no longer being fearful of falling at home and feels more satisfied with his life. He has increased his strength, cardiovascular endurance, balance, flexibility, and posture.

Recommended Readings

Brienesse, L and Emerson, M. Effects of resistance training for people with Parkinson's disease: a systematic review. *J Am Med Dir Assoc* 14:236-241, 2013.

Dibble, L, Addison, O, and Papa, E. The effects of exercise on balance in persons with Parkinson's disease: a systematic review across the disability spectrum. *J Neurol Phys Ther* 33:14-26, 2009.

Falvo, M, Schilling, B, and Earhart, G. Parkinson's disease and resistive exercise: rationale, review, and recommendations. *Mov Disord* 23(1):1-11, 2008.

Goodwin, V, Richards, S, Taylor, R, Taylor, A, and Campbell, J. The effectiveness of exercise interventions for people with Parkinson's disease: a systematic review and meta-analysis. *Mov Disord* 23(5):631-640, 2008.

Lima, LO, Scianni, A, and Rodrigues-de-Paula, F. Progressive resistance exercise improves strength and physical performance in people with mild to moderate Parkinson's disease: a systematic review. *J Physiother* 59(1):7-13, 2013.

MUSCULAR DYSTROPHY

Muscular dystrophy (MD) is a group of progressive muscular disorders characterized by damage to the muscle's structure and progressive muscle weakness. Some authorities argue that there are more than 30 types of MD, but most agree that there are 9 primary types. The two most common types are Duchenne (DMD) and Becker (BMD) (68). In both DMD and BMD, there is a dysfunction with the muscle protein dystrophin (174). Dystrophin is responsible for keeping the muscle cells intact. Individuals with DMD have a complete lack of dystrophin, while those with BMD have dystrophin but it only partially functions properly. Both DMD and BMD are X-linked recessive disorders, which means that they must be inherited from a mother who is a carrier of the disease. The two types affect boys almost exclusively (150); the rate of inheriting DMD and BMD is 1 in 3,500 and 1 in 20,000 per live male births, respectively (157).

Pathology and Pathophysiology of Muscular Dystrophy

The first signs of DMD or BMD include muscle weakness and clumsiness (41). In DMD, these signs are first seen in boys between the ages of 1 and 4 years (23). A parent or teacher may notice that the boy is not keeping up with his male peers, for example in running, jumping, stair climbing, and even rising from the floor. These boys often develop a modified strategy using their arms to get up from the floor, called Gowers' sign (31). They may also develop large calf muscles, called **pseudohypertrophy**, not because the muscle is really enlarged but rather because it has been replaced with scar tissue (146). These children may also have poor balance and walk with a wider than normal stance. The first muscles that are affected are muscles of the hip, pelvis, thigh, and shoulder; later, the muscles of the arms, legs, and trunk are also involved, including the muscles of the heart and lungs (146). The signs and symptoms seen in BMD are similar to those in DMD but develop later in life, between ages 5 and 10, and progress more slowly (109). Individuals with BMD also experience muscle cramps (234). Boys with DMD and BMD eventually need to use wheelchairs for locomotion. They also tend to have lower than average IQs, cognitive impairments, and learning disabilities (267). Boys with DMD used to survive only into their teens due to complications with the heart and respiratory muscles, but with advances in medical care are now living into their 30s; boys with BMD survive into mid or late adulthood (128, 188).

The most common adult form of MD is myotonic (MMD) (99). Myotonic MD affects women and men equally, is inherited, occurs in 1 in 8,000 live births, and is usually seen in people between 20 and 30 years old (162). There are two types of MMD, type 1 and type 2, named for two different gene abnormalities (243). Individuals with MMD are unable to relax their muscles and have the highest rate of mental retardation; their disease progresses slowly (190). People with MMD also have contractures, breathing and swallowing problems, cataracts, heart problems, and insulin resistance (217).

The six other types of MD are congenital, Emery-Dreifuss, facioscapulohumeral, limbgirdle, distal, and oculopharyngeal (57). In order to diagnose MD, a neurologist first performs a physical examination looking for muscle weakness. The physician also tests the blood for elevated levels of the enzyme creatine kinase, performs genetic testing of the DNA, and performs a muscle biopsy (158).

Common Medications Given to Individuals With Muscular Dystrophy

Currently, no pharmaceutical approaches have been shown to be effective in reversing MD. However, corticosteroids, specifically prednisone, are commonly prescribed to people with MD in order to minimize symptoms and slow disease progression. These medications (e.g., prednisone and methylprednisolone) have the potential side effects of high glucose levels, depression, and anxiety, which may limit the capacity of some persons with MD to participate in regular exercise training.

Also, individuals with MD tend to develop heart conditions; therefore, they may be taking some type of heart medication depending on their symptoms and pathology. Common heart medications include various ACE (angiotensin-converting enzyme) inhibitors and β-blockers, which may reduce the ability of the individual to participate in exercise training due to reductions in circulation that lead to side effects such as dizziness, low blood pressure, drowsiness, and weakness. See medications table 8.3 near the end of the chapter for a summary of medications used in the treatment of MD.

Effects of Exercise in Individuals With Muscular Dystrophy

Overall, little controlled research has examined the efficacy of exercise in people with MD; most published works regarding exercise recommendations are expert opinions or case studies or are based on rodent models (139, 147). The use of exercise in persons with MD is somewhat controversial (77), but most experts recommend that those with DMD and BMD not perform traditional resistance training (221).

In 2012, Alemdaroglu and colleagues examined the acute hemodynamic responses and fatigue levels in relation to three different types of exercise in ambulatory boys with DMD (2). The three exercise interventions were 3-minute stair climbing; 40-minute cycling; and 40 minutes of combined stretching, strengthening, and aerobic activity. Heart rate increased significantly after stair climbing and combined exercise, but not with cycling. All three exercise interventions increased fatigue directly following activity, but did not negatively affect activities of daily living within the day following the intervention. There was an acute decrease in strength following cycling and an increase in strength following stair climbing, no change in acute strength following the combined intervention. Time to rise from the floor increased following the cycling and the combined intervention. Overall this study demonstrated that prolonged cycling may acutely fatigue the quadriceps muscles, which will negatively affect strength; 3 minutes of stair climbing may warm up the lower extremity muscles for future strength tasks; and combined strengthening, stretching, and aerobic activities with rest breaks may be best for those with DMD.

In 1979, DeLateur and Giaconi examined the effects of submaximal isokinetic quadriceps training in four boys with DMD. The boys strengthened only one leg for four or five days per week for six months. Over the course of training and two years following the intervention, the strength-trained leg was able to produce more force than the untrained leg until the disease progressed to the point at which the boys were not able to exert enough force to extend their knees. No adverse effects of the intervention were reported; however, all the boys eventually lost their strength as the disease progressed.

Sveen and colleagues (233) examined the effects of aerobic training in men with BMD compared to men without BMD. All subjects cycled for 30 minutes at 65% of their $\dot{V}O_2$ max for a total of 50 times over a 12-week period. Those with BMD improved their $\dot{V}O_2$ max more than the control group; cyclists with BMD also improved the strength of their quadriceps muscles. Individuals with BMD did not exhibit increased plasma creatine kinase levels or display any other adverse effects. This study suggests that cycling at a submaximal work level is safe and effective for those with BMD.

Tollback and colleagues (237) examined the effects of a high-intensity resistance training program in adults with MMD. The program included three sets of 10 repetitions of knee extensions with one leg at 80% of 1RM, performed three times per week for 12 weeks; the other leg served as the control. After the 12-week intervention, 1RM strength was significantly greater in the trained leg, and no adverse effects were noted. This investigation provides some evidence of the safety and efficacy of high-intensity resistance training in adults with MMD.

Exercise Recommendations for Clients With Muscular Dystrophy

Children with MD will most likely be receiving some type of physical therapy or exercise intervention at school, in their homes, or at an outpatient center. Exercise professionals should be aware of the activities that a child with MD is already involved in and his weekly schedule. These clients are susceptible to fatigue and increased muscle damage, so if they are already exercising elsewhere or have a busy weekly schedule, they may not qualify for an additional exercise intervention.

Program design guidelines for clients with MD are summarized in table 8.3. Clients who are not exercising elsewhere can benefit from a light exercise program including submaximal aerobic activity and flexibility training. The light aerobic activity can be performed either in a warm-water pool, on a stationary recumbent bicycle, or on an arm–leg ergometer. Aerobic training should be performed initially with one weekly session of 15 to 20 minutes in duration. Over time, training duration may be increased slowly to 30 minutes per session and volume to two or three training sessions per week (160). In addition, these clients can benefit from a light stretching program of all major muscle groups, especially their calf muscles.

The benefits of resistance training in persons with MD have been demonstrated in a number of scientific investigations (2, 49). However, other researchers have expressed concerns regarding resistance training (particularly eccentric muscle actions) potentially exacerbating progression of the MD processes (137). Therefore, at this time it is recommended that participation of persons with MD in resistance training be limited to light-intensity training using isokinetic or pneumatic training equipment that provides concentric resistance without eccentric stresses. Resistance training should be initiated with one set of several multijoint movements, with low levels of concentric resistance performed one time weekly. Resistance levels and training volume may be increased very slowly as tolerated.

Exercise Modifications, Precautions, and Contraindications for Clients With Muscular Dystrophy

Clients with MD are very susceptible to muscle damage and fatigue; therefore, they should never be encouraged to exercise maximally. The exercise professional should also listen to clients' subjective reports of fatigue or pain and stop the activity at their request. All stretches should be performed slowly and held for at least 60 seconds. In addition, clients with MD should not perform eccentric resistance training. Their daily activities are already causing some muscle damage (77, 136, 137), and it is important not to increase the rate of damage. Because each case is so individual, a case study is not included for this condition.

Table 8.3 Program Design Guidelines for Clients With Muscular Dystrophy

Type of exercise	Frequency	Intensity	Volume
Resistance training			

Modes of training*
  a. Weight training machines (e.g., isokinetic or pneumatic)
  b. Elastic tubing
	Begin with one session per week.
	Progress to 4 days per week, split routine, as tolerated.
		Initially 8-10 exercises with resistance of 40-60% 1RM, emphasizing multijoint approach.	Start with 1 set per exercise of 10-12 reps.
			Possibly increase to 2-3 sets per exercise.
			If multiple sets, then have 1-2 min between sets.

Aerobic training			

Modes of training
  a. Walking
  b. Cycling
  c. Rowing
  d. Reciprocal press–pull exercise
	Begin with one session per week.
	Progress to 2 or 3 days per week.
		Begin with light to moderate intensity of 30% to <60% $\dot{V}O_2$ or heart rate reserve, 55% to <75% MHR, or RPE of 9-13 on Borg 6- to 20-point scale. Increase intensity gradually.	Begin with 15- to 20-min sessions.
			Gradually increase to 30-min sessions.

*Minimize (or, ideally, eliminate) the eccentric component of resistance training exercises.

References: (77, 136, 137)

Recommended Readings

Eagle, M. Report on the muscular dystrophy campaign workshop: exercise in neuromuscular diseases Newcastle, January 2002. *Neuromuscul Disord* 12:975-983, 2002.

Gianola, S, Pecoraro, V, Lambiase, S, Gatti, R, Banfi, G, and Moja L. Efficacy of muscle exercise in patients with muscular dystrophy: a systematic review showing a missed opportunity to improve outcomes. *PLoS One* 8(6):e65414, 2013.

Grange, R and Call, J. Recommendations to define exercise prescription for duchenne muscular dystrophy. *Exerc Sport Sci Rev* 35(1):12-17, 2007.

Markert, C, Ambrosio, F, Call, J, and Grange, R. Exercise and Duchenne muscular dystrophy: toward evidence-based exercise prescription. *Muscle Nerve* 43:464-478, 2011.

Markert, C, Case, L, Carter, G, Furlong, P, and Grange R. Exercise and Duchenne muscular dystrophy: where we have been and where we need to go. *Muscle Nerve* 45:746-751, 2012.

CEREBRAL PALSY

Cerebral palsy (CP) is a group of nonprogressive, permanent neurological disorders that are caused by a variety of birth injuries. These disorders affect the CNS and are primarily characterized by limitations in motor control affecting body movement and posture. While the disorder of CP is considered "static," as the condition is expected to remain relatively stable throughout life, the symptoms due to the disorder may alter over time, either improving or worsening. States of **hypertonia** (excessive muscle tone) and **spasticity** (excessive muscle tone with increased tendon reflexes) are exhibited in almost half of the cases of CP (13, 50). Motor deficits commonly displayed by persons with CP include a lack of motor coordination with volitional movements (**ataxia**); tight muscles; exaggerated reflexes (spasticity); and a number of gait abnormalities including crouched gait, scissoring gait, and walking on the toes (64, 241). The motor effects of CP range from slight clumsiness to impairments that prevent almost all coordinated movements (88). Individuals with CP also exhibit a number of complications aside from motor control, which may include epilepsy, communication disorders, and impaired cognition (74).

Pathology of Cerebral Palsy

There are several forms of CP, including spastic, ataxic, and athetoid–dyskinetic variations. Spastic CP is the most common form, occurring in about 75% of all cases (252a). A hypertonic state is evident with spastic CP, as this form develops from damage that interferes with the uptake of GABA (gamma-aminobutyric acid), the primary inhibitory neurotransmitter (107). Limitations in GABA uptake interfere with "normal" control of neural excitability and muscle tone. Depending on the extremities affected, spastic CP may present in conditions of spastic **hemiplegia**, spastic diplegia, or spastic tetraplegia (198). Spastic hemiplegia affects one side of the body, with damage to one side of the brain resulting in deficits in the opposite side of the body. These persons are generally ambulatory but often require assistive devices (e.g., ankle–foot orthoses) to assist gait on the affected side (154). Persons with spastic diplegia present deficits in the lower extremities with little or no upper extremity spasticity (66). These individuals are usually fully ambulatory but exhibit a scissoring gait pattern with some degree of flexed knees and hip during gait. Spastic **tetraplegia** affects all four extremities, thereby being the most restrictive to independent gait due to excessive muscle tone and tremors that interfere with energy-efficient movements (25).

The second primary type of CP is ataxic CP. This variation is caused by damage to the cerebellum and is less common (less than 10% of all CP cases) (183). Individuals with ataxic CP tend to display limitations in movement coordination with decreased muscle tone. Functional deficits may include problems with writing or typing or upright balance, particularly during gait.

The third and final form of CP is athetoid or dyskinetic, which occurs in about 25% of all cases (177). Athetoid CP is characterized by mixed muscle tone, which limits the ability to hold upright sitting or walking postures (201). This CP condition also may limit the ability to hold and control items such as pencils.

Pathophysiology of Cerebral Palsy

Cerebral palsy is caused by complications during early development of the brain. These complications may arise during pregnancy, during childbirth, or during infancy and up to three years of life (169). During pregnancy, a number of factors can influence neurological development of the fetus leading to development of congenital CP. First, infections, including rubella (German measles) and toxoplasmosis (caused by a parasite carried in cat feces and undercooked meat), may damage the developing nervous systems (212). Secondly, congenital CP can be caused by jaundice in the fetus or newborn as a result of Rhesus (Rh) factor incompatibility between the mother and fetus that destroys the blood cells of the fetus (18). However, in the majority of cases, it is not possible to determine the specific cause of congenital CP (1).

During the process of childbirth, a number of events may also occur that result in a state of CP. The very process of birthing involves a degree of physical and metabolic stresses that may in some cases result in physical damage to the still-developing nervous systems (175). In particular, oxygen deprivation and head trauma during the labor process have been associated with increased incidence of permanent brain damage and CP (62). While brain damage from lack of oxygen in the developed CNS is generally limited to the cerebral cortex, anoxic injury in the developing brain may likely affect development of the entire cerebrum and result in loss of gray and white matter (3).

Common Medications Given to Individuals With Cerebral Palsy

Persons with CP are generally prescribed medications for treatment of the secondary complications associated with the disease. As seizures or the tendency for seizures is apparent in approximately 60% of persons with CP (268), antiseizure medications are commonly used (118). A depressant effect on the CNS is produced with most antiseizure drugs, which may have a limiting effect on exercise capacity as well as producing states of mental confusion, irritability, or dizziness (78). Antispasmodics and muscle relaxers are also commonly prescribed to persons with CP as they reduce muscle tone, which may otherwise interfere with efficient performance of daily activities (263). However, these medications may increase a sense of lethargy and drowsiness, thereby introducing a limiting effect of these drugs on the performance of daily activities, including the capacity for exercise training. See medications table 8.4 near the end of the chapter for a summary of medications used in the treatment of CP.

Effects of Exercise in Individuals With Cerebral Palsy

The need for exercise in persons with CP was demonstrated by the early work of Lundberg (131), in which the exercise capacity and aerobic power of children with spastic diplegia were compared with findings in peers without physical disability. Results indicated that the children with CP displayed physical work capacity less than half that of their age-matched peers. Peak values of $\dot{V}O_2$, heart rate, ventilation rate, and blood lactate concentrations were also significantly lower. Fernandez (63) examined the effects of an eight-week training program with two exercise sessions weekly, consisting of 30 minutes of training with an arm and leg cycle ergometer at work intensities of 40% to 70% of $\dot{V}O_2$ peak (peak oxygen uptake). The eight-week training program produced significant enhancement of $\dot{V}O_2$ peak (12%). However, the authors also noted that only one of the seven study participants continued with the exercise activities after the formal research program finished. The authors concluded that while the population of persons with CP presents very poor fitness levels and that their study demonstrated the ability to significantly enhance fitness, participation in such programming appears to be limited by a number of barriers, including availability of resources, transportation, cost, and medical concerns.

The application of resistance training in persons with CP has been scientifically justified by associations between muscular strength and endurance with important functional outcomes (216, 235). There is a direct relationship between lower extremity strength (particularly of the knee extensors) and gait efficiency and gross motor capabilities (216). Similarly, upper extremity muscular strength and endurance are highly associated with both anaerobic and aerobic wheelchair propulsion (151).

Resistance training in persons with CP produces gains in strength, muscular endurance, and power similar to those exhibited in persons without physical disability (40, 149, 153, 184, 200, 215). Furthermore, programs of resistance training have been shown to produce gains in fitness levels that are matched by enhancements in measures of functional abilities (126, 251). For example, resistance training has been shown to improve gait capabilities in ambulatory persons with CP.

Exercise Recommendations for Clients With Cerebral Palsy

Persons with CP exhibit significantly lower levels of exercise capacity, including lower muscular strength and endurance as well as reduced $\dot{V}O_2$peak values. Motor limitations also restrict gait efficiency, requiring considerably more energy uptake during ambulation than in persons who do not have disability. Strength training programs have been shown to be effective at increasing gait capabilities in persons with CP. Thus, both resistance training and upright mobility activities, such as treadmill training and walking over ground, may be used in programs designed to promote increased performance of upright activities including independent ambulation. However, it is also beneficial to include exercise activities that do not require substantial gross motor coordination in order to provide exercise conditioning effects without the limitations associated with lack of coordination. Cycling, steppers, and elliptical devices may provide a means of cardiovascular training without the limitations associated with more complicated gait tasks.

Exercise conditioning for clients with CP should be based on the same general recommendations as set forth for the overall population. Aerobic training should begin with an intensity equivalent to 30% to <60% of $\dot{V}O_2$peak or heart rate reserve for 15- to 20-minute training sessions with one to two sessions weekly. However, if the client is limited in her ability to perform continuous exercise, then the aerobic training may be divided into multiple shorter bouts of exercise, performed either in the same training session with a recovery period between bouts or in separate training sessions.

Specific recommendations for resistance training by clients with CP are not well established. The limited amount of work in this area does not lend itself to general recommendations, as most evidence is based on children with CP and the disease process includes a diverse group of disorders with a variety of levels of functioning. Therefore, the general recommendations for adults are appropriate, with two modifications. First, the use of free weights may not be indicated for many with this disease due to limitations in static and dynamic balance. It is generally held that single-joint movements are appropriate for initial training. Secondly, resistance intensity should be established based on the individual client's functional capacity, as many with CP display reduced exercise efficiency. Initial resistance training intensity for clients with CP may begin at a lower level than the general recommendations of 60% to 80% 1RM for 8 to 12 repetitions. In many cases, initial intensity levels of 50% to 60% 1RM are appropriate. Program design guidelines for clients with CP are summarized in table 8.4.

Exercise Modifications, Precautions, and Contraindications for Clients With Cerebral Palsy

Persons with CP who are ambulatory may be capable of exercising with standard exercise devices such as stationary bicycles, steppers, and elliptical devices. Arm exercise devices, such as arm crank devices or recumbent steppers with arm levers, are appropriate for cardiovascular training of clients

Table 8.4 Program Design Guidelines for Clients With Cerebral Palsy

Type of exercise	Frequency	Intensity	Volume
Resistance training			
Modes of training a. Weight training machines b. Bodyweight resistance c. Elastic tubing	Begin with one or two sessions per week. Possibly progress to 4 days per week, split routine.	Begin with four to eight exercises with resistance of 50-60% 1RM, emphasizing single-joint approach.	Start with 1 set per exercise of 10-12 reps. Possibly increase to 2-3 sets per exercise. If multiple sets, then 1-2 min between sets.
Aerobic training			
Modes of training a. Cycling b. Rowing c. Seated arm–leg cycling	Begin with one or two sessions per week. Progress to three to five sessions per week.	Begin with light to moderate intensity of 30% to <60% $\dot{V}O_2$ or heart rate reserve, 55% to <75% MHR, or RPE of 9-13 on Borg 6- to 20-point scale. Increase intensity gradually.	Begin with 15- to 20-min sessions. Gradually increase to 30-min sessions. Can be performed in multiple shorter bouts if unable to complete continuously.

References: (14, 159)

with CP who use a wheelchair for locomotion. The selection of the exercise device should be based on the program goals. If the goals are to enhance upright mobility via improved gross coordination, then less stabilized systems, such as treadmill or overground walking, may be appropriate. Programs emphasizing training volume may be more effective using more supportive equipment such as recumbent cycles.

It may be necessary to use specialized apparatus in order for some persons with CP to effectively and safely use standard exercise equipment. For example, it may be appropriate to strap the feet onto foot pedals or the hands onto level handles in order to provide a stable supported point of contact with the equipment. Care should be taken to ensure that the limbs are capable of the range of motion dictated by the device. Movement should never be forced against a muscle under spasm.

Key Point

Spasticity is a condition of excessive muscle tone or stiffness, with increased tendon reflexes, that may interfere with movement and may be a result of damage within the CNS. Muscles under spasm activity should never undergo forced movement against the spasm.

Case Study

Cerebral Palsy

Gloria is a 13-year-old with CP. She is able to walk with a cane and wears bilateral ankle–foot orthoses. Gloria works with a physical therapist at school but not during the summertime. Gloria's sister is taking gymnastics lessons at a fitness center, and Gloria's parents would like her to work with an exercise professional while her sister is at gymnastics. Gloria's parents signed her up for three 1-hour sessions per week for the summer.

Gloria's neurologist provided clearance for her to participate in the program. She has no other medical contraindications for exercise. Gloria's sessions began with a cardiovascular warm-up on the recumbent bicycle. She required slight assistance to get on and off the bicycle safely. Next, she participated in strength training using weighted balls, BOSU balls, and resistance bands. All major muscle groups were trained using a circuit to keep Gloria engaged. After resistance training, Gloria practiced balance while playing catch. The exercise professional would guard Gloria from falling while her father would toss her the ball. Gloria also participated in balance training using a BOSU ball. She was closely and carefully spotted by the exercise professional as she completed various standing tasks on the BOSU. All sessions ended with static stretching.

Gloria expressed that she had a lot of fun exercising at the fitness center this summer and would like to come back next year. Her parents were very pleased with her sessions. She was able to maintain all strength and range of motion that she had previously achieved.

Recommended Readings

Damiano, DL, Vaughan, C, and Abel, MF. Muscle response to heavy resistance exercise in children with cerebral palsy. *Dev Med Child Neurol* 37:731-739, 1995.

Fernandez, JE and Pitetti, KH. Training of ambulatory individuals with cerebral palsy. *Arch Phys Med Rehabil* 74(5):468-472, 1993.

Kramer, J and MacPhail, H. Relationships among measures of walking efficiency, gross motor ability, and isokinetic strength in adolescents with cerebral palsy. *Pediatr Phys Ther* 10:3-8, 1994.

MyChild at CerebralPalsy.org: The Ultimate Resource for Everything Cerebral Palsy. www.cerebralpalsy.org. Accessed May 24, 2016.

TRAUMATIC BRAIN INJURIES

A **traumatic brain injury** (TBI) is an acquired injury to the brain that takes place when a sudden traumatic force causes damage to the brain tissue. Traumatic brain injuries can occur due to an external force striking the head or as a result of the head traumatically making contact with an object. If the trauma does not result in the skull being fractured or penetrated, then the injury is referred to as a closed head injury. Closed head injuries tend to result in damage to the brain that is relatively widespread or diffuse. Open head injuries are TBIs in which the skull is penetrated by an object, causing damage to specific regions of the brain tissue.

Pathology of Traumatic Brain Injury

Traumatic brain injuries can be classified based on severity ranging from mild to moderate and severe (214). Brain injuries are usually graded in the emergency room based on whether the injury caused unconsciousness and if so how long unconsciousness lasted, and the individual's verbal, motor, and eye-opening responses to stimuli (67). A physician may also order computed tomography scans or magnetic resonance imaging scans of the brain to determine the extent of the injury.

With mild TBIs, including concussions, either a loss of consciousness did not result or the individual was unconscious for 30 minutes or less. Symptoms typically present at, or soon after, the injury but may not develop for weeks afterward. When an individual appears dazed or confused or loses consciousness, a mild TBI is diagnosed. The injury is classified as a concussion when a change in mental status is observed.

Moderate TBIs result in loss of consciousness for more than 20 minutes but less than 6 hours. The symptoms of moderate TBIs are similar to those of mild TBIs but are more serious and last longer. The individual may be confused for a period of days to weeks. Physical, cognitive, and behavioral performance may be impaired for months and potentially for life. Severe TBIs are generally a result of dramatic head wounds, both closed head injuries and penetrating injuries to the head, resulting in unconsciousness lasting more than 6 hours. These more severe injuries result in significant damage to the brain tissue with a range of physical and behavioral outcomes involving most aspects of daily life. Outcomes of moderate to severe TBIs are determined by a number of factors including the severity of the initial insult, the nature of the functional deficits, the significance of the outcomes to the individual, and the resources available for rehabilitation. Moderate to severe TBIs commonly result in deficits in cognition, speech and language, and sensory awareness. Physical issues include the potential for muscular paralysis and spasticity that may affect the performance of many important daily tasks. A number of emotional and behavioral concerns such as increased irritation, aggression, depression, lack of motivation, or dependency may become primary issues of concern.

Although there is a continuum for classifying the severity of brain injuries, all brain injuries are serious medical emergencies. Even concussions, which often go undiagnosed, can result in serious brain dysfunction (56). For this reason, some professional groups, such as the National Athletic Training Association (NATA), recommend not relying heavily on grading systems in the treatment of persons with TBI (27). According to the Centers for Disease Control and Prevention, in 2010 approximately 2.5 million people sustained TBIs, with concussion as the most common type (29).

Pathophysiology of Traumatic Brain Injury

The most common causes of TBIs are falls, motor vehicle accidents, being struck by objects, and assaults (236). The effects of any brain injury depend on the cause of the injury, the location of the injury, and the severity of the injury. Injuries that result in contusions, lacerations, or intracranial hemorrhage tend to produce focal damage of the brain (115). In contrast, injuries producing intense acceleration and deceleration of the brain are associated with axonal injuries and brain swelling, resulting in more diffuse damage of the brain tissue (266).

There are two distinct phases of TBI, each affecting brain integrity and function (110). First, the injury impact is considered as the source of primary mechanical damage to the brain. Secondary damage develops as a result of altered cranial mechanisms subsequent to the initial trauma. Ischemia of the brain and intracranial hypertension are examples of secondary insults that may significantly alter brain blood flow (hyper- or hypoperfusion), brain metabolism, and brain oxygenation. The composite of direct tissue damage and altered circulatory patterns commonly produces further damage and inflammation leading to neuronal cell death (110).

Primary mechanical damage from TBIs can be affected by preventive means but is not appreciably responsive to therapeutic measures (104). In contrast, the secondary damage from TBI, from limited circulation or inflammation, tends to be more responsive to therapeutic treatments (7).

Common Medications Given to Individuals With Traumatic Brain Injury

There are no medications to treat the actual brain injury; however, physicians prescribe a variety of medications to treat patients' specific symptoms. See medications table 8.5 near the end of the chapter for a summary of medications given to individuals with TBI. Patients may be prescribed analgesics for pain management, anticoagulants to prevent blood clots, antispasticity drugs, or anticonvulsants to prevent seizures. Side effects of opioid analgesics include nausea, drowsiness, urinary retention, and orthostatic hypotension, which could in some cases limit exercise capacity (170). Anticoagulants, such as warfarin, carry a risk of increased bleeding, so some would recommend avoiding high-contact sports and activities that put the individual at high risk for injuries. Anticonvulsants, also known as antiseizure medications, have known side effects including fatigue, digestive disorder, dizziness, and blurred vision. If a patient is having psychological dysfunction, he may be prescribed anti-anxiety, antipsychotic, or antidepressant medications. A patient may also be prescribed muscle relaxants, sedatives, or stimulants. All of these medication categories have the potential to limit exercise capacity and balance.

Effects of Exercise in Individuals With Traumatic Brain Injury

The safety of aerobic training in people with postconcussion syndrome (PCS) was demonstrated by Leddy and associates (122). The Balke treadmill test was used to effectively monitor headache symptoms in concussed persons who were asymptomatic at rest. Test results were used to determine the appropriate submaximal aerobic training zone for persons with PCS. The same research group (123) also later reported the safe and effective application of the Buffalo Concussion Treadmill Test to prescribe aerobic exercise following a concussion.

Bhambhani and colleagues (17) demonstrated the effects of a 12-week circuit training program on cardiorespiratory responses and body composition in individuals with moderate to severe TBI. Individuals performed 1 hour of aerobic and resistance exercise three times per week. At the completion of the study, there were no differences in body composition, but the peak values of power output, oxygen uptake, and ventilation rate were all significantly greater following the aerobic and resistance training program.

In 2009, Hassett and colleagues compared the effects of a fitness center exercise program and a home exercise program for individuals with TBI (83). Both groups performed strength and aerobic training three times per week for 12 weeks in a similar fashion, with only the location and supervision being different. After completing the program, both groups improved their 20-m shuttle time, with no difference between groups. This study demonstrates the benefits of exercise in individuals with TBI regardless of supervision.

The effects of aerobic exercise on depression and quality of life in persons with TBIs were examined by Wise and associates (262). Subjects performed one weekly 30-minute session of aerobic exercise with an exercise professional for 10

weeks and received exercise information with instructions to perform four additional 30-minute training sessions each week without supervision. During the supervised weekly session, the participants were also provided encouragement. Following the 10-week aerobic training program, scores on the Beck Depression Inventory were significantly improved, indicating less depression. These findings are important because many people who sustain TBIs also experience alterations in mood and depression (218).

Although many concussion programs use resistance training in their return to play protocol, at this time there are no published research studies in support of or against this training.

Exercise Recommendations for Clients With Traumatic Brain Injury

Many people who have sustained a TBI lead sedentary lifestyles and exhibit low levels of aerobic and muscular endurance, which further limit their ability to perform important activities of daily living and may subsequently lead to increased incidences of secondary disabilities such as heart disease and diabetes. Therefore, participation in well-designed exercise programs may provide a means to enhance physical fitness levels as well as abilities to engage in more challenging life activities.

While specific recommendations for exercise training have not been established for persons who have sustained a traumatic head injury, general recommendations for the older population may be modified for this population. Aerobic training should start with a light intensity of 55% to <65% MHR for 15- to 20-minute bouts of exercise in one or two weekly sessions (155). As tolerated, exercise duration may be increased to 20 to 40 minutes per session for three or four sessions per week. Persons with brain injury may have limitations in upright stability, both seated and standing, and stationary cycling and rowing may be appropriate modes of training in such cases.

Resistance training has been shown to provide significant benefits to persons with brain injuries. Unfortunately, specific resistance training protocols have not been developed for this population. Therefore at this time, resistance training for persons with TBI should be based on modified versions of recommended programming for the general population. Program design guidelines for clients with TBI are summarized in table 8.5.

Exercise Modifications, Precautions, and Contraindications for Clients With Traumatic Brain Injury

Although recent evidence has demonstrated the safety and efficacy of exercise in patients with PCS and TBI, it is not recommended that exercise professionals train these clients until they receive full clearance to exercise from their physician or other health care professional. After receiving clearance, clients who sustained TBIs may participate in both resistance training and cardiovascular training. Often people who have sustained head injuries, regardless of the severity, have cognitive or processing deficits; therefore, instructions should be especially clear and possibly be given multiple times.

These clients may also have motor impairments, and adjustments to exercise will have to be made on an individual level. For example, if a client has poor balance or coordination, she may benefit from seated machine exercises as opposed to free weight activities. Clients who have sustained TBIs may display autonomic system dysfunction and heart rate variability; therefore, heart rate is not a good measure of exercise intensity in this population.

Table 8.5 Program Design Guidelines for Clients With Traumatic Brain Injury

Type of exercise	Frequency	Intensity	Volume
Resistance training			

Modes of training
  a. Weight training machines
  b. Bodyweight resistance
  c. Elastic tubing
	Begin with one or two sessions per week.
	Possibly progress to 4 days per week, split routine.
		Initially do four to eight exercises with resistance of 50-60% 1RM, emphasizing single-joint approach.	Start with 1 set per exercise of 10-12 reps.
			Possibly increase to 2-3 sets per exercise.
			If multiple sets, then have 1-2 min between sets.

Aerobic training			

Modes of training
  a. Cycling
  b. Rowing
  c. Reciprocal press–pull exercise
  d. Circuit training
  e. Walking
	Begin with one session per week.
	Progress to 3 or 4 days per week.
		Begin with light intensity of 55 to <65% MHR or RPE of 9-11 on Borg 6- to 20-point scale.
		Increase intensity gradually.
			Begin with 15- to 20-min sessions.
			Gradually increase to 20- to 40-min sessions.

References: (14, 155)

Case Study

Traumatic Brain Injury

Mr. G, a 35-year-old businessman, was involved in a serious motor vehicle accident two months ago. He sustained a moderate TBI and received inpatient physical therapy before moving back to live with his parents. He is unable to drive or return to work and currently uses a wheelchair. Mr. G has access to a bus, made available by the city to those with disabilities, in order to access a nearby fitness facility associated with a medical clinic. Mr. G's neurologist has cleared him to exercise under the supervision of an exercise professional, and he is enrolled in a program of three sessions per week of 1 hour each.

Mr. G's neurologist has provided instructions that he should exercise only at light intensity so as to keep his heart rate and blood pressure responses to low levels; he should avoid the Valsalva maneuver and should remain seated for all exercise. Before his accident Mr. G had a BMI of 27; however, at the start of his outpatient exercise program, it was 33. He also is prediabetic and has been diagnosed with depression. He is currently taking an anticonvulsant, an antidepressant, ibuprofen, and baclofen (a medication that affects the chemical balance in the motor system of the brain) to control bodily movements.

Mr. G started his sessions with a light-intensity warm-up on a recumbent bicycle followed by mild partner-assisted mobility exercises. He then completed 15 minutes of aerobic recumbent arm–leg ergometry at light intensity (55% to <65% MHR) followed by low-intensity static stretching for each major muscle group. Over four months Mr. G progressed to 30 minutes per session of aerobic exercise on various seated ergometers, three times per week, and one weekly session of light machine weights. Mr. G was closely supervised and spotted during all activities.

After three months of training, Mr. G was able to walk small distances with the assistance of a roller walker and increased his ability to perform upper body activities of daily living. He decreased his body weight and increased his self-esteem. While Mr. G is not yet able to live independently, his progress toward his goals has motivated him to continue his exercise program.

Recommended Readings

Archer, T. Influence of physical exercise on traumatic brain injury deficits: scaffolding effect. *Neurotox Res* 21:418-434, 2012.

Archer, T, Svensson, K, and Alricsson, M. Physical exercise ameliorates deficits induced by traumatic brain injury. *Acta Neurol Scand* 125:293-302, 2012.

Griesbach, G. Exercise after traumatic brain injury: is it a double-edged sword? *Am Acad Phys Med Rehabil* 3:S64-S72, 2011.

Hassett, L, Moseley, A, Tate, R, and Harmer, A. Fitness training for cardiorespiratory conditioning after traumatic brain injury. *Cochrane Database Syst Rev* 2:CD006123, 2009.

Mossberg, K, Amonette, W, and Masel, B. Endurance training and cardiorespiratory conditioning after traumatic brain injury. *J Head Trauma Rehabil* 25(3):173-183, 2010.

STROKE

A **stroke** is a serious vascular event involving a loss of neurological functions related to an acute interruption of blood flow to the brain. Stroke is also commonly known as a cerebrovascular accident (CVA), named for the disrupted vascular flow to brain structures. The two main variations of stroke are ischemic stroke, in which blood flow is interrupted by a physical blockage, and hemorrhagic stroke, which occurs as a result of bleeding in the brain. Approximately 80% of all strokes are ischemic and 10% to 15% are hemorrhagic in origin (161). The remaining cases of stroke are transient ischemic attacks (TIAs), which are referred to as "mini-strokes" and are a result of temporary blood clots.

Pathology of Stroke

Interruption of blood flow prevents the necessary delivery of oxygen and vital nutrients, including glucose, to the network of brain tissues. The brain uses glucose as the primary energy source, and as glucose is not stored in the brain, the time of ischemic blockage is critical. The outcomes of stroke are also related to the location of the blockage of blood flow and to the amount of brain tissue influenced. A right-side stroke generally produces paralysis on the left side of the body, visual limitations, and memory loss (173). A stroke to the left side of the brain commonly results in paralysis of the right side of the body, limitations in speech, and memory loss (117). Paralysis, total or partial, of one side of the body as a result of a disease or injury to the CNS is referred to as hemiplegia.

Pathophysiology of Stroke

A number of controllable and uncontrollable risk factors are associated with the development of strokes. Controllable risk factors of stroke represent life habits that can be altered in order to reduce risk. Factors that increase the risk of stroke include smoking, high blood pressure, arterial disease, diabetes, abnormal lipid profiles, inactive lifestyles, and obesity (226, 252). Reversing any of these controllable risk factors will presumably reduce the risk of developing a stroke. Some risk factors of stroke are not controllable, including age, sex, heredity, race, and history of prior stroke (113). While a stroke can occur in persons with a wide range of these factors, the risk of stroke is greater if the person is older, male, or African American or if the person or an immediate family member has a history of stroke (91, 113, 119).

Ischemic strokes are caused by three primary mechanisms, including thrombosis, embolism, and global ischemia. Thrombotic strokes are produced by blockage of an artery by a clot (thrombus) that forms on blood vessels of the brain (246). Fatty deposits and cholesterol build up on the inner lining of blood vessels, creating an irritating influence that stimulates the formation of clots. A focal embolic stroke is caused when a blood clot that is formed somewhere in the body other than the brain, such as the heart, travels to the brain via the bloodstream (254). If the clot, known as an **embolus**, makes it to the brain via the bloodstream, it may block the flow of blood through an arterial structure, thus causing damage to the brain tissue supplied with blood, oxygen, and nutrients by that artery. Global ischemic stroke occurs if blood flow to the entire brain is interrupted by a systemic restriction such as myocardial infarction. Damage to brain tissue is related to the time the brain is deprived of oxygen and glucose. Global ischemic stroke can also be caused by particularly low blood pressures produced by drug overdoses and adverse reactions that limit blood flow to the brain (90, 239).

Hemorrhagic strokes are caused by the rupture of a blood vessel due to damage to the vascular structure, such as cerebral aneurysms or chronic high blood pressure (225). **Aneurysms** are areas of ballooning on a blood vessel due to weakening of the vessel wall. Over time, particularly with high blood pressure, the bulging area may rupture, causing bleeding into the brain.

Common Medications Given to Individuals Who Have Had a Stroke

Individuals who have had a stroke are prescribed medications that may assist with recovery and that may help prevent another stroke from occurring. Two types of blood thinner medications are used to lower the risk of the formation of blood clots. Antiplatelet drugs reduce the aggregation or clumping together of blood platelets (245). Blood clots are formed when blood platelets stick together. Anticoagulant medications also reduce the formation of blood clots but through different chemical actions (80). While these medications are quite effective in reducing the risk of subsequent strokes by reducing blood viscosity or "thickness," they also increase the risk of bleeding complications (92). Some physicians may recommend that the individual on anticoagulants avoid vigorous physical activity or contact sports. Side effects of antiplatelet and anticoagulant medications include nausea and upset stomach, which may limit the ability to participate in exercise training sessions.

Individuals who have sustained a stroke are commonly prescribed different types of medications to reduce high blood pressure, which is a primary risk factor for experiencing subsequent strokes. Hypertensive medications frequently used by stroke patients include angiotensin II receptor blockers, ACE inhibitors, β-blockers, calcium channel blockers, and diuretics, each of which exhibit different mechanisms of action for reducing high blood pressure but also may reduce the ability of the individual to engage in stressful exercise due to side effects such as dizziness, drowsiness, tiredness, and fatigue.

Persons who are poststroke will likely also need to treat other multiple morbidities commonly associated with strokes. For example, many persons who have sustained a stroke also present with hypertension, high cholesterol, diabetes, or some combination of these (129, 255). Thus, when developing an exercise program for these individuals, it is vital to consider all comorbidities and their respective medications, side effects, and effects on exercise responses. Refer to the applicable chapters in this book for further information. See medications table 8.6 near the end of the chapter for a summary of medications given to individuals who have had a stroke.

Effects of Exercise in Individuals Who Have Had a Stroke

Following stroke, the primary causes of death are recurrent strokes and coronary arterial disease (CAD). Additionally, between 25% and 50% of these persons require assistance in the performance of activities of daily living (179). This inability to perform basic daily tasks has been related to physiological deconditioning, preexisting cardiovascular disease, or dramatically reduced efficiency of gait and other upright activities (54, 196). Individuals with stroke hemiplegia exhibit energy uptake during walking that is two to three times greater than that of the general population walking at the same pace (101). They also exhibit peak values of oxygen uptake that are approximately 50% of those displayed by healthy persons of the same age (111, 132). These issues tend to limit activity in the lifestyles of persons following stroke, leading to further physical deconditioning, particularly of the cardiovascular system (231).

The rehabilitation process following stroke was traditionally limited to the first six to nine months following the acute episode based on the assumption that most, if not all, motor recovery would take place within that period (19, 35). The primary rehabilitation goals include increasing activity levels, particularly with regard to activities of daily living, reducing the incidence of recurring strokes, and improving aerobic fitness. In the clinical setting, aerobic fitness has commonly been addressed with task-specific activities rather than generalized exercise conditioning. Research has indicated that structured physical conditioning programs past the nine-month window can provide continued enhancement of aerobic fitness, strength, and functional capacity (264).

Aerobic exercise training has been shown to be capable of enhancing peak oxygen uptake and workload while reducing submaximal blood pressures with both cycle ergometry training and various forms of treadmill training. Potempa (194) reported that a 10-week program of cycle ergometry in 43 persons with hemiplegia produced enhancement of cardiovascular fitness similar in magnitude to that commonly shown in people without disability participating in similar programming.

Treadmill training has been shown to provide similar increases in values of peak oxygen uptake during gait, with reduced energy cost at submaximal-effort walking indicating improved gait efficiency (133). Following treadmill training, persons with hemiplegic gait displayed significantly faster overground walking in a 6-minute walk test with enhanced values of peak oxygen consumption. Interestingly, Macko and associates (133) reported significant associations between treadmill training velocity and peak values of $\dot{V}O_2$, while duration of treadmill training per session was significantly related to performance of the 6-minute walk test. Treadmill training therefore may provide a means of exercise training that transfers directly to gait pace and aerobic endurance.

The treadmill also provides a means of upright gait training for persons unable to do this over ground with full bodyweight loading. With the use of handrails for weight shifting and loading support and through the use of bodyweight unloading systems (harnesses attached to overhead support), the amount of loading can be reduced. Training intensity can be increased with either greater treadmill speed or increased treadmill elevation; the latter may be useful in increasing intensity with a comfortable pace of walking. Treadmill bodyweight support systems also reduce, or eliminate completely, the need for arm support–unloading, thereby providing the ability to coordinate the upper and lower extremity reciprocal movements important to coordinated gait.

Limitations in gait efficiency and motor coordination of many important daily tasks were traditionally attributed, to a great degree, to the state of hypertonia or spasticity common in persons following stroke (37). Because a vital goal of rehabilitation in this population is the improvement of the control and quality of movement, control of spasticity was seen as the principal issue to address. However, research has shown that spasticity is not the primary impairment following stroke; rather, muscular weakness is the principal limitation to function poststroke (180). For example, muscular weakness is significantly associated with decreased gait velocity and performance of important activities of daily living, such as bodyweight transfer during walking.

More recent research in this area has shown that resistance training of the lower extremities does provide significant improvements of muscle strength, power, and endurance in both the affected and nonaffected limbs of persons with hemiplegia poststroke. Lee and colleagues (124) reported that 12 weeks of high-intensity resistance training resulted in improvements in muscular strength, power, and endurance, while three 30-minute cycle ergometry training sessions per week for 12 weeks produced no significant changes in muscle function. Resistance training consisted of two sets of 80% 1RM for the movements of hip extension and flexion, knee extension and flexion, and ankle plantar flexion in each of the three weekly sessions.

The effects of an intensive training program consisting of high-intensity resistance training, body weight–supported treadmill training, aerobic exercise, and functional training were described by Jorgensen and associates (102). Resistance training movements included semiseated leg press, leg extension, leg curl, and seated leg press, with relative training intensity increasing weekly from 12RM to 4- to 8RM levels during the 12-week program. Training was performed unilaterally for three to five sets per exercise with recovery periods of 90 seconds between sets. The findings of this study included improvements of the agonist muscle neurological activation with enhanced twitch torque, which were associated with increased muscular strength during concentric, eccentric, and static contractions with enhanced gait performance. The reduced neurological activation at baseline was highly related to muscular weakness. The hamstring muscles

of the paretic limb were found to be particularly weakened at baseline, suggesting that specific attention should be given to the knee flexors with training in order to achieve greater levels of knee extension and improved gait ability.

Exercise Recommendations for Clients Who Have Had a Stroke

The body of literature supports the use of aerobic training in persons following stroke using exercise of the legs, arms, or combined arm and leg activities. Recommended training intensity for this population is 40% to <60% of $\dot{V}O_2$peak or heart rate reserve. Training frequency is recommended at three to seven days per week, with training duration ranging from 20 to 60 minutes per session. Intermittent programs of treadmill training (multiple shorter bouts per session) may prove particularly beneficial in more deconditioned clients until they are capable of completing longer sessions.

Research also suggests that resistance training following stroke in persons with hemiparesis should be similar to programming for persons who are elderly. Recommendations for resistance training poststroke include 8 to 10 exercises performed three times weekly. Training intensity should begin with 50% to 60% 1RM and progress to 60% to 85% 1RM. In order to place appropriate stresses on the paretic limb, it is advisable to concentrate on unilateral movements.

Most persons who have sustained a stroke also present with other special conditions or comorbidities and are likely taking medications for those conditions. For example, many, if not most, of these clients (poststroke) also have CAD and hypertension (47, 176). When designing the individualized exercise program, it is vital to consider and plan for potential compounded effects of the multiple special conditions, as well as possible interactions of the respective medications.

It is common for persons who have sustained a stroke to have limitations in communication and mental processing. A significant number of these clients have problems with written communication (writing and reading) as well as trouble with speech and understanding verbal cues (222). It is necessary to provide these clients with multiple means of communication, including verbal cues as well as visual examples of the exercise techniques. Program design guidelines for clients who have had a stroke are summarized in table 8.6.

Exercise Modifications, Precautions, and Contraindications for Clients Who Have Had a Stroke

A common outcome following stroke is paralysis or limitations in motor control. Paralysis generally occurs on one side of the body (i.e., the side opposite the side of the brain in which the stroke occurred). For example, damage to the right side of the brain may affect the left-side arm, left leg, or the entire left side of the body. The limitations in motor control may be accompanied by reduced or a total lack of sensation from the paralyzed region (87). Reduced visual awareness on the affected side is not uncommon, which reduces the ability of the individual to respond to changes in the environment in that field of view.

Limitations in motor control and sensory awareness on one side of the body necessitate the inclusion of unilateral exercise movements in the exercise program. Training the affected side of the body independent of the unaffected side will ensure conditioning of the region or regions that are most compromised. The affected and unaffected sides of the body can be trained independently or with alternating bilateral movements. Exercise equipment that allows reciprocal movements of the right and left limbs provides a particularly useful means of exercise training in many persons poststroke. The reciprocating pushing–pulling upper extremity actions of the arm levers on some arm and leg cycle ergometers or recumbent steppers provide a means by which the affected limb can be guided through the exercise range of motion by the nonaffected limb. Specialized mitts and gloves can be used to increase grip of the affected hand. Similarly, recumbent cycles and steppers can be used for conditioning affected lower extremities. When using this strategy, it is important to make sure that the client's affected limb is fully capable of moving passively through the range of exercise motion.

Limitations in motor control and sensory awareness can also affect body stability, especially if the lower extremities and torso are affected (171). With reduced ability to self-stabilize, it is imperative to use exercise equipment that provides external stabilization. For example, recumbent cycles would be preferred over upright stationary cycling. The use of exercise machines with stable back support may prove advantageous, especially in early phases of training, compared to training with free weights without body support. That said, a goal of the exercise program may be to gradually strengthen the weakened stroke-affected

Table 8.6 Program Design Guidelines for Clients Who Have Sustained a Stroke

Type of exercise	Frequency	Intensity	Volume
Resistance training			
Modes of training a. Weight training machines b. Bodyweight resistance c. Elastic tubing	Begin with one or two sessions per week. Possibly progress to 4 days per week, split routine.	Begin with 8-10 exercises with resistance of estimated 50-60% 1RM (and progress to 60-85% 1RM), emphasizing multijoint approach.	Start with 1 set per exercise of 10-12 reps. Possibly increase to 2-3 sets per exercise. If multiple sets, then have 1-2 min between sets.
Aerobic training			
Modes of training a. Cycling b. Rowing c. Arm crank exercise d. Reciprocal press–pull exercise e. Treadmill walking	Begin with one session per week. Progress to 2 or 3 days per week.	Begin with light to moderate intensity of 30% to <60% $\dot{V}O_2$ or heart rate reserve, 55% to <75% MHR, or RPE of 9-13 on Borg 6- to 20-point scale. Increase intensity gradually.	Begin with 15- to 20-min sessions. Gradually increase to 30-min sessions.

References: (14, 180, 189)

muscles in order to enhance the ability to self-stabilize. The amount of external stabilization must be very gradually reduced, if possible, in order to safely progress. For example, when using a resistance training selectorized machine, the exercise sessions may start with a snug torso support (chest strap) wrapped around the client and back support, moving gradually to less snug and then loosened support, and then eventually progressing to use of the exercise station relying on the back support without a chest strap.

Case Study

Stroke

Mr. H, 45 years old, is a former college football lineman who had a large stroke six months ago. Mr. H had both in- and outpatient physical therapy but no longer has insurance benefits. He currently cannot drive, is not able to return to work, and can walk unsteadily with a cane but refuses to use a walker. Mr. H can take the bus to the fitness center, and his wife signed him up to work with an exercise professional. She registered him for three sessions per week for 1 hour each. Mr. H agreed to the training sessions and stated that he would like to do powerlifting as he had in the past to prepare for football.

Both Mr. H's cardiologist and neurologist cleared him to exercise at the fitness center with supervision. They both stated that the patient should not hold his breath; they also noted that care was warranted because Mr. H had poor balance. Mr. H had a BMI of 35, hypertension, diabetes, and depression. He took the following medications: insulin, an ACE inhibitor, a β-blocker, a statin, an anticoagulant, and an antidepressant.

Mr. H's sessions started with a warm-up on a recumbent bicycle, recumbent arm–leg ergometry, or an upright elliptical holding on with both hands. After the warm-up, Mr. H reviewed rhythmic breathing and exhaling during resistance training before starting his strengthening program. At first, all strengthening exercises were performed with resistance machines; however, over time Mr. H was able to progress to upright activities with light free weights. He required close supervision and spotting during all activities. After resistance training, he was instructed in balance activities on even and uneven surfaces. Sessions ended with stretching activities. In view of Mr. H's balance limitations, the initial stretching was proprioceptive neuromuscular facilitation (PNF) with instructor assistance and gradually introduced controlled passive stretching.

After three months of training, Mr. H was able to walk without his cane more steadily. He decreased his body weight and the amount of insulin that he needed, and increased his balance and self-esteem. He is still working toward his goals of powerlifting and driving.

Recommended Readings

Billinger, SA, Arena, R, Bernhardt, J, Eng, JJ, Franklin, BA, Johnson, CM, MacKay-Lyons, M, Macko, RF, Mead, GE, Roth, EJ, Shaughnessy, M, and Tang, A. Physical activity and exercise recommendations for stroke survivors: a statement for healthcare professionals from the American Heart Association/American Stroke Association. *Stroke* 45:2532-2553, 2014.

Eng, JE. Fitness and Mobility Exercise (FAME) Program for stroke. *Top Geriatr Rehabil.* 26(4):310-323, 2011.

National Stroke Association. HOPE: A Stroke Recovery Guide. Chapter 4, Movement and Exercise. www.stroke.org/sites/default/files/resources/NSA-Hope-Guide.pdf. Accessed December 19, 2016.

Pak, S and Patten, C. Strengthening to promote functional recovery poststroke: an evidence-based review. *Top Stroke Rehabil.* 15(3):177-199, 2008.

SPINAL CORD INJURIES

Spinal cord injury (SCI) is an injury or disease process of the spinal cord that results in altered motor, sensory, or autonomic functioning (or some combination of these). Injuries to the spinal cord can limit motor ability and sensation to differing degrees depending on the location and severity of damage to the cord. The spinal cord is the primary conduit for all neural communication between the brain and most of the rest of the body (except the optic nerve). In general, the higher the level of SCI in the vertebral column, the more widespread the damage, as such injuries commonly affect all tissues with more distal nerve roots (238). Injuries of the cervical region affect the upper and lower extremities as well as the trunk, producing a state of tetraplegia (in the past referred to as **quadriplegia**). Persons with **paraplegia** have sustained a spinal injury at the thoracic or lumbar vertebral levels, causing impairment in the lower extremities and some portion of the trunk. While these two terms are useful, more specific terminology provides increased accuracy of communication regarding specific neurological capabilities.

The number of persons in the United States living with SCI was estimated by the National Spinal Cord Injury Statistical Center in 2012 (168) to be between 236,000 and 327,000 individuals. According to statistics generated by data from regional SCI centers, approximately 80.6% of persons with SCI were male, with the highest rates of SCI between the ages of 16 and 30 years. The average age at SCI was 41 years. About 57% of persons with SCI were considered paraplegic (21.6% complete, 21.4% incomplete), with 43% of new injuries classified as tetraplegia (40.8% incomplete, 15.8% complete).

Pathology of Spinal Cord Injuries

Spinal cord injuries are commonly described using a system denoting both the functional level of the spinal lesion and the relative degree of functional deficit, referred to as "completeness" (148). First, the level of SCI indicates the last descending nerve root associated with exhibited full function of movement and sensation. If a SCI results in total loss of volitional movement (paralysis) and total loss of sensory functions, then the injury is deemed "complete," while "incomplete" SCIs are those in which there is some preservation of sensory or motor function below the spinal lesion. Thus, a person characterized as having motor-complete tetraplegia at the C5 level is expected to show strong elbow flexors without volitional control of wrist extensors or elbow extensors or any muscles of legs or torso.

Accurate assessment of the motor and sensory functioning following SCI is typically performed within the clinical setting by a physician or more likely a physical therapist. The exercise professional should not attempt to determine the level of SCI himself, but rather work with the clinician's assessment. Certainly, documentation of the clinical motor-sensory–based classification of the SCI provides a vital perspective on which all subsequent goals and programming should be based. The level of SCI inherently refers to the specific musculature and the associated movements that are significantly affected, thereby influencing total and regional work capacity, incidence of joint imbalances and instabilities, and the ability to proximally stabilize. Autonomic dysfunctions in tissues below full CNS control include altered circulatory patterns, central hemodynamic functioning, and thermoregulatory responses, all of which should be considered when one is developing exercise programming for persons with SCI. A state of **autonomic dysreflexia**, a serious potentially life-threatening condition, may be exhibited by persons with SCI (220).

Autonomic dysreflexia develops when noxious stimuli applied below the point of spinal lesion at the T4 level or above produce quite intense increases of heart rate and blood pressure. Thus, clinical determination of SCI level provides a needed component for the activities of the exercise professional.

Pathophysiology of Spinal Cord Injuries

The spinal cord is a large complicated bundle of nerves that carries neural impulses between the brain and the rest of the body. The cord itself is surrounded by a series of bony rings, the vertebrae, which make up the spinal column. This arrangement allows considerable protection of the spinal cord while also allowing a good amount of motion as a function of the summation of movement between multiple vertebral spaces. However, traumatic injuries and disease processes can introduce mechanical stresses that produce damaging effects on the spinal cord, whether or not there is vertebral body injury. The cord can be partially or completely cut (transected) or can be contused (bruised) by trauma. Secondary damage of the spinal cord may also result from edema, or swelling, which restricts circulatory flow into the region.

The most common cause of SCI is motor vehicle related (39%), followed by falls (28%) and acts of violence (15%) (168). Approximately 8% of SCI are attributed to sport activities. Acts of violence, now the third highest cause of SCI nationally, are the primary source of SCI in several major urban cities.

Common Medications Given to Individuals With Spinal Cord Injury

No pharmaceutical treatment has been shown to be effective in the reversal of the damage from a SCI. However, medications are commonly prescribed for the negative symptoms, such as both orthopedic and neurogenic pain, spasticity, bladder control, and depression. See medications table 8.7 near the end of the chapter for a summary of medications given to individuals with SCI. Nonsteroidal anti-inflammatory drugs (NSAIDs) are commonly prescribed for joint pain associated with overuse from manual wheelchair locomotion and other activities of daily living performed with the upper extremities. Persons with SCI also experience neurogenic pain, which is usually treated with medications such as tricyclic drugs and selective serotonin and norepinephrine reuptake inhibitors. These medications are known to frequently produce side effects including nausea, drowsiness, sedation, light-headedness, dizziness, and muscle weakness, which may significantly reduce the ability of the individual to exercise vigorously or to maintain balance.

Individuals with SCI may also be prescribed medications for bladder control and depression, as well as for autonomic dysreflexia. Bladder control medications such as Ditropan may produce states of dizziness, drowsiness, and weakness, which would presumably limit the capability to exercise intensely. Depression medications such as Prozac, Zoloft, and Wellbutrin may also make the client dizzy, drowsy, fatigued, or nauseous and should be viewed as potentially negatively affecting exercise performance. Persons with SCI may exhibit the serious life-threatening condition of autonomic dysreflexia, in which intense increases of heart rate and blood pressure are produced. The individual may be prescribed medications such as sublingual Nitrostat or Catapres, which reduce hemodynamic stresses. In the case of autonomic dysreflexia, the remainder of the exercise session should be immediately cancelled and immediate medical support should be acquired.

Effects of Exercise in Individuals With Spinal Cord Injury

It is well established that persons with SCI can engage in purposeful exercise activities using the intact musculature above the point of spinal lesion (69, 95). However, several factors tend to limit the physiological responses to volitional upper extremity exercise with SCI, thereby reducing peak exercise capacity (95). First, depending on the level of SCI, less active muscle mass is available to contribute to the force generation and stabilization involved in exercise. Secondly, ascending levels of SCI are also associated with greater levels of autonomic dysfunctions, thereby limiting exercise capacity due to reduced hemodynamic responses to upper extremity exercise.

There is also a well-established association between the level of SCI and the upper extremity work capacity as determined with $\dot{V}O_2$peak. This association between level and severity of SCI with exercise capacity is the basis for the classification used in Paralympic sport competition (120). Persons with complete SCI above the T4 level are devoid of sympathetic cardio-acceleration processes, with elevation of HR limited to withdrawal of parasympathetic influences, thereby limiting

HRpeak to approximately 120 to 125 beats/min (81, 247). Thus, persons with cervical-level SCI (tetraplegia) exhibit dramatically reduced work capacity due to restrictions in available active musculature, as well as reduced cardiac output, thereby limiting delivery of oxygen and nutrients to the exercising muscles. Persons with SCI below the T6 level generally do exhibit sympathetic drive and HRpeak similar to persons without physical disability (134). However, people with paraplegia also display decreased venous return from the paralyzed lower limbs, limited cardiac end-diastolic volumes, and reduced levels of stroke volume (209). Even with a compensatory elevation of HR, persons with SCI paraplegia exhibit a state of circulatory hypokinesis in which a reduced cardiac output is seen for a given level of oxygen uptake ($\dot{V}O_2$), thus requiring a greater degree of oxygen extraction at any given level of cardiac output, leading to earlier local muscle fatigue (94).

It may seem intuitive that resistance training would prove beneficial for the persons with SCI due to the increased reliance on upper extremity work efforts. Wheelchair locomotion, transfers, and weight shifts are necessary activities in the lives of this population, thereby establishing a need for the generation of high forces in the upper body in order to carry out basic activities of daily living. Over 40 years ago, Nilsson and associates (172) reported significantly elevated $\dot{V}O_2$ with increased triceps strength in a group of persons with SCI paraplegia following a seven-week conditioning program. More recently, Davis (44) examined the effects of an arm cranking intensity of 70% $\dot{V}O_2$ peak for 20-minute training sessions as contrasted with 40-minute sessions at 40% $\dot{V}O_2$ peak. Strength gains were limited to the moderate-intensity condition and to the shoulder extensors and elbow flexor muscles, indicating that arm cranking is not an appropriate mode of training for functional strength as the gains were not reflected in the muscles most commonly used in activities of daily living.

Circuit resistance training (CRT) was examined in persons with paraplegia in a program of high-intensity resistance exercises performed in agonist–antagonist pairs (e.g., shoulder press, lat pulldown) alternated with periods of high-paced, low-intensity arm cranking (96). Three circuits of CRT, each circuit consisting of three pairs of resistance exercises (1 minute each) and three 2-minute bouts of arm cranking, were performed three times weekly over a 16-week training period. Circuit resistance training produced significant enhancement of muscular strength (13-40%) and $\dot{V}O_2$ peak (29%) with improvements in lipid profiles.

The specific effects of resistance training and aerobic endurance training in persons with paraplegia have been compared. Jacobs and associates (93) assigned matched pairs of persons with paraplegia to either aerobic endurance training or resistance training for three weekly sessions over a 12-week period. The aerobic endurance training program consisted of 30 minutes of arm cranking at 70% to 85% of HRpeak. The resistance training group performed three sets of 10 repetitions at six exercise stations with intensity ranging from 60% to 70% of 1RM. The aerobic endurance training group displayed 11.8% gain of $\dot{V}O_2$ peak with no significant changes observed in muscular strength or power. Conversely, muscular strength and power significantly increased in the resistance training group for all exercise maneuvers, with $\dot{V}O_2$ peak increasing 15.8%. The results of this investigation indicate that resistance training is a means of training for persons with SCI that provides significant enhancement of cardiorespiratory functioning as well as significant increases in muscular strength and power.

Exercise Recommendations for Clients With Spinal Cord Injury

The general exercise recommendations for persons with SCI do not vary dramatically from those established for the general population in terms of training intensity, duration, frequency, or specificity. Exercise programming recommendations for persons with SCI should be in accordance with those set forth by the U.S. Department of Health and Human Services (244): 150 minutes a week of aerobic training at a moderate intensity or 75 minutes a week at a combination of moderate and vigorous intensity. Initial sessions, though, should be at a light to moderate intensity (30% to <60% $\dot{V}O_2$ or heart rate reserve) for 15 to 20 minutes. Intensity and duration should be increased gradually, with duration increasing to 30-minute sessions for two or three weekly sessions. Resistance training should be performed with all major muscle groups available on two or more days per week, initially with light intensity (40-60% 1RM). Resistance training intensity may be increased progressively to 60% to 85% 1RM.

Persons with SCI are limited to exercise of the muscle groups under volitional control, usually the muscle groups innervated by nerve roots above the point of spinal lesion. Aerobic training is commonly limited to arm cranking exercise or wheelchair propulsion activities. Resistance training is best performed using well-stabilized weight training machines. Specialized weight machines have been developed for exercise from the wheelchair, which is the preferential mode for this population. The alternative, transferring the client to and from general resistance training equipment, carries a substantial risk to both the client and the exercise professional and should be performed only with additional specialized training on the transfer process. Resistance training can also be undertaken in the wheelchair using handheld weights and with resistance bands and tubing. Program design guidelines for clients with SCI are summarized in table 8.7.

Exercise Modifications, Precautions, and Contraindications for Clients With Spinal Cord Injury

Conditioning of persons with SCI requires revisions in the training environment in order to provide a safe and efficacious training setting. Spinal cord injuries alter functioning of several major body systems, requiring modifications of the exercise movements and strategies from those appropriate for the general population.

The most notable characteristic of a motor-complete SCI is the total lack of volitional control of muscles below the point of the spinal injury (i.e., muscular paralysis). Exercise conditioning of persons with SCI is generally limited to those muscle groups innervated by nerve roots arising above the injury point. Persons with paraplegia are capable of exercising with the arms and much of the torso (depending on injury level), while persons with tetraplegia are limited to muscular actions within the upper extremities (see figure 8.1). Thus, exercise capacity is dramatically lower in clients with SCI compared to the general public and is related to the level and completeness of injury.

Table 8.7   Program Design Guidelines for Clients With Spinal Cord Injury

Type of exercise	Frequency	Intensity	Volume
Resistance training			
Modes of training a. Weight training machines and free weights b. Bodyweight resistance c. Elastic tubing	Begin with one or two sessions per week. Possibly progress to 4 days per week, split routine.	Begin with 8-10 exercises with resistance of 40-60% 1RM, emphasizing multijoint approach. Intensity may be increased to 60-85% 1RM as tolerated.	Start with one set per exercise of 10-12 reps. Possibly increase to 2-3 sets per exercise. If multiple sets, then have 1-2 min between sets.
Aerobic training			
Modes of training a. Arm crank exercise b. Reciprocal press–pull exercise	Begin with one session per week. Progress to 2 or 3 days per week.	Begin with light to moderate intensity of 30% to <60% $\dot{V}O_2$ or heart rate reserve, 55% to <75% MHR, or RPE of 9-13 on Borg 6- to 20-point scale. Increase intensity gradually.	Begin with 15- to 20-min sessions. Gradually increase to 30-min sessions.

References: (95, 242)

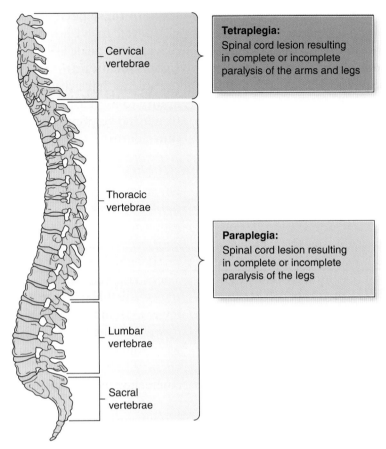

Tetraplegia:
Spinal cord lesion resulting in complete or incomplete paralysis of the arms and legs

Paraplegia:
Spinal cord lesion resulting in complete or incomplete paralysis of the legs

Figure 8.1 Vertebral ranges for tetraplegia and paraplegia.

With a reduced amount of muscle mass under volitional control and available for exercise training, it might seem appropriate to increase the volume of work applied to those muscle groups available. However, this is not appropriate and would eventually result in overtraining and increased risk of injuries. Similarly, it would be prudent to concentrate the most intense exercise efforts on those muscle groups used by people in wheelchairs during daily life activities, including wheelchair propulsion, wheelchair transfers, and weight shifts. It is vital to consider that those movements can be relatively intense and are performed repetitively on a daily basis, because emphasizing the major muscle groups that contribute to those movements (anterior deltoid, pectorals, triceps) with substantial training volume and intensity could introduce serious overuse syndromes with potential for injury. Thus it is recommended that resistance training programs for persons with SCI initially concentrate on antagonist movements in wheelchair propulsion, wheelchair transfers, and weight shifts (i.e., pulling actions).

Many upper body exercise activities are effectively performed in the general population using stabilization forces generated by the lower extremities and torso. Persons with lower limb paralysis are unable to produce such steadying effects and would be unsafe in many generalized exercise positions. Thus it is often necessary to use strapping around the torso and weight machine or wheelchair in order to establish a safe and effective base of support for more intense training.

Partial or complete paralysis of the lower arms and hands dramatically reduces gripping force. Persons with cervical-level SCI may exhibit quite limited gripping abilities but retain the ability to generate substantial forces in the more proximal musculature such as the biceps and deltoid muscles. Specialized mitts and gloves with attaching straps have been developed to provide gripping in those unable to grip independently. Likewise, wrist straps (similar to those used with shrugs and deadlifts by powerlifters) can be used for these purposes. While these devices can provide a means to increase work efforts in persons with SCI, it is important that the exercise professional supervise exercise at all times, as these devices are usually not appropriate for independent use.

Persons with SCI also exhibit dysfunction of the autonomic nervous system. People with SCI paraplegia present significantly reduced levels of venous return from the paralyzed lower extremities. This limits the magnitude of ventricular filling and therefore stroke volume, as well as reducing the stretch of the cardiac chamber and subsequently the effects of the Frank-Starling law. Persons with SCI tetraplegia exhibit even greater deficits in venous return associated with the proportionally greater amount of paralyzed muscle mass (75).

Sympathetic neural drive is dramatically limited or absent in persons with SCI above the T4 level. In these persons, heart rate acceleration is limited to withdrawal of parasympathetic drive, with peak HR values restricted to 120 to 125 beats/min. Thus, persons with SCI tetraplegia have dramatic limitations in their ability to increase cardiac output and delivery of needed oxygen and nutrients to exercising musculature.

Persons with cervical SCI or with paraplegia above T4 are also at risk of autonomic dysreflexia, which can be life threatening. In this case, noxious stimuli arising from below the spinal lesion are inappropriately processed, resulting in dangerous cardiovascular responses such as dramatic increases of HR and blood pressure (220). These noxious stimuli can range from blisters to overfilled bladder or bowels or injuries of the lower extremities. If the source of the autonomic dysreflexia cannot be immediately identified, with adjustments eliminating the problem, the client should be immediately transported to an emergency medical facility.

Case Study

Spinal Cord Injury

Mr. L, 26 years old, sustained a SCI as a result of an automobile accident four years ago. His spinal injury was classified as a motor-sensory–complete SCI at the T8 level. John lives independently, drives his car with hand controls, and uses a manual wheelchair. He is currently not employed. Since discharge from the rehabilitation hospital about three years ago, he has been relatively inactive. Before his injury, Mr. L was quite active, having participated in high school and community recreational sports and training regularly at the community fitness center. Mr. L has experienced shoulder and elbow pain, which increases the challenges associated with wheelchair locomotion and transfers. He is taking Ditropan, a prescription medication for control of involuntary muscle spasms. He measured 69 inches (1.75 m) in height and 186 pounds (84 kg) in weight.

Mr. L's rehabilitation physician approved him for exercise training without restriction. The exercise professional discussed exercise training with him and determined that Mr. L was not interested in a "special" program but would prefer training in a manner as similar to what he perceived as "normal" as possible. He explained that before his SCI, he enjoyed a program consisting of a cardiovascular warm-up, followed by static stretching and then a series of resistance training exercises. Based on his experiences and his preferences, the exercise professional designed an appropriate program.

Mr. L's training program initially included two sessions weekly, with each session comprising a cardiovascular training period, a flexibility period, and a resistance training segment. His cardiovascular training was carried out with a NuStep ergometer, which allowed reciprocal upper extremity press–pull movements. Initial cardiovascular sessions were 15 minutes. Flexibility training was carried out with static stretching movements with assistance from the exercise professional. Emphasis was placed on the anterior deltoids and pectoral muscles. Resistance training was performed with a circuit of wheelchair-accessible weight training machines. One set of 8 to 12 repetitions each of chest press, seated row, shoulder press, lat pulldown, biceps curl, and triceps extension was completed.

After four weeks, the NuStep cardiovascular training had increased to 30 minutes daily with resistance training load increased to three sets of each resistance training session. After three months of exercise training, Mr. L reported little to no shoulder or elbow pain. He expressed a great deal of appreciation for the opportunity to engage in what he had always enjoyed: exercise.

Recommended Readings

Jacobs, PL and Beekhuizen, KS. Appraisal of physiological fitness in persons with spinal cord injury. *Top Spinal Cord Inj Rehabil* 10(4):32-50, 2005.

Jacobs, PL and Nash, MS. Exercise recommendations for individuals with spinal cord injury. *Sports Med* 34(11):727-751, 2004.

Turbanski, S and Schmidbleicher, D. Effects of heavy resistance training on strength and power in upper extremities in wheelchair athletes. *J Strength Cond Res* 24(1):8-16, 2010.

EPILEPSY

Epilepsy is not a single disorder, but a collection of disorders with the common characteristic of recurring seizure activity. A **seizure** is a sudden surge in the electrical activity of the brain that may affect an individual's appearance or actions for a short period. Epilepsy is now considered a disease and is defined by any of the following (59):

- At least two unprovoked (or reflex) seizures occurring more than 24 hours apart.

- One unprovoked (or reflex) seizure and a probability of further seizures similar to the general recurrence risk (at least 60%) after two unprovoked seizures, occurring over the next 10 years.

- Diagnosis of an epilepsy syndrome. This means that epilepsy is considered resolved for individuals who had an age-dependent epilepsy syndrome but are now past the applicable age, or those who have remained seizure-free for the last 10 years, with no seizure medicines for the last 5 years.

Epilepsy is caused by an excessive electrical discharge in the brain that disrupts the normal pattern of brain electrical activity. This is seen when the brain releases more excitatory signals than inhibitory signals. The threshold between excitatory and inhibitory signals that the brain can withstand before the consequence of a seizure is genetically predetermined. The outcomes of the seizures depend on where and how much of the brain was affected. The durations of seizures range from seconds to minutes, often with disorientation after the seizure ends. Seizure activity also ranges in severity. More severe seizures exhibit signs such as uncontrolled and uncoordinated movements or convulsions, which affect various physical and mental functions and may lead to unconsciousness (58). Less severe seizures may be characterized by blank staring, lip smacking, and jerking movements of the arms and legs (182).

Pathology of Epilepsy

People with epilepsy can experience one or more types of seizures. Seizures are now classified into two general types: primary generalized and partial–focal (16). Primary generalized seizures involve both sides of the brain, while partial seizures affect only part of the brain. In addition to classification of epilepsy by seizure type, it can also be classified into seizure syndromes, taking more variables into account. There are many subtypes of seizures, and exercise professionals are encouraged to consult with their client's physician or other health care professional and the Epilepsy Foundation (www.epilepsy.com) for more information on the specific type of seizures that are affecting their client. In diagnosing epilepsy, physicians order a battery of tests including a combination of blood work, medical history, neurological examination, positron emission tomography (PET) scans, computed tomography (CT) scans, and magnetic resonance imaging (MRI). The best means of diagnosing epilepsy is monitoring using an electroencephalogram for one or two days, as well as videotaping seizures in order to determine what type of seizures a person has and subsequently the treatment.

Although most seizures cannot be foreseen, there are a few things that people with epilepsy can avoid because they are considered seizure triggers. The most important thing a person with epilepsy can do to avoid seizures is to take medications as prescribed. Other triggers include eating or drinking certain foods, changes in hormone levels, stress, sleep patterns, and photosensitivity (sensitivity to flashing lights at certain intensities) (76, 135, 191, 229, 250).

Although there is no central database that keeps track of either the incidence or prevalence of seizure activity or epilepsy, epidemiologists have made estimates using a variety of sources. Epilepsy is estimated to affect more than 3 million Americans, with the greatest incidence rates occurring during the first year of life and in those 55 years and older (78). African Americans have a higher chance of developing epilepsy than Caucasians; however, it is more common for a Caucasian to have uncontrolled epilepsy (34, 71, 105).

Pathophysiology of Epilepsy

Epilepsy is caused by abnormal brain function. Some suggested causes include head injury, brain damage during or before birth, brain tumors,

genetics, lead poisoning, and infections (meningitis or encephalitis) (208). While the exact physiological cause of epilepsy cannot be determined in the majority of cases, it is important to determine what may be causing the seizures in the individual before designing a treatment plan in order to maximize its effectiveness.

Common Medications Given to Individuals With Epilepsy

See medications table 8.8 near the end of the chapter for a summary of medications given to individuals with epilepsy. These medications are known to have potential side effects such as fatigue, digestive disorder, dizziness, and blurred vision (51, 156, 203). They have also been associated with behavioral changes, depression, and suicidal ideation (156). While these side effects may have serious adverse influences on the ability to perform exercise, it is vital that people never discontinue their medication without notifying their physician or other health care professional, as this could increase seizures and place them at increased risk. The primary issue is to maintain the medication at particular levels in the blood to control seizure activity. If the goals of the exercise conditioning program include loss of body weight, then the medication dosage may need to be adjusted if a side effect is weight gain. However, the supervising physician should always coordinate adjustment of medication levels.

Cases of epilepsy that do not respond to drug treatment are termed intractable, and other treatment options may be attempted, including special diets, complementary therapy, vagus nerve stimulation (VNS), or surgery (15, 125, 229). If a person is diagnosed with underlying brain damage that causes seizures, surgery may be an option (86).

People with epilepsy often suffer from depression or mood disorders caused directly or indirectly by their seizures, in addition to the potential for depression from the antiseizure medications. Depression can also stem from the challenges associated with leading a normal life with epilepsy (106, 156). Further, depression may be initiated by seizure activity caused by damage to the area of the brain that is responsible for emotion (20).

Effects of Exercise in Individuals With Epilepsy

The safety and efficacy of exercise in persons with epilepsy have been demonstrated in two studies from the same research group in Brazil (46, 248). Physiological and electroencephalographic (EEG) responses to acute exhaustive cardiorespiratory treadmill testing in individuals with both juvenile myoclonic epilepsy and temporal lobe epilepsy were compared with those in control cohorts without epilepsy. It was found that people with epilepsy exercised less and had a significantly lower resting metabolic rate and resting oxygen consumption compared to control groups. Individuals with epilepsy also had decreased EEG activity during and following exercise as compared to before exercise. These studies not only demonstrate the positive effect that exercise has on EEG activity, but also highlight the importance of exercise to maintain a healthy BMI in persons with epilepsy due to their lower resting metabolism.

McAuley and colleagues (145) demonstrated the efficacy of a 12-week exercise intervention in persons with epilepsy. Subjects were assigned to either a control group or an exercise intervention group that participated in strength, aerobic, and flexibility training three days per week. Results indicated that exercise did not affect seizure frequency in those with active seizures. Quality of life as well as strength, peak oxygen consumption, aerobic endurance time, and body composition were, however, improved in the exercise group.

Exercise Recommendations for Clients With Epilepsy

Persons with epilepsy have traditionally been discouraged from active participation in programs of exercise training due to the misconception that increased activity may induce seizure activity or increase the frequency of seizures. Actually, exercise-induced seizures are rare, and increased levels of activity have been associated with reduced seizure frequency, with the expected benefits of improvements in cardiovascular and psychological health (8).

The primary concern for the exercise professional when working with a client who has epilepsy is the potential for seizure activity during or following training sessions. As the association of seizures and exercise is very low, training programs for persons with epilepsy are similar to programming recommended for persons without disability (227). Resistance training should begin with one set each of 8 to 10 exercise movements with emphasis on multijoint movements. Training intensity should be progressed from 50% to 60% 1RM (initial loading) to 60% to 85% 1RM, and volume should be increased to three or four weekly sessions as tolerated. Aerobic training should start with one 15-minute session weekly with light to moderate intensity (30% to <60% $\dot{V}O_2$ or heart rate reserve) and should be increased progressively to two or three weekly 30-minute sessions. Program design guidelines for clients with epilepsy are summarized in table 8.8.

Exercise Modifications, Precautions, and Contraindications for Clients With Epilepsy

The Epilepsy Foundation advocates physical activity and exercise. Exercise in most cases does not trigger seizures unless the client is overly fatigued or overheated (8, 192). If this is the case, precautions should be taken to give the client adequate breaks, and exercise should be performed in a cool environment. Otherwise sport participation and exercise are strongly encouraged for those with well-managed epilepsy.

When working with a person who has epilepsy, it is important to know first aid procedures in case a seizure occurs. In most cases, seizures do not last long; they end naturally, and the exercise professional should not try to stop them (or any subsequent movements) (32). Important first aid tips include not putting anything in the victim's mouth, protecting the head from further injury during the seizure, loosening tight-fitting clothing, and securing the area from anything the victim's head might hit. In addition, do not give the

Table 8.8 Program Design Guidelines for Clients With Epilepsy

Type of exercise	Frequency	Intensity	Volume
Resistance training			
Modes of training a. Weight training machines and free weights b. Bodyweight resistance c. Elastic tubing	Begin with one or two sessions per week. Possibly progress to 4 days per week, split routine.	Begin with 8-10 exercises with resistance of 50-60% 1RM, emphasizing multijoint approach. Increase intensity gradually to 60-85% 1RM as tolerated.	Start with one set per exercise of 10-12 reps. Possibly increase to 2-3 sets per exercise. If multiple sets, then have 1-2 min between sets.
Aerobic training			
Modes of training a. Walking b. Cycling c. Rowing d. Arm crank exercise e. Reciprocal press–pull exercise	Begin with one session per week. Progress to 2 or 3 days per week.	Begin with light to moderate intensity of 30% to <60% $\dot{V}O_2$ or heart rate reserve, 55% to <75% MHR, or RPE of 9-13 on Borg 6- to 20-point scale. Increase intensity gradually.	Begin with 15- to 20-min sessions. Gradually increase to 30-min sessions.

References: (227)

victim anything to eat or drink or any medications until the person is fully conscious. After a seizure has occurred, victims tend to be disoriented or tired and describe having a headache. Recovery can take minutes to hours, and the person should be allowed sufficient time to rest before being expected to move.

During tonic–clonic seizures (person loses consciousness, muscles stiffen, and convulsions occur), clients may stop breathing during the tonic phase but are often able to breathe again during the clonic phase. If they do not resume breathing, cardiopulmonary resuscitation (CPR) or rescue breathing should be started immediately. Clients may also vomit and have incontinence during a tonic–clonic seizure. To prevent choking and aid in breathing, positioning the victim on the left side may be beneficial.

The following are reasons to call for emergency medical services during any type of seizure: having difficulty breathing, a seizure lasting longer than 5 minutes, two seizures in a row without regaining of consciousness, and a seizure in water. One should call for emergency medical services also if the person is pregnant or is injured

or has diabetes. A status event (nonstop seizures) is always a medical emergency. Also, seeking further care for individuals who just experienced their first seizure is advisable.

If a person experiences frequent seizures, certain types of exercise, such as lifting free weights and upright treadmill exercises, are contraindicated. It should be up to all clients and their physician or other health care professional to weigh the risk and benefits associated with the expected gains from particular types of exercise against the danger of possibly having a seizure while performing this type of exercise.

Swimming is generally a good form of exercise for persons with epilepsy; however, it can be very dangerous if someone has a seizure or becomes unconscious in the water. To be safe, people with epilepsy should always swim in an area with a lifeguard. Finally, contact sports are potentially dangerous; a participant can hit the head and sustain a concussion, which could trigger a seizure. People with epilepsy should discuss participation in contact sports with their physician or other health care professional before participation is permitted (205).

Epilepsy

Mr. W is a 62-year-old retired firefighter who began experiencing epileptic seizures with no other health-related issues. He reported reduced consciousness in a variety of settings, with concerns regarding safety while driving his car. He also shared that his wife had observed that during conversations he had been tending to ramble on confusedly. He had no history of sustaining a head injury.

Neurological examination revealed that Mr. W had abnormal electrical discharges of the right temporal lobe of his brain. Magnetic resonance imaging findings were negative. Mr. W responded well to the prescription medicine Tegretol, which controlled the seizure activity. Mr. W had been relatively inactive since retiring from the fire department at the age of 58. He was 6 feet (183 cm) tall and weighed 232 (105 kg) pounds. He was aware that he should return to his previous active lifestyle especially as a means to control his body weight. However, he was tentative regarding exercising with epilepsy without supervision or guidance. Mr. W sought out the assistance of an exercise professional with advanced certification in working with persons with special conditions.

The exercise professional gained the approval of the supervising physician to carry out exercise training. The physician cleared Mr. W to exercise based on general recommendations as long as seizure activity was not observed to increase in frequency or severity. Mr. W participated in three weekly exercise sessions, with each session including a cardiovascular training segment, a flexibility segment, and a strengthening segment. The cardiovascular training began with 15-minute treadmill walks, with duration increased gradually to 20- to 30-minute segments of treadmill, stationary biking, or rowing. Flexibility training included 20-second stretches of major muscle groups for one or two sets each. The strengthening segments began with one set of 8 to 12 repetitions of four to eight exercises per session. Training volume was increased gradually to three sets of five to eight repetitions at 70% to 85% 1RM with eight exercises per session.

After 12 weeks of training with the exercise professional, Mr. W had reduced his body weight by 7 pounds (3 kg). He also reported a significantly increased energy level and increased ability to carry out his daily tasks. He did not report any seizure activity since beginning the Tegretol medication and the exercise training.

Recommended Readings

Arida, RA, Cavalheriro, EA, da Silva, AC, and Scorza, FA. Physical activity and epilepsy. *Sports Med* 38(7):607-615, 2008.

Arida, RA, Guimarães de Almeida, AC, Cavalheiro, EA, and Scorza, FA. Experimental and clinical findings from physical exercise as complementary therapy for epilepsy. *Epilepsy Behav* 26:273-278, 2013.

Dubow, JS and Kelly, JP. Epilepsy in sports and recreation. *Sports Med* 33(7):499-516, 2003.

Fountain, NB and May, AC. Epilepsy and athletics. *Clin Sports Med* 22(3):605-616, 2003.

Howard, GM, Radloff, M, and Sevier, TL. Epilepsy and sports participation. *Curr Sports Med Rep* 3(1):15-19, 2004.

CONCLUSION

It is well established that active lifestyles, specifically participation in well-designed exercise programs, provide significant benefits across populations regardless of chronological age, sex, training status, and current health condition. These benefits include important health benefits as well as enhanced functional performance of daily activities. Unfortunately, persons with physical disability or chronic disease are known to be less active than persons without disability or disease (85). The lack of active participation is commonly related to limited background in exercise training in general and specific concerns related to the person's particular disability or disease. People with neurological disorders commonly exhibit characteristics that require condition-specific recommendations for exercise, as well as appropriate precautions and contraindications, in order to experience effective and safe training. This chapter provides an overview of the most common neurological disorders, with discussions of their pathology and pathophysiology, in order to give readers a basic understanding of the unique physiological functioning of persons with the given condition (with emphasis on how this differs from what is seen in the general apparently healthy population). Specific recommendations for exercise activities as well as precautions and contraindications have also been provided for each condition.

Key Terms

aneurysm
ataxia
autonomic dysreflexia
bradykinesia
cerebral palsy
demyelination
diplegia
embolus
epilepsy
exacerbation
flare-up
hemiplegia
hypertonia

multiple sclerosis
muscular dystrophy
myelin
paraplegia
Parkinson's disease
pseudohypertrophy
quadriplegia
remission
seizure
spasticity
stroke
tetraplegia
traumatic brain injury

Study Questions

1. Which of the following is a nonprogressive neurological disorder?

   a. cerebral palsy

   b. multiple sclerosis

   c. Parkinson's disease

   d. muscular dystrophy

2. Which of the following is a symptom of demyelination?

   a. joint pain

   b. persistent bleeding

   c. pseudohypertrophy

   d. reduced muscle coordination

3. A client with cerebral palsy is ambulatory, but walks stiffly with flexed hip and knees in both legs. There is no obvious deficit in upper body coordination. Which form of CP is the client likely suffering from?

    a. ataxic

    b. spastic hemiplegia

    c. athetoid

    d. spastic diplegia

4. Which of the following is true regarding resistance training programming for a client with traumatic brain injury?

    a. Perform only machine exercises, no free weights.

    b. Treadmill walking is preferred to cycling or rowing.

    c. Rest period between sets should be at least 2 to 3 minutes.

    d. There are currently no consistent, specific recommendations for resistance training in TBI patients.

Medications Table 8.1   Common Medications Used to Treat Multiple Sclerosis

Drug class and names	Mechanism of action	Most common side effects	Effects on exercise
Disease-modifying drugs			
interferon β-1a (Avonex, Rebif, Plegridy)	Anti-inflammatory and immunomodulatory effects potentially via inhibition of T-cell activation and proliferation, apoptosis of autoreactive T cells, induction of regulatory T cells, inhibition of leukocyte migration across blood–brain barrier, cytokine modulation, and potential antiviral activity	Associated with injection sites: redness, itching, skin dimpling	Potential for reduced exercise capacity and balance Potential for reduced recovery between training sessions
interferon β-1b (Betaseron, Extavia)	Same as above	Flu-like symptoms: aches, fatigue, fever, chills	Same as above
glatiramer acetate (Copaxone, Glatopa)	Exact mechanisms are unknown but believed to modify immune responses via specific suppressor T cells	Potential for reduced white blood cells with increased risk of infections	Same as above
teriflunomide (Aubagio)	Inhibit synthesis of dihydroorotate dehydrogenase, thereby reducing production of activated T and B lymphocytes	Diarrhea, abnormal liver tests, nausea, and hair loss; potential for liver problems and birth defects	Potential for reduced exercise capacity
natalizumab (Tysabri)	Bind to white blood cells and prevents them from crossing blood–brain barrier and attacking the CNS	Linked with progressive multifocal leukoencephalopathy (PML), a rare viral disease of the brain	Potential for reduced exercise capacity
mitoxantrone (Novantrone)	Chemotherapy that suppresses the immune system; suppresses the production of T cells, B cells, and macrophages; reduces proinflammatory cytokines; inhibits macrophage-mediated myelin degradation	Heart damage, leukemia	Potential for reduced exercise capacity
Corticosteroids			
prednisone (Deltasone), methylprednisolone (Solu-Medrol), dexamethasone (Decadron)	Reduce inflammation of the CNS	High blood glucose levels, depression, anxiety	Potential for reduced exercise capacity
Antispasticity, muscle relaxants			
baclofen (Kemstro, Gablofen, Lioresal)	Inhibit reflexes at the spinal level	Drowsiness, muscle weakness, dizziness, headache, low blood pressure, anxiety, numbness or tingling, digestive discomfort, fever	Potential for reduced exercise capacity, muscle strength, power, and balance
tizanidine (Zanaflex)	Increase presynaptic inhibition of motor neurons	Same as above	Potential for reduced exercise capacity, muscle strength, power, and balance

Drug class and names	Mechanism of action	Most common side effects	Effects on exercise
Sedatives			
diazepam (Valium), clonazepam (Klonopin)	Enhance the inhibitory effects of GABA, supraspinal sedative effects	Drowsiness, sleepiness, reduced coordination, slurred speech, loss of appetite, blurred vision, headache	Potential for reduced exercise capacity, muscle strength, power, and balance
Fatigue-relieving			
amantadine (Symmetrel), modafinil (Provigil), armodafinil (Nuvigil)	The exact mechanism of action of amantadine and modafinal is not known. May be associated with antiviral activity, immune-mediated activity, or an amphetamine-type effect.	Drowsiness, dizziness, blurred vision, nausea, nervousness, trouble sleeping, headache	Potential for reduced exercise capacity, muscle strength, power, and balance
Antidepressants			
fluoxetine (Prozac), sertraline (Zoloft), bupropion (Wellbutrin)	The exact mechanism of action is not known. Believed to be associated with inhibition of serotonin uptake by CNS.	Insomnia, dizziness, drowsiness, fatigue, tremor, nausea, headache, loose stools, dyspepsia, anorexia	Potential for reduced exercise capacity
Bladder control			
oxybutynin (Ditropan), tolterodine (Detrol)	Competitive antagonist of acetylcholine at postganglionic muscarinic receptors	Insomnia, loose stools, dizziness, drowsiness, weakness, sleep problems, dyspepsia, nausea, headache, paresthesia, decreased libido and ejaculation, anorexia	Potential for reduced exercise capacity and body awareness

References: (43, 163, 257)

Medications Table 8.2   Common Medications Used to Treat Parkinson's Disease

Drug class and names	Mechanism of action	Most common side effects	Effects on exercise
levodopa–carbidopa (Sinement)	Levodopa converts to dopamine in the brain. Carbidopa prevents conversion of levodopa into dopamine in the bloodstream, allowing more of it to get to the brain.	Dizziness, light-headedness, nausea, vomiting, sleep problems, headache	Potential for reduced balance and exercise capacity
Dopamine agonists			
pramipexole (Mirapex), ropinirole (Requip)	Activates dopamine receptors to mimic the function of dopamine in the brain	Nausea, hallucinations, sedation including sudden sleepiness and light-headedness due to low blood pressure	Potential for reduced exercise capacity and balance
COMT (catechol-O-methyl transferase) inhibitors			
entacapone (Comtan)	Prolongs the effect of dopamine by blocking breakdown by enzymatic actions	Risk of dyskinesia (involuntary movements), diarrhea	Potential for reduced exercise capacity and balance
MAO-B (monoamine oxidase B) inhibitors			
rasagiline (Azilect), selegiline (Eldepryl, Zelapar)	Reduce breakdown of dopamine in the brain via inhibition of the brain enzyme monozmine oxidase B (MOA-B), which metabolizes brain dopamine	Nausea, insomnia, dry mouth, light-headedness, constipation; confusion and hallucinations can occur in elderly persons with PD	Potential for reduced exercise capacity
amantadine (Symmetrel)	Indirect dopamine-releasing actions and direct stimulation of dopamine receptors	Drowsiness, hallucinations, purple skin mottling, ankle swelling	Potential for reduced exercise capacity
Anticholinergics			
benztropine (Cogentin), trihexyphenidyl (Trihex)	Restore balance of dopamine and acetylcholine in the brain by reducing the amount of acetylcholine	Can impair memory and cognitive processes	Potential for reduced balance and exercise capacity
apomorphine (Apokyn)	Acts as a nonselective dopamine agonist and an agonist of adrenergic receptors	Nausea, vomiting, headache, increased sweating, dizziness, drowsiness, yawning, runny nose, hand or foot swelling, pale skin, flushing	Potential for reduced balance and exercise capacity

References: (43, 186, 256)

Medications Table 8.3   Common Medications Used to Treat Muscular Dystrophy

Drug class and names	Mechanism of action	Most common side effects	Effects on exercise
Corticosteroids			
prednisone (Deltasone), methylprednisolone (Solu-Medrol), dexamethasone (Decadron)	Reduce inflammation of the CNS	High blood glucose levels, depression, anxiety	May limit exercise capacity
ACE inhibitors			
benazepril (Lotensin), captopril (Capoten), enalapril (Vasotec), lisinopril (Prinivil), quinapril (Accupril), ramipril (Altace)	Slow the activity of the enzyme ACE, thereby decreasing the production of angiotensin II and allowing vascular dilation	Cough, elevated blood potassium levels, low blood pressure, dizziness, headache, drowsiness, weakness	Potential for reduced exercise capacity and balance
β-blockers			
acebutolol (Sectral), propranolol (Inderal), atenolol (Tenormin), bisoprolol (Zebeta), metoprolol (Lopressor), nadolol (Corgard), timolol (Blocadren), sotalol (Betapace), nebivolol (Bystolic)	Act as competitive agonists to block receptor sites for epinephrine and norepinephrine	Fatigue, nausea, cold hands, headache, upset stomach, constipation, diarrhea, dizziness, shortness of breath	May significantly limit exercise capacity and balance

References: (43, 141, 261)

Medications Table 8.4 Common Medications Used to Treat Cerebral Palsy

Drug class and names	Mechanism of action	Most common side effects	Effects on exercise
Antispasmodics			
baclofen (Kemstro, Gablofen, Lioresal)	Inhibit reflexes at the spinal level	Drowsiness, muscle weakness, dizziness, headache, low blood pressure, anxiety, numbness or tingling, digestive discomfort, fever	Potential for reduced exercise capacity and balance
tizanidine (Zanaflex)	Increase presynaptic inhibition of motor neurons	Same as above	Potential for reduced exercise capacity and balance
botulinum toxin (Botox)	Block release of acetylcholine from nerve endings	Allergic reactions, rash, itching, muscle stiffness, shortness of breath, diarrhea, stomach pain, loss of appetite, weakness, fever, cough, injection site reactions	Potential for reduced exercise capacity and balance
diazepam (Valium)	Exert the following types of effects: anxiolytic, sedative, muscle relaxant, anticonvulsant, and amnestic	Memory issues, drowsiness, dizziness, muscle weakness, restlessness, nausea, drooling, blurred or double vision, skin rash, loss of libido	Potential for reduced exercise capacity and balance
clonidine (Catapres)	Agonist of alpha-2 adrenergic system	Dry mouth, drowsiness, irritability, mood issues, sleep problems, headache, ear pain, fever, constipation, diarrhea, increased thirst, loss of libido	Potential for reduced exercise capacity and balance
Anticonvulsants			
lamotrigine (Lamictal), oxcarbazepine (Trileptal)	Mechanisms of anticonvulsant effects are unknown; known to inhibit voltage-sensitive sodium channels	Dizziness, tremors, loss of coordination, headache, double or blurred vision, nausea, vomiting, dry mouth, back pain, menstrual irregularities, sleep problems	Potential for reduced exercise capacity and balance
Anticholinergics			
benztropine (Cogentin), trihexyphenidyl (Trihex)	Restore balance of dopamine and acetylcholine in the brain by reducing the amount of acetylcholine	Can impair memory and cognitive processes	Potential for reduced exercise capacity and reduced capacity for independent exercise training

References: (43, 140, 258)

Medications Table 8.5 Common Medications Used by Persons With Traumatic Brain Injuries

Drug class and names	Mechanism of action	Most common side effects	Effects on exercise
Anticonvulsants			
sodium valproate (Depakote), gabapentin (Neurontin), topiramate (Topamax), carbamazepine (Tegretol)	Block voltage-dependent sodium channels and augment brain levels of GABA	Hair loss, amnesia, anorexia, ataxia, confusion, double vision, drowsiness, speech issues, insomnia, nausea, diarrhea, tremor, vomiting, weight gain	Potential for reduced exercise capacity and balance
Antidepressants			
citalopram (Celexa), amitriptyline (Elavil), paroxetine (Paxil), sertraline (Zoloft)	Inhibit the CNS reuptake of serotonin in the brain	Blurred vision, cardiac palpitations, confusion, constipation, dizziness, drowsiness, dry mouth, hypotension, insomnia, numbness, seizures, skin rashes, sweating, tremor, urinary retention	Potential for reduced exercise capacity and balance
Antipsychotics			
quetiapine (Seroquel)	Mechanism not known but proposed as an agonist of dopamine type 2 and serotonin type 2 receptors	Blurred vision, dizziness, dry mouth, dystonia, headache, hypotension, parkinsonism, tremor, urinary retention, weight gain	Potential for reduced exercise capacity and balance
Pain management			
acetaminophen, ibuprofen, naproxen sodium	Inhibit the activity of cyclooxygenase-1 (COX-1) and cyclooxygenase-2 (COX-2) and therefore reduce synthesis of prostaglandins and thromboxanes	Burning sensation, constipation, dizziness, gastrointestinal irritation and bleeding, heartburn, nausea, sedation, tingling, vomiting	Potential for reduced exercise capacity and balance
Motor system medications			
caclofen (Gablofen, Lioresal)	Inhibit reflexes at spinal level	Abdominal cramps, confusion, constipation, depression, diarrhea, dizziness, dyskinesia, euphoria, fatigue, headache, nasal congestion, nausea, psychotic episodes, vomiting	Potential for reduced exercise capacity and balance
tizanidine (Zanaflex)	Increased presynaptic inhibition of motor neurons	Dry mouth, upset stomach, dizziness, drowsiness, fatigue, tiredness, constipation, nausea, headache	
cyclobenzaprine (Amrix)	Mechanism is unknown	Dry mouth, dizziness, fatigue, constipation, nausea, dyspepsia, sleepiness	Potential for reduced exercise capacity and balance
Anti-anxiety			
alprazolam (Xanax), chlordiazepoxide (Librium), clanozepam (Klonopin)	Bind to the gamma subunit of the GABAA receptor, increasing the frequency of channel opening, increasing chloride ion conductance and inhibition of action potentials	Abnormal sleep patterns, sedation, drowsiness, altered cognition, weakness, unsteadiness	Potential for reduced exercise capacity and balance

References: (28, 43, 143)

Medications Table 8.6 Common Medications Used to Treat Stroke

Drug class and names	Mechanism of action	Most common side effects	Effects on exercise
Anticoagulant			
warfarin (Coumadin)	Prevent blood clots from forming and existing clots from getting larger	Nausea, loss of appetite, stomach–abdominal pain, risk of serious bleeding	
Antiplatelet medicines			
aspirin, clopidogrel (Plavix)	Keep platelets in the blood from sticking together	Nausea, upset stomach, stomach pain, diarrhea, rashes, itching	
Angiotensin II receptor blockers (ARBs)			
candesartan (Atacand), eprosartan (Teveten), irbesartan (Avapro), losartan (Cozaar), olmesartan (Benicar), telmisartan (Micardis), valsartan (Diovan)	Act to block type I angiotensin receptors, thereby reducing vasoconstriction	Dizziness, headache, drowsiness, nausea, vomiting, diarrhea, cough, elevated potassium levels, low blood pressure, muscle or bone pain, rashes	Potential for reduced exercise capacity and balance
ACE inhibitors			
benazepril (Lotensin), captopril (Capoten), enalapril (Vasotec), lisinopril (Prinivil), quinapril (Accupril), ramipril (Altace)	Inhibit the production of angiotensin II, a vasoconstrictor that also promotes sodium and water retention	Dizziness, headache, drowsiness, diarrhea, low blood pressure, weakness, cough, rashes	Potential for reduced exercise capacity and balance
β-blockers			
acebutolol (Sectral), propranolol (Inderal), atenolol (Tenormin), bisoprolol (Zebeta), metoprolol (Lopressor), nadolol (Corgard), timolol (Blocadren), sotalol (Betapace), nebivolol (Bystolic)	Block receptor sites for epinephrine and norepinephrine on adrenergic beta receptors of sympathetic nervous system, thereby decreasing descending sympathetic nerve drive	Fatigue, cold hands, headache, upset stomach, constipation, diarrhea, dizziness, shortness of breath	Potential for reduced balance and exercise capacity
Calcium channel blockers			
amlodipine (Norvasc), diltiazem (Cardizem, Dilacor, Tiazac), nicardipine (Cardene), nifedipine (Procardia), nisoldipine (Sular), verapamil (Calan, Verelan)	Interfere with voltage-operated calcium channels in cell membrane, thereby promoting vasodilatory activity	Light-headedness; low blood pressure; slower heart rate; drowsiness; constipation; swelling of feet, ankles, and legs; increased appetite; gastroesophageal reflux disease (GERD)	Potential for reduced exercise capacity and balance
Diuretics			
chlorothiazide (Diuril), chlorthalidone (Thalitone), hydrochlorothiazide (Microzide)	Suppress the sodium chloride cotransporter leading to inhibition of NaCl reabsorption in the distal convoluted tubules of kidneys	Dizziness, light-headedness, blurred vision, loss of appetite, itching, stomach upset, headache, weakness	Potential for reduced exercise capacity and balance
furosemide (Lasix), torasemide (Demadex)	Inhibit the Na+/K+/2Cl– transporter protein in walls of ascending loop of Henle; reabsorption of NaCl	Dizziness, light-headedness, blurred vision	Potential for reduced exercise capacity and balance

Drug class and names	Mechanism of action	Most common side effects	Effects on exercise
Diuretics *(continued)*			
spironolactone (Aldactazide, Aldactone), triamterene (Dyrenium, Dyazide, Maxzide)	Block entry of aldosterone into collecting duct and distal tubule of nephron, thereby preventing retention of sodium and water	Dizziness, light-headedness, loss of appetite, diarrhea, nausea, vomiting, headache, gas, stomach pain, rashes	Potential for reduced exercise capacity and balance
metolazone (Zaroxolyn)	Inhibit sodium reabsorption; increased sodium delivery to distal tubular exchange site produces increased potassium excretion	Dizziness, spinning sensation, drowsiness, tiredness, depression, muscle or joint pain, numbness, tingling, nausea, stomach pain, loss of appetite, diarrhea, constipation, headache, heart palpitations	Potential for reduced exercise capacity and balance

References: (43, 144, 259)

Medications Table 8.7 Common Medications Used With Spinal Cord Injury

Drug class and names	Mechanism of action	Most common side effects	Effects on exercise
Pain management			
Nonsteroidal anti-inflammatory drugs (NSAIDs), acetaminophen, aspirin, ibuprofen, naproxen sodium	Inhibit the activity of cyclooxygenase-1 (COX-1) and cyclooxygenase-2 (COX-2) and therefore reduce synthesis of prostaglandins and thromboxanes	Stomach problems, kidney problems, anemia, dizziness, swelling in legs, abnormal liver blood tests, headaches, heartburn, nausea, easy bruising	Potential for reduced exercise capacity and balance
pregabalin (Lyrica)	The precise mechanism of action for neuropathic pain is not known, but this drug is a GABA analogue that binds to a subunit of voltage-gated calcium channels in the CNS.	Dizziness, sleep disorders, peripheral edema, ataxia, fatigue, weight gain, tremor, blurred or double vision, dry mouth	Potential for reduced exercise capacity and balance
tramadol (Tramal), oxycodone (Percocet), morphine (MS Contin, Morphine Sulphate ER, Kadian), fentanyl (Sublimaze, Actiq, Duragesic, Fentora, Abstral, Lazanda), methadone (Dolophine), codeine	Act on presynaptic receptors to inhibit neurotransmitter release	Constipation, nausea, vomiting, drowsiness, sedation, light-headedness, dizziness, sweating	Potential for reduced exercise capacity and balance
Tricylic drugs			
amitriptyline (Elavil), imipramine (Tofranil), clomipramine (Anafranil), doxepin (Sinequan), nortriptyline (Sensoval), desipramine (Norpramin)	Act as serotonin–norepinephrine reuptake inhibitors (SNRIs), thereby raising neurotransmitter concentrations	Dry mouth, blurred vision, constipation, drowsiness, increased appetite leading to weight gain, orthostatic hypotension, increased sweating	Potential for reduced exercise capacity and balance
Selective serotonin–norepinephrine reuptake inhibitors (SSNRIs)			
desvenlafaxine (Pristiq), duloxetine (Cymbalta), venlafaxine (Effexor), venlafaxine XR (Effexor XR), milnacipran (Savella), levomilnacipran (Fetzima)	Inhibit reuptake of serotonin and norepinephrine	Nausea, dizziness, sweating, tiredness, constipation, insomnia, anxiety, headache, loss of appetite	Potential for reduced exercise capacity and balance
Antispasmodics			
baclofen (Kemstro, Gablofen, Lioresal)	Inhibit reflexes at the spinal level	Drowsiness, muscle weakness, dizziness, headache, low blood pressure, anxiety, numbness or tingling, digestive discomfort, fever	Potential for reduced exercise capacity and balance
tizanidine (Zanaflex)	Increase presynaptic inhibition of motor neurons	Same as above	Potential for reduced exercise capacity and balance
botulinum toxin (Botox)	Block release of acetylcholine from nerve endings	Allergic reactions, rash, itching, muscle stiffness, shortness of breath, diarrhea, stomach pain, loss of appetite, weakness, fever, cough, injection site reactions	Potential for reduced exercise capacity and balance

Drug class and names	Mechanism of action	Most common side effects	Effects on exercise
Antispasmodics			
diazepam (Valium)	Exert the following types of effects: anxiolytic, sedative, muscle relaxant, anticonvulsant, and amnestic	Memory issues, drowsiness, dizziness, muscle weakness, restlessness, nausea, drooling, blurred or double vision, skin rash, loss of libido	Potential for reduced exercise capacity and balance
clonidine (Catapres)	Agonist of alpha-2 adrenergic system	Dry mouth, drowsiness, irritability, mood issues, sleep problems, headache, ear pain, fever, constipation, diarrhea, increased thirst, loss of libido	Potential for reduced exercise capacity and balance
Bladder control			
oxybutynin (Ditropan), tolterodine (Detrol)	Competitive antagonist of acetylcholine at postganglionic muscarinic receptors	Insomnia, loose stools, dizziness, drowsiness, weakness, sleep problems, dyspepsia, nausea, headache, paresthesia, decreased libido and ejaculation, anorexia	Potential for reduced exercise capacity and balance
Autonomic dysreflexia			
sublingual nitrates (Nitrostat)	Form free radical nitric oxide (NO), which activates guanylate cyclase, which increases cyclic GMP resulting in vasodilation	Headache, dizziness, light-headedness, nausea, flushing, tingling under tongue	Potential for reduced exercise capacity and balance
clonidine (Catapres)	Stimulate alpha-adrenoceptors of brain stem, thereby reducing sympathetic outflow	Dizziness, orthostatic hypotension, dry mouth, headache, fatigue, skin reactions, hypotension	Potential for reduced exercise capacity and balance
trimethaphan camsylate (Arfonad)	Inhibit transmission between preganglionic and postganglionic neurons in the autonomic nervous system	Urinary retention, orthostatic hypotension, tachycardia, precipitation of angina, anorexia, nausea, vomiting, dry mouth, extreme weakness, restlessness, vision problems, hives, itching	Potential for reduced exercise capacity and balance
Antidepressants			
fluoxetine (Prozac), sertraline (Zoloft), bupropion (Wellbutrin)	The exact mechanism of action is not known. Believed to be associated with inhibition of serotonin uptake by CNS.	Insomnia, dizziness, drowsiness, fatigue, tremor, nausea, headache, loose stools, dyspepsia, anorexia	Potential for reduced exercise capacity and balance

References: (33, 43, 142)

Medications Table 8.8 Common Medications Used to Treat Epilepsy

Drug class and names	Mechanism of action	Most common side effects	Effects on exercise
Anticonvulsants			
carbamazepine (Carbatrol, Tegretol)	Mechanism of action remains unknown.	Fatigue, vision issues, nausea, dizziness, rash	Potential for reduced exercise capacity and balance
diazepam (Valium), lorazepam (Ativan), clonazepam (Klonopin)	Bind to benzodiazepine receptors, which increase GABA affinity to coupled GABAA receptors, leading to opening of chloride channels and hyperpolarization	Tiredness, unsteady gait, nausea, depression, loss of appetite	Potential for reduced exercise capacity and balance
eslicarbazepine (Aptiom)	Block the voltage-gated sodium channel	Dizziness, nausea, headache, vomiting, fatigue, vertigo, ataxia, blurred vision, tremor	Potential for reduced exercise capacity and balance
lamotrigine (Lamictal)	Inhibit voltage-sensitive sodium channels, calcium channels, or both, leading to release of glutamate and aspartate	Dizziness, insomnia, rashes	Potential for reduced balance
levetiracetam (Keppra)	Bind to a synaptic vesicle glycoprotein, SV2A, and inhibit presynaptic calcium channels, thereby reducing neurotransmitter release	Tiredness, weakness, behavioral issues	Potential for reduced exercise capacity
oxcarbazepine (Oxtellar XR, Trileptal)	Block voltage-sensitive sodium channels	Dizziness, sleepiness, headache, vomiting, double vision, balance issues	Potential for reduced balance
perampanel (Fycompa)	Act as a selective noncompetitive antagonist of AMPA receptors, the major subtype of ionotropic glutamate receptors	Serious effects including irritability, aggression, anger, anxiety, paranoia, euphoria, agitation, altered cognition	Potential for reduced exercise capacity
phenobarbital	Inhibits GABAA postsynaptic receptors leading to synaptic inhibition	Sleepiness, behavioral issues	Potential for reduced exercise capacity
phenytoin (Dilantin)	Block voltage-sensitive sodium channels	Dizziness, fatigue, slurred speech, acne, rash, increased hair growth	Potential for reduced balance
pregabalin (Lyrica)	Reduce release of several neurotransmitters, apparently by binding to alpha-2-delta subunits	Dizziness, sleepiness, dry mouth, blurred vision, edema, weight gain, concentration issues	Potential for reduced exercise capacity and balance
tiagabine (Gabitril)	Block GABA uptake into presynaptic neurons, increasing postsynaptic receptor binding	Dizziness, fatigue, weakness, irritability, confusion	Potential for reduced exercise capacity and balance
topiramate (Topamax)	Block voltage-dependent sodium channels, augment GABA activity, inhibit carbonic anhydrase	Sleepiness, dizziness, speech issues, nervousness, memory and vision issues, weight loss	Potential for reduced exercise capacity and balance
zonisamide (Zonegran)	Block sodium and T-type calcium channels, act as a weak carbonic anhydrase inhibitor	Drowsiness, dizziness, unsteady gait, kidney stones, headache, rashes	Potential for reduced exercise capacity and balance

References: (43, 204, 260)

Cognitive Conditions and Disorders

William J. Kraemer, PhD, CSCS,*D, FNSCA

Brett A. Comstock, PhD, CSCS

James E. Clark, MS, CSCS

After completing this chapter, you will be able to

◆ describe the range of cognitive disorders and their respective etiologies;

◆ recognize the importance of individualization in the exercise prescription process;

◆ discuss the importance of encouragement, fun, and the environment in the exercise setting for people with cognitive disorders; and

◆ explain the difference between dementia and Alzheimer's disease.

Cognitive disorders encompass a wide range of challenges and difficulties, including but not limited to impaired brain function, anxiety and panic disorders, and dementia. This chapter focuses on specific considerations concerning health and fitness maintenance within some current major cognitive disorders. At the outset, it is important to stress that these discussions emphasize the individuals involved rather than the disorders. Thus, one speaks of a young girl with Down syndrome, not a Down syndrome girl. This focus has been a great challenge over the past many years and shows the respect needed for individuals who experience such demands in their lives.

In addition to affecting brain properties before and after birth, many cognitive disorders are accompanied by various motor function impairments. This chapter focuses on those disorders that primarily affect the cognitive abilities of the person but, when appropriate, also addresses motor impairments. These cognitive disorders fall into two primary categories: developmental disorders and neurodegenerative diseases. Within the vast list of diagnosable developmental disorders, the chapter discusses autism spectrum disorder (ASD), Down syndrome (trisomy 21), and intellectual disability (ID). (Please note that even though intellectual disability has been referred to elsewhere and in the literature as *mental retardation*, that terminology is not used in reference to these individuals.) From a similar vast list of diagnosable neurodegenerative diseases, this chapter discusses dementia and Alzheimer's disease. These disorders were primarily chosen on the grounds of previously established impact and the recently noted increasing prevalence and the effect on individuals within the general population of the United States.

While reading this chapter, it is important to keep in mind that each of these disorders has varying levels of manifestations and subsequent cognitive and physical disabilities. This variation of presentation is based on severity of the disorder and individual differences within populations of those who are affected. Each of these disorders is individually presented, with useful information concerning implementation of exercise programs for the persons involved. The necessary background information about each disorder is provided, including a summary of the disorder, etiology and epidemiology, a review of benefits that can be derived from utilization of exercise, and finally general recommendations for exercise prescription that should be used in training. It is important to note that within the context of exercise and its various positive benefits, information concerning some of these cognitive disorders is limited. The authors used the best available data to make recommendations, yet a great deal of future study is needed and could provide significant benefit to individuals and practitioners within these populations.

In the United States, according to the Centers for Disease Control and Prevention, there is greater risk for obesity in children and adults with mobility issues or learning or intellectual disabilities than in individuals who do not have a chronic condition (9, 19, 29). In many cases this includes children and adults with cognitive disorders. This may be manifested by decreased opportunities for physical activity as recess and gym class are taken out of school curriculums; other factors include decreases in physical activity as age increases and a meteoric increase in sedentary pursuits. Poor food choices, poor economic conditions, and a lack of cognitive understanding can also be major contributors to the obesity epidemic in such populations. Individuals with cognitive disorders may be more vulnerable to these issues due to even fewer opportunities for regular physical activity. This is also true for children outside of a school setting, in part due to the needed supervision and instruction by qualified professionals, which can make all the difference when available (37, 68). Other factors affecting opportunities for physical activity include the previously mentioned shortage of knowledge on how to individualize an exercise program, as well as the common practice of "preoccupying" individuals with movies, TV, or other technology (56). However, a real concern is the volunteering of well-meaning adults trying to take the place of trained professionals in providing exercise and sport-related activities.

GENERAL EXERCISE CONSIDERATIONS FOR CLIENTS WITH COGNITIVE DISORDERS

Before presenting general exercise recommendations for working with persons who have special needs and then the individual disorders and accompanying considerations for exercise, it is appropriate to discuss general considerations appropriate for all of the cognitive disorders within this chapter. These considerations focus on individualization of training session design to allow for the person to tolerate and consistently complete workouts. While beyond the scope of this chapter, considerations for proper nutrition and hydration are vital for optimal exercise and adaptive changes. In addition, the program needs to account for the client's ability to learn and safely execute the exercises, as matching abilities and program design is vital from a motor learning perspective. In other words, everyone may not learn a movement or skill in the same manner (e.g., with the exercise professional showing the movement and expecting the client to replicate it). This approach assumes that all neural brain functioning, from vision imaging to spatial movement replication, is possible.

The ability to tolerate exercise is typically diminished based on the unique characteristics of each of the disorders, but four considerations will guide the recommendations for each population. These considerations are related to individualization, use of machines when beginning resistance training, progressive overload during resistance training, and the use of aerobic endurance exercise.

Individualization is the first general consideration and should be central to the total program design. This modification needs to take into account not only the cognitive disabilities in the client but also any anatomic limitations to exercise. By considering cognitive and biomechanical characteristics of the client, one can design an exercise program to allow the person to be able to tolerate the metabolic demand of the training session. Tolerance is developed through exercise

selection, as well as through the implementation of varying lengths of rest between sets of each exercise and rest between exercises within a training session. The selection of exercise should focus on all major muscle groups of the body within each exercise session. This exercise selection should also use a progressive pattern of periodization over the length of the training program, while rest time should be at least 2 to 3 minutes in length but ultimately is based on the client's tolerance for the exercise itself.

Key Point

To individualize exercise programs for people with cognitive disabilities, exercise professionals should consider not only the cognitive abilities of the client but also any anatomic limitations to exercise.

Although free weights may be ideal for many populations, cognitive, anatomic, and biomechanical issues may limit their effectiveness for special populations. The second general consideration is that the use of weight machines should be a starting point for the choice of exercise equipment when one is beginning a resistance training program with clients who have cognitive disabilities (figure 9.1). Learning can be made easier because the client can be "locked" into a set pattern of movement that can be safely and easily replicated throughout a workout session. The benefits of using machines when training these populations are valid only if care is taken to "fit" the piece of equipment to the client and the movement. Thus, one can progress to heavier resistance more quickly due to fewer demands on the motor capabilities needed to learn the exercise movement, as well as coordination. In addition, adequate amounts of time should be taken for progression of the program, with special attention to motor capabilities within the exercise movements as well as the metabolic demands of each exercise. The proper use of machines for these clients will allow for an improvement of strength within primary patterns of movement and can allow for the client to work toward an increased workload (a hallmark of a progressive resistance training program).

Additionally, increase in the person's strength may lead to a carryover of strength to other patterns of movement, allowing for improved functionality and independence of the person throughout everyday life. Variations of free weight and machine exercises can be found in a number of books, for example, *Strength Training for Young Athletes, Second Edition,* or *Designing Resistance Training Programs, Fourth Edition* (31, 32).

The third general consideration is that the resistance training program should be a progressive program, with additional levels of resistance or increase of exercise intensity used to meet an increased tolerance of the metabolic demand of the workout. This progression typically starts with one set and later expands to two or three sets per exercise using a varied range of 8 to 12 repetitions in a periodized format. The progressive resistance training program needs to take into account the ability to tolerate the metabolic demands of the exercise program before adding either repetitions, sets, or amount of resistance. Additionally, the progression of the resistance training program should take into account the need or requirement for individual supervision of each exercise session and the total number of persons needed to supervise the client or group of clients.

The last general consideration addresses aerobic endurance exercise. Much like the limitations noted regarding resistance training are limitations related to aerobic endurance training. Because of the cognitive, anatomic, and biomechanical limitations that persons with these disorders exhibit, a general rule of thumb is that use of standard aerobic endurance training equipment may not be the best choice. Long-duration, repetitive activities may not suit the client's preferences and could create negative attitudes toward this type of exercise. Instead, the creative use of various alternative physical activities, such as dancing to music, swimming, or water aerobics, may allow for greater tolerance to the exercise. As a function of being more enjoyable, the use of alternatives may lead to completion of more aerobic endurance exercise sessions, although this is speculation deserving of further study.

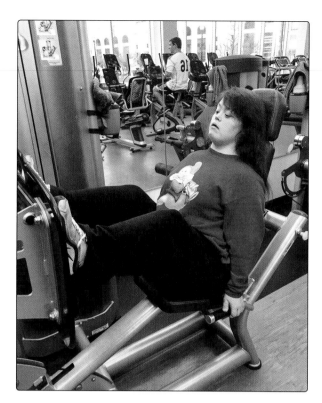

Figure 9.1 Machine exercises can be used to stabilize the exercise movement to help strengthen body parts, and they require little if any balance or motor coordination. Even if balance and functional skills are not developed, complementary exercises based on each client's motor capabilities should be used in the choice of exercises. Weight machines can be used for strengthening when free weight exercises demand too much skill and coordination.

© William Kraemer

EXERCISE RECOMMENDATIONS FOR CLIENTS WITH COGNITIVE CONDITIONS AND DISORDERS

There are few specific recommendations for exercise in persons with cognitive disorders due to limited controlled studies in this area. For context of what is usually done when working with clients who have special needs, exercise professionals can consult the general guidelines adopted by the U.S. Department of Health and Human Services (DHHS) (72) for developing exercise workouts and programs for healthy adults. However, the actual exercise prescription must be individualized and the exercise progression tolerated for successful development of health, fitness, and function. Exercise prescriptions need to be carefully monitored when one is working with diverse clients who have various cognitive and intellectual challenges. In cases in which the general recommendations are unattainable due to limitations, a lower frequency or intensity (or both) can be selected.

Clients with cognitive conditions and disorders should begin their aerobic training program by performing one or two 10- to 20-minute sessions a week at a light to moderate intensity (30% to <60% $\dot{V}O_2$ or heart rate reserve). As a person progresses, he or she can strive to meet the DHHS recommendations of at least 150 minutes of moderate-intensity (40% to <60% $\dot{V}O_2$ or heart rate reserve) aerobic exercise per week (72). This can be attained with 30 to 60 minutes of moderate-intensity exercise (five days per week) or 20 to 60 minutes of vigorous-intensity ($\geq$60%-90% $\dot{V}O_2$ or heart rate reserve) exercise (three days per week).

For resistance exercise it is recommended that clients train each major muscle group two or three days each week, and that using very light or light intensity is best for older persons or previously sedentary adults starting exercise, with two to four sets of each exercise to help adults improve strength and power. These exercise recommendations are appropriate as guidance for exercise programming for clients with cognitive disorders. The response to exercise acutely and over time does not vary dramatically due to a cognitive condition.

Proper progression in a periodized format from a base program starting at one set of 8 to 12 repetitions with regard to resistance and sets can be implemented as fitness levels increase. Also, if the recommended duration of a single exercise bout is not tolerable, enjoyable, or practical, then accumulating these amounts throughout the day is permitted. This flexibility is a necessity, as any opportunity for physical activity within these populations is far more beneficial to health and quality of life than acquiescing to the trend of an increasingly sedentary existence. Program design guidelines for clients with cognitive conditions and disorders are summarized in table 9.1.

Table 9.1   Program Design Guidelines for Clients With Cognitive Conditions and Disorders

Type of exercise	Frequency	Intensity	Volume
Resistance training			
Modes of training a. Weight training machines and free weights b. Bodyweight resistance c. Elastic tubing	Begin with one or two sessions per week Increase to two or three weekly sessions as tolerated	Begin with very light to light intensity and slowly and progressively increase to 8-10RM Recovery periods of 2-4 min	Start with 1 set per exercise of 8-12 reps and increase to 2-4 sets per exercise as appropriate If multiple sets, then rest 1-2 min between sets
Aerobic training			
Modes of training a. Treadmill walking b. Cycling c. Arm and leg cycling d. Rowing e. Aquatic exercise f. Aerobic dance	Begin with one session per week	Begin with light to moderate intensity (30% to <60% $\dot{V}O_2$ or heart rate reserve)	Begin with 10- to 20-min sessions
	PROGRESS TO		
	Five sessions/week OR Three sessions/week	Moderate intensity (40% to <60% $\dot{V}O_2$ or heart rate reserve) OR Vigorous intensity ($\geq$60%-90% $\dot{V}O_2$ or heart rate reserve)	30- to 60-min/session OR 20- to 60-min/session

AUTISM SPECTRUM DISORDER

Autism spectrum disorder (ASD) is a complex group of conditions that are behaviorally defined and have multiple etiologies with varying levels of severity (33). This group of disorders is characterized by deficits in social communication and social interaction and restrictive repetitive behaviors, interests, and activities. These include sensitivity to sensory stimuli of all kinds (taste, touch, smell, sound, and sight); stereotyped behaviors, including various physical actions like body rocking, hand clapping, and echolalia or repetitive vocalizations; obsession with an object or topic of interest; and an insistence on sameness.

Pathology of Autism Spectrum Disorder

The conditions included in ASD are pervasive developmental disorder—not otherwise specified (PDD-NOS), childhood disintegrative disorder (CDD), Asperger's syndrome, and classical autism (6). **Classical autism** can be either mildly severe (high functioning) or very severe (low functioning) (33). Individuals with **Asperger's syndrome** mainly have detriments in social interaction but have normal to above-average cognitive function. **Childhood disintegrative disorder (CDD)** (also known as Heller's syndrome) is characterized by a loss of previously acquired language, social skills, and various motor skills. **Pervasive developmental disorder—not otherwise specified (PDD-NOS)** differs from the other conditions in being the most difficult form of ASD to diagnose. Autism spectrum disorders are usually diagnosed anywhere from after the first 14 months to three years of life and persist through adulthood (57). An emerging body of evidence supports the efficacy of early, intense behavioral and cognitive intervention strategies to improve language and social function, which provide the most successful outcomes possible to those diagnosed with ASD (34, 42).

The core deficiencies of ASD are impairments in communication and social interactions, and engagement in repetitive or stereotypic behaviors (39, 53, 61). In addition to these symptoms, other symptoms pertaining to sensory cues are also key players in the behavior of children and adolescents with ASD (39, 42, 57). It is worth noting that children and adolescents with ASD, in some situations, can exhibit outbursts and cause physical harm to themselves or to others. This usually happens if a sudden change is forced upon them, if frustration builds from not being able to communicate properly, or if they have a sensitivity issue with their sensory system (39, 42, 53, 61).

History and Demographics of Autism Spectrum Disorder

The Centers for Disease Control and Prevention (CDC) reported in 2012 that 1 in 68 births in the United States had ASD (21). This represented the fastest-growing disability, as the prevalence increased by 6% to 15% each year from 2002 to 2010. It is estimated that 3.5 million people live in the United States with ASD, with a greater rate in boys (1 in 42) compared with girls (1 in 189) (16).

The numbers of ASD diagnoses are undeniably on the rise from past estimates. However, it is unclear how much of this increase is due to a true increase in prevalence or to a broadening of the diagnostic criteria. When assessing whether or not a child has ASD, medical and allied health (i.e., psychologists) professionals consult the diagnostic criteria set forth by the *Diagnostic and Statistical Manual of Mental Disorders: DSM-5* (6), and it should be noted that previous editions did not include Asperger's or PDD-NOS with ASD (4, 5, 7). With these two disorders included in the ASD diagnosis, there is a good chance that prevalence rates are on the rise because populations are being accounted for that have not previously been included in the estimates (33, 34, 61). In addition to the inclusion of the spectrum of disorders, the increase in prevalence may be in part due to the increase in public awareness of ASD (33, 34, 61).

Pathophysiology of Autism Spectrum Disorder

Children and adolescents with and without ASD are more likely to be overweight or obese due to the trend of decreasing physical activity as age increases (26, 54). This is most likely attributable to decreased opportunities for physical activity as recess and gym class are taken out of school curriculums and sedentary pursuits increase. Children and adolescents with ASD are susceptible to this same trend; however, they may be more vulnerable to it because of the small number of opportunities for physical activity outside of school, a shortage of programs tailored to their needs, and the common practice of preoccupying them with movies, TV, or other media (54).

Common Medications Given to Individuals With Autism Spectrum Disorder

It is important to understand that there are no medications that can cure ASD or even treat the main symptoms of ASD. Medications are used to help some people deal with some of the related symptoms (e.g., to help manage high energy levels, the inability to focus, depression, or seizures) (51). The two main categories of medications used include selective serotonin reuptake inhibitors (SSRIs) and antipsychotic agents. The SSRIs, such as citalopram, fluoxetine, and sertraline, are used to address depression, anxiety, and obsessive behaviors. Side effects of these medications can include insomnia, increased agitation, and weight gain. Persons with ASD may also be prescribed antipsychotic medications such as haloperidol, risperidone, or thioridazine. These medications alter effects of brain chemicals and have been shown, in many cases, to reduce aggressive or self-harming behavior. Antipsychotic medications can have side effects such as sleepiness, tremors, and weight gain.

Effects of Exercise in Individuals With Autism Spectrum Disorder

The benefits of regular physical activity are well documented, and seemingly, the overall effects of exercise are no different for individuals with and without ASD (8, 44, 55, 66).

These effects include increased cardiovascular health, increased lean body mass, decreased adiposity, weight control, increased strength, increased balance and coordination, decreased risk of musculoskeletal injury, increased cognitive function, and decreased risk factors for cardiovascular disease (i.e., obesity and overweight), among others. In children with ASD, exercise has been shown to have positive effects. For instance, cognitive function and time spent doing learning activities improve in children and adolescents with ASD after an exercise bout. The major cause of this increase in cognitive function is the decrease in stereotypic behaviors (40, 60) that occurs in a dose–response relationship. This results in greater academic engagement because increased physical activity leads to decreased anxiety and stress reactivity (40, 60). It has also been shown that multiple exercise bouts and vigorous intensity produce greater and longer-lasting reductions in stereotypic behavior in this population (40).

In the general population, there exists a trend for adolescents to be more sedentary than children, either due to decreased opportunity for physical activity or because of increased sedentary pursuits (54). Children and adolescents with ASD are not apart from this trend (10, 26). Being habitually active can lead to increased weight control, which can decrease the risk of health problems associated with inactivity, such as hypertension, obesity, and diabetes. Since a trend of these health concerns exists in this population, increasing the amount of physical activity in youth with ASD should be a primary goal for health, wellness, and medical professionals.

Training Considerations for Clients With Autism Spectrum Disorder

Based on the available evidence with this population, the following recommendations might be a starting point for an exercise training program (43). It is recommended that exercise training with persons with ASD include a variety of activities that are enjoyable and developmentally appropriate for the client based on a behavioral model for teaching. Many exercises are difficult to perform, from basic jumping to walking, pulling, pushing, and so on, due to ASD. Thus, each workout program must be developed within the scope of the client's ability to progress. However, the option is open for use of all the typical activities if they can be properly taught by the exercise professional and achieved by the client challenged with ASD.

A basic progressive resistance training program for persons with ASD may be initiated with one set each of several movements for 8 to 12 repetitions per set. If possible and with time, up to three sets may be performed using a varied program with different intensities from 8 to 12 repetitions in a periodized format. Two or three exercise sessions should be performed per week. Tolerance of the workout will be determined by progressive addition of sets for a particular muscle group; however, not all exercises need to be performed for the same number of sets in a workout.

Exercise should be performed with moderate intensity (physical activity that noticeably increases breathing, sweating, and heart rate) to vigorous intensity (physical activity that substantially increases breathing, sweating, and heart rate), with the understanding that gaining intensity in an exercise may be challenging. The progression should be matched with behavioral strategies to pique and maintain interest. Thus, the exercise programming for someone with ASD should be creatively and individually prescribed. The initial recommendation is to include 20 to 30 minutes of moderate-intensity aerobic activity accumulated over the day for three days a week (66). The activity can also incorporate several different modalities to maintain interest and enjoyment.

The rest periods used should allow for complete recovery between sets, as too short a rest period increases physiological stress. This has to be interfaced with behavioral learning approaches as well. Typically, 2 to 3 minutes between sets and exercises is a starting point to make sure the client can tolerate the exercise (e.g., showing no signs of nausea or dizziness and ready to take on the next set or exercise without extreme fatigue).

Many clients with ASD have significant gait and posture disorders, and exercise activities may not be of obvious interest, thus requiring behavioral modifications in teaching.

Verbal exchanges between an instructor and a youth with ASD should be emotionally neutral (no up and down intonations), free of jargon, and free of sarcasm and rhetoric (63, 75) so as to make communication no more difficult than it already is for youths with ASD. This will minimize frustration and distraction during conversations, which can lessen the possibility of outbursts and potentially increase learning ability (63, 75). To further minimize the sensory stimulation, the room and clothing should be kept as neutral as possible as well (75).

Key Point

When working with clients with ASD, it is ideal if the environment (room, clothing, music) and verbal exchanges are kept as neutral as possible. Verbal exchanges should be emotionally neutral and free of jargon, sarcasm, and rhetoric.

Case Study

Autism Spectrum Disorder

Maria is an exercise professional at the local health club, which has started to provide classes for special populations, including ASD, to help with basic fitness and strength development. She has a solid understanding of exercise training and holds appropriate certification for generalized fitness training (Certified Personal Trainer) and an advanced certification for exercise training of special populations (Certified Special Population Specialist).

Laura is a 15-year-old female with ASD and has the expected gross motor imbalances and posture issues. Coach Maria anticipates that it may be difficult to teach the leg press movement, as it may not be seen by Laura as interesting or fun; she may rather do some other activity that catches her attention, such as bouncing on the big pink Swiss ball. Using a behavioral strategy, Coach Maria has explained to Laura that once she completes a set of leg press exercises she can then bounce on the pink Swiss ball. Pairing the leg press—or for that matter any weight training exercise—with another activity that Laura liked proved to be an effective way to motivate and engage her with a basic workout. Coach Maria's goal was to teach the exercise so that Laura could do a set of 10 repetitions with a light load to begin with over the first several weeks. Coach Maria will look for other activities Laura might find interesting in the weight room to serve as a behavioral pairing with another exercise.

Coach Maria also knows that verbal praise for the exact thing Laura did correctly with the exercise is vital and knows not to use general praise like "Good going, way to go" but rather "Great job pushing the weight up with your legs." She knows that depending on Laura's cognitive capabilities, getting her set in the seated leg press machine and showing her how to grab the handles and then push out with her legs is not simple. Coach Maria also knows that when she practices the movement with Laura with no load she may need to help by guiding her leg movement with her hands so Laura feels the correct movement. However, as with coaching any client, it is important for the coach to ask if it is okay to touch the client and to explain why before doing so. In the case of Laura, since she is 15 years old, it is also important to discuss this with her parents to ensure that they provide consent before any training is initiated. As Laura learns the exercise, prompts can be gradually withdrawn so she can complete the activity independently. Once the exercise is taught and other exercises are progressively added to the workout routine, gradual loading can be added, making sure that the exercise techniques are correct and that the toleration of the movement is acceptable. Again, Coach Maria knows that verbal encouragement and careful observation as to acceptability and effectiveness of the reward pairing need to be constantly assessed.

Recommended Readings

Autism Speaks. Sports, exercise, and the benefits of physical activity for individuals with autism. 2009. www.autismspeaks.org/science/science-news/sports-exercise-and-benefits-physical-activity-individuals-autism. Accessed November 29, 2016.

Lochbaum, MR and Crews, DJ. Exercise prescription for autistic populations. *J Autism Dev Disord* 25:335-336, 1995.

Pardo, CA and Eberhart, CG. The neurobiology of autism. *Brain Pathol* 17:434-447, 2007.

Zhang, J and Griffin, AI. Including children with autism in general physical eduation: eight possible solutions. *JOPERD* 78:33-50, 2007.

DOWN SYNDROME

Down syndrome (DS) is a genetic disorder that results in a trisomy (three copies) of the 21st human chromosome (52). The fundamental basis is that individuals with DS have 47 chromosomes instead of the usual 46. This third chromosome, which constitutes the genotype of the individual, can have highly varied effects on expression of the phenotype of an individual characteristic (e.g., heart structure, cognitive capabilities, and other pathologies). There are cases of very rare forms of DS (less than 6%) called Translocation Down syndrome or Mosaic Down syndrome in which not all of the chromosome is triplicated or not all cells of the body carry the extra chromosome. The distinctive facial look, such as flat face and slanting eyes, and delays in growth are characteristic of DS.

Down syndrome can be associated with delays in growth and lower cognitive and intellectual capabilities. The range is wide, with some individuals having very low IQs and others much higher (35). Interestingly, the average reported IQ of those with DS has increased in the past few years. The average IQ of an adult with DS is approximately 50, with about 40% in the mild intellectual disability range of 50 to 70. An IQ of

50 matches the mental age of an 8- to 9-year-old, and average IQ in the general adult population ranges from 70 to 130. Recently it has been shown that DS can be combined with ASD, complicating many aspects of behavioral and developmental capabilities. Down syndrome is not curable and is not related to race, nationality, religion, or socioeconomic status.

Pathology of Down Syndrome

The most common origin of the genetic causes of DS occurs during the formation of the egg (meiosis of the gamete) within the ovary (74). Although there is some debate over the cause of the development of the trisomy, the only established relationships between the mother and a child with DS are advanced age of the mother (>35 years old) and a younger mother who is a heavy smoker (13). Interestingly, since there are more births among younger women, 80% of newborns with DS in the United States are born to mothers under 35 years old (17). As already noted, individuals with DS have a wide range of symptoms from mild to severe, including delays in both mental and physical development (13, 28, 74).

Demographics of Down Syndrome

According to the CDC, approximately one in every 700 babies in the United States is born with DS (i.e., almost 6,000 babies per year), making DS the most commonly diagnosed chromosomal condition in the United States (27). Some epidemiological evidence has indicated that DS is one of the most commonly identified causes for developmental delay in children (74).

Pathophysiology of Down Syndrome

Characteristics of individuals with DS include a delay in mental maturation (see section on intellectual disability); muscle weakness (hypotonia); short stature; cardiac anomalies; flat face profile with short and low-set ears and upslanting of the palpebral fissures that is accompanied by a protruding, broad, and furrowed tongue; curved fifth finger and a single palmar crease; and a gap between the hallux and the second toe (74). These characteristics of individuals with DS often lead to difficulties with early childhood motor patterns and learning of both generalized social and self-care skills (see section on intellectual disability) throughout childhood and into adulthood (74).

Common Medications Given to Individuals With Down Syndrome

There is no drug treatment for DS itself; however, individual care by a physician or other health care professional who understands the syndrome is vital, as other conditions such as dementia, epilepsy, and mental health issues have been associated with DS, particularly in children (50). A variety of supplements (i.e., amino acids and antioxidants) and pharmaceutical interventions (e.g., drugs that affect brain activity) have been used, but they have largely yielded negative, inconclusive, and even some adverse results (50).

Effects of Exercise in Individuals With Down Syndrome

Because of the developmental delay in both mental and physical maturation, the population of individuals with DS presents special cases for the development and design of exercise programs, which can be complicated by additional ASD. Individuals with DS have generalized muscle weakness, poor cardiovascular fitness, impaired motor coordination, and poor exercise economy, which leads to an inability to perform exercise for prolonged periods of time (22, 64). These physical limitations (6, 22, 64) diminish the ability to perform many activities of daily living. To complicate these issues, DS to a certain extent hinders cognitive function in most individuals with the syndrome, which may impede compliance with necessary exercise programs.

Most exercise programs for individuals who have DS focus on increasing cardiovascular fitness and aerobic endurance along with an increase in muscle strength through incorporation of various exercise paradigms (6, 22, 64). By increasing cardiovascular fitness and generalized muscle strength, the person will have increased economy of movement and increased time to fatigue, which will in turn increase functional independence (22, 64). Most of this increase in functional independence is achieved through musculoskeletal adaptations resulting from the incorporation of structured resistance training or aerobic endurance training programs, normally within group or community training settings (6, 22, 64).

Resistance exercise has been shown to be effective in improving leg strength and functional performance (e.g., stair ascent and descent) in adults with DS compared to subjects who did not train over a 10-week period (25). The combination of resistance and aerobic endurance training has also shown aerobic fitness improvements in adults with DS (45). A 12-week program included three sessions per week of aerobic endurance training performed for 30 minutes per session at 65% to 85% of peak oxygen consumption. Additionally, resistance training was performed two days a week and consisted of two rotations in a circuit of nine exercises at a 12-repetition maximum (12 RM) resistance load. Improvements in peak oxygen consumption and walking speed were observed. Thus, resistance training is an important modality to include in an exercise program for individuals with DS.

Exercise Recommendations for Clients With Down Syndrome

The following recommendations are made based on the available evidence for this population; they include aerobic exercise as well as resistance training in programming for clients with DS (45). Although it is important for all individuals, proper drinking behavior before, during, and after exercise is vital to maintain needed hydration levels in people with DS. This is even more important due to potential limitations in the capability of the sweat glands in those with DS to adequately cool the body during exercise. Thus, careful attention to environmental conditions, exercise demands, and symptoms of heat illness is needed.

The aerobic endurance training should use activities such as walking or jogging patterns to assist with independence of the client with DS following training. Walking in most clients without orthopedic issues can serve as an important cardiovascular activity that is effective in maintaining or improving cardiovascular function (14). However, as previously noted, there may be a better choice for aerobic endurance training through the use of dancing to music, swimming, and water aerobics for these clients. Research has shown that music and dance is a universal medium for exercise activities and DS (67) and can provide the external motivation for movement as well as add an important social element to exercise programming. The only concern for such group activities is that some clients with DS have noise sensitivity and may need headsets to dampen the noise to acceptable levels.

It is recommended that exercise programming for persons with DS include three days per week of aerobic endurance training using creative modalities and an interesting environment to stimulate interest. Aerobic training intensity for higher-functioning clients should be 50% to 70% of $\dot{V}O_2$ peak. The duration for aerobic endurance training should be between 15 and 30 minutes per session. This time may be broken into smaller units such that completion of small and easier tasks can be acknowledged through verbal recognition or physical reward for accomplishment of a goal; also psychological encouragement can help the person move toward the next task to be achieved within the exercise session.

Two or three days of resistance training per week are recommended for exercise programming of persons with DS. The resistance program should be designed to enhance muscle strength and function and should include major muscle group exercises to stimulate the body's musculature. Initially standard resistance training exercises can be used, with determinations made on an individual basis, for example, if motor control is of the proficiency needed to use free weights or machines. Loading is also individualized based on understanding and tolerance of the increased load. Again, metabolic intensity needs to be carefully monitored and addressed with rest periods from 2 to 3 minutes between sets and exercises to provide adequate recovery and reduce any symptoms of undue fatigue, as the primary goal is to increase muscular strength. It is recommended that resistance training sessions for clients with DS be no more than 45 minutes in length.

Cognitive learning capabilities related to each exercise movement must be individually assessed.

Motor capabilities for a particular exercise must be kept in mind, and in some cases weight machines can assist in reducing balance and control issues and thereby lead to faster development of strength. Incorporating free weight exercises is important to help develop motor capabilities more related to real-world demands. As previously stated, progression, periodization, and individualization of programs are needed and often can follow the basic concepts of training for younger athletes due to similarities in cognitive function (31). A variety of exercises can be used, including both free weights and machines, but they should address each body part and include some multi-joint exercises.

Exercise Modifications, Precautions, and Contraindications for Clients With Down Syndrome

Because of the cognitive impairments, successful exercise programs for persons with DS have needed to incorporate the following modifications into program designs: a high ratio of instructors to exercise participants and the utilization of various reward programs for participation (64). Secondary to the rewards system is a need to understand that using general guidelines for exercise testing may not apply within this population, as actual $\dot{V}O_2max$ for these clients may be only 80% of predicted $\dot{V}O_2max$; the most likely cause for this discrepancy stems from poor economy of exercise (6, 22, 64). For this reason, it has been recommended that if exercise testing is used, $\dot{V}O_2peak$ should be of greater importance than $\dot{V}O_2 max$ in determining heart rate intensity for training (22).

As with individuals with ASD, one has to work to make sure that the client with DS can learn and mimic the movement patterns of the exercise. Due to limitations in translation of information, one cannot assume that visual demonstration can be replicated. It is important to understand that in DS, informational processing in the brain is different and time delays exist.

Care is needed to monitor potential issues with heat tolerance as DS can affect the normal functioning of sweat glands; thus the environmental challenges and the exercise intensity interactions are important factors to carefully monitor in any exercise program.

Key Point

Exercise professionals should carefully monitor participants for overheating, as some clients with Down syndrome do not sweat as much as the typical population.

Case Study

Down Syndrome

Coach James, an exercise professional, works as a fitness instructor at a tennis club that started offering recreational sessions for children and adults with DS. Each session used courts dedicated to different skill levels and motor capabilities, and accordingly, four groups of clients were created after a period of assessments. The groups reflected the differential abilities of each client to perform basic skills in tennis and the level of motor function each exhibited. An adapted physical education teacher provided "teaching" seminars and educated the tennis coaches who volunteered to work with these special clients. It was clear that not all individuals with DS learn in the same way and that some were much higher functioning than others. But the goal was to encourage activity, movement, socialization, and fun with the sport of tennis.

Having experience with special populations and holding the appropriate professional specialized certifications in strength training, Coach James wanted to add a fitness component to the tennis program for persons with DS. He designed a modified program based in part on the basic circuit weight training program in the tennis club's fitness facility. With the tennis groups already divided based on motor skill functions and learning aptitudes, he knew which of the groups would need additional coaches to help administer the group workouts. In this case he decided he would use the same approach the tennis program used: a coaching buddy for each client during the circuit weight training program.

The first task was to ensure that each exercise station had appropriate equipment (a machine, Swiss ball, or free weight) for each client. Coach James tested each program participant through the circuit individually to determine the appropriate exercise choices and the ability to properly perform the exercises. He noted which exercises presented greater learning challenges to each client (e.g., if someone could not stand with a barbell without having balance issues). Appropriate substitutions or modifications to the equipment were then made. Eventually, the goal was for each coach to take each client through the circuit weight training workout without loading.

Coach James had understood that getting a client ready to do a circuit weight training workout would take practice involving lead-up activities and motivational encouragement to promote and maintain interest in doing the workout. This was a big challenge, and rewards played a role. Once this preparatory phase was completed, the workout started; light or no weights (12 to 15 repetitions) were used to create the first workout. A 2- to 3-minute rest was used between the exercises, and careful monitoring of the clients' tolerance was needed. To begin, only one circuit was performed. Over time some of the major muscle group exercises were progressed to heavier loads in the circuit (6 to 8 repetitions) with rest periods monitored. The coach also varied the circuits for loading and progressively changed the exercises, but was careful to always monitor technique and toleration of each client.

The circuit weight training program followed the tennis practices that included a lot of running and balance activities in the warm-ups. All of the clients took a 20-minute rest and hydration break after the tennis activity before the circuit training workout. As with the indoor tennis session, water and hydration were stressed as being important during and after all activities. The clients with DS all reported that they enjoyed the program and felt that they were "getting in good shape." Eventually Coach James plans to make the circuit training program available for times away from the tennis activity to spread the activity profile over the week. The program would have to provide more available time options and proper supervision to be successful, but Coach James is up to the task to improve the fitness and health of individuals with DS.

Recommended Readings

Cowley, P, Ploutz-Snyder, L, Baynard, T, Heffernan, K, Jae, S, Hsu, S, Lee, M, Pitetti, K, Reiman, M, and Fernhall, B. The effect of progressive resistance training on leg strength, aerobic capacity and functional tasks of daily living in persons with Down syndrome. *Disabil Rehabil* 33:2229-2236, 2011.

Dodd, KJ and Shields, N. A systematic review of the outcomes of cardiovascular exercise programs for people with Down syndrome. *Arch Phys Med Rehabil* 86:2051-2058, 2005.

Li, C, Chen, S, Meng How, Y, and Zhang, AL. Benefits of physical exercise intervention on fitness of individuals with Down syndrome: a systematic review of randomized-controlled trials. *Int J Rehabil Res* 36:187-195, 2013.

Mendonca, G, Pereira, F, and Fernhall, B. Effects of combined aerobic and resistance exercise training in adults with and without Down syndrome. *Arch Phys Med Rehabil* 92:37-45, 2011.

Shields, N, Taylor, N, and Dodd, K. Effects of a community-based progressive resistance training program on muscle performance and physical function in adults with Down syndrome: a randomized controlled trial. *Arch Phys Med Rehabil* 89:1215-1220, 2008.

Stratford, B and Ching, EY. Responses to music and movement in the development of children with Down's syndrome. *J Ment Defic Res* 33:13-24, 1989.

INTELLECTUAL DISABILITY

Intellectual disability (ID), also known as general cognitive disabilities or mental retardation (see note at beginning of chapter), typically develops before a child reaches the age of 18 years (48). Delay in cognitive (mental) maturation is characteristic of ID, resulting in significantly below-average scores on tests of mental ability, or intelligence, and further characterized by limitations in the ability to function in areas of daily life—that is, communication skills, ability to perform activities of self-care, and ability to perform appropriately within social situations including school activities (48).

Pathology of Intellectual Disability

Even though there is a delay in mental maturation, individuals with ID can and do learn new skills; however, they develop these skills at a much slower rate than do children with average intelligence (48). Intellectual disability can be caused by injury, disease, or a brain abnormality during gestation or soon after birth. The following are some of the most common known causes (18):

- Down syndrome
- Fetal alcohol syndrome
- Fragile X syndrome
- Genetic conditions (e.g., cri-du-chat syndrome, Prader-Willi syndrome)
- Infections (e.g., congenital cytomegalovirus)
- Birth defects that affect the brain (e.g., hydrocephalus or cortical atrophy)
- Asphyxia during the birthing process
- Metabolic conditions, such as phenylketonuria (PKU), galactosemia, and congenital hypothyroidism

Demographics of Intellectual Disability

Data from the U.S. Census Bureau (71) indicate that the number of people with disabilities is on the rise, with 56.7 million people having a disability in 2010, an increase of 2.2 million since 2005. Interestingly, despite the increase in disability prevalence, the percentage of people with all impairments remains about the same at 18.7%. Recent statistics indicated that approximately 0.5% of Americans, or about 1.2 million people aged 15 years and older, and 4.5% or 1.7 million children aged 6 to 15 years, had an ID (70, 71). Additionally, 944,000 adults had other developmental disabilities including autism and cerebral palsy.

Pathophysiology of Intellectual Disability

Intellectual disability does not have a singular cause. The mechanisms by which ID manifests are specific to the syndromes that accompany it. Our physiological understanding of these mechanisms is in its relative infancy and is a fertile area of research. Although we have already noted the outcomes of ID in a general way, the causes can be genetic or neurobiological in origin. The proper development of the brain, neurons, and synapses is vital to proper function and cognition. Anatomic malformations and defects in the control of synaptogenesis are underlying causes of many forms of ID. The particulars of the cutting-edge understanding of ID are complex and require in-depth examination, which is somewhat out of the scope of this book, but are discussed by Picker and Walsh (58).

Common Medications Given to Individuals With Intellectual Disability

Any medications prescribed for individuals with ID reflect the growing concept in medicine of a "personalized approach." No cures exist for the multitude of IDs. New drugs are being developed on a continuous and regular basis for specific facets of specific IDs, but exercise therapy is one aspect that has shown promise for improving physical and neurological function. It is important for the professionals who work with special populations to ensure that their participants are cleared by a physician or other health care professional and to be aware of medical aspects that may affect physical exercise and performance. Additionally, musculoskeletal exams are important before activity to ensure that the exercise will not compromise function or safety (e.g., orthotic needs for foot, knee, or spine issues may exist).

Effects of Exercise in Individuals With Intellectual Disability

Individuals with ID are able to achieve health benefits from exercise similar to those for the general population. Research suggests that exercise can temporarily enhance neural activity and cognitive performance in individuals with ID, but the long-term meaning of this enhancement is generally unknown (24, 38, 41). Also, although there are developmental disorders in the brain and its connections, skeletal muscle is usually developed normally (15). Thus, adaptations and benefits of muscular stimulation, along with its downstream effects on different levels of physiological systems, should occur similarly to those for an individual without ID (65). In general, persons with ID have been shown to improve cardiovascular fitness (62, 73), muscular strength (59), balance (69), and quality of life (36). However, it should be noted that there are relatively few controlled studies on the exercise effects in this population. Also, many studies on individuals with ID and exercise include participants with DS, as well as very general exercise regimens. Although this serves as a good foundation, future study designs should use a greater range of ID types and exercise modalities. These modalities should be creative yet safe, should account for individual physical limitations, and should attempt to incorporate traditional exercise modalities and techniques.

Training Considerations for Clients With Intellectual Disability

General training considerations for clients with ID follow the basic principles already discussed with regard to all persons with cognitive disorders, and are similar to those for clients with DS. Exercise prescription for persons with ID should be individualized to meet people's specific needs for different target goals to improve physical function, health, and fitness. The exercise programming should be developed with appreciation of the challenges each client with ID must deal with in everyday life.

Aerobic endurance exercise for persons with ID can be performed three or four days a week using a variety of modalities, from walking to dance, step aerobics, water aerobics, or stationary cycling, with the goal of improving cardiovascular function and health. Resistance training should be based on a progressive program that includes major muscle group exercises to stimulate the body's musculature. As such, resistance training should use multiple sets and should be periodized, with the loading and stress of the workouts adapted to each client's specific challenges and capabilities. Persons with ID should engage in resistance training a minimum of two days a week in order to achieve significant benefits, with three days of training per week for persons capable of the increased training volume.

Exercise Modifications, Precautions, and Contraindications for Clients With Intellectual Disability

Exercise activities for persons with ID should be modified according to the client's particular intellectual capabilities. As basic movement patterns may be limited in association with cognitive limitations, more complicated activities may not be appropriate. Exercise tasks may be simplified in order to allow safe success in the most basic movement patterns, with exercise technique gradually but progressively adjusted in complexity as tolerated. The relatively simplified nature of weight training machines and cycling equipment provides an appropriate initial training option for many persons with ID. Some clients with ID may be capable of incorporating free weight training, which may be more beneficial to the development of strength and transfer to real-life tasks.

Key Point

In work with clients who have intellectual disability, care must be taken to ensure that the person can perform the exercises correctly. Movement patterns may need to be simplified, and the person should be able to perform the movements properly before increasing load or volume.

Determining the ability to perform the exercise movements properly is vital before any loading. The process of learning the correct execution of exercise movements may be enhanced through the use of a part–part–whole teaching process in which more complicated movements are reduced to simpler movement segments. Progressively, the exercise movement segments may be combined to produce complete exercises. Similarly, initial training may consist of one set of a few movements, progressing to multiple sets of the same movements, and potentially progressing to circuit training with the learned movements. Loading, rest periods, and exercise should be balanced to create a tolerable stress and to strengthen muscles with the goal of enhancing locomotion and movements in everyday life. Verbal recognition or physical reward for accomplishment of a goal, as well as psychological encouragement to move toward the next task, should be incorporated into all exercise sessions.

Case Study

Intellectual Disability

Mr. J is a 24-year-old man diagnosed with ID since birth. He lives with his parents and two younger sisters and is employed as a grocery carryout person. Other than his work-related duties, Mr. J had been relatively inactive most of his life. Due to his sedentary lifestyle and appreciation of pizza, his body weight progressively increased to over 275 pounds (125 kg) with a body mass index (BMI) value of 41.8. Mr. J began experiencing low back pain and needed to take frequent breaks at work. Family and friends regularly suggested exercise and diet programs, but Mr. J was not interested.

Mr. J had always been a big sports fan, closely following the local professional and college teams. Recently, he had been invited to participate in the Special Olympics program. After very careful consideration, Mr. J decided that he was interested in bowling and archery (two sports not requiring a great amount of movement). After his first competition, he became very committed to his new sport pursuits, with a new interest in a more active lifestyle. However, he was clear that his interest was in improved sport performance and that he was not concerned with weight loss.

Mr. J's parents had a family membership at the local fitness center and knew that one of the exercise professionals, Rudy, had a specialized certification in training of persons with special conditions. Rudy met with Mr. J and determined that his program should be as independent as possible. Again, Mr. J stressed that he was interested in sport performance for his Special Olympics competitions and "not just working out." The initial exercise program Rudy designed included two sessions per week with both aerobic and anaerobic components. The initial sessions began with comfortable treadmill walking with no incline for 10 minutes, gradually increasing pace and elevation per session for up to 30 minutes. Following the treadmill walking, Mr. J completed a series of eight machine weight training exercises emphasizing large multijoint movements. Resistance was adjusted to allow for one circuit of 8 to 12 repetitions per exercise. The load was increased to two sets per exercise in week 3.

After the first month of training, Mr. J reported virtually no low back pain and increased energy in his workplace. Body weight had decreased only 2 pounds (1 kg) with this first month of exercise training. Rudy met with Mr. J and discussed his progress and goals at this point. Mr. J stated that he was ready to make an increased effort with the goal of significant improvements in the next six months to prepare for a big Special Olympics competition. Together, they revised the training program to include three weekly gym sessions and increased training volume to three circuits of the resistance training series per session. Mr. J agreed that his performance in bowling and archery might improve if he was able to reduce his body weight. Rudy helped him make an appointment with a nutritionist for guidance in that area. Mr. J shared with Rudy that his competitions and training had changed his life and given him an increased sense of his own potential.

Recommended Readings

Bartlo, P and Klein, PJ. Physical activity benefits and needs in adults with intellectual disabilities: systematic review of the literature. *Am J Intellect Dev Disabil* 116:220-232, 2011.

Chapman, DP, Williams, S, Strine, T, Anda, R, and Moore, M. Dementia and its implications for public health. *Prev Chronic Dis* 3:A34, 2006.

Podgorski, C, Kessler, K, Cacia, B, Peterson, D, and Henderson, C. Physical activity intervention for older adults with intellectual disability: report on a pilot project. *Ment Retard* 42:272-283, 2004.

Rimmer, J, Heller, T, Wang, E, and Valerio, I. Improvements in physical fitness in adults with Down syndrome. *Am J Ment Retard* 109:165-174, 2004.

DEMENTIA AND ALZHEIMER'S DISEASE

Dementia is an umbrella term for a collection of symptoms relating to a loss of memory and brain function that interferes with daily life (18). Dementia can be caused by a number of disorders affecting the brain, including Alzheimer's disease and other pathological states such as Huntington's disease, Parkinson's disease, and Creutzfeldt-Jakob disease, or can result from a vascular stroke. It is estimated that over half of cases with dementia are related to Alzheimer's disease (2). A medical diagnosis for dementia occurs only when two or more of the following cognitive functions are significantly impaired without loss of consciousness: memory, language skills, ability to focus attention, reasoning and judgment, and visual perception. Some causes (e.g., vitamin deficiencies, drug interactions) of dementia can be treated and the condition may be reversible. Accurate diagnosis is needed so appropriate treatments can be initiated to mitigate the problems and avoid misdiagnosis. For example, while dementia is frequently thought to be related to Alzheimer's disease, this may not be correct. Without a medical diagnosis, the situation can be confusing, particularly as an individual starts to realize some of the symptoms.

Currently, despite ongoing research every year, Alzheimer's disease is degenerative and incurable. This pathology progressively worsens over time, whereas dementia may be more static. Working with individuals who have Alzheimer's disease or dementia is challenging based on their functional understanding and on how much impairment exists at the time of an initial intervention and over time.

Pathology of Dementia and Alzheimer's Disease

Individuals with cognitive impairments can have significantly impaired intellectual functioning that interferes with normal activities and social relationships, and may eventually lead to a loss of the ability to solve both simple and complex problems and is thereby defined by the National Institutes of Health as dementia (49). The progression of dementia can lead to an inability to maintain emotional control; and individuals may eventually experience various behavioral problems, that is, agitation, delusions, or hallucinations, which over time can develop into personality changes. Although dementia is associated with aging, there is no age delineation regarding when it occurs within the life span (23).

Alzheimer's disease (AD) is an irreversible, progressive brain disease that slowly and progressively destroys memory and thinking skills, eventually including the ability to carry out the simplest tasks (49). This disease is tiered into a tri-level diagnosis (mild, moderate, or severe) that is based on the severity of memory and cognitive difficulties along with a loss of self-care skills that occur over the lifetime. It is known that both younger and older people are at risk for the development of AD; however, the disease usually begins after age 60, and the risk progressively increases with age (23). While there is no definitively known cause for AD, a combination of risk factors and causes for its development appears to be present. These may include a genetic predisposition for the disease (modification of the APOE gene) along with limitation in one or more components of an "active lifestyle" (i.e., being physically active, participating in mentally stimulating activities, and having frequent social interactions) (20). Additionally, there is growing support for associations between the onset of AD and age of the individual, a family history of AD, high blood pressure, high total cholesterol, and a history of diabetes (23).

Demographics of Dementia and Alzheimer's Disease

The prevalence of dementia within the overall population varies with age. There is a 13.5% prevalence in the U.S. population for individuals 80 to 84 years old, 30.8% for those aged 85 to 89 years, 39.5% for those aged 90 to 94 years, and 52.8% for those older than 94 years (23). The percent of new cases of dementia reported per year ranges from 6% for the population from 80 to 84 years up to 20.7% among those over 94 years old.

The development of AD with aging is not typical or normal, albeit the greatest known risk factor for the disease is increased age (most common with 65+ years of age), followed by genetic factors. However, an estimated 5% of people with AD have early-onset Alzheimer's, which is also known as younger-onset disease; this can occur in individuals in their 40s or 50s. The CDC estimates that as many as 5 million Americans have some level of AD. It is further estimated that about 5% of the population between 65 and 74 years old has some level of AD and that nearly half of those aged 85 and older may have the disease (23).

Pathophysiology of Dementia and Alzheimer's Disease

The development and causes of AD are not known but are thought to be associated with neural degradation due to the buildup of proteins by amyloid plaques (between neurons) and neurofibrillary tangles (within neurons). Amyloid plaque builds up when the normal process of breaking down and eliminating amyloid protein fragments is faulty. Alzheimer's disease is also related to neurofibrillary tangles in which tau protein, a critical factor in the integrity of the neural microtubules, degenerates into tangles of filaments. While the accumulation of amyloid plaque and neurofibrillary tangles is part of the normal aging process, with AD the rate of accumulation is much greater, leading to progressive and accelerated decline in cognitive function compared to normal. Oxidative stress, or damage to cellular structures by toxic oxygen molecules called free radicals, is also regarded as a pathology characteristic of AD.

Those who develop AD and dementia tend to have poor lifestyle and general fitness (3). However, there is no known causal relationship between either disease and trained status of the individual. Research indicates that cardiovascular disease and related risk factors increase the risk of dementia and AD. Behavioral and psychological interventions are often used before medications, due to efficacy issues (3). Exercise is among the treatments that can improve dementia or slow its progression, as well as possibly benefitting cognitive function in populations with AD. In general, exercise can improve brain structure and function through improvements in vascular health (for a detailed review, see Tarumi and Zhang, 2014).

Common Medications Given to Individuals With Dementia and Alzheimer's Disease

Currently, there is no cure or means to prevent the progression of AD. However, there are medications commonly prescribed for reduction of symptoms, such as memory loss (49). Cholinesterase inhibitors are prescribed to individuals with AD for symptoms such as memory loss, confusion, and reasoning problems (49). These medications (Aricept, Exelon, Razadyne) slow the breakdown of acetylcholine and have been shown to delay the progression of symptoms for up to a year in approximately half of those with AD (1). Potential side effects of cholinesterase inhibitors include nausea, vomiting, and loss of appetite.

Another class of medication, memantine (Namenda), is generally prescribed to persons with moderate to severe AD for the symptoms related to memory, reasoning, and attention and the performance of simple tasks (46, 49). Memantine regulates glutamine activity and may temporarily slow symptom development. This medication can produce side effects including headaches, confusion, and dizziness (49). Cholinesterase inhibitors and memantine may limit exercise performance primarily in relation to symptoms such as nausea, confusion, and dizziness.

Effects of Exercise in Individuals With Dementia and Alzheimer's Disease

The ability of someone with dementia to safely and effectively participate in exercise activities is affected by where the individual is on the spectrum of the disorder. In the early phases of dementia and AD, more conventional exercises may be realistic, while in later stages, exercise may be achieved only in a wheelchair or in bed. Although exercise has been purported to enhance cognitive function throughout the life span, the specific mechanisms through which this occurs are still a topic of intense investigation. In general, exercise can have conflicting effects on dementia and AD, most likely due to the stage of the disease or the rate of progression. With higher-functioning patients, improvement may occur in executive function, memory, cognitive function, and rating of functional status; but with lower-functioning individuals, little if any change may be detected (47). Additionally, exercise may indirectly affect cognition by improving stress levels and sleep quality, as well as reducing elements of chronic disease that can affect cognitive function (12). Also, specific to the type of exercise performed, improvements in cardiovascular fitness, muscular strength, balance, and other determinants of functional independence can be expected in this population. Studies incorporating specific manipulations of the program variables of intensity, duration, volume, exercise choice, and others should be conducted to elucidate which programs better enhance cognitive function, physical health, and function.

Key Point

In the early phases of dementia and Alzheimer's disease, more conventional exercises may be realistic; but as the conditions progress, significant modifications may be necessary, and the exercise professional may need to consult with the individual's physical therapist, physician, or other health care professional.

Training Considerations for Clients With Dementia or Alzheimer's Disease

Exercise may well improve cognitive and age-related losses in many clients with dementia, yet highly individual variation is to be considered (11). Exercise recommendations for persons with dementia or AD are related to the functional state of the client whether in a home-based program, a specialized nursing care facility, or a hospital program. With early phases of the pathologies, more conventional guidelines and programs with well-established resistance and aerobic exercise components can be applied (30). However, as the conditions progress, many clients with dementia or AD will need significant modifications to this programming. For example, while in some cases group activities may be appropriate, most people require individual implementation with consults from their physical therapist, physician, or other health care professional due to the progressive decline in cognitive function and associated physical capacities. Behavioral issues stemming from anger and agitation may also require creative approaches for maintaining participation. The exercise professional should be prepared to handle any outburst of anger or aggression with the understanding that these are reflections of a disease process and not a personal attack. This may mean having adequate support in the exercise environment or unit to support the calming of the situation, including the known caregiver at certain states of the disease. The loss of memory can make each day a new one that requires repetition of directions, encouragement, and evaluation of status.

Case Study

Alzheimer's Disease

Jayden had been working with a group of patients with Alzheimer's disease at a novel center for aging run by a special unit from the local hospital. Most of the patients were not oriented to their surroundings, and each had differential physical abilities in relation to normal movements. Jayden found that he had to divide his patients into those needing individual exercise therapy and those who could exercise with a group with similar functionalities. He worked with the physical therapist to develop individual stretching and movement programs with light weights and rubber tubing. He regularly needed to answer the same questions relating to the purpose and techniques of the exercise, as many patients had limited recall day to day. Jayden realized that each session was unique to the day, and he knew instruction and explanations would need to differ each day.

Some of the higher-functioning patients walked from 20 to 40 minutes for cardiovascular adaptations, and in other individuals Jayden worked to incorporate activity into the entire day, implementing different exercise breaks so that daily activity totals could be achieved. However, he was aware that for many of his patients in more advanced stages of AD, the early parts of the day were better times to exercise because AD patients can exhibit a condition called "**sundowning**," showing greater agitation and fatigue at the end of the day. Jayden arranged training schedules around these individual factors but generally attempted to provide two or three training sessions per week.

Jayden used the center's fitness facility for patients who could work with the various weight machines and seated exercise bikes. With other patients, he found that flexibility exercises along with light weights and rubber band exercises worked to challenge their muscle function. Jayden was aware that depression could be an issue with some of the patients and always tried to make the exercise process enjoyable, using encouragement, using music they liked, and regularly seeking feedback about what aspects the patients enjoyed. Jayden realized early in the development of his program that individual supervision and individualization of the exercise programs, creation of a fun environment, persistence, and understanding the characteristics of AD would be key to the program's success.

Recommended Readings

Bherer, L, Erickson, KI, and Liu-Ambrose, T. A review of the effects of physical activity and exercise on cognitive and brain functions in older adults. *J Aging Res* 2013:657508, 2013.

Chapman, DP, Williams, S, Strine, T, Anda, R, and Moore, M. Dementia and its implications for public health. *Prev Chronic Dis* 3:A34, 2006.

Eshkoor, S, Hamid, T, Mun, C, and Ng, C. Mild cognitive impairment and its management in older people. *Clin Interv Aging* 10:687-693, 2015.

National Institute on Aging. *Alzheimer's Disease Medications Fact Sheet.* Bethesda, MD: U.S. Department of Health and Human Services, 2016.

Tarumi, T and Zhang, R. Cerebral hemodynamics of the aging brain: risk of Alzheimer disease and benefit of aerobic exercise. *Front Physiol* 5:6, 2014.

PHILOSOPHY OF EXERCISE PROGRAMMING FOR CLIENTS WITH SPECIAL NEEDS

Prescribing a general exercise program to be used by the special populations discussed here without appropriate modifications, precautions, or contraindications would be irresponsible and ineffective, due to each disorder's unique characteristics and wide range of individual symptom presentations. All programs must be individualized and carefully monitored for alterations depending on functional and disease changes, whether they are increasing or decreasing. Some of this variety will affect motor function, while other components address cognitive function without motor impairment. Therefore, the exercise program should be written and implemented so that the client is able to tolerate it. Tolerance of exercise will be dictated by the cognitive, physiological, and biomechanical deficits expressed by the person.

Special consideration is warranted for supervision and monitoring of exercise sessions and workout progression for the client with cognitive disorders. These considerations will ensure that the person can properly execute the exercise, can complete the appropriate number of sets and repetitions, has sufficient rest within the session to complete each workout, and is intrinsically motivated and extrinsically rewarded. The rewards and motivation can be either verbal encouragement or a physical reward for the completion of the exercise, leading to a sense of satisfaction and perhaps a noticeable increase in functionality and independence for the client. Reward systems are their own area of study, and discussions pertaining to these are outside the context of this chapter.

The chapter has emphasized that programs for individuals with cognitive disorders need to be highly adapted to their unique abilities and limitations. Further, getting to know the individual through copious personal interaction should allow the exercise professional to become familiar with the person's mannerisms, personality, and background, because specific home life, environmental, and sensory factors can dictate an individual's attitude and ultimately the success of any exercise program. Additionally, extra caution and patience are in order in dealing with individuals who have cognitive disorders, as frustration may become evident even with simple tasks. One should also consider the sensory sensitivity of some people, especially when they are first learning a movement or activity. Clutter, noise, sunlight, and even shirt logos, no matter how subtle, can cause distractions, particularly for youths with certain conditions (75). Controlling the environment to minimize these distractions can make each session more productive.

Lastly, verbal exchanges between an instructor and clients with a cognitive disorder should be emotionally neutral (no up and down intonations), free of jargon, and absent of sarcasm and rhetoric (63, 75), and should be used in such a way as to make communication no more difficult than it may already be for these clients. By communicating in this way, the exercise professional is able to minimize the distractions and frustrations that can develop during conversations and minimize possibilities for detrimental outbursts, which helps allow for increases in the learning of exercises (60). Additionally, although the evidence is anecdotal, enthusiasm of the instructor during the task is essential (especially with persons who have developmental disorders). Being able to balance the aforementioned considerations regarding ease of communication and enthusiasm is a part of the art of training these clients.

CONCLUSION

Developing exercise programs for people with the wide range of cognitive disorders is highly individual. While standard recommendations for exercise program frequency, intensity, volume, and approach can be used as a marker for what is used in the general population, deviations from these standard recommendations are needed in most cases. Functional limitations and cognitive inhibitions may not allow for the learning and movement capabilities needed to stimulate physiological adaptations to the level of a person without these challenges. The goal should be to provide effective exercise training within the context of fun, with reinforcement of individual progress. New data in neuroscience studies show the importance of even minimal exercise programs like walking on brain development, so having some type of exercise program for people with cognitive disorders is a positive influence in their lives. Optimizing the movement capabilities of each person is the initial goal for every program, and then progressing to

maximize the gains possible for each individual. Thus, the training program of the person with a cognitive disorder should be individually based, with progressive increases of training stressors and complexity according to the person's particular abilities.

Key Terms

Alzheimer's disease
Asperger's syndrome
autism spectrum disorder
childhood disintegrative disorder (CDD)
classical autism
dementia

Down syndrome
intellectual disability
pervasive developmental disorder—not
    otherwise specified (PDD-NOS)
sundowning

Study Questions

1. Which of the following is one reason that weight machines are preferred to free weights for individuals with cognitive disabilities?

    a. There is a wider variety of machine exercises than free weights.

    b. Free weights may be too difficult or intense for these individuals.

    c. Machines can stabilize the body, allowing progressive increases in workload.

    d. Machines are more likely to fit a variety of different body types than free weights.

2. Which of the following aspects of a training program for a mildly autistic child might be contraindicated?

    a. participation in water aerobics

    b. using a variety of aerobic exercises

    c. use of an exercise bike instead of outdoor walking

    d. using a brightly colored and decorated room for workouts

3. Which of the following is the most accurate statement regarding training individuals with Down syndrome?

    a. They are resistant to change, so consistency in programming is very important.

    b. Free weights are contraindicated, due to decreased coordination and safety concerns.

    c. Exercise economy is less than average; therefore shorter bouts may be more effective to prevent fatigue.

    d. Persons with Down syndrome typically have above-average strength and can tolerate moderate to heavy loads early in a training program.

4. Alzheimer's disease is thought to be caused by

    a. vitamin deficiencies

    b. amyloid plaques in the brain

    c. history of brain injury at an early age

    d. cardiovascular disease risk factors such as high blood pressure and cholesterol

10

Cancer

Alejandro F. San Juan, PhD, PT

Steven J. Fleck, PhD, CSCS, FNSCA

Alejandro Lucia, MD, PhD

After completing this chapter, you will be able to

♦ define cancer and the general principles of its staging,

♦ describe the pathophysiology and the treatments for tumoral cells,

♦ recognize the side effects of cancer treatment in each patient and be able to adjust the personal exercise prescription for each patient, and

♦ develop exercise recommendations for cancer patients.

Cancer is a major public health concern worldwide. The term *cancer* is a synonym for **malignant neoplasm** and has eight biological capabilities during the multistep development of human tumors. These capabilities include sustained proliferative signaling, evading growth suppressors, resisting cell death, enabling replicative immortality, inducing angiogenesis, activating invasion and metastasis (occurrence of the cancer at a distant site), reprogramming of energy metabolism, and evading immune destruction (53). Unregulated cell growth without invasion is a feature of benign neoplasms.

PATHOLOGY OF CANCER

Cancer mortality and survival rates have improved over the years (4), and more people are able to successfully return to their daily tasks and improve their quality of life (QoL) after cancer. Physical activity has been demonstrated to play a preventive role in terms of the risk of developing cancer (e.g., breast, colon, prostate, lung, endometrial) (44, 153). But, as discussed throughout this chapter, physical activity is also emerging as a major tool to improve the QoL and survival of patients with cancer.

Untreated cancers cause serious illness and invariably lead to death. The American Cancer Society (4) reports that today, one in four deaths occurring in the United States is due to cancer and that it is the second leading cause of death in the United States after heart disease (it was estimated that 600,000 Americans would die of cancer in 2016). About 1,685,210 new cancer diagnoses were expected in 2016. Moreover, 14.5 million people in the United States with cancer (diagnosed and under treatment or survivors with no current evidence of cancer) were alive in 2014 (4). In the United States, 86% of all cancers are diagnosed in people 50 years of age or older (4). In women, breast (29%), lung and bronchus (13%), and colorectal cancer (8%), were estimated as the most prevalent in 2016. In men, prostate (21%), lung and bronchus (14%), and colorectal cancer (7%) were estimated as the most prevalent in 2016 (4).

Approximately 595,690 deaths due to cancer were expected in 2016. The tumors with the highest number of deaths in both sexes are lung (27%), colorectal (8%), and pancreas cancer (7%) (4). In women, lung and bronchus (26%), breast (14%), and colorectal cancer (8%) had the highest estimated mortality in 2016. Similarly in men, lung (27%), prostate (8%), and colorectal cancer (8%) were estimated as the tumors with the highest number of deaths in 2016 (4). For these main cancer sites (lung, colorectal, breast, and prostate), mortality rates continue to decrease (4).

Cancer is also the second leading cause of death among children between the ages of 1 and 14 years in the United States (4). Leukemia (particularly acute lymphocytic leukemia) is the most common cancer (30%) in children, followed by brain and other central nervous system tumors (26%) (4). The survival rate in children for all types of cancer combined improved from 58% in 1975 through 1997 to 80% for children diagnosed from 1996 to 2003 (114), and it continued to increase to 83% in the most recent time period for which data are available (2005-2011) (4). The American Cancer Society (4) reports that childhood cancers are rare, representing less than 1% of all new cancer diagnoses in the United States. Unfortunately, childhood cancer incidence rates increased slightly, by 0.6% per year, from 1975 until 2016 (4).

PATHOPHYSIOLOGY OF CANCER

Most cancers appear sporadically; others occur more frequently in families that carry a germline mutation in genes that contribute to the development of cancer (42). Inherited cancer syndromes account for only a small percentage of all cancers. The current view is that cancer is a genetic disease that develops in various adult cells (somatic cells) through a series of DNA alterations that lead to uncontrolled cell proliferation (53). Most of these alterations involve changes to the DNA itself, and this is called a **mutation**. For example, mutation occurs due to random DNA replication errors, either spontaneously or due to exposure to carcinogens (e.g., radiation). Other mutations may occur when certain genes whose gene products regulate DNA replication or repair are mutated (e.g., *p53* gene).

SPECIFIC MANAGEMENT AND TREATMENT OF INDIVIDUALS WITH CANCER

The management and treatment of a patient with cancer depend on the type and stage (i.e., how widespread the cancer is) of the cancer. Thus, determining the type and stage of cancer is essential for selecting the treatment that will be most effective. Several classification schemes exist to stage a cancer process. The **TNM (Tumor, Node, Metastasis) system** gives three key pieces of information and is currently the method most commonly used (4):

- T: Reflects the size of the tumor and is ranked as T_0 (no tumor) to T_4 (tumor invasion of a vital organ such as the heart or lungs)
- N: Reflects whether the lymph nodes are affected by the cancer; this factor is scored as N_0 (no invasion of the lymph nodes) to N_3
- M: Reflects the presence or absence of cancer metastasis to other organs of the body and is designated M_0 (no metastasis) or M_1 (metastases present)

For example, a tumor staged as $T_1N_0M_0$ is a very small tumor that has not spread to the lymph nodes or metastasized. Once the TNM descriptors of a given tumor have been defined, they are combined together in an overall stage grouping comprising a simple set of stages (stage 0 to IV). In brief, the lower stage numbers (e.g., stage I) are used to describe a small primary tumor and no metastases, and higher numbers (e.g., stage IV) to describe a cancer that has metastasized, or spread, to other organs or throughout the body.

After receiving treatment for cancer, the patient may undergo a period of remission lasting several weeks to many years, when the cancer is responding to treatment or is under control. When the cancer is characterized as being in complete remission, all signs and symptoms of the disease have disappeared. However, in some patients the tumor is said to be in partial remission; symptoms improve but do not completely disappear. If the cancer returns (known as recurrence or relapse), further treatment often leads to another period of remission (4).

Currently, there are four main types of treatment for cancer: surgery, radiation, chemotherapy, and biological therapies. More than one kind of therapy may be combined to treat cancer.

Radiation therapy is usually a local form of treatment and is targeted only at the area of the tumor so there is little effect elsewhere (4). It uses special equipment to deliver high-energy particles or waves to destroy or damage cancer cells (e.g., x-rays or gamma rays). It prevents the growth and division of the cancer cell by breaking apart the DNA molecule inside the cell. It can be delivered in two ways:

- *External radiation.* A machine delivers a high-energy ray to the cancer site and surrounding tissue. Usually this treatment is given daily (five days a week) for five to eight weeks. The newer machines (e.g., three-dimensional conformal radiation therapy [3D-CRT], intensity-modulated radiation therapy [IMRT]) provoke less damage to surrounding normal tissues and deliver higher doses to the tumor.
- *Internal radiation or brachytherapy.* This type of radiation is delivered in one of two ways:
  - A small container is placed inside the tumor or in the area of the incision after surgery to act as a radioactive source, killing or damaging the tumor cells.
  - Another mode of internal radiation therapy involves the administration of radioactive drugs (radiopharmaceuticals) by mouth or by injection.

Chemotherapy involves delivering chemotherapy drugs into the bloodstream to treat cancer cells that have metastasized to other parts of the body. Chemotherapy treatment may last from several months to even years (i.e., hematologic cancer usually requires chemotherapy treatment for two to three years), and is given in cycles followed by a recovery period (4). Chemotherapy duration depends on different factors including the kind of tumor, tumor phase, patient's tolerance to chemotherapy, and the patient's general condition (4). Chemotherapy can significantly reduce the risk of cancer recurrence after surgery. Chemotherapeutic drugs have many modes of action, including disruption of DNA replication and disruption of normal cellular architecture necessary for cell shape and structure; more recently, drugs target specific enzymatic functions in cancer cells that control growth (called "targeted" therapies) (4).

Biological therapy (which includes immunotherapy, biotherapy, or biological response modifier therapy) uses a variety of large molecules (usually protein molecules) to fight cancer or to lessen the side effects of some cancer treatments (4). This form of treatment usually interferes with cancer cell growth, acts directly to help healthy immune cells control cancer in certain therapies, or helps to repair normal cells damaged by other forms of cancer treatment.

Bone marrow transplantation is another common therapy used to treat blood cancers such as leukemia, Hodgkin lymphoma, and others (4). In this type of treatment, diseased bone marrow is ablated (destroyed) using large doses of chemotherapeutic agents, radiation, or both. The patient's blood-forming system is then replaced with either bone marrow cells from the patient when in remission (autologous bone marrow transplant) or a tissue antigen-matched donor (allogeneic).

Hormonal therapy uses drugs to modify body hormones (e.g., stopping their synthesis, changing their effects on specific cells) with the final objective of blocking the tumoral growth (141). There are some tumors that are hormone dependent; these tumors have hormonal receptors in their cells, and their growth depends on hormones. These types of tumors are termed *hormone receptor positive* and can be treated with hormone therapy. In cancers that are hormone receptor negative, this kind of treatment is not helpful (4). The tumors that are hormone receptor positive are essentially breast and prostate cancer, but there are other cancers that can also be treated with hormonal therapy (e.g., endometrium cancer, neuroendocrine tumors) (141):

- **Breast cancer:** The hormone estrogen increases tumor growth of breast cancers that are hormone receptor positive. Approximately 66% of breast cancers are hormone receptor positive.

These tumors have hormone receptors for estrogen (ER-positive cancers), progesterone (PR-positive cancers), or both. The objective of hormone therapy for breast cancer is to lower estrogen levels as much as possible (4).

- **Prostate cancer:** The androgen hormones (male hormones) increase the tumor growth of prostate cancer. The objective of the hormone therapy for prostate cancer is to lower androgen levels (e.g., testosterone) as much as possible (4). The hormone therapy for prostate cancer is also called androgen deprivation therapy.

Side Effects of Cancer Treatment

Normal healthy cells, tissues, and body functions may be affected by cancer treatment. The side effects suffered by a patient depend on the type of radiation or drugs, the amounts given, and the length of treatment. **Early side effects** are experienced during or shortly after treatment and usually include nausea and vomiting, temporary hair loss, increased chance of infections, fatigue, skin changes, loss of appetite, pain, hemorrhagic and thromboembolic complications, and allergic reactions (4).

Late side effects are those that take months or years to develop, and some are often permanent. Severe side effects include toxicities in many body systems and organs. These toxic effects impair health-related QoL and include hematologic and immune system toxicity (e.g., anemia, leukopenia, lymphocytopenia) (79, 139, 140, 148); cardiovascular toxicity (e.g., high blood pressure, cardiomyopathy) (12, 55, 79, 83, 104, 138); pulmonary toxicity (e.g., pulmonary fibrosis, diminished diffusion capacity, impaired aerobic capacity) (79, 119, 140, 148); musculoskeletal alterations (e.g., muscle weakness, muscle atrophy, diminished range of motion, osteopenia–osteoporosis) (33, 52, 66, 79, 84, 86, 99, 117, 119, 124, 148, 161, 162); gastrointestinal system toxicity (e.g., intestinal fibrosis, ulceration) (79, 139); endocrine toxicity (e.g., alterations to the thyroid, hypothalamus, and pituitary) (79, 86, 139); hepatic toxicity (e.g., hepatocyte necrosis, steatosis) (79, 139); nephrotoxicity (e.g., gout, kidney and bladder abnormalities) (79, 139); and neural toxicity (e.g., pain, impaired gross and fine motor control) (11, 52, 79, 117, 124, 140, 147, 161, 162).

Cancer-Related Fatigue

Cancer-related fatigue is the most common side effect of cancer and cancer treatment. It differs from the normal fatigue of everyday living activities and affects up to 70% of cancer patients during chemo- and radiotherapy and after surgery (31, 79). Patients are usually advised to rest and downregulate their level of activity, but rest does not improve cancer-related fatigue because inactivity promotes muscular catabolism, and extended periods of rest may lead to chronic fatigue (31, 79). Moreover, several researchers have reported that 30% to 50% of cancer survivors claim that their fatigue lasts for months or even years after the end of treatment (79). In severe cases, patients may develop cachexia, or muscle-wasting disease (79).

Key Point

> Many cancer patients experience fatigue during and after treatment. Exercise can reduce muscular deconditioning and break the cycle of fatigue.

Cancer patients characterize fatigue as the most distressing side effect of cancer and its treatment (more distressing than pain, nausea, vomiting, or depression), probably because it seriously impairs a person's QoL (79). The American Cancer Society (4) defines cancer-related fatigue as feeling tired (physically, mentally, and emotionally). It can be caused by the cancer itself or by cancer treatment or other factors, and can last a long time, making the patient's daily living activities difficult. It usually increases in severity as treatment continues.

The causes of cancer-related fatigue are multifactorial (79) and still poorly understood. Anemia, pain, emotional distress (i.e., depression and anxiety), sleep disturbances, nutritional problems, a low level of physical activity, medicines, and other medical problems (e.g., infection, diminished thyroid function, lung disease) are some factors related to cancer or its treatment that may produce fatigue. Many adult patients report fatigue as a physical disturbance and loss of functionality during daily tasks involving physical activity,

such as walking a short distance, climbing a few stairs, or completing household tasks (79). Child patients complain of early fatigue in childhood games with the consequence of feeling frustrated and unhealthy (121, 122). Severe activity-limiting fatigue is caused by extreme muscular deconditioning related both to the illness and treatment and also to sedentary habits (79).

Cancer-related fatigue is mainly caused by the illness itself, the treatment, and inactivity resulting in deconditioning. Moreover, the sedentary habits usually recommended by the biomedical staff and the family to protect the patient may lead to the development of the **self-perpetuating fatigue cycle** (figure 10.1) (79), which results in a higher and higher level of catabolic processes at all levels (i.e., physical, emotional, social). Physical training breaks this downward cycle and diminishes cancer-related fatigue (79). The American Cancer Society (4) recommends physical activity as a major ancillary treatment to break the cycle of self-perpetuating fatigue and to combat fatigue. The **Big Team**—physicians, nurses, social workers, physical therapists, nutritionists, exercise professionals, and psychologists as well as other health care professionals—needs to be involved. The work of the Big Team is a patient necessity because fatigue is often caused by more than one problem, and also because the patient needs the strength of the entire health team to help cope with her particular fatigue. This help must take the form of a treatment prescription tailored to the particular needs of a given patient—for example, treating different patient problems (e.g., sleep disturbances, nutrition problems, anemia, muscle atrophy) with biomedical solutions (e.g., diet, exercise program, blood transfusion, psychological support).

The net balance is that the cumulative effects of the disease, its treatment, and reduced physical activity will have repercussions on the musculoskeletal and cardiorespiratory systems. Thus, the cancer patient and the cancer survivor find that daily activities take much more effort and demand more effort than previously. A number of studies have shown that exercise training improves cancer-related fatigue in adult patients and survivors with the outcome of improved health, well-being, and QoL (15, 28, 30, 32-34,

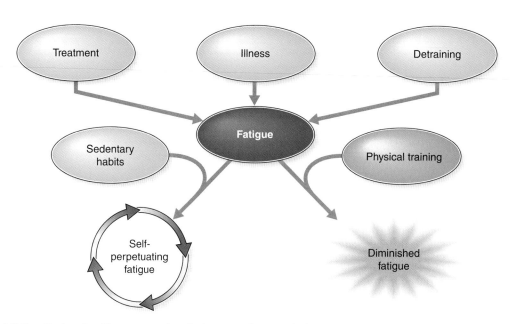

Figure 10.1 Cycle of self-perpetuating fatigue. Sedentary habits can transform cancer-related fatigue into chronic fatigue.

Adapted from *Lancet Oncology*, Vol 4, A. Lucia, C. Earnest, and M. Perez, "Cancer-related fatigue: How can exercise physiology assist oncologists?" pgs. 616-625. Copyright 2003, with permission of Elsevier.

38, 64, 81, 106, 133, 149). Some authors have even reported that exercise can improve the survival rate after diagnosis of breast cancer (65, 103) and prostate cancer (9, 10, 45). The explanation for this could be improved oxygen transport to the muscles, cardiac dynamics, and muscle function (i.e., increased mitochondrial density, improved muscle fiber vascularization, cardiac ejection fraction, muscular efficiency) (79).

Lymphedema

In cancer patients, lymphedema can occur after lymphadenectomy (surgical removal of lymph nodes) or after radiotherapy that affects lymph nodes. Treatment procedures (lymphadenectomy, radiotherapy) produce partial blockage of the lymph system because of a lower number of lymph nodes or a diminished lymph flow or both. These abnormal conditions usually result in accumulation of interstitial fluid and cause inflammation and swelling due to lymph fluid buildup, in turn caused by blockage of the lymph system in the extremities (upper, lower, or both). This pathological dysfunction in the lymphatic system is called **lymphedema**.

Chronic lymphedema in the upper extremities is a common secondary effect in breast cancer, but the incidence data of lymphedema after breast cancer are not consistent (101), possibly due to differences in some study variables (e.g., diagnosis, patient characteristics, inadequate follow-up). These differences in study variables result in the prevalence of arm lymphedema ranging from 8% to 56% at two years postsurgery (85, 98, 108, 143). Lower extremity lymphedema has the highest incidence in uterine cancer, prostate cancer, lymphoma, or melanoma (101), with the highest prevalence (36%) in vulvar cancer survivors (7).

Lymphedema may occur within days and up to 30 years after breast cancer treatment (137). Approximately 80% of women with lymphedema experience its onset within three years after axillary lymph node dissection (ALND) surgery. For women without lymphedema for three years after ALND surgery, the ongoing risk of developing lymphedema is about 1% per year for at least 20 years (109). A recent surgical technique called sentinel lymph node biopsy (SLNB) is used to diminish the prevalence of lymphedema. A sentinel lymph node is the node to which tumor cells are most likely to spread from a primary tumor

(101). It is determined whether postsurgery tumor invasion of the sentinel lymph node is occurring, and if this is not the case, only one lymph node needs to be removed and the risk of lymphedema is lowered. If the sentinel node is invaded, lymphadenectomy usually must be performed, and the risk of lymphedema is increased. Celebioglu and colleagues (18) observed an incidence of lymphedema of 20% in an ANLD group compared with an incidence of 0% in a SLNB group. The rate of breast cancer lymphedema after SLNB ranges from 5% to 17%, depending on the diagnostic threshold and length of follow-up (68, 152), and most lymphedema diagnosed is mild (43).

Breast cancer lymphedema usually affects the ipsilateral hand or arm as a result of dissection and irradiation of the axillary lymph nodes (97). Health care professionals often warn patients that they should avoid intense upper body exercise due to concern about causing lymphedema (71), but to date there are no data to support a link between upper body exercise and breast cancer–related lymphedema (21, 54, 89). In fact, the incidence of upper body limb swelling is similar, the severity of self-reported lymphedema reduced, and the incidence of lymphedema exacerbations lower in breast cancer patients performing resistance training (including upper body resistance training) compared to a control group performing no training (129). The reduction in lymphedema may be due to several physiological changes associated with long-term exercise (i.e., increased sympathetic outflow, increased muscular contractions, increased ventilation) that could favor lymph return to the blood (88) and lymphangiogenesis or recruitment of dormant lymph vessels as possible outcomes of exercise training (76).

COMMON MEDICATIONS GIVEN TO INDIVIDUALS WITH CANCER

As previously discussed, there are four main types of treatment for cancer: surgery, radiation, chemotherapy, and biological therapies. In this section we focus on the most common medications used during cancer treatment and their side effects—first chemotherapy medications and then hormone therapy. See medications table 10.1 near the end of the chapter, which lists the most common medications used to treat cancer, along with those medications' most common side effects and effects on exercise.

Chemotherapy Medications

Tumors are dependent on their own cell reproduction capacity (i.e., to grow, to disseminate), so drugs that interfere with enzyme function or substrate utilization related to DNA synthesis or function can interfere with tumor growth. Chemotherapy drugs are divided into groups differentiated by the mechanism of action that interferes with tumor growth (4, 93, 101).

Alkylating Agents

These drugs work in all phases of the cell division cycle by bonding to DNA nucleotides, preventing the normal processes of replication, gene transcription, and translation. They are used to treat many different cancers (e.g., leukemia, lymphoma, Hodgkin disease, multiple myeloma, sarcoma, lung, breast, ovarian). However, they can produce long-term side effects to bone marrow; and in rare cases, acute leukemia may develop with high doses. Alkylating agents are divided into several types (4):

- Nitrogen mustards (e.g., mechlorethamine, chlorambucil, cyclophosphamide [Cytoxan], ifosfamide, and melphalan)
- Nitrosoureas (e.g., streptozotocin, carmustine [BCNU], lomustine)
- Alkyl sulfonates (e.g., busulfan)
- Triazines (e.g., dacarbazine [DTIC], temozolomide [Temodar])
- Ethylenimines (e.g., thiotepa, altretamine [hexamethylmelamine])
- Platinum drugs: sometimes grouped with alkylating agents because they have the same mechanism of action (e.g., cisplatin, carboplatin, oxaliplatin); these drugs have a lower risk of leukemia development

Antimetabolites

These drugs work during the S phase, when the cell's chromosomes are being copied (4). They block purine and pyrimidine synthesis and distort the normal synthesis of DNA and RNA. They are used to treat many different cancers (e.g., leukemia, breast, ovarian, intestinal tract) and are the drug most used to treat cancer (4): 5-fluorouracil (5-FU), 6-mercaptopurine (6-MP), capecitabine (Xeloda), cytarabine (Ara-C), floxuridine, fludarabine, gemcitabine (Gemzar), hydroxyurea, methotrexate, and pemetrexed (Alimta).

Antitumor Antibiotics

These drugs are different from antibiotics used to treat infections. They function by being interspersed among DNA base pairs, preventing normal function, and block cell growth and multiplication. They are divided into several types (4):

- Anthracyclines: These interfere with enzymes involved in DNA replication and work in all phases of the cell division cycle. They are extensively used to treat most cancers (4). However, they have dangerous side effects because in high doses they can produce permanent heart damage (4). Daunorubicin, doxorubicin (Adriamycin), epirubicin, and idarubicin are the drugs in this class most often used (4).

- Other antitumor antibiotics (not anthracyclines): Actinomycin-D, bleomycin, mitmycin-C, and mitoxantrone work as a toposomerase II inhibitor.

Topoisomerase Inhibitors

These drugs interfere with topoisomerases (enzymes), which help separate the strands of DNA to be copied during the cellular S phase (4). They are used to treat many different cancers (e.g., certain leukemias, lung, ovarian, gastrointestinal) and are divided in two types depending on the enzyme they affect (4):

- Topoisomerase I inhibitors: Topotecan, irinotecan (CPT-11).

- Topoisomerase II inhibitors: May augment the risk of a second cancer (acute myelogenous leukemia [AML]). Etoposide (VP-16), teniposide, and mitoxantrone (also work as an antitumor antibiotic) are the most frequently used of this type of drug (4).

Antimitotic or Mitotic Inhibitors

These drugs interfere with the structure and function of cellular microtubule apparatus. They stop mitosis in the cellular M phase and also can damage cells in all phases of cell replication by slowing enzymes necessary to synthesize proteins needed for cell reproduction (4). They are used to treat many different cancers (e.g., breast, lung, myelomas, lymphomas, leukemias), but may cause nerve damage (4). This class of drugs is divided in many types; these are some examples (4):

- Taxanes: paclitaxel (Taxol) and docetaxel (Taxotere)
- Epothilones: ixabepilone (Ixempra)
- Vinca alkaloids: vinblastine (Velban), vincristine (Oncovin), and vinorelbine (Navelbine)
- Estramustine (Emcyt)

Corticosteroids

These are hormones with a powerful anti-inflammatory effect useful in the treatment of many types of cancer and other diseases. They are used in patients with cancer to help before chemotherapy in the prevention of severe allergic reactions and after chemotherapy in the prevention of nausea and vomiting (4). As catabolic agents, they can produce long-term side effects in all body tissues (e.g., muscle atrophy, osteopenia–osteoporosis, immunosuppression) (102). Examples of corticosteroids are (4) prednisone, methylprednisolone (Solu Medrol), and dexamethasone (Decadron).

Other Chemotherapy Drugs

These drugs do not fit into the previous categories. Examples of these drugs (4) are L-asparaginase (enzyme) and proteasome inhibitor bortezomib (Velcade).

Hormone Therapy

As previously discussed, hormone therapy is a frequently used treatment for some types of cancer, especially breast and prostate cancer (141).

Hormone Therapy Against Breast Cancer

The objective of hormone therapy for breast cancer is to lower estrogen levels as much as possible (4). Following are the most important hormone therapy drug groups (4, 101):

Drugs that block estrogen:

- **Selective estrogen receptor modulators (SERMs):** These work as estrogen antagonists in some tissues and as agonists in others (e.g., tamoxifen blocks estrogen in breast tissue but works like estrogen in the uterus and bone tissue). Side effects include (4, 101) fatigue, hot flashes, vaginal dryness in women, impotence in men, mood changes, depression, loss of libido, cataracts, increased risk of endometrial and uterine cancer, increased risk of blood clots especially in lungs and lower extremities (e.g., pulmonary embolism, deep venous thrombosis), heart attack, stroke, and bone loss in premenopausal women; but these drugs often have a positive effect on bone health in postmenopausal women. The following are the most commonly used drugs in this class of drugs (101): tamoxifen (Nolvadex), raloxifene (Evista), toremifene (Fareston).
- **Other anti-estrogen drugs:** These drugs work by temporarily blocking the estrogen receptors in all tissues (4). Side effects include (4, 101) hot flashes, night sweats, mild nausea, gastrointestinal symptoms, loss of strength, fatigue, pain, bone loss (sometimes resulting in osteopenia–osteoporosis and fractures). The most common anti-estrogen drug is fulvestrant (Faslodex) (101).

Treatments to lower estrogen levels:

- **Aromatase inhibitors (AIs):** These drugs block the enzyme aromatase in fat tissue. Fat tissue in postmenopausal women produces a small quantity of estrogen. Aromatase inhibitors cannot block the normal estrogen production of the ovaries, so they are effective only in women with nonfunctioning ovaries due to menopause or to treatment for ovarian suppression (see the next point). Side effects include (4, 101) mood changes, depression, heart attack, angina, heart failure, hypercholesterolemia, muscle and joint pain, joint stiffness, and bone loss (sometimes resulting in osteopenia–osteoporosis and fractures). The most common drugs in this class are (101) letrozole (Femara), anastrozole (Arimidex), and exemestane (Aromasin).
- **Ovarian suppression or ablation:** In premenopausal women, the ovaries are the main source of estrogens. One way to suppress estrogen is to remove the ovaries or prevent them from producing estrogen. Permanent ovarian suppression or ablation can be done surgically (oophorectomy, removal of the ovaries). However, in most instances, drugs resembling luteinizing hormone-releasing hormone (LHRH) are used to suppress the ovaries' production and release of estrogen. After ovarian suppression, the woman is in a postmenopausal state, and this allows other hormone therapies to be more beneficial. Side effects include (4, 101) hot flashes, night sweats, vaginal dryness, mood changes, depression, loss of libido, and bone loss (sometimes resulting in osteopenia–osteoporosis and fractures). The most common drugs used in ovarian suppression are (101) goserelin (Zoladex) and leuprolide (Lupron).

Hormone Therapy Against Prostate Cancer

The objective of hormone therapy for prostate cancer is to lower androgen levels (e.g., testosterone) as much as possible (4). The principal androgen source in men is the testes; a small quantity is also produced by the adrenal glands, and prostate cancer tissue can produce testosterone as well (4, 111). The most important hormone therapy drug groups to treat prostate cancer are as follows (4, 101).

Hormone therapy that lowers androgen levels:

- **Orchiectomy:** This is a surgical procedure in which one or both testicles are removed; this reduces blood testosterone levels by 90% to 95% (116). In a procedure termed subcapsular orchiectomy, only the tissue that produces androgens is removed, rather than the entire testicle (101).

- **Luteinizing hormone-releasing hormone (LHRH):** These drugs are termed LHRH agonists, LHRH analogues, or gonadotropin-releasing hormone (GnRH) agonists. These drugs are synthetic proteins that bind to the LHRH receptor in the pituitary gland, which decreases the production of luteinizing hormone, resulting in less production of testosterone and lowering testosterone levels. Initially LHRH analogues result in a phenomenon termed "flare," in which testosterone levels increase briefly; they then decrease to low levels. Men with metastases to bone may have bone pain during flare, in which case antiandrogen drugs can be given to reduce the pain. The most common drugs in this class are leuprolide (Lupron, Eligard), goserelin (Zoladex), triptorelin (Trelstar), and histrelin (Vantas) (101).

- **LHRH antagonists:** These are also termed GnRH antagonists and work as LHRH analogues. These drugs decrease testosterone levels faster and without flare compared to LHRH agonists. The most commonly used drug in this class is degarelix (Firmagon) (101).

- **Abiraterone (Zytiga):** This is an androgen biosynthesis inhibitor. Even when testicle secretion of androgens is under control, other cells can produce small amounts of androgens (e.g., adrenal glands, prostate cancer tissue). Abiraterone blocks the enzyme CYP17 and significantly reduces androgen production by other cells (4, 111). Other less used androgen synthesis inhibitors are ketoconazole and aminoglutethimide (101).

Drugs that stop androgens from working:

- **Antiandrogens:** These drugs block androgen binding to androgen receptors (4). Treatment with antiandrogens in combination with orchiectomy or a LHRH agonist is termed combined, complete, or total androgen blockade (101). The drugs most commonly used in this class are flutamide, enzalutamide, bicalutamide, and nilutamide (101).

- **Enzalutamide (Xtandi):** This is an antiandrogen that stops androgens from binding to coactivator proteins after being transported into the cell, a needed step for the androgen to cause protein synthesis. Antiandrogens can help diminish tumors and augment survival in men with advanced prostate cancer (4).

These are the common side effects of hormone therapy (orchiectomy, LHRH analogues, and LHRH antagonists) in prostate cancer: hot flashes, loss of libido, changes in mood, depression, erection problems, growth (gynecomastia) and tenderness of breast tissue, shrinkage of testicles and penis, muscle atrophy, reduced muscle strength, bone loss (sometimes resulting in osteopenia–osteoporosis and fractures), anemia, high cholesterol, weight gain, lower mental sharpness, fatigue, and increased risk of hypertension, diabetes, liver damage, stroke, heart attack, and death from heart disease (4, 101).

EFFECTS OF EXERCISE IN INDIVIDUALS WITH CANCER

Exercise both during and after treatment is an effective tool to improve functional capacity ($\dot{V}O_2$max), strength, functional mobility (i.e., improving balance will lower the risk of falls and fractures), fatigue, psychological well-being (i.e., reducing the risk of anxiety and depression), and health-related QoL in cancer patients and survivors (21, 46, 50, 72, 79, 90, 123). However, the benefits of physical training may vary according to the type of cancer and treatment; the stage of disease; the mode, intensity, and duration of the exercise program; and the current lifestyle of the patient (72). Most studies on this topic conducted on adults have focused on patients with breast cancer (13, 20, 26, 27, 41, 62, 63, 67, 73, 75, 81, 89, 95, 105, 115, 125, 127, 131-135, 144, 150, 155, 156, 164), prostate cancer (14, 22, 23, 47, 48, 70, 78, 136, 146, 154, 157, 158), and a few other types of cancer (1, 2, 8, 17, 33-37, 39, 56-59, 91, 92, 94, 100, 110, 112, 113, 151, 159). Studies performed in children have included pediatric leukemia (40, 74, 82, 121, 122) and other cancer types (19, 69, 120). There is still, however, much research needed in this area.

Key Point

Both resistance training and aerobic endurance training provide a number of benefits for cancer patients related to health, physical conditioning, and quality of life.

Resistance Training Research

Some research has examined the positive effects of resistance training alone on patients' health and QoL (13, 47, 92, 105, 112, 113, 125-129, 136, 157, 158). Also some studies have assessed the benefits of combined aerobic and resistance training (1, 14, 20, 22, 36, 62, 67, 73, 82, 110, 120-122, 144), and some have compared aerobic to resistance training (27, 125, 126, 150). Currently there is no information concerning the effect of changes in specific training variables (i.e., volume, intensity or load, duration of rest periods, frequency of training, and training velocity) on training outcomes, so more research is needed to address these issues.

During treatment (see table 10.1) and after treatment (see table 10.2), resistance training and combined aerobic and resistance intervention studies in cancer patients and survivors, in both adults and children, have reported improvements in many areas:

- Functional capacity ($\dot{V}O_2$max) or aerobic performance (1, 20, 22, 23, 36, 48, 57, 62, 73, 112, 120, 122, 144, 150)
- Muscular strength (1, 20, 22, 23, 27, 47, 48, 57, 62, 73, 82, 92, 105, 120-122, 127-129, 136, 144, 150, 157)
- Functional mobility (8, 13, 22, 47, 48, 62, 120-122, 150)
- Physical activity level (23, 67, 115)
- Flexibility–ROM (range of motion) (20, 73, 82, 91, 92)
- Bone mineral density (47, 113)
- Body composition (19, 22, 23, 27, 56, 62, 105, 127)
- Total energy expenditure (56)
- Weight loss (115)
- Weight gain (19)
- Total cholesterol: high-density lipoprotein cholesterol ratio (22)

- Pain (67, 91, 92, 150)
- Fatigue (22, 36, 112, 125, 136, 144)
- Psychological well-being (20, 22, 27, 105, 110)
- Quality of life (14, 20, 58, 62, 73, 105, 120, 125, 136)
- Resting systolic pressure (73, 115)
- Prostate-specific antigen (PSA) levels (136)
- Sexual function (22)
- Insulin-like growth factor (IGF)-II levels (which are significantly reduced) (127)

Studies of resistance training and combined aerobic and resistance intervention studies in cancer patients and survivors have also reported lower incidence or recurrence of breast cancer–related lymphedema (128, 129), lower severity of breast cancer–related lymphedema (129), no delayed immunologic recovery (19, 59), and improved chemotherapy completion rates (27).

Follow-up after an exercise program intervention (two to six months) was completed by a few researchers (26, 48, 63, 122, 150), and some of these studies indicate sustained improvement in functional capacity ($\dot{V}O_2$max) or aerobic performance (48, 122), muscular strength (48, 63, 122), functional mobility (48, 63, 122), and psychological well-being (26, 48) and QoL (63) compared to baseline. Most of these findings could be the consequence of the high level of deconditioning of cancer patients and survivors, such that any small stimulus such as a short exercise program (e.g., eight weeks) may lead to the partial recovery of the patient's normal physiological and psychological characteristics. However, more work is needed to elucidate the long-term beneficial effects of resistance exercise training in cancer patients and survivors.

Aerobic Training Research

A number of exercise interventions in cancer patients and survivors have focused on aerobic training (17, 24, 33, 34, 37-39, 41, 69, 70, 74, 95, 132, 135, 155, 156, 164).

During treatment (see table 10.3) and after treatment (see table 10.4), aerobic intervention studies in adult and child cancer patients and survivors have indicated a reduction in nausea (155), improved functional capacity ($\dot{V}O_2$max)

Table 10.1 Summary of Examples of Supervised Resistance Training and Combined Exercise Interventions Conducted During Cancer Treatment

Study	Type of cancer	No. of patients, age	Duration (weeks)	Frequency	Exercise program	Intensity	Results
Kolden et al. 2002 (73)	Breast	40 W 45-76 years	16	3/week	AET (walking, cycling, step) RET Flexibility	Unspecified	↑ 15.4% $\dot{V}O_2$max ↑ ≈35% strength ↑ Flexibility ↑ Quality of life ↓ RSBP
Adamsen et al. 2003 (1)	Leukemia, breast, colon, ovary	23 M&W 18-63 years	6	4/week	AET (cycling)	60-100% MHR	↑ 16% $\dot{V}O_2$max ↑ 32.5% strength ↑ Quality of life
					RET (3 sets, 5-8 reps)	85-95% 1RM	
					Relaxation		
Segal et al. 2003 (136)	Prostate	155 M 68 years	12	3/week	RET (2 sets, 12 reps)	60-70% 1RM	↑ ≈39% strength ↔ PSA ↓ Fatigue ↑ Quality of life
Hayes et al. 2003, 2004 (56-58)	Peripheral blood stem cell transplant	12 M&W 16-64 years	12	2-3/week	AET (walking, cycling)	70-90% MHR	↑ $\dot{V}O_2$peak ↑ Strength ↑ Fat-free mass ↓ % body fat ↑ Total energy expenditure ↑ Quality of life
					RET	20- to 8RM	
					Flexibility		
Galvão et al. 2006 (47)	Prostate	10 M 59-82 years	20	2/week	RET (2-4 sets, 12 reps)	12- to 6RM	↑ 40-96% strength ↑ >100% muscular endurance ↑ Functional mobility ↑ Balance ↔ Lean body mass ↔ Body fat ↔ BMD and BMC ↔ PSA ↔ Testosterone ↔ Hemoglobin
Courneya et al. 2007 (27)	Breast	242 W 25-78 years	17-24	3/week	AET (walking, cycling, elliptical)	60-80% $\dot{V}O_2$max	↔ $\dot{V}O_2$peak ↔ Body fat ↑ Self-esteem
					OR		
					RET (2 sets, 8-12 reps)	60-70% 1RM	↑ Strength ↑ Lean body mass ↑ Self-esteem ↑ Chemotherapy completion rate

Study	Type of cancer	No. of patients, age	Duration (weeks)	Frequency	Exercise program	Intensity	Results
San Juan et al. 2007 (122)	Acute lymphoblastic leukemia	7 M&W 4-7 years	16	3/week	AET (cycling, games)	50-70% MHR	↑ $\dot{V}O_2$peak ↑ Strength ↑ Functional mobility
					RET (1 set, 8-15 reps)	15- to 8RM	
San Juan et al. 2008 (120)	Bone marrow transplant	8 M&W 8-16 years	8	3/week	AET (cycling, games)	50-70% MHR	↑ $\dot{V}O_2$peak ↑ Strength ↑ Functional mobility ↑ Quality of life
					RET (1 set, 8-15 reps)	15- to 8RM	

Abbreviations: 1RM, one repetition maximum; M, men; W, women; AET, aerobic exercise training; RET, resistance exercise training; MHR, maximal heart rate; $\dot{V}O_2$max, maximal oxygen consumption; $\dot{V}O_2$peak, peak oxygen consumption; RSBP, resting systolic blood pressure; PSA, prostate-specific antigen; BMD, bone mineral density; BMC, bone mineral content.

Table 10.2 Summary of Examples of the Results of Resistance Training and Combined Exercise Interventions Conducted After Cancer Treatment

Study	Type of cancer	No. of patients, age	Duration (weeks)	Frequency	Exercise program	Intensity	Results
Herrero et al. 2007 (63)	Breast	16 W 50 years	8	3/week	Aerobic cycling	70-80% MHR	↑ $\dot{V}O_2$peak ↑ Lower body strength ↑ Functional mobility ↑ Muscle mass ↓ % body fat ↑ Quality of life
					RET (2-3 sets, 8-15 reps)	12- to 8RM	
Ohira et al. 2006 (105)	Breast	79 W 53 years	24	2/week	RET Stretching	Unspecified	↑ Upper strength ↑ Lean body mass ↑ Psychosocial ↑ Quality of life
McNeely et al. 2008 (92)	Head and neck carcinoma	52 M&W 32-76 years	12	2-3/week	RET (2 sets, 10-15 reps) Therapeutic exercise	25-70% 1RM	↑ Upper extremity strength and muscular endurance ↓ Shoulder pain ↑ Shoulder ROM

Abbreviations: 1RM, one repetition maximum; M, men; W, women; RET, resistance training; MHR, maximal heart rate; $\dot{V}O_2$peak, peak oxygen consumption; ROM, range of motion.

Table 10.3 Summary of Examples of the Results of Several Aerobic Exercise Interventions Conducted During Cancer Treatment

Study	Type of cancer	No. of patients, age	Duration (weeks)	Frequency	Exercise program	Intensity	Results
Yang et al. 2015 (164)	Breast	47 W 50 years	6	3/week	Aerobic walking	40-65% MHR	↓ Fatigue
Alibhai et al. 2015 (2)	Myeloid leukemia	83 M&W 59 years	4-6	4-5/week	Mixed modalities	50-75% HRR	↑ Quality of life ↓ Fatigue ↑ Aerobic fitness ↑ Lower body strength ↑ Grip strength
Jones et al. 2014 (70)	Prostate	46 M 59 years	24	3-5/week	Aerobic walking	55-65% V̇O₂peak	↑ 9% V̇O₂peak
Windsor et al. 2004 (154)	Prostate	65 M 69 years	4	3+/week	Aerobic walking	60-70% MHR	No ↑ in fatigue from radiotherapy ↑ Physical functioning ↑ Distance walked
Dimeo et al. 1998 (34)	Bronchial, breast	5 M&W 18-55 years	6	5/week	Aerobic walking	3 mmol/L (LC) 80% MHR	↑ MAP ↓ Lactate concentration

Abbreviations: M, men; W, women; MAP, maximal aerobic performance; MHR, maximal heart rate; HRR, heart rate reserve; LC, lactate concentration; V̇O₂peak, peak oxygen consumption.

Table 10.4 Summary of Examples of the Results of Several Aerobic Exercise Interventions Conducted After Cancer Treatment

Study	Type of cancer	No. of patients, age	Duration (weeks)	Frequency	Exercise program	Intensity	Results
Daley et al. 2007 (29)	Breast	108 W 51 years	8	3/week	Aerobic walking	65-85% MHR	↑ Quality of life ↑ Aerobic fitness
Carlson et al. 2006 (17)	Postallogeneic hematopoietic stem cell transplant	12 M&W 28-55 years	12	3/week	Aerobic cycling	VT-1 to VT-2 +20 Watts	↑ V̇O₂peak ↑ Power at VT-2 ↓ Fatigue
Thorsen et al. 2005 (142)	Lymphomas or breast, gynecologic, or testicular cancer	111 M&W 39 years	14	2+/week	Aerobic walking, cycling, aerobics, skiing	RPE 13-15 or 60-70% MHR	↑ V̇O₂max ↓ Fatigue
Courneya et al. 2003 (24)	Breast	52 W 59 years	15	3/week	Aerobic cycling	70-75% V̇O₂peak	↑ V̇O₂peak ↑ Quality of life ↑ Body weight and composition

Abbreviations: M, men; W, women; MHR, maximal heart rate; LC, lactate concentration; V̇O₂peak, peak oxygen consumption; MAP, maximal aerobic performance; RPE, rate of perceived exertion on a 6- to 20-point scale; VT-1, ventilatory threshold 1; VT-2, ventilatory threshold 2; V̇O₂peak, peak oxygen consumption; V̇O₂max, maximum oxygen consumption.

or aerobic performance (2, 17, 29, 35, 39, 70, 81, 135, 142, 154), greater functional mobility (34, 95, 132, 134), improved body composition (156), reduced fatigue (2, 17, 34, 95, 132, 133, 142, 164), increased psychological well-being (29, 37, 95), and improved hematologic and immune system variables (33, 39, 41, 74, 100).

EXERCISE RECOMMENDATIONS FOR CLIENTS WITH CANCER

Although resistance and aerobic training guidelines can be postulated from the research performed to date, more research is needed to develop more defined training guidelines. Thus, the training guidelines presented should be considered not definitive, and, as is standard practice, they should be modified to meet the needs and medical condition of individual cancer patients.

The goals of an exercise program designed for healthy people similarly apply to cancer patients and survivors, and any individualized exercise program should be safe, effective, and enjoyable for the person for whom it is intended. The components of the exercise prescription (i.e., the mode, frequency, intensity, duration, and progression) depend on the type of cancer and the health and treatment status of the cancer patient or survivor. In short, however, the most important guideline is to avoid inactivity (96, 145).

Physical exercise programs are safe and well accepted by cancer patients, even those who have undergone hematopoietic stem cell transplantation (5, 46, 49, 72, 76, 79, 90, 96, 123, 160). For clients who do not have impaired physical functioning, begin the exercise program with light to moderate walking at a self-selected intensity based on the person's exercise tolerance, and gradually progress to more vigorous walking or other large muscle group activities. The initial exercise duration is what the client can tolerate, but the goal, over a four-week period, is to gradually increase to 40 minutes (20 minutes if the aerobic workout is combined with a resistance training workout) (96). Progression should be more gradual for deconditioned clients or those

who are experiencing severe treatment side effects (25, 79, 123).

Key Point

Physical exercise programs are safe and well accepted by cancer patients. In fact, inactivity should be avoided.

As usual, the exercise session should be divided into a warm-up (i.e., light aerobic exercise and stretching of all major muscle groups), a main exercise period (i.e., aerobic exercise, resistance training, or both), and a cooldown period (i.e., light aerobic exercise and stretching again). The exercise program should focus on physical activities that use large muscle groups rather than small groups, since most daily living tasks depend on these large muscle groups. Session design and exercises must be modified according to the acute or chronic treatment effects of surgery, chemotherapy, or radiotherapy. For example, if the client shows signs of fatigue during the session, then it should be divided into shorter periods of exercise with frequent rest periods.

Based on the cancer exercise guidelines available in the literature (5, 25, 46, 49, 51, 60, 92, 96, 123, 130) and the experience of the authors of this chapter (6, 19, 61-63, 79, 80, 119-122), the recommendation can be made for an individually supervised combined (aerobic, resistance, and flexibility training) exercise program for adults (see table 10.5) or children (see table 10.6). A program should be targeted at improving strength, functional mobility, flexibility, body composition, and aerobic conditioning, as well as psychological well-being and physical-related QoL.

Special Considerations in Cancer Training Prescription

Cancer patients and survivors should always check with their physician or other health care professional before starting any exercise program. This is especially important when the client is receiving treatment that affects the lungs (e.g., bleomycin, chest radiation therapy) or heart (e.g., doxorubicin, epirubicin, anthracycline) or when the client has a risk of lung or heart disease. More

Table 10.5 Exercise Guidelines for Adult Cancer Patients and Survivors Based on the Recommendations in the Literature

Exercise	Intensity	Frequency	Volume	Dosage
Aerobic exercise	Begin at a self-selected intensity (e.g., talk test) and increase intensity over time as tolerated (e.g., RPE of 3-5 on a 1-10 scale)	4-5/week	Any duration (as tolerated) and progress to 40 min	Begin with walking and progress to include other large muscle group activities
Resistance exercise	30-80% 1RM	2-3/week	8-10 exercises for major muscle groups 1-3 sets per muscle group	15- to 8RM Rest 1-3 min between exercises and sets
Flexibility exercise	Lower than discomfort level	≥3/week	2-4 sets per muscle area	10-30 s

Abbreviations: RPE, rate of perceived exertion; RM, repetition maximum.

References: (5, 25, 46, 49, 62, 63, 79, 92, 96, 130)

Table 10.6 Exercise Guidelines for Child Cancer Patients and Survivors Based on the Recommendations in the Literature

Exercise	Intensity	Frequency	Volume	Dosage
Aerobic exercise	50-90% MHR* 40-85% HRR	3-5/week	10-30 min	Continuous or intermittent (i.e., walking, cycling, running, group games)
Resistance exercise	30-80% 1RM	2-3/week	8-10 exercises (major muscle groups) 1 set per muscle group	15- to 8RM Rest 1-3 min between exercises and sets
Flexibility exercise		≥3/week	2-4 sets per muscle area	10-30 s

Abbreviations: MHR, maximal heart rate; HRR, heart rate reserve; RM, repetition maximum.

*Note: Heart rate reserve is the best guideline if maximal heart rate is estimated rather than measured.

References: (80, 118, 120-123)

research is needed to establish the minimum platelet count and hemoglobin levels needed to ensure safety of training interventions, especially for inpatients. Preliminary data from Chamorro-Viña and colleagues (19) suggest that training during the neutropenic phase in childhood solid tumor treatment following hematopoietic stem cell transplant with a neutrophil count <0.5×10^9/μL does not increase risk of adverse events. So far, no detrimental effects of exercise training in cancer patients and survivors have been reported (5, 46, 60, 72, 79, 90, 123). However, in some established conditions, certain precautions must be taken when prescribing exercise in certain types of clients (see table 10.7).

The conditions listed in table 10.7 can lead to more physical problems if they are not taken into account when planning an exercise program. Moreover, side effects caused by the disease and treatment (e.g., nausea, extreme fatigue or muscle weakness or both, dyspnea, pain) may make it difficult for the client to complete the training during an exercise session. In this situation, the client is told to reduce the intensity of exercise or cease immediately depending on the side effects, and to consult with his physician or other health care professional as soon as possible.

Table 10.7 Precautions to Take in Exercise Prescription for Cancer Patients

Pathology or condition	Precaution
• Fever (temperature >104°F [>40°C]) • Severe anemia (hemoglobin <8 g/dl) • Severe neutropenia (neutrophil count <0.5 × 10⁹/μL) • Severe thrombocytopenia (platelet count <50 × 10⁹/μL) • Severe cachexia (loss of over 35% premorbid weight) • Cardiotoxicity induced by anthracyclines	Avoid all types of exercise but not activities of daily living. Avoid sedentary behavior during the day as much as possible.
• Fever (temperature >100.4°F [>38°C]) • Low to moderate anemia • Low to moderate cachexia	Avoid intense and strenuous exercise (i.e., high intensity). Do light-intensity and progressive exercise.
• Primary or metastatic bone cancer (increased risk of bone fractures) • Low to moderate thrombocytopenia (increased risk of hemorrhage)	Avoid high-impact exercise, contact sports, activities that have high risk of impact and falls. Use a controlled quilted environment with soft material (i.e., soft balls).
• Low to moderate neutropenia (increased risk of bacterial infection) • Patients with nephrostomy tubes, central venous access or urinary bladder catheters	Avoid swimming. Aseptic environment. Do light-intensity and progressive exercise.
Patients with ataxia, dizziness, or peripheral neuropathy (impaired balance and coordination and increased risk of falls)	Avoid high-impact exercise, contact sports, activities that have high risk of impact and falls, or that require additional balance and coordination (e.g., treadmill walking, outdoor cycling). Use controlled quilted environment with soft material (i.e., soft balls). Walk re-education and physical therapy treatment of neuropathy are recommended.
Breast cancer survivors	Be aware of increased risk for fracture. Watch for arm or shoulder symptoms and lymphedema.
Prostate cancer survivors	Be aware of increased risk for fracture. Pelvic floor exercises are recommended for patients with radical prostatectomy.
Colon cancer survivors with an ostomy	Resistance exercise: Start with low intensity and progress the resistance in small increments to avoid herniation in the stoma. Contact sports: Physician permission is recommended (due to the risk of a blow to the stoma site), and modifications may be needed (e.g., additional protection such as a stoma guard). Swimming: modifications may be needed (e.g., a stoma cap or a mini drainable pouch).

References: (5, 79)

Cancer-Related Lymphedema: Special Considerations

Exercise, and more specifically resistance training, is safe for breast cancer survivors with and at risk of lymphedema (5, 21, 107, 128, 129). However, vigorous upper body exercise should be performed with caution: Reduce resistance or stop specific exercises according to symptom response (128, 129). Precautions such as wearing compression sleeves, lifting the arm above the head after exercise, and active light recovery may facilitate lymph return after exercise (76, 128, 129).

There are no data on safety of resistance training in lower limb lymphedema secondary to a gynecologic cancer, and it is not possible to extrapolate the exercise knowledge on upper limb lymphedema. So proceed with caution (i.e., reduce resistance or stop specific exercises according to symptom response) if lymphedema occurs with lower limb exercise (128, 129).

Program Design Guidelines for Clients With Cancer

For a healthy person not accustomed to physical exercise, embarking on an exercise program can be difficult, and this is even more difficult if the person has a chronic illness such as cancer.

Alternative forms of physical activities (e.g., yoga, tai chi, dancing, soccer) in which exercises are performed in the company of others often help encourage training consistency and exercise performance and improve the physical and psychological well-being of cancer patients and survivors (16, 77, 146, 163).

In clients undergoing high-dose treatment (chemo or radiotherapy) or a recent hematopoietic stem cell transplant, exercise sometimes has a strong physical stabilization effect (i.e., maintaining physical performance and decreasing some of the detrimental physical effects of treatment) and has been related to greater positive effects than exercise performed during periods of lower treatment intensity or after treatment (91, 96, 131, 160).

The exercise program should be individually supervised (96) since previous research has identified greater strength gains in a supervised program in healthy clients (87). In addition, research has revealed significantly greater gains in aerobic, muscle, and QoL variables (120-122) in supervised programs (96) than in home-based exercise programs in the same type of patient population (82). It is also recommended that supervised exercise programs be a part of the routine intrahospital therapy administered to cancer patients, even those in the initial stages of a hematopoietic transplant (120). Once the patient has left the hospital, continuing with a supervised exercise program during treatment and once treatment is complete can help the client fight the later effects of the disease and treatment by adopting healthy habits that can improve physical performance, fatigue, well-being, QoL (26, 62, 122), and rate of survival (10, 65, 103). Although physicians and oncologists could set up a small intrahospital exercise facility for patients, it may be more efficient to refer patients to exercise professionals with qualifications in clinical exercise who could conduct an exercise program with this patient population (96).

As previously explained, aerobic training should begin with walking and should later consist of any type of exercise that is easily accessible, such as walking, cycling, or gardening (96) or, in the case of children, aerobic games. Resistance training should consist of at least one exercise for all major muscle groups. Progression of exercise volume and intensity should be gradual and individualized. For clients severely affected by their condition, medical treatments, or both, or those who are highly deconditioned, an exercise program should begin at a lower level and make gradual progressions as tolerated (see table 10.8) since there can be very large fluctuations in a client's physical functioning from day to day (96).

Table 10.8 Example of an Exercise Program for Very Deconditioned Adult Cancer Patients and Survivors

Program stage	Week	AEROBIC TRAINING			RESISTANCE TRAINING		
		Frequency	Intensity	Volume	Frequency	Intensity	Volume
Starting period*	1-2	3/week	40% HRR	10-15 min	2/week	30% 1RM	1 set
	3-5	3-4/week	40-50% HRR	12-15 min	2/week	30-40% 1RM	1-2 sets
	5-7	3-4/week	45-55% HRR	15-20 min	2/week	40-50% 1RM	1-2 sets
Progression	8-10	3-4/week	50-60% HRR	15-20 min	2-3/week	50% 1RM	1-2 sets
	11-14	3-4/week	55-65% HRR	20 min	2-3/week	50-60% 1RM	1-2 sets
	15-18	3-4/week	60-70% HRR	20-25 min	2-3/week	50-60% 1RM	2 sets
	19-22	4-5/week	65-75% HRR	25 min	2-3/week	60-70% 1RM	2-3 sets
	23-26	4-5/week	70-80% HRR	25-30 min	2-3/week	65-75% 1RM	2-3 sets
	27-30	4-5/week	70-85% HRR	30 min	2-3/week	70-80% 1RM	2-3 sets
Maintenance period	+30	4-5/week	70-85% HRR	30-45 min	2-3/week	70-80% 1RM	2-3 sets

Abbreviations: HRR, heart rate reserve; 1RM, one repetition maximum.

*Or whatever is tolerated, especially to begin the program.

Case Study

Cancer

Mrs. O is a 50-year old postmenopausal woman with breast cancer in her last phase of treatment. She had a tumor T1N1M0. The oncologist removed the tumor surgically and Mrs. O underwent chemotherapy. The oncologist recommends she start an individualized physical exercise program to become more physically fit to improve her overall health and QoL. She is very deconditioned ($\dot{V}O_2$max of 15 ml $\cdot$ kg^{-1} $\cdot$ min^{-1}) and is overweight with a body mass index of 27 kg/m². She has no relevant side effects except slight anemia, thrombocytopenia, and fatigue.

Mrs. O must begin her exercise program with light exercise because she has anemia and cancer-related fatigue. It is also recommended that she avoid physical activities with a high risk of falling and contact (i.e., contact sports, mountain biking).

Her program should start with light-intensity activity three times a week. The initial intensity should be lower than recommended for cancer patients, and she will progress as her physical condition, health, and psychological status allow. The aerobic part of training will start at 50% MHR (or lower, based on what she can tolerate) for a duration of 10 minutes in a safe environment (e.g., walking). If it is necessary due to the patient's fatigue, she can divide the 10 minutes into smaller segments (e.g., two intervals of 5 minutes, five intervals of 2 minutes). The strength training will start with eight exercises or fewer of the major muscle groups at 30% 1RM and one set per muscle group. The flexibility exercise will start with two sets per muscle area during 10 to 30 seconds.

Recommended Readings

American Cancer Society. Cancer Facts & Figures. www.cancer.org. Accessed October 28, 2016.

American College of Sports Medicine, Schmitz, KH, Courneya, KS, Matthews, C, Demark-Wahnefried, W, Galvão, DA, Pinto, BM, Irwin, ML, Wolin, KY, Segal, RJ, Lucia, A, Schneider, CM, von Gruenigen, VE, and Schwartz AL. American College of Sports Medicine roundtable on exercise guidelines for cancer survivors. *Med Sci Sports Exerc* 42:1409-1426, 2010.

Courneya, KS and Friedenreich, CM. Physical activity and cancer: an introduction. In *Physical Activity and Cancer*. Berlin, Heidelberg: Springer, 1-10, 2010.

Irwin, M. *ACSM's Guide to Exercise and Cancer Survivorship*. Champaign, IL: Human Kinetics, 2012.

Moore, G, Durstine, JL, Painter, P, American College of Sports Medicine. 2016. *ACSM's Exercise Management for Persons With Chronic Diseases and Disabilities*. 4th ed. Champaign, IL: Human Kinetics, 2016.

CONCLUSION

Exercise programs for cancer patients and survivors are safe and necessary in order for them to recover their health and quality of life, with multiple studies showing that exercise has positive effects on multiple relevant variables (i.e., muscle strength, cardiorespiratory fitness, and quality of life). Exercise during the first and more intense treatment phases should be supervised and preferably located at a hospital. Once cancer patients have progressed into later phases of treatment, community physical activity programs supervised by health and exercise professionals, or, if this is not possible, home-based physical activity programs, are recommended. Cancer patients should always be encouraged to follow an active lifestyle.

Key Terms

Big Team
biological therapy
bone marrow transplantation
cancer
cancer-related fatigue
chemotherapy
early side effects
hormonal therapy

late side effects
lymphedema
malignant neoplasm
mutation
radiation therapy
self-perpetuating fatigue cycle
TNM (Tumor, Node, Metastasis) system

Study Questions

1. Which of the following is a unique characteristic of benign tumors?

    a. angiogenesis

    b. resisting cell death

    c. reprogramming of energy metabolism

    d. unregulated cell growth without metastasis

2. All of the following are components of a classification scheme to stage a cancer process except

    a. node

    b. tumor

    c. mutation

    d. metastasis

3. Which of the following is most likely to be classified as a late side effect of cancer treatment?

    a. nausea

    b. hair loss

    c. loss of appetite

    d. pulmonary fibrosis

4. Which of these statements on exercise guidelines for cancer patients is most accurate?

    a. Resistance exercise should be done no more than once per week.

    b. Duration of a flexibility exercise should be only 5 seconds per repetition.

    c. Aerobic exercise should begin as tolerated and progress to 40 minutes.

    d. Rest between sets of resistance exercises should be 5 minutes or greater.

Medications Table 10.1 Most Common Medications Used to Treat Cancer

Drug class and names	Mechanism of action	Most common side effects	Effects on exercise
Alkylating agents	Work in all phases of the cell division cycle; join to DNA nucleotides preventing the normal processes of replication, gene transcription, and translation		
busulfan (Busulfex), carmustine (Bicnu), lomustine (Ceenu)		Pulmonary function (i.e., fibrosis, interstitial pneumonitis, restrictive or obstructive lung disease), psychosocial function (i.e., social withdrawal, difficulty learning, depression, anxiety, posttraumatic stress)	Low functional capacity ($\dot{V}O_2$peak), fatigue
ifosfamide (Ifex)		Renal function (i.e., glomerular toxicity, tubular dysfunction, renal insufficiency, hypertension), psychosocial function (i.e., social withdrawal, difficulty learning, depression, anxiety, posttraumatic stress)	Fatigue
cyclophosphamide (Cytoxan)		Urogynecologic function (i.e., hemorrhagic cystitis, bladder fibrosis, neurogenic bladder, bladder malignancy), psychosocial function (i.e., social withdrawal, difficulty learning, depression, anxiety, posttraumatic stress)	Fatigue
cisplatin (Platinol), carboplatin (Paraplatin)		Peripheral nervous system function (i.e., peripheral sensory or motor neuropathy), psychosocial function (i.e., social withdrawal, difficulty learning, depression, anxiety, posttraumatic stress)	Fatigue, higher risk of falling, lower motor control and strength
Antimetabolites			
mercaptopurine (Purinethol), thioguanine (Tabloid)	Work during S phase of cell division cycle when the cell's chromosomes are being copied to block purine and pyrimidine synthesis and distort the normal synthesis of DNA and RNA	Hepatic function (i.e., hepatic dysfunction, veno-occlusive disease, hepatic fibrosis, cirrhosis, cholelithiasis), psychosocial function (i.e., social withdrawal, difficulty learning, depression, anxiety, posttraumatic stress)	Fatigue

Drug class and names	Mechanism of action	Most common side effects	Effects on exercise
Antimetabolites *(continued)*			
methotrexate (Trexall)	Interferes with the rapid growth of cancer cells	Hepatic function (i.e., hepatic dysfunction, veno-occlusive disease, hepatic fibrosis, cirrhosis, cholelithiasis), renal function (i.e., glomerular toxicity, tubular dysfunction, renal insufficiency, hypertension), hematologic function (i.e., anemia, leukopenia, neutropenia, thrombocytopenia), bone function (i.e., osteopenia–osteoporosis, osteonecrosis), neurocognitive function (i.e., neurocognitive deficits [attention, memory processing speed, visual–motor integration], learning deficits, diminished intellectual quotient), central nervous system function (i.e., leukoencephalopathy, spasticity, ataxia, dysarthria, dysphagia, hemiparesis, seizures, motor and sensory deficits), psychosocial function (i.e., social withdrawal, difficulty learning, depression, anxiety, posttraumatic stress)	Fatigue; increased risk of infection, bleeding, fracture, and falling
Antitumor antibiotics	Are interspersed among DNA base pairs preventing normal function and blocking cell growth and multiplication		
Anthracycline agents: doxorubicin (Doxil), daunorubicin (Cerubidine)		Cardiac function (i.e., cardiomyopathy, congestive heart failure, arrhythmia), psychosocial function (i.e., social withdrawal, difficulty learning, depression, anxiety, posttraumatic stress)	Decreased functional capacity ($\dot{V}O_2$peak), fatigue
Other antitumor antibiotics: bleomycin (Blenoxane)		Pulmonary function (i.e., fibrosis, interstitial pneumonitis, restrictive or obstructive lung disease), psychosocial function (i.e., social withdrawal, difficulty learning, depression, anxiety, posttraumatic stress)	Decreased functional capacity ($\dot{V}O_2$peak), fatigue
Topoisomerase inhibitors			
Topoisomerase I inhibitors: irinotecan (Camptosar) Topoisomerase II inhibitors: etoposide (Etopophos), teniposide (Vumon)	Interfere with the topoisomerases (enzymes), which helps separate the strands of DNA to be copied during the cellular S phase	Hematologic function (i.e., anemia, leukopenia, neutropenia, thrombocytopenia), psychosocial function (i.e., social withdrawal, difficulty learning, depression, anxiety, posttraumatic stress)	Increased infection and bleeding risk, fatigue

(continued)

Medications Table 10.1 *(continued)*

Drug class and names	Mechanism of action	Most common side effects	Effects on exercise
Antimitotic or mitotic inhibitors			
Vinca alkaloids: vinblastine (Velban), vincristine (Oncovin)	Stop mitosis M phase and damage cells in all cell division phases by slowing enzymes necessary for protein synthesis, slowing cell reproduction	Peripheral nervous system function (i.e., peripheral sensory or motor neuropathy), psychosocial function (i.e., social withdrawal, difficulty learning, depression, anxiety, posttraumatic stress)	Decreased motor control, increased risk of falling, decreased strength, fatigue
Corticosteroids			
prednisone, methylprednisolone (Solu-Medrol), dexamethasone (Decadron)	Catabolic hormones with a powerful anti-inflammatory effect useful in the treatment of many types of cancers and other diseases	Bone function (i.e., osteopenia–osteoporosis), immune function (i.e., immunosuppression), muscle function (i.e., muscle atrophy, low muscle strength), psychosocial function (i.e., social withdrawal, difficulty learning, depression, anxiety, posttraumatic stress)	Increased fracture and infection risk, decreased strength, fatigue
Other chemotherapy drugs			
L-asparaginase	Stop the production of asparagine (essential to cell life) in the body; cancer cell cannot produce it and dies	Neurologic function (i.e., confusion, excessive somnolence, agitation, disorientation, coma), hematologic function (i.e., higher risk of blood clots or bleeding), psychosocial function (i.e., social withdrawal, difficulty learning, depression, anxiety, posttraumatic stress)	Decreased motor control, increased risk of bleeding and falling, decreased strength, fatigue
Hormone therapy for breast cancer			
Selective estrogen receptor modulators (SERMs): tamoxifen (Nolvadex), raloxifene (Evista), toremifene (Fareston)	Decrease estrogen levels that control cancer growth	Urogynecologic function (i.e., higher risk of developing endometrial and uterine cancer, vaginal dryness in women, impotence in men), cardiovascular function (i.e., pulmonary embolism, deep venous thrombosis, heart attack, stroke), muscle function (i.e., muscle atrophy and lower strength), bone function (i.e., osteopenia–osteoporosis), endocrine and metabolic function (i.e., weight gain), psychosocial function (i.e., social withdrawal, difficulty learning, depression, anxiety, posttraumatic stress)	Decreased functional capacity ($\dot{V}O_2$peak), increased fracture risk, increased weight, decreased strength, fatigue
Aromatase inhibitors (AIs): letrozole (Femara), anastrozole (Arimidex), exemestane (Aromasin)	Decrease estrogen levels that control cancer growth	Cardiovascular function (i.e., heart attack, angina, heart failure, hypercholesterolemia), muscle function (muscle pain), skeletal function (joint pain, joint stiffness), bone function (i.e., osteopenia–osteoporosis, higher risk of fractures), psychosocial function (i.e., social withdrawal, difficulty learning, depression, anxiety, posttraumatic stress)	Decreased functional capacity ($\dot{V}O_2$peak), increased fracture risk, increased weight, decreased strength, fatigue

Drug class and names	Mechanism of action	Most common side effects	Effects on exercise
Hormone therapy for prostate cancer			
LHRH analogues: leuprolide (Lupron, Eligard), goserelin (Zoladex), triptorelin (Trelstar), istrelin (Vantas) LHRH antagonists: degarelix (Firmagon)	Decrease androgen levels, which control cancer growth	Hepatic function (i.e., liver damage), urologic function (i.e., erection problems, growth [gynecomastia] and tenderness of breast tissue; testicles and penis become smaller), cardiovascular function (i.e., hypertension, stroke, heart attack), muscle function (i.e., muscle atrophy and lower strength), bone function (i.e., osteopenia–osteoporosis), hematologic function (i.e., anemia), endocrine and metabolic function (i.e., higher cholesterol, weight gain, diabetes), psychosocial function (i.e., social withdrawal, difficulty learning, depression, anxiety, posttraumatic stress)	Decreased functional capacity ($\dot{V}O_2$peak), increased fracture risk, increased weight, decreased strength, fatigue

References: (3, 4, 101, 102)

Children and Adolescents

Avery D. Faigenbaum, EdD, CSCS, CSPS, FNSCA

After completing this chapter, you will be able to

- ◆ recognize the impact of physical inactivity on disease risk and lifetime health;

- ◆ understand the fundamental principles of pediatric exercise science;

- ◆ explain the benefits of regular physical activity on health and fitness performance in school-age youth; and

- ◆ design an exercise program for children and adolescents that is safe, effective, and developmentally appropriate.

Physical activity is essential for normal growth and development in children and adolescents. In addition to enhancing cardiovascular fitness, musculoskeletal strength, metabolic health, and mental well-being, participation in games, sports, and free play provides youth with an opportunity to make friends, have fun, and learn something new (55). From a developmental perspective, children who are physically active early in life have an opportunity to develop and reinforce prerequisite motor skills and physical abilities that underlie participation in health-enhancing physical activity later in life (20, 23). Furthermore, an emerging body of evidence suggests a positive association between physical activity and cognitive performance in school-age youth (21, 34, 54).

Global health recommendations state that children and adolescents should accumulate at least 60 minutes of moderate to vigorous physical activity (MVPA) daily as part of play, sports, transportation, recreation, physical education, and planned exercise (100). Since children are not simply miniature adults anatomically, physiologically, or developmentally, physical activity programs for younger populations need to be developmentally appropriate, sustainable, and enjoyable if the health and fitness benefits are to be realized and long-lasting. Adult exercise programs and training philosophies are suboptimal for school-age youth, who are active in different ways and for different reasons than older populations. Exercise professionals need to be aware of the physical and psychosocial uniqueness of younger populations and mindful of the special needs of children and adolescents with medical ailments.

In order to create and sustain an infrastructure that promotes physical activity for all youth, particularly those who are at risk for physical inactivity, it is important to recognize the impact of physical inactivity on long-term health and well-being, understand the fundamental principles of pediatric exercise science, and appreciate the multiple benefits of MVPA for physical, mental, and cognitive health. This chapter reviews contemporary trends in physical activity behavior among youth, benefits of regular MVPA, basic growth and development cycles, and physiological responses to exercise in children and adolescents. Specific exercise recommendations and strategies for implementing youth programs are also explored. In this chapter, the term **children** refers to boys and girls who have not yet developed **secondary sex characteristics** (roughly up to the age of 11 years in girls and 13 years in boys), and the term **adolescence** refers to a period of time between childhood and adulthood. Secondary sex characteristics are features that appear at sexual maturity and include growth of body hair, breast development in girls, and increased muscle mass in boys. The terms *youth* and *pediatric* are broadly defined to include both children and adolescents.

TRENDS IN YOUTH PHYSICAL ACTIVITY

Although children tend to be more active than adults, the volume and intensity of daily physical activity among youth have declined over the past few decades (8, 55, 94). Fewer children walk or bike to school, and free-time physical activity participation prevalence is decreasing in children and adolescents (66, 98). The decline in physical activity seems to emerge around age 6 (74, 95), and children with disabilities engage in even less physical activity than their peers who do not have disability (67). Despite the effectiveness of quality physical education, nearly half of school administrators in the United States report cutting significant amounts of time from physical education in order to increase time for reading and mathematics (55). In view of the health, economic, environmental, and social consequences of physical inactivity among youth, this global health issue has been described as a pandemic (57).

A notable corollary of these troublesome trends in physical inactivity is a low level of muscular fitness and **fundamental movement skill** competence among school-age youth. Fundamental movement skills are basic movements or skills that can be categorized into three groups: locomotor skills (e.g., running and jumping), object control skills (e.g., throwing and catching), and stability skills (e.g., balancing and twisting). Researchers examined 10-year secular trends in muscular fitness in children and found declines in bent arm hang, sit-up performance, and hand-grip strength over the study period (25). Others described 13-year trends in children's fundamental movement skill competency and reported a consistent and clear association between low competency in fundamental movement skills (especially kicking and throwing) and inadequate levels of cardiorespiratory fitness (53). These findings highlight the importance of enhancing muscular fitness and motor skill performance in youth in order to alter physical activity trajectories and improve health outcomes.

Contemporary trends in youth physical inactivity have become the biggest public health problem of the 21st century (14), and changes in our current approach to managing this condition are needed to counteract this crisis. In 1961, Kraus and Raab coined the term **hypokinetic disease** and said that insufficient movement or exercise, particularly in children, was an independent risk factor for the development and progression of chronic diseases including obesity, diabetes, and heart disease (58). They said that physicians need to recognize the harmful effects of *underexercise* to prevent "motion deficiency" in their young patients (58). The negative consequences of physical inactivity on lifelong health and well-being are so compelling that the term **exercise deficit disorder** (EDD) (60) was recently introduced to characterize a condition of reduced levels of MVPA that are inconsistent with current public health recommendations (46, 70, 89). Use of the term exercise deficit disorder may help to raise public awareness and convey a modern-day view of this health care concern. Qualified professionals should identify boys and girls who do not meet daily recommendations for MVPA and subsequently initiate strategies to prevent the upsurge in high-risk behaviors during this critical period of life. Since there are no medications to treat deficiencies in physical activity, age-related exercise interventions that begin early in life are

needed to develop healthy habits and optimize health and fitness outcomes. Screening children and adolescents for EDD will encourage early detection and promote intervention before they become resistant to behavior modification, pharmacotherapy, and expensive medical procedures.

BENEFITS OF PHYSICAL ACTIVITY FOR CHILDREN AND ADOLESCENTS

Regular participation in MVPA is recognized as a powerful marker of health, and numerous benefits have been reported in the literature (55, 75, 90). Significant gains in measures of health and physical fitness, as well as improvements in psychosocial health outcomes, have been observed following regular participation in exercise and sport programs. Daily physical activity helps to reduce body fat, build skeletal tissue, strengthen muscle, improve blood lipids, enhance aerobic fitness, and reduce symptoms of anxiety and depression in children and adolescents (4, 17, 90). Regular participation in meaningful physical activity also has cognitive effects that can positively influence social self-efficacy and academic attainment in youth (54, 77, 79).

Because many "adult diseases" are influenced by lifestyle habits established during the growing years, it is important to identify and treat physical inactivity early in life before youth develop bad habits and increase their risk for disease (30, 89). This view is supported by the observation that nearly half of children who become obese between the ages of 5 and 14 years were already overweight when they entered kindergarten (29). Children who are exposed to an environment with opportunities to participate in physical activity early in life are more likely to be active later in life (93). While these observations highlight the significance of establishing healthy behaviors during the growing years, it is important to consider the type of physical activity that provides the foundation for a lifetime of recreation, fitness, and sport. Research indicates that proficiency in fundamental movement skills during childhood best predicts subsequent physical activity and fitness performance later in life (20, 80, 87).

Key Point

Modern-day youth are not as active as they should be, and the decline in physical activity tends to start early in life. Evidence-based strategies and public health policies are needed to identify youth at risk for physical inactivity and promote positive lifestyle choices.

Since muscular strength is an essential component of motor skill performance (40, 63), the importance of performing resistance exercise along with fundamental movement skills should not be overlooked in the design of youth programs.

New insights in the field of pediatric exercise science have highlighted the importance of integrating strength-building and skill-enhancing activities into youth programs to alter physical activity trajectories and reduce associated injury risks (36, 37, 69). Suboptimal levels of physical activity may increase the risk of injury during free play, youth sports, and physical education. In a prospective study that described risk factors associated with injuries in a large group of children, the steepest increase in injury risk was found for the quartile of youth with the lowest habitual physical activity, and the cutoff for this level was 5 hours per week of physical activity (15). These observations are consistent with those of others who noted that young athletes are at greater risk of a sport-related injury if they do not possess adequate muscular strength and physical conditioning (32, 96). While public health actions call for increasing physical activity across the life span (55, 100), participation in MVPA should evolve out of preparatory fitness conditioning that is consistent with the needs and abilities of growing children and adolescents.

GROWTH, MATURATION, AND PHYSICAL ACTIVITY

Measures of health and fitness in children and adolescents are in a constant state of change, which makes it more challenging to distinguish maturational differences in physiological measures from training-induced gains in physical fitness. Muscular power, for example, normally improves throughout childhood and adolescence even without participation in a structured training program. Comparing the vertical performance of an 8-year-old child to that of a 16-year-old adolescent supports the premise that physical measures improve over time as a result of growth and maturation. But if an 8-year-old child participates in a well-designed fitness program, jumping performance will improve beyond gains due to growth and maturation.

Understanding the influence of growth and maturation on measures of physical fitness and possible outcomes of exercise training assists in the design and progression of youth programs. There are considerable interindividual differences in physical development among youth of the same age, and exercise professionals should be mindful of maturity-associated variation in growth and performance. For example, a 12-year-old girl can be taller and more physically skilled than a 12-year-old boy, and two 14-year-old adolescents can have considerable differences in body mass and muscle strength. These differences are related to the timing of puberty, which can vary from 8 to 13 years of age in girls and from 9 to 15 years of age in boys. **Puberty** is a process of physical changes related to sexual maturation in which a child's body matures into an adult body. During this period, the biological and physical changes that occur can influence measures of physical fitness. Although the onset of puberty is typically two years later in males than in females, the age at which puberty begins is influenced by genetics as well as environmental factors, including nutrition, exercise habits, and socioeconomic conditions (63).

Biological maturation can be assessed in terms of skeletal age, somatic (physique) maturity, or sexual maturity. In females, **menarche** (first menstrual cycle) is a marker of sexual maturation, whereas in males the best indicators of sexual maturity are physical features called secondary sex characteristics. Secondary sex characteristics can be used to describe pubertal maturation in terms of different stages. The most common staging system was proposed by and named for J.M. Tanner and includes a sequence of stages that progress from Tanner stage 1 (preadolescence) to Tanner stage 5 (mature adult) (92). Criteria for each stage are based on pubic hair growth and breast and genital maturation, and ratings are ordinarily made by observation at a clinical examination. Because of the invasive nature of direct observation of Tanner staging, self-assessment techniques have been used that require children to compare their own sexual characteristics to those of reference drawings or photographs (65).

Although it is not possible to assess the onset of puberty with body measurements, longitudinal data for height can provide useful information to mark the age at onset of the adolescent growth spurt and the age at the maximum rate of growth (termed **peak height velocity** or PHV) (63). On average, the age of PHV is about 12 years in girls and 14 years in boys. The age at PHV is an indicator of somatic maturity and can also provide a landmark for other measures of sexual maturation. For example, menarche occurs after PHV in girls (63). Exercise professionals need to be sensitive to interindividual differences in physical appearance and abilities when teaching children and adolescents because considerable variability exists in the age at which youth pass through developmental stages. Boys and girls advanced in maturity are, on average, taller and heavier than their peers who are average (on time) or delayed (late) in maturity status (63). Individual differences in maturity status can influence body size as well as the performance of tasks that require strength, power, and speed. In contact sports, player grouping strategies that are based on physical size or biological maturity may help to protect smaller, later-maturing players as they progress through adolescence. However, emotional and cognitive factors need to be considered when one is asking a player to train or compete with younger or older athletes (64).

Key Point

Knowledge of growth and maturation can help to explain fluctuations in fitness performance during the growing years and optimize the design of training programs to maximize performance and reduce the risk of injury.

EFFECTS OF EXERCISE IN CHILDREN AND ADOLESCENTS

Anatomical, physiological, and developmental differences between children and adults influence the responses and adaptations to exercise training. Because children are less mature than adults, the principles of pediatric exercise science have practical implications for exercise professionals who design, implement, and assess youth programs. The information in table 11.1 provides a comparison of physiological performance measures in children and adults.

Age-Related Differences in Performance

Perhaps the most visible difference between children and adults relates to the relative lack of metabolic specialization in younger populations.

Table 11.1 Comparison of Physiological Measures in Children and Adults

Measure	Comparison		
Maximal heart rate	Children	>	Adults
Stroke volume	Children	<	Adults
Cardiac output	Children	<	Adults
Tidal volume	Children	<	Adults
Breathing frequency	Children	>	Adults
Absolute $\dot{V}O_2$	Children	<	Adults
Relative $\dot{V}O_2$	Children	>	Adults
Glycolytic activity	Children	<	Adults
Exercise lactate	Children	<	Adults
Anaerobic performance	Children	<	Adults
Absolute muscle strength	Children	<	Adults
Exercise recovery	Children	>	Adults

Adapted, by permission, from A. Faigenbaum, 2015, Children and adolescents. In *Exercise physiology,* edited by J.P. Porcari, C.X. Bryant, and F. Comana (Philadelphia, PA: FA Davis), 692.

Unlike adults, who tend to specialize in sports such as weightlifting or long-distance running, children tend to be "metabolic nonspecialists" with regard to their exercise performance (11). A child who is the strongest in class is likely to be a leader in an aerobic endurance run as well. Laboratory data support the concept that children with a relatively high level of aerobic fitness also have superior performance on anaerobic tests (81). The metabolic uniqueness of children is just one reason why it is important to expose youth to a variety of sports during the growing years. Children who specialize in one sport year-round at the exclusion of other sports may be at increased risk for burnout, social isolation, and overuse injury (32, 71).

Although our relative understanding of exercise metabolism in youth is limited, a review of early findings based on muscle biopsy data suggests that adenosine triphosphate (ATP) and creatine phosphate (CP) levels at rest are similar to those of adults (33). In terms of exercise-related differences in anaerobic metabolism, children appear to have a faster rate of intramuscular CP resynthesis than adults, which suggests that the capacity of children to perform high-intensity exercise for less than 10 seconds is not impaired (50). However, glycolytic activity appears limited in children as compared to adults (6). Thus, less mature subjects should not be expected to perform as well as adults on short-burst, high-energy activities lasting 30 to 120 seconds. Age-related differences in muscle characteristics (e.g., muscle mass and muscle enzyme activity) as well as hormonal changes during puberty could explain these observations.

Children typically demonstrate lower levels of blood lactate than adults during submaximal and maximal exercise, which supports the contention that youth have a depressed capacity for glycolytic metabolism (16). However, the rate of elimination of lactate after exercise is the same in youth and adults (50). While different physiological factors may explain child–adult differences in recovery, it is possible that youth may recover faster from high-intensity bouts of physical exertion because they have less to recover from. That is, a lower level of absolute work in children as compared to adults may yield less potential for an absolute

reduction in performance. These findings have practical implications for the design of youth programs because, in addition to the training goals, the length of the rest interval between bouts of physical exertion may need to be age related. Research indicates that children may require rest intervals of only 1 minute between sets of resistance exercise to minimize loading reductions and attain the highest possible training volume (48).

Differences in the cardiorespiratory responses to exercise between children and adults are observable when adults play with children. While resting heart rates are similar between youth and adults, children and adolescents exhibit higher heart rates and lower stroke volumes at all exercise intensities than older populations (81). Since children and adolescents have smaller hearts than adults, and therefore smaller left ventricles, it is not surprising that youth have lower stroke volumes. The higher heart rates children typically exhibit when exercising with an adult are probably an attempt to compensate for the smaller ventricular size and lower stroke volume. However, the heart rate compensation during exercise is somewhat incomplete, as youth show smaller increases in cardiac output at all exercise intensities as compared to adults (81). Maximal heart rates (MHR) do not change appreciably during childhood and early adolescence, and it is not uncommon for a child's heart rate to exceed 200 beats/min during vigorous physical activity. Therefore, the estimation of MHR by age-based equations is inappropriate for youth under 15 years of age. For older adolescents who want to estimate their MHR, the following formula has been recommended: MHR = 207 – (0.7 × age) [7].

The total amount of air a person breathes per minute is called **minute ventilation**, and this measure is a product of **tidal volume** and **respiratory rate**. The tidal volume is the amount of air inspired or expired in a single breath, and respiratory rate refers to the number of breaths per minute. Children and adolescents have a lower tidal volume and higher breathing frequency than adults at all exercise intensities (81). It is normal for healthy children and adolescents to breathe rapidly during vigorous activity because they process a relatively smaller amount of air in absolute terms per minute. However, during maximal exercise, minute ventilation expressed per kilogram of body weight is equal between youth and adults (81). No compelling evidence indicates that the cardiorespiratory responses to exercise in healthy children and adolescents limit exercise performance.

Trainability of Children and Adolescents

A widely recognized measure of aerobic fitness in youth is termed **peak oxygen uptake** (peak $\dot{V}O_2$), which can be expressed in absolute (L/min) or relative (ml $\cdot$ kg^{-1} $\cdot$ min^{-1}) terms. In adults, peak $\dot{V}O_2$ is closely linked to cardiorespiratory fitness and is an established measure of one's ability to perform prolonged periods of aerobic endurance exercise. In children, peak $\dot{V}O_2$ reflects the physiological functioning of the cardiorespiratory system, but is only weakly related to objectively measured physical activity and aerobic endurance performance (31, 81). Peak $\dot{V}O_2$ per kilogram body weight remains relatively stable over time during the growing years, yet performance on standard field tests such as the 1-mile (1.6 km) run consistently improves. Moreover, during childhood, training-induced gains in peak $\dot{V}O_2$ (about 5-10%) are significantly less than gains typically observed in older populations, which suggests that physiological adaptations to aerobic training in children are maturity dependent (10, 81). For these reasons, exercise professionals who assess endurance performance in younger populations need to be aware of age-related factors when monitoring changes in performance over time. While regular exercise training can enhance aerobic fitness in youth, the influence of age, maturation, and sex on training-induced adaptations during the growing years should not be overlooked.

Observable gains in muscular strength and muscular power are expected in healthy children and adolescents due to growth and maturation. Although boys and girls do not follow the same rate of change, performance on tests such as the push-up and vertical jump increases from childhood through adolescence for both sexes. In addition to growth-related gains in muscle size, neuromuscular changes in motor unit firing rate, recruitment, or conduction velocity, as well as alterations in muscle pennation angle, contribute to qualitative changes in muscle function during childhood and adolescence (63).

Following regular participation in a well-designed and -implemented resistance training program, children and adolescents can improve their strength and motor skill performance above and beyond gains due to growth and maturation (38, 61). Of note, relative strength gains of roughly 30% are typically observed following short-term (8 to 20 weeks) resistance training in untrained youth (38). During childhood, training-induced gains in muscular fitness are primarily due to neuromuscular factors (37, 38, 47). However, during puberty, testosterone secretion in males is associated with gains in fat-free mass following resistance training, whereas smaller amounts of testosterone in females limit the magnitude of training-induced increases in muscle hypertrophy (63). Knowledge of the qualitative and quantitative responses and adaptations to exercise training, along with an understanding of realistic outcomes, is important for exercise professionals who monitor changes in performance over time.

Key Point

Measures of physical fitness are in a constant state of change throughout childhood and adolescence, which makes it more challenging to distinguish maturational differences in performance from training-induced gains in health and fitness.

EXERCISE RECOMMENDATIONS FOR CHILDREN AND ADOLESCENTS

Children and adolescents are active in different ways and for different reasons than older populations. Enhancing one's peak $\dot{V}O_2$ or improving one's blood lipid profile may be a important motivating factor for adults, but most children want to have fun, build friendships, and improve physical skills. Thus, exercise professionals should focus on creating an enjoyable experience whereby youth have an opportunity to learn meaningful content with age-appropriate instruction.

The dynamic relationship between motor skills, muscular fitness, and physical activity should be reinforced over time with qualified instruction, enthusiastic leadership, and adequate practice time. This concept is consistent with a positive feedback loop whereby youth who gain competence and confidence in their muscular fitness and motor skill abilities will be better prepared to participate in lifetime activities with energy and vigor (41). In turn, this will continue to drive their abilities and willingness to engage in health-, skill-, and performance-enhancing physical activities. Exercise professionals should genuinely appreciate the long-lasting value of enhancing physical literacy, which encompasses an individual's motivation, competence, and confidence to engage in purposeful physical pursuits (99). The importance of designing programs that provide an opportunity for all youth to enhance their movement repertoire early in life has been proposed in several developmental models of lifetime physical activity (62, 88).

Global health recommendations state that youth should accumulate at least 60 minutes of MVPA throughout the day (100), yet a continuous bout of sustained physical activity at a predetermined intensity may not be appropriate for most youth. While continuous activity is not physiologically harmful, most youth tend to enjoy nonsustained activities or games that vary in volume and intensity (9). Continuous MVPA without rest or recovery is rare among children. Exercise professionals should carefully design and sensibly progress youth programs that are characterized by alternate bouts of moderate and vigorous physical activity with brief periods of rest and recovery as needed. Age-related circuit training activities that alternate lower-effort and higher-effort segments and integrate both health- and skill-related components of physical fitness have proven to be beneficial (26, 36, 37). Health- and skill-related components of physical fitness are outlined in table 11.2.

Key Point

Circuit training activities are a feasible, effective, and time-efficient approach for incorporating moderate- and vigorous-intensity physical activities into youth exercise programs.

Table 11.2 Components of Physical Fitness

Health related	Skill related
Aerobic fitness	Agility
Muscular strength	Balance
Muscular endurance	Coordination
Flexibility	Speed
Body composition	Power
	Reaction time

Exercise Guidelines for Children and Adolescents

A prerequisite for the development and administration of safe, effective, and enjoyable youth exercise programs is an understanding of established training principles and an appreciation for the developmental uniqueness of children and adolescents (35). Not only does qualified and enthusiastic instruction enhance participant safety and enjoyment, but direct supervision of youth programs can improve program compliance and optimize outcomes (28, 91). Qualified supervision and basic education on proper exercise technique, skill-based progression, and age-related training principles should be part of all youth exercise programs. Although there is no minimum age requirement at which children can begin exercise training, all participants must be mentally and physically ready to comply with instructions and undergo the stress of an exercise program. In general, most 7- and 8-year-old boys and girls are ready for participation in some type of structured recreation or sport activity (38).

Exercise professionals who work with adults need to modify exercise guidelines for children and adolescents to better match the physical and psychosocial characteristics of youth. The standard means of assessing aerobic exercise intensity in adults is heart rate monitoring. In one respect, heart rate monitoring is problematic for children who have great difficulty finding and counting their pulse rate during exercise. Moreover, as noted earlier, there is little need for healthy children to monitor their heart rate response because target heart rate formulas are designed for older populations. Generally, observations by the exercise professional may be sufficient for determining children's physical exertion during their training sessions.

The aerobic segment of youth programs should include a variety of fundamental movement skills (e.g., balancing, jumping, kicking, and throwing), as well as activities that involve apparatus including hoops, ropes, cones, and playground balls. In addition, physically active but less competitive games can keep children moving and motivated without fear of failure. Inactive youth can begin with 20 or 30 minutes and gradually accumulate at least 60 minutes or more on all or most days of the week. When appropriate, vigorous bouts of activity should be systematically incorporated into the exercise session to optimize training adaptations.

The importance of integrating resistance training exercises with movement skill activities should not be overlooked. Research demonstrates that resistance training can be a safe and effective way to enhance motor performance in youth provided that age-appropriate training guidelines are followed (13, 39, 45). Bodyweight exercises and different types of equipment, including free weights (i.e., barbells and dumbbells), child-size machines, elastic bands, and medicine balls, can be used in youth resistance training programs. It is important to incorporate multijoint movements in youth programs because these exercises require the coordinated action of many muscle groups. Also, the importance of strengthening the abdominal muscles, hips, and lower back should not be overlooked because low back pain in youth is becoming a public health concern (19). Rest periods of about 1 minute between sets and exercises should suffice for most children, but this may need to be increased if the training intensity increases or if the exercises require a high degree of technical skill (e.g., weightlifting movements) (61).

Exercise professionals typically recommend a percentage of an individual's one repetition maximum (1RM) to prescribe an appropriate resistance training intensity. Research indicates that strength and power testing are safe and reliable for children and adolescents when standardized protocols are followed (43, 44). For youth without resistance training experience, the initial program should use a low volume (one or two sets) and a light training intensity (40-60% 1RM) for a range of exercises. Once youth develop basic exercise technique, the resistance training program can be progressed, for example, to two or three sets with a light to moderate training intensity (40-80% 1RM). As youth gain experience resistance training and as exercise technique improves, youth can be introduced to periodic phases of higher external loads (≥80% 1RM) on the proviso that technical competency remains (61). Exercise professionals should observe and monitor participants throughout the resistance training session to minimize the risks associated with fatigue-induced decrements in exercise performance, which may increase the risk of injury. If 1RM testing is not performed, a simple approach is to first establish the repetition range and then determine the appropriate load that can be handled for the prescribed number of repetitions. Youth resistance training guidelines are as follows (38), and program design recommendations are outlined in table 11.3:

- Provide qualified instruction and supervision.

- Ensure that the exercise environment is safe and free of hazards.

- Review proper training procedures and sensible starting loads.

- Focus on correct exercise technique rather than the amount of weight lifted.

- Perform one to three sets of 6 to 15 repetitions on a variety of strength exercises.

- Perform one to three sets of 3 to 6 repetitions on a variety of power exercises.

- Increase the resistance gradually (5% to 10%) as performance improves.

- Begin resistance training two or three times per week on nonconsecutive days.

- Monitor progress and establish realistic expectations.

- Systematically vary the training program to maintain interest and optimize adaptations.

- Encourage youth to ask questions and state their concerns.

Table 11.3 Program Design Guidelines for Children and Adolescents

Type of exercise	Frequency	Intensity	Volume
Aerobic games and skill-building activities	Daily	Moderate to vigorous with rest and recovery as needed	≥60 min
Resistance training	2-3 times/week	Begin with a light training intensity (40-60% 1RM) on a variety of exercises; progress to a higher intensity on more advanced exercises as technical competency improves	≥20-40 min
Static and dynamic flexibility	≥2-3 times/week	Controlled movements throughout the range of motion for all muscle groups	≥5-10 min

Key Point

Supervised exercise interventions that include resistance training are needed to target deficits in muscular fitness and enhance resistance training skill competency. Youth should receive constructive feedback to ensure safe and correct movement skill development.

While flexibility is a well-recognized component of health-related fitness, long-held beliefs regarding the traditional practice of warm-up static stretching have been questioned. An acute bout of static stretching can have a negative influence on muscle performance, and static stretching immediately before exercise has no significant effect on injury prevention (12, 85). This is not to suggest that children and teenagers should avoid regular static stretching, but rather that exercise professionals should consider the immediate impact of an acute bout of static stretching on performance. The cooldown may actually be the ideal time to perform static stretching exercises because the muscles are already warmed up and participants need to recover from the exercise session with less intense activities. Static stretches should be held for 10 to 30 seconds and repeated two to four times (73).

Since there is not sufficient scientific evidence to endorse preevent static stretching in youth fitness programs, there has been a rising interest in warm-up procedures that involve the performance of dynamic movements designed to elevate core body temperature, enhance motor unit excitability, improve kinesthetic awareness, maximize active ranges of motion, and develop motor skills (42). This type of preevent protocol is referred to as **dynamic warm-up** and typically includes low-, moderate-, and high-intensity hops, skips, jumps, lunges, and various movement-based exercises for the upper and lower body. And since equipment is not needed, dynamic warm-up protocols are a cost-effective method for enhancing movement skills that are the basic components of games and sports.

A well-designed dynamic warm-up can set the tone for the session and establish a desired tempo for the upcoming activities. This concept of *instant activity* satisfies the need for children, after sitting in school all day, to move when they enter the gymnasium or fitness center and helps to focus their attention on listening and learning (52). In addition, dynamic warm-up activities that are active, engaging, and challenging provide an opportunity for participants to gain confidence in their abilities while practicing a variety of motor skills. A 5- to 10-minute dynamic warm-up typically consists of 8 to 12 movements that progress from less intense to more intense. Participants can perform selected movements in place or can perform each dynamic movement for about 10 yards (about 9 m), rest about 5 to 10 seconds, and then repeat the same exercise for 10 yards as they return to the starting point. Examples of these dynamic movements include high knee lift, woodchopper, torso twist, lunge walk, and lateral shuffle.

It is important to remember that the goal of children's exercise programs should not be limited to time spent in MVPA. Teaching children and adolescents proper exercise technique, enhancing performance on a variety of movement skills, and fostering healthy behaviors in a supportive environment are equally important. Consequently, in addition to monitoring the quantity of MVPA, the quality of the "exercise dose" should be carefully prescribed (76). This is where the art and science of developing youth programs come into play, because the principles of pediatric exercise science and skill development need to be coupled with effective learning, mental engagement, and making friends.

Table 11.4 outlines a sample exercise program for a group of healthy children in an after-school fitness program. Every class begins with dynamic warm-up activities. During the warm-up, children can perform basic locomotor movements (e.g., skipping, jumping, and lateral shuffling), as well as different exercises with lightweight medicine balls (1 to 2 kg), to reinforce proper movement patterns. If space is limited, modified dynamic warm-up activities can be performed while standing in place. While brief recovery periods between movements are needed, the transition time between movements should be short to maintain interest and reduce the likelihood of off-task behaviors.

The exercise segment includes a fundamental integrative training (FIT) circuit that is designed to enhance both health- and skill-related components of fitness using different types of equipment, including medicine balls, exercise bands, agility ladders, fitness ropes, punch balloons, and bodyweight exercises (18). While there are literally hundreds of exercises that can be performed, youth programs should follow a simple progression so participants can experience small successes every class. Begin with 30 seconds at 8 to 10 exercise stations and periodically make the movements more challenging as competence and confidence improve. Provide adequate opportunity for participants to perform each exercise correctly at each station before moving to the next station during a short transition period. Once participants master basic skills, allow them to create new exercises so they can apply the skills learned in a positive manner. Play background music during the lesson, and encourage all students to focus on personal improvements while encouraging some to try their best.

By identifying the health- and skill-related components of physical fitness that are developed at each station, participants have an opportunity to learn about different fitness components and apply movement concepts to future lessons. For less skilled children, use basic exercise movements that enhance movement patterns and spatial awareness. For example, animal activities such as bear crawls, seal walks, kangaroo hops, and inchworms provide an opportunity for youth to explore their environment while developing physical abilities. Children are still learning how to manipulate both their body and objects through space; and activities with colorful punch balloons slow down each movement to a controllable level so young children can master new skills and achieve success. The exercise lesson can end with child-friendly games and cooldown stretching activities. Of note, exercise professionals should allow time for feedback and reflection after every session. Detailed descriptions of age-related exercises and activities are available elsewhere (22, 49, 68).

Table 11.4   Sample Exercise Lesson for Children

Session phase	Time	Sample exercises
Dynamic warm-up with medicine ball (1-2 kg)	5-10 min	Jog while catching ball, moving ball side to side, pressing ball overhead, rolling ball on the floor; lateral shuffles, giant steps; walking with high knees.
Movement preparation	5 min	Review daily lesson and safety concerns; demonstrate proper exercise technique on new exercises.
Fundamental integrative training circuit	20-25 min	8-12 exercise stations using body weight, medicine balls, elastic bands, fitness ropes, punch balloons, agility ladders, balance boards, and other modalities.
Games and activities	5 min	Aerobic games and skill-building activities
Cooldown and review	5 min	Aerobic games and skill-building activities

Special Considerations for Children and Adolescents Who Are Overweight

The epidemic of pediatric obesity and associated comorbidities has become a critical public health threat with far-reaching health, economic, and social consequences (29, 78). While there is not one program of proven efficacy that professionals can use to manage this condition, multifaceted interventions that include physical activity, nutrition education, and behavior modification offer the best chance for success (3). Although aerobic-type activities are efficacious for reducing percent body fat (56), resistance training has been found to improve insulin sensitivity, enhance self-concept, and reduce abdominal fat in overweight youth (59, 84, 86, 97).

A major objective of youth exercise programming is for physical activity to become a habitual part of children's lives and hopefully persist into adulthood. With this objective in mind, exercise professionals must strive to increase participants' perceptions of their physical abilities and target deficiencies in muscle strength and movement patterns to foster participation in regular physical activity. Most overweight youth find resistance training enjoyable because this type of exercise is not aerobically taxing and provides an opportunity for all youth to experience success and feel good about their performance. This is particularly important for youth who are overweight because they often lack the skills, confidence, and motivation to engage in aerobic exercise (24).

Since youth tend to be more physically active when in the presence of peers and when relationships are positive and rewarding, resistance training provides a unique opportunity for companionship and recreation. Overweight youth spend more time alone and tend to be more sensitive to any type of peer interaction than nonoverweight youth (83). Therefore, exercise classes that include activities that enhance muscular fitness and promote social networking can provide youth who are overweight with an opportunity to form social networks while gaining confidence in their abilities to be physically active. Thus, the first step in encouraging overweight youth to exercise regularly may be to increase their confidence in their ability to be physically active in a socially supportive environment; this, in turn, may lead to an increase in regular physical activity, an improvement in body composition, and hopefully, exposure to a form of exercise that can be carried over into adulthood.

Exercise Modifications, Precautions, and Contraindications

There is no scientific evidence to suggest that the risks and concerns associated with exercise in healthy youth are greater than those associated with free play and structured fitness activities. However, children and adolescents with diseases and disabilities including asthma, diabetes mellitus, obesity, cystic fibrosis, and cerebral palsy should have their exercise prescription tailored to their specific needs, abilities, symptoms, and medical condition (2). Medical clearance is recommended for youth with preexisting medical concerns (1).

While exercise programs for children and adolescents should be supervised by qualified exercise professionals and take place in a well-lit and clean environment, it is important to be aware of risk factors for exercise-related injuries and injury prevention strategies. Exercise training injuries in youth are most often the result of accidents that could be preventable with increased supervision and adherence to safety guidelines. For example, researchers reported that two-thirds of exercise training–related injuries sustained by 8- to 13-year-old patients who reported to emergency departments in the United States were to the hand and foot, and most were related to "dropping" and "pinching," according to the injury descriptions (72). These observations highlight the importance of close supervision and qualified instruction on the proper use of exercise equipment.

While an understanding of the fundamental principles of pediatric exercise science is valuable, a key issue is to know how to provide youth with the skills, knowledge, attitudes, and behaviors that lead to a lifetime of physical activity. Exercise professionals need to respect children's feelings while appreciating the fact that their thinking is different than that of an adult. Exercise programs should be consistent with individual needs and abilities, and the challenges associated with promoting youth fitness should be met with enthusiastic leadership, creative programming, and age-related teaching strategies. Youth should be taught how to perform each exercise correctly and should receive constructive feedback every class. Exercise professionals should provide clear demonstrations of every exercise and regularly remind participants of proper training guidelines and safety rules (e.g., proper footwear, shoes tied, no gum chewing). Modifiable risk factors associated with exercise-related injuries in youth that can be reduced or eliminated with qualified supervision and instruction are outlined in table 11.5 (47).

Key Point

The focus of youth exercise programs should be on positive learning experiences in which participants have an opportunity to make friends and learn something new while gaining competence and confidence in their physical abilities.

Another concern involves thermoregulation for the exercising child or adolescent. During exercise, heat production increases and the body must increase blood flow to the skin for heat removal. Children and adolescents have a larger surface area–to–mass ratio than adults, which allows for greater heat exchange (51). When the environmental temperature is lower than body temperature (e.g., in a swimming pool), more heat is dissipated. However, when the environmental temperature is higher than body temperature (e.g., during summer sport practice), less heat will be lost. Failure to effectively remove body heat during strenuous exercise in conditions of high ambient temperature and humidity can result in a decrement in performance and an increased risk for heat-related illness (5, 51).

In addition to poor hydration status, other determinants of reduced performance and exertional heat illness risk in youth during exercise and sport in a hot environment include undue physical exertion, insufficient recovery between repeated exercise bouts, and inappropriate clothing (27). Exercise professionals need to be aware of thermoregulatory concerns and make the necessary modifications to reduce the likelihood of exertional heat illness. Of note, since youth tend to underestimate the amount of fluid they need to stay hydrated during prolonged periods of exercise, they should be encouraged to consume adequate fluid before, during, and after every exercise session (82).

Table 11.5   Modifiable Risk Factors in Youth Exercise Programs

Risk factor	Modification by exercise professional
Unsafe exercise environment	Adequate training space and proper equipment layout
Incorrect use of equipment	Proper instruction and adherence to safety rules
Improper equipment storage	Safe and secure storage of exercise equipment
Inadequate warm-up	Proper dynamic warm-up before training
Excessive load and volume	Gradual progression of training load and volume
Poor exercise technique	Proper instruction of exercise movements
Poor trunk control	Targeted core training
Muscle imbalances	Focus on appropriate muscle balance around joints
Previous injury	Communicate with treating clinician and modify program
Dehydration	Adequate fluid before, during, and after exercise training
Sex-specific growth	Modify training to address specific needs and abilities
Chronic fatigue	Consider lifestyle factors such as proper nutrition, adequate sleep, and recovery between training sessions

Adapted, by permission, from A. Faigenbaum et al., 2011, "Injury trends and prevention in youth resistance training," *Strength and Conditioning Journal* 33: 36-41.

Case Study

Children and Adolescents

Damien is 10 years old and attends a primary school that offers physical education only one day per week. Because Damien does not play any sports, his parents were concerned that he wasn't getting enough physical activity. They learned about an after-school fitness program for primary school students and enrolled Damien in it. The exercise professional directing the program understands that while youth sport programs are available in most communities, not all boys and girls enjoy intense competition, and the musculoskeletal system of today's youth may not be prepared for the demands of sport practice and competition. Consequently, Damien's exercise program should provide him with an opportunity to enhance muscular strength, master fundamental movement skills, and improve movement mechanics while gaining confidence in his abilities to be physically active. In the long run, youth programs that enhance basic motor skills and fitness proficiency while augmenting competence and confidence in one's abilities are more likely to spark an interest in physical activity as an ongoing lifestyle choice. Focusing only on sport skills at an early age not only limits the ability of children to succeed at tasks outside a narrow physical spectrum, but also discriminates against children whose motor skills are not as well developed.

The program Damien participates in uses the general structure shown earlier in tables 11.3 and 11.4. Each session is 45 to 60 minutes long and consists of a dynamic warm-up, a FIT circuit, games and activities, and a cooldown. The FIT circuit includes stations using body weight, medicine balls, elastic bands, and other implements and modalities. The games and activities segment generally involves games with beach balls, variations of soccer or hockey, and tag games.

Following regular participation in the after-school program, Damien made observable gains in muscular fitness; his ability to perform movement skills that required agility, balance, and coordination improved. As the exercise program progressed, Damien was able to perform advanced skills and understand the fundamental concepts of a fitness workout. He made new friends and developed a keen interest in playing soccer during game activities. He now enjoys playing outside with his friends and riding his bike. Due to the remarkable improvements in his physical competence and perceived competence, Damien wants to continue in the after-school program and plans to join a community-based soccer team next season. With ongoing support from his parents, friends, and exercise professionals who enjoy daily MVPA, Damien will develop the fundamental skills, positive attitudes, and prerequisite knowledge needed for participation in exercise and sport for a lifetime.

Recommended Readings

Chu, D and Myer, G. *Plyometrics.* Champaign, IL: Human Kinetics, 2013.

Faigenbaum, A, Lloyd, R, and Myer, G. Youth resistance training: past practices, new perspectives and future directions. *Pediatr Exerc Sci* 25:591-604, 2013.

Institute of Medicine. *Educating the Student Body: Taking Physical Activity and Physical Education to School.* Washington, DC: National Academies Press, 2013.

Lloyd, R and Oliver, J. *Strength and Conditioning for Young Athletes.* London: Routledge, 2014.

Malina, R, Bouchard, C, and Bar-Or, O. 2004. *Growth, Maturation and Physical Activity.* 2nd ed. Champaign, IL: Human Kinetics, 2004.

CONCLUSION

Throughout childhood and adolescence, the developing body is evolving physically and psychosocially into a mature adult body. Markers of fitness are in a constant state of change, and exercise professionals need to be cognizant of the developmental diversity among youth. Regular participation in free play and structured exercise activities can offer observable health and fitness value to children and adolescents provided that the games and activities are consistent with the needs, interests, and abilities of youth. Developing fundamental movement skills and enhancing muscular fitness early in life are important for ongoing participation in games and sports. The challenges associated with sparking a lifelong interest in daily physical activity should be met with enthusiastic leadership, creative programming, and effective teaching strategies.

Key Terms

adolescence
children
dynamic warm-up
exercise deficit disorder
fundamental movement skills
hypokinetic disease
menarche
minute ventilation

peak height velocity
peak oxygen uptake
puberty
respiratory rate
secondary sex characteristics
tidal volume

Study Questions

1. Throwing and catching are fundamental skills that are further classified as
    a. hand–eye skills
    b. propulsion skills
    c. ball-control skills
    d. object-control skills

2. Which of the following is true regarding physiological differences between children and adults?
    a. Relative $\dot{V}O_2$ is higher in adults.
    b. Maximal heart rate is greater in children.
    c. Breathing frequency is greater in adults.
    d. Maximal stroke volume is greater in children.

3. Which of the following is true regarding the use of peak $\dot{V}O_2$ as a measure of cardiorespiratory fitness in children?
    a. Peak $\dot{V}O_2$ relative to body weight increases steadily as children grow.
    b. Peak $\dot{V}O_2$ is weakly correlated with aerobic endurance performance.
    c. Influences of age, maturation, and sex on peak $\dot{V}O_2$ are similar to those of mature adults.
    d. Training-related improvements in peak $\dot{V}O_2$ are similar to those measured in mature adults.

4. Proper training parameters for children and adolescents with no prior training history include

    a. 1 set per exercise, 80% 1RM

    b. 2 sets per exercise, 50% 1RM

    c. two times per week with 4 or 5 sets per exercise

    d. four times per week with 1 day off between training days

12

Older Adults

Wayne L. Westcott, PhD, CSCS

After completing this chapter, you will be able to

◆ explain the detrimental effects of inactive aging on muscle, bone, and metabolism;

◆ explain the beneficial effects of resistance training on muscle, bone, and metabolism in older adults;

◆ describe the health-related advantages of performing combined resistance training and aerobic endurance exercise with respect to osteoporosis, obesity, type 2 diabetes, hypertension, hypercholesterolemia, and cognitive decline;

◆ design an age-appropriate program of resistance training for older adults, including exercise selection, exercise sets, exercise repetitions, training frequency, training progression, movement speed, movement range, and breathing pattern;

◆ design an age-appropriate program of aerobic endurance training for older adults, including training frequency, exercise duration, exercise intensity, and exercise selection; and

◆ describe effective teaching techniques for educating and motivating older adults with respect to beginning and maintaining a productive exercise program.

The aging process is accompanied by a variety of physiological changes, all of which present some degree of challenge to health and fitness, including both physical and mental performance. The two primary purposes of this chapter are to examine those physiological aging factors that may be favorably modified by resistance training and aerobic endurance training, and to present the most effective exercise training programs for enhancing health and fitness in older adults. The following areas are addressed, with emphasis on practical application for exercise professionals: physiological changes associated with aging; effects of resistance training and aerobic endurance training on aging factors; and recommended training protocols, procedures, and instructional strategies for older adults.

EXERCISE RECOMMENDATIONS FOR OLDER ADULTS

Aging is accompanied by degenerative responses in essentially all body tissues and systems. With respect to health and fitness, three major areas of concern for older adults are the muscular system, cardiorespiratory system, and brain and nervous system. Muscle loss, which averages 5% to 10% per decade after age 50, is closely associated with bone loss (10% to 30% per decade), as well as metabolic rate reduction (2% to 3% per decade) that typically leads to fat gain and related health issues. Undesirable changes in the aging cardiorespiratory system may result in reduced aerobic capacity (95) and cardiovascular function (111), as well as increased risk of coronary disease (157).

Key Point

Adults over age 50 who do not perform resistance exercise can lose muscle mass at the rate of 5% to 10% per decade and bone mass at the rate of 10% to 30% per decade. Resistance training is effective for reversing the muscle loss and metabolic decline that accompany inactive aging.

Muscular System

Muscle plays a major role in health and fitness. Muscle is essential for movement, and without regular movement, health, fitness, and quality of life deteriorate at a rapid rate (153). A lesser-known fact about muscle tissue is that it produces and releases **myokines** (hormone-like substances) that have endocrine effects on other body organs (141, 142) and may contribute to exercise-induced protection against several chronic diseases (141). Muscular fitness has a profound and pervasive influence on physical function (80, 94), which is especially relevant during the older adult period of life. Research also indicates that muscular fitness may have a positive effect on mental and emotional health in older adults (22, 27).

After age 30, muscle tissue is lost at the rate of 3% to 8% each decade for people who do not perform resistance training (52). Muscle mass decreases more rapidly after age 50, averaging 5% to 10% each decade (121). By age 60, individuals who do not resistance train may forfeit approximately 1 pound (0.45 kg) of muscle every year of life (135). This reduction in muscle mass adversely affects a variety of metabolic risk factors, including obesity, dyslipidemia, type 2 diabetes, and cardiovascular disease (161).

Muscle is very metabolically active tissue, even at rest, and therefore has a major influence on resting metabolic rate. In untrained muscle, ongoing protein breakdown and synthesis uses approximately 5 to 6 calories per pound of muscle every day (187). Consequently, the age-related reduction in muscle mass has a direct relationship with the age-related decline in resting metabolic rate, which averages 2% to 3% per decade in adults (103). Because 65% to 75% of the calories used on a daily basis by older adults are attributed to resting metabolism, muscle loss and subsequent metabolic slow-down are almost always accompanied by fat gain (187). Unfortunately, approximately 80% of men and 20% of women over age 60 are overweight or obese (54). Research reveals that increased fat weight is associated with increased risk of elevated blood pressure, undesirable blood lipid profiles, type 2 diabetes, and cardiovascular disease (119, 161, 185). Aging is also associated with increased **intra-abdominal fat** deposits, which is an independent risk factor for diabetes (35, 106) and cardiovascular disease (3).

Muscle loss may more directly increase the risk of type 2 diabetes and cardiovascular disease (52). The reason is that muscle tissue is the principal site for both glucose and triglyceride disposal (44, 161). In light of predictions that one of three adults will have diabetes by the middle of this century (19), it would be prudent for people to maintain as much muscle tissue as possible during the older adult years.

Muscle loss (**sarcopenia**) is closely associated with bone loss (**osteopenia**), and the aging process is accompanied by progressive deterioration of the musculoskeletal system. However, the rate of bone loss exceeds the rate of muscle loss. Whereas muscle mass may decrease as much as 10% each decade (121), bone mass may decrease as much as 30% each decade (range of 1% to 3% reduction in bone mineral density each year) (100, 135, 177). The National Osteoporosis Foundation reports that 35 million American adults have osteopenia, characterized by reduced bone mass and weak bones, and that 10 million American adults (8 million women) have **osteoporosis**, characterized by low bone mass and frail bones (134). According to the U.S. Department of Health and Human Services (173), osteoporosis will be responsible for bone fractures in almost one of three women and one of six men.

Musculoskeletal decline presents challenges for activities of daily living, including rising from seated positions, walking, climbing stairs, and carrying objects, as well as maintaining desirable posture and dynamic balance (77, 80, 94). Of particular concern is the increased risk of falling (12, 179), as morbidity and mortality rates are greater in older adults who have suffered a fall (63).

Although all physical performance factors are adversely affected with aging, the rate of decrease is greater in some activities than others. This is due to the disproportionately higher rate of atrophy (size reduction) in **Type II** (fast-twitch) **muscle fibers** compared to **Type I** (slow-twitch) **muscle fibers** (46, 104). As a consequence, muscle power, which is more closely associated with Type II muscle fibers than Type I muscle fibers,

decreases at a faster rate than muscle strength (70, 89, 118, 123, 124, 128). Conversely, muscle endurance, which is more closely associated with Type I muscle fibers than Type II muscle fibers, decreases at a slower rate than muscle strength (33, 59, 110, 166). Thus, while skeletal muscle enables movement and enhances many physiological functions in the body, muscle loss associated with aging predisposes people to diminished health, fitness, and physical abilities.

Cardiorespiratory System

The heart, lungs, blood vessels, and blood compose the cardiorespiratory system (120). Similar to what occurs in the muscular system, the aging process adversely affects all of the cardiorespiratory components and increases the risk of cardiovascular disease. Maximal heart rate, stroke volume, and cardiac output decrease progressively throughout the aging process (156). Additionally, aging is associated with thickening of the heart (left ventricle wall) and arteries, as well as a stiffening of the lungs resulting in a reduced aerobic capacity (37, 53).

The pervasive risk factors for cardiovascular disease are elevated resting blood pressure (systolic or diastolic) and undesirable blood lipid profiles (high triglycerides, high total cholesterol, high low-density lipoprotein [LDL] cholesterol, or low high-density lipoprotein [HDL] cholesterol) (48). Among American adults, approximately 35% experience elevated blood pressure (hypertension) (138), and approximately 45% have blood lipid profiles outside of the recommended ranges (116). Although these coronary risk factors increase with age, there are exercise interventions that can reduce the probability of cardiovascular decline and disease. These are addressed in a later section of this chapter.

Brain and Nervous System

Like all other body systems, the brain and nerves experience gradual deterioration during the aging process. Age-associated changes in the brain and nervous system are responsible for a variety of mental and physical performance problems in aging adults, ranging from delayed response time to Alzheimer's disease. Some of the mental health issues in this domain are poor physical self-concept and self-esteem, general mood disturbance, depression, high tension and anxiety, and reduced cognitive abilities (4-7, 137). Physical health problems that affect the brain and nervous system include the chronic discomfort associated with osteoarthritis, fibromyalgia, and low back injuries that often accompany aging (137).

A major nervous system problem associated with aging is a progressive decline in motor skills and performance of physical tasks (160). Aging is accompanied by gradual deterioration of eye function (154) leading to less accurate visual input (93) for eye–limb coordination (66); gradual deterioration of ear functions including impaired hearing and balance (149); and gradual deterioration of musculoskeletal feedback from sensory mechanisms in the muscles (**muscle spindles** sensitive to movement range) and in the joints (**Golgi tendon organs** sensitive to movement force) (39, 81). These sensory input issues make it more challenging for older adults to perform physical activity in general and standard exercise programs specifically.

COMMON MEDICATIONS GIVEN TO OLDER ADULTS

Many older adults take a variety of medications for a number of health conditions, including high blood pressure, high blood cholesterol, high blood sugar, arthritis, low back pain, osteoporosis, and depression. Older adults take more prescriptions, over-the-counter (OTC) medications, and supplements than any other age group in the United States (50); and the probability of filling a prescription increases as a person gets older (50), with 87% of those aged 62 through 85 years taking at least one prescription medication (152). As a result, older adults commonly have more than one physician who is prescribing a medication and more than one pharmacy filling a prescription (184), which makes it difficult to be aware of harmful drug–drug interactions. Even mixing OTC medications such as aspirin, ibuprofen, or other nonsteroidal anti-inflammatory drugs (NSAIDs) with medications commonly taken by older adults (e.g., warfarin, a blood thinner to pre-

vent blood clots) can have unwanted side effects (e.g., an increased risk of severe gastrointestinal problems) (132).

Although most of the common medications that older adults take are not contraindicated with respect to physical activity, some do affect heart rate response to exercise (i.e., artificially slow it down) and require recommendations from a physician or other health care professional for training intensity. The most prevalent of these are cardiovascular medications known as β-blockers. Examples include acebutolol (Sectral), atenolol (Tenormin), bisoprolol (Zebeta), metoprolol (Lopressor, Toprol-XL), nadolol (Corgard), nebivolol (Bystolic), and propranolol (Inderal LA, InnoPran XL) (78).

In general, it is recommended that older adults who list medications on their medical history form obtain approval from their physician or other health care professional and advisement for their exercise program design, especially the training intensity. More specifically, the reader should refer to chapters in this book that address particular conditions, such as cardiovascular conditions, osteoarthritis, and depression. An exercise professional should know the medications an older adult client is taking and fully understand the possible side effects and their impact on the client's ability to exercise.

EFFECTS OF EXERCISE IN OLDER ADULTS

Resistance training has been shown to significantly increase lean muscle mass and resting energy expenditure and to significantly decrease fat weight, including intra-abdominal fat. Research also indicates that resistance training is effective for preventing and managing type 2 diabetes. Resistance training further appears to enhance cardiovascular health by reducing resting blood pressure, improving blood lipid profiles, decreasing fat stores, increasing glycemic control, and lowering the risk of metabolic syndrome. Resistance training has also demonstrated significant bone mineral density (BMD) increases in men and women of all ages, thereby promoting a strong musculoskeletal system that facilitates improved physical function in activities of daily living. Mental health benefits associated with resistance training include improved cognitive abilities, enhanced self-concept, and reduced symptoms of depression. In addition, resistance training has demonstrated significant reversal of specific aging factors in skeletal muscle.

Aerobic endurance training increases **maximal oxygen uptake**, generally referred to as **aerobic capacity**, which enables individuals to perform large-muscle physical activities at higher energy levels and for longer durations. These beneficial physiological adaptations include an increase in the pumping capacity of the heart and a decrease in resting heart rate (122), and they are associated with reduced resting blood pressure (120) and improved blood lipid profiles (lower LDL levels, higher HDL levels, lower triglyceride levels) (133, 140).

Aerobic endurance activity is effective at reducing body fat and with respect to long-term weight maintenance (133, 172). Aerobic endurance activity is also beneficial for people with type 2 diabetes, as it has been shown to improve glycemic control and increase insulin sensitivity (11).

Muscle Mass

Muscle and associated strength losses are among the most persistent and pervasive problems associated with the aging process. During the adult years for those who are sedentary, muscle mass decreases by about 5 pounds (2.3 kg) per decade, and during the older adult years, muscle loss increases to up to 10 pounds (4.5 kg) per decade (52, 56, 57, 121, 135). It is therefore encouraging to learn that regular resistance training can attenuate muscle loss in adults of all ages. Numerous research studies have shown significant increases in muscle mass through relatively brief exercise sessions (15 to 35 minutes, two or three nonconsecutive days per week) (24, 51, 69, 84, 135, 148, 179). For example, in a study with more than 1,600 participants (21 to 80 years of age), 10 weeks of standard resistance training (one set of 12 machine exercises, two or three days per week) produced a mean lean (muscle) weight increase of 3.1 pounds (1.4 kg) (182). The two training frequencies resulted in identical average lean weight gains (3.1 pounds [1.4 kg]), and the responses were similar for all of the age groups (20s through each decade of life including the 70s).

Resting Energy Expenditure

Resistance training elicits an increase in muscle protein turnover, which enhances resting energy expenditure in two ways. The immediate (acute) effect of resistance training is muscle tissue **microtrauma**, which necessitates relatively high energy expenditure for muscle remodeling processes (68, 76). Several studies have shown significant increases in resting energy expenditure (averaging approximately 7%) after several weeks of resistance training (21, 24, 84, 114, 148, 175). Interestingly, more recent research has revealed that a single resistance training session may increase resting energy expenditure between 5% and 9% for 72 hours following the workout (68, 76). In a study by Heden and associates (76), beginning exercisers performed either a low-volume resistance training session (one set of 10 exercises in 15 minutes) or a moderate-volume resistance training session (three sets of 10 exercises in 35 minutes). Both training protocols resulted in a 5% average elevation in resting energy expenditure (approximately 100 calories a day) for three days after the training session. In a similar study by Hackney and colleagues (68), beginning and advanced exercisers completed a high-volume resistance training session (eight sets of eight exercises); and over the next three days, the beginning exercisers averaged a 9% increase in resting energy expenditure while the advanced exercisers averaged an 8% increase. The findings from these studies indicate that a moderate- to high-effort resistance training session may elevate resting energy expenditure by 100 or more calories per day (68, 76).

The more chronic effect of progressive resistance training is a gradual increase in muscle mass (**muscle hypertrophy**). As stated earlier, every pound (0.5 kg) of untrained skeletal muscle uses approximately 5 or 6 calories per day for ongoing protein breakdown and synthesis (187). However, every pound (0.5 kg) of resistance-trained skeletal muscle uses approximately 9 calories per day for tissue maintenance and remodeling processes (161). Consequently, a person who increases his muscle mass by 5 pounds (2.3 kg) through chronic resistance training may experience an additional resting energy expenditure of approximately 45 calories per day. Combining the acute metabolic effect of regular resistance training (more than 100 calories per day) with the chronic metabolic effect of 5 additional pounds (2.3 kg) of muscle tissue (approximately 45 calories per day), the total increase in resting energy expenditure approaches 150 calories per day.

Body Fat

Progressive resistance training is widely accepted as the best means for systematically building muscle in older adults (181). However, resistance training is also an effective activity for reducing body fat. For example, more than 1,600 individuals following a resistance training program experienced an average lean weight gain of 3.1 pounds (1.4 kg) and an average fat weight loss of 3.9 pounds (1.8 kg) after 10 weeks (182). Several other studies with older adults showed similar reductions in fat weight after approximately three months of resistance training (24, 84, 148, 179).

As indicated in the previous section, the increased resting energy expenditure associated with resistance training may account for a larger percentage of the fat loss than the calories used during the actual exercise sessions. Consider that a 20-minute circuit resistance training program may use approximately 200 calories during each workout and up to 50 additional calories during the hour following the exercise session (71). Over a one-month period, 12 strength workouts (three sessions per week × four weeks) would therefore expend approximately 2,400 calories (200 calories per session × 12 sessions) not including the immediate postexercise period. Assuming an increased resting energy expenditure of only 100 calories per day, the total monthly calorie cost of three weekly 20-minute circuit resistance training sessions would be approximately 5,400 calories (2,400 calories from exercise and 3,000 calories from elevated resting energy expenditure). Other things being equal, this could average about a 1.5-pound (0.7 kg) fat loss per month or almost 4 pounds (1.8 kg) over a 10-week training period (182).

More specifically, resistance training has been shown to reduce intra-abdominal fat in older men (88, 169) and older women (83, 168). This is an important effect of resistance training, as the accumulation of intra-abdominal fat appears to be associated with insulin resistance in aging adults (35, 106). In conjunction, excessive body fat also increases the risk of experiencing one or more risk factors (elevated blood pressure, elevated blood cholesterol, elevated blood glucose) associated with type 2 diabetes and cardiovascular disease (119, 161, 185).

Aerobic endurance exercise is also an effective means for reducing body fat, as large-muscle activities such as walking, jogging, running, cycling, swimming, rowing, stepping, and dancing burn relatively large numbers of calories. For example, walking on level ground at 3 miles per hour (4.8 km/h) requires approximately 3 metabolic equivalents (METs) of energy expenditure, which uses between 4 and 5 calories per minute depending on body weight (1). Running on level ground at 6 miles per hour (9.7 km/h) requires approximately 10 METs of energy expenditure, which uses between 11 and 12 calories per minute depending on body weight (1).

Key Point

Resistance training and aerobic endurance exercise are effective for reducing body fat and the risk of associated health problems such as type 2 diabetes, elevated blood pressure, undesirable blood lipid profiles, and cardiovascular disease.

Type 2 Diabetes

In addition to reducing total body-fat stores and intra-abdominal fat accumulation, resistance training provides other benefits related to preventing and managing type 2 diabetes (162). Several studies have shown significant improvements in insulin resistance and glycemic control as a result of resistance training (28, 29, 42, 47, 62, 79). Research indicates that resistance training may be preferable to aerobic activity for increasing insulin sensitivity (23, 47) and for decreasing glycosylated hemoglobin (23). These beneficial resistance training adaptations appear to be associated with increases in lean body mass, muscle cross-sectional area, and glucose transporter type-4 density (144). A comprehensive review on aging, resistance training, and diabetes prevention (52) concluded that resistance training may provide an effective intervention for counteracting age-associated declines in insulin sensitivity and for preventing the onset of type 2 diabetes.

Resting Blood Pressure

Elevated resting blood pressure, a major risk factor for cardiovascular disease (48), is experienced by approximately 35% of American adults (138). Aerobic endurance exercise has long been recognized as an effective means for reducing resting systolic and diastolic blood pressure (122). However, many people do not realize that properly performed resistance training results in similar blood pressure responses. Whether performed alone (29, 87, 97, 159) or in conjunction with aerobic activity (96, 182), standard and circuit-style resistance training have been shown to reduce resting systolic or diastolic blood pressure or both. In a 10-week study (182), more than 1,600 participants between ages 21 and 80 performed 20 minutes of resistance training and 20 minutes of aerobic endurance exercise two or three days a week. Twice-a-week training significantly reduced resting blood pressure by an average of 3.2 mmHg systolic and 1.4 mmHg diastolic, whereas training three days per week significantly reduced resting blood pressure by an average of 4.6 mmHg systolic and 2.2 mmHg diastolic. In another 10-week study (180), prehypertensive adults over age 60 who performed resistance exercise and followed a sensible nutrition plan experienced an average resting blood pressure reduction of 5.8 mmHg systolic and 3.6 mmHg diastolic.

A 2000 meta-analysis of randomized controlled trials by Kelley and Kelley (98) determined that resistance training is an effective means for reducing resting blood pressure. In support of these findings, a 2005 meta-analysis of randomized controlled trials by Cornelissen and Fagard (36) also reported that resistance training was associated with an average systolic blood pressure reduction of 6.0 mmHg and an average diastolic blood pressure reduction of 4.7 mmHg. These favorable blood pressure changes were similar to those associated with aerobic activity (36). In addition to reducing resting blood pressure, resistance training may also be beneficial for people who remain hypertensive, as research reveals that higher levels of muscle strength are associated with lower risk of all-cause mortality (8).

Blood Lipid Profiles

An undesirable blood lipid profile, another major risk factor for cardiovascular disease (48), is experienced by approximately 45% of American adults (116). As with resting blood pressure, aerobic endurance exercise has been shown to improve blood lipid profiles including lower total cholesterol and LDL cholesterol levels, lower triglyceride levels, and higher HDL cholesterol levels (3). Although there are notable exceptions (107, 159), numerous studies have shown significant improvements in blood lipid profiles subsequent to participation in resistance training programs (18, 69, 99, 164, 171, 174). Older women (ages 70 to 87 years) experienced significant reductions in triglyceride and LDL cholesterol levels and increases in HDL cholesterol levels as a result of resistance training (49). More specifically, resistance training has been shown to increase HDL cholesterol by 8% to 21%, decrease LDL cholesterol by 13% to 23%, and reduce triglycerides by 11% to 18% (3, 49, 69, 91). Some research indicates that resistance training and aerobic activity are almost equally effective for improving blood lipid profiles (16, 159), but the combination of resistance training and aerobic activity appears to produce more favorable blood lipid changes than either exercise performed alone (146).

Cardiovascular Health

People can definitely improve cardiovascular health by performing regular aerobic endurance exercise. The training benefits include lower resting blood pressure and more desirable blood lipid profiles, as well as increased blood volume, plasma volume, red blood cell volume, and capillary density (122). Resistance training may also enhance cardiovascular health by reducing resting blood pressure and improving blood lipid profiles, as well as by decreasing total body fat, mobilizing intra-abdominal fat, and improving glycemic control (161). Several studies have shown that resistance training reduces the risk of metabolic syndrome, which is a predisposing condition for cardiovascular disease (86, 92, 162, 186). A 2011 research review by Strasser and Schobersberger (161) concluded that resistance training is at least as effective as aerobic endurance training in reducing some major cardiovascular disease risk factors. However, the combination of resistance and aerobic training is recommended for maximizing cardiovascular health benefits (20).

Bone Mineral Density

Approximately 35 million American adults have insufficient bone mass (osteopenia), and about 10 million others have frail bones (osteoporosis) (134). Older adults who do not perform resistance training lose 10% to 30% of their BMD every decade of life (100, 135, 177). Bone loss is associated with age-related muscle and strength loss (sarcopenia) (2, 14, 85). It therefore makes sense that the same resistance training programs that increase muscle mass also increase BMD to some degree. Although some research has not demonstrated improvements in bone condition consequent to resistance training (31, 136), many longitudinal studies have shown significant increases in BMD following several months of certain types of resistance exercise, typically higher intensity strength training (38, 41, 61, 101, 117, 129, 135, 176, 189).

Earlier research reviews indicated that resistance training is positively associated with high BMD in both younger and older adults (113, 188) and that resistance training may have a more potent effect on bone density than other types of physical activity such as aerobic and weight-bearing exercise (67). More recent studies by Cussler and colleagues (38) and by Milliken and colleagues (129) further support the role of resistance exercise for bone remodeling in postmenopausal women. A 2009 research review by Going and Laudermilk (60) revealed BMD increases between 1% and 3% in postmenopausal women who participated in resistance training programs. In a two-year study of postmenopausal women, the resistance-trained group increased BMD by 2%, whereas the nontraining control group experienced a reduction in BMD (101). The resistance training program consisted of eight exercises performed for three sets of eight repetitions each, with resistance increase whenever nine repetitions were completed.

Key Point

Resistance training is effective for increasing bone mineral density in older adults.

Physical Function

The ability to perform activities of daily living decreases during older adult years. This progressive reduction in physical function is largely due to the gradual loss of muscle mass and strength (181). Resistance training has been shown to reverse many of the physical issues associated with inactive aging in older adults (51, 69, 167, 179). In a study of nearly 90-year-old nursing home residents, 14 weeks of resistance training (six exercises, one set, 8 to 12 repetitions, two sessions/week) resulted in an average strength gain of 60%, an average lean weight gain of 3.9 pounds (1.8 kg), and an average improvement in their **Functional Independence Measure (FIM®)** score of 14% (179). More specifically, resistance training studies with older adults have demonstrated improvements in movement control (12), physical performance (77, 84), and walking speed (155). Aerobic endurance training is the best means for increasing functional capacity of the cardiorespiratory system, thereby enabling improved performance of sustained large-muscle activities, such as walking or jogging at a faster pace for a longer distance (122).

Mental Health

Research studies have revealed many mental health benefits for older adults who perform resistance training (137). Older individuals who do not have severe mental health issues may experience enhanced self-esteem and improved cognitive abilities; reduced fatigue, anxiety, and depression; and decreased discomfort from osteoarthritis, fibromyalgia, and low back pain (15, 55, 70, 75, 90, 112, 115, 137, 151).

Aerobic endurance training has also demonstrated benefits in the areas of mental and emotional health, especially in adults over 55 years of age (74). For example, in a study of complex cognitive function, older men (age 60 and above) who had relatively high levels of aerobic fitness performed significantly better than their peers who had relatively low levels of aerobic fitness (43). Other psychological benefits of aerobic endurance exercise include reductions in stress, anxiety, and depression (74).

Studies by Annesi and colleagues (6) have shown that 10 weeks of combined resistance and aerobic training can significantly improve psychological measures of physical self-concept, total mood disturbance, depression, fatigue, positive engagement, revitalization, tranquility, and tension in older adults (4-7). With respect to depression, 10 weeks of resistance training significantly reduced symptoms of depression in more than 80% of the older adults who were clinically depressed at the start of the research study (158).

Studies with older adults have also shown that resistance training is associated with significant improvements in cognitive abilities (22, 27, 109). Based on meta-analysis results, resistance training appeared to enhance the cognitive improvements attained from aerobic activity alone when both types of exercise were performed concurrently (34).

Aging Factors

The aging process is typically accompanied by a progressive deterioration of skeletal muscle **mitochondria**, which function as a major energy source for cellular activity (147). Both circuit training, characterized by brief rests between successive exercises, and standard resistance training have been shown to increase muscle tissue mitochondrial content and oxidative capacity (139, 143, 147, 165). A classic study by Melov and associates (126) examined the effects of resistance training on the mitochondrial deterioration that accompanies the aging process. Following six months of standard resistance training, older adults experienced favorable changes in 179 genes associated with age and exercise, while concurrently, mitochondrial characteristics in the older adults (mean age 68 years) revealed a modified genetic fingerprint similar to the mitochondrial gene expression of young adults (mean age 24 years). The researchers concluded that resistance training has the potential to reverse certain aging factors in skeletal muscle, supporting the findings of previous studies.

EXERCISE RECOMMENDATIONS FOR OLDER ADULTS

For older adults who are apparently healthy, the recommendations for resistance training and aerobic endurance training are comparable to the guidelines for adults in general. For those clients who have a current health or medical condition, are at risk for a condition, or both, the exercise professional should refer them to a physician or other health care professional for an evaluation before beginning any type of exercise program.

Resistance Training

Established resistance training recommendations (181) call for a variety of both **single-joint exercises** and **multiple-joint exercises** that involve the major muscle groups, including the quadriceps, hamstrings, gluteals, pectoralis major, latissimus dorsi, deltoids, biceps, triceps, erector spinae, and rectus abdominis.

According to these guidelines, older adults should perform two or three resistance training sessions per week on nonconsecutive days. Although the authors present a resistance range of 60% to 90% of the one repetition maximum (1RM), they recommend using a resistance that permits between 10 and 15 repetitions of each exercise during the initial training period. They suggest increasing the resistance by approximately 5% whenever 15 repetitions can be completed. For strength development, older adults are advised to perform resistance exercises with a controlled movement speed (4 to 6 seconds per repetition) and a complete movement range with the exception of painful positions.

The following section presents research-based recommendations for older adults who perform resistance exercises. This more specific information should be useful for designing older adult resistance training programs that maximize exercise effectiveness and efficiency while minimizing injury risk.

Frequency

Resistance training studies with older adults reveal different results with respect to exercise frequency. Research by Hunter and associates (82) revealed no significant differences in strength development among training frequencies of one, two, and three nonconsecutive days per week. However, Westcott and colleagues (182) found that resistance training two days per week and three days per week produced similar increases in lean weight that were significantly greater than lean weight gains attained by training one day per week. A study by DeMichele and associates (40) also showed similar and significant strength gains from two and three resistance training sessions per week, but no significant increases in strength from one weekly workout. It is therefore recommended that older adults schedule resistance training sessions two or three nonconsecutive days each week.

Sets

Over the past several years, three major reviews have examined more than 160 research studies that compared the effects of various exercise sets on strength development. The review by Carpinelli and Otto (25) concluded that single-set resistance training is as effective as multiple-set resistance training for increasing muscle strength and hypertrophy. The meta-analysis by Rhea and associates (150) indicated that two exercise sets were more effective than one exercise set, that three exercise sets were more effective than two exercise sets, and that four exercise sets were more effective than three exercise sets. They concluded that multiple-set training was more productive than single-set training, and that four sets per muscle group elicited the greatest strength gains. Krieger's (108) meta-regression also found multiple-set training to be more effective than single-set training. His analyses showed similar effects from performing one set per exercise and four sets per exercise, as well as similar effects from performing two sets per exercise and three sets per exercise, which produced greater strength gains than single-set training. On the other hand, a 2013 research study revealed significantly greater increases in both muscle mass and strength from one high intensity exercise set than from three sets of each exercise (45).

A general guideline for previously untrained older adults is to begin with one set of each exercise. As the client increases her muscle strength, muscle endurance, and enthusiasm for resistance exercise, the fitness professional may increase the training volume by progressively transitioning to two or more sets of selected exercises (10). Older adults should rest 2 to 3 minutes between successive training sets to facilitate muscle recovery and energy replenishment before each exercise bout (130).

Repetitions and Resistance

There is an inverse relationship between the resistance used for an exercise and the number of repetitions that can be completed. The majority of studies reporting significant positive adaptations in older adults incorporated training protocols of 8 to 12 repetitions with a resistance that produced temporary muscle fatigue within this repetition range (51, 58, 105, 127, 135, 148, 179, 182). However, many other studies with adult and older adult participants have revealed similar results with lower (4 to 8) and higher (12 to 16) repetition ranges (13, 30, 72, 102, 163, 175). Older adults without prior experience in resistance exercise may begin training with 10 to 15 repetitions at a light intensity (approximately 40% to 60% 1RM). As they become accustomed to resistance training, they may progress to 10 to 15 repetitions at 60% to 70% 1RM. When this exercise protocol becomes comfortable, older adults may train safely and effectively with higher intensity resistance and repetition protocols, such as 8 to 12 repetitions with 70% to 80% 1RM, and even 4 to 8 reps at 80% to 90% 1RM (181). Whether or not 1RM testing is performed, the recommended repetition ranges will typically correspond with the suggested resistance ranges when muscle fatigue is experienced by the end of the exercise set.

Key Point

Older adults are advised to perform resistance exercise for all of the major muscle groups, two or three days a week, beginning with a resistance that permits 10 to 15 controlled repetitions.

Progression

The key to increasing muscle strength, size, and function is progressive resistance training that systematically stresses the skeletal muscles. While this can be accomplished to some degree with bodyweight training (performing more repetitions with the same weight), training with external resistance (such as free weights, weight stack machines, and elastic bands) enables older adults to gradually increase the exercise resistance as their muscles become stronger. When the exercise resistance is progressively increased within the prescribed repetition range, training protocols using 6 to 15 repetitions have resulted in significant and similar strength gains in older adults (72). Whatever repetition range is used (4 to 8 reps, 8 to 12 reps, or 12 to 16 reps), when the end number of repetitions can be completed with correct form, the resistance should be raised by approximately 5% (181). For example, an older adult performing two sets of the vertical chest press exercise with 100 pounds (45 kg) using an 8 to 12 repetition protocol may be encouraged to increase the exercise resistance to 105 pounds (48 kg) when 12 repetitions can be properly performed in both sets. Training should continue with 105-pound (48 kg) vertical chest presses until 12 repetitions can again be correctly completed, at which point the resistance should again be raised by about 5%. By first increasing the number of repetitions within the training range and then increasing the resistance, older adults experience a double progressive protocol for safely and effectively increasing the muscle-building stimulus (10).

Selection

It is recommended that adults and older adults perform a resistance training program that addresses the major muscle groups (181). If trained with single-joint movements, the following example provides 10 different machine exercises that independently work 10 major muscle groups:

- Quadriceps—leg (knee) extension
- Hamstrings—leg (knee) curl
- Pectoralis major—pec deck (butterfly)
- Latissimus dorsi—pullover
- Deltoids—lateral raise
- Triceps—triceps pushdown
- Biceps—biceps curl
- Erector spinae—low back extension
- Rectus abdominis—abdominal curl
- Upper trapezius—shoulder shrug

If trained with multiple-joint movements, which involve more muscle mass for greater strength gains than single-joint exercises, the following example provides four different free weight exercises that collectively work eight of these major muscle groups:

- Quadriceps and hamstrings—dumbbell squat
- Pectoralis major and triceps—dumbbell bench press
- Latissimus dorsi and biceps—one-arm dumbbell row
- Deltoids, upper trapezius, and triceps—dumbbell shoulder press

It is therefore recommended that older adults perform at least four multiple-joint exercises each training session to address the major muscle groups. However, it may be advisable for older adults to perform a combination of multiple-joint and single-joint movements during most training sessions, as not all muscles are worked equally in multijoint movements (32). When training in this manner, older adults should perform multiple-joint exercises that use more muscle mass and higher resistance (e.g., leg press, vertical chest press, lat pulldown) before they do single-joint exercises that use less muscle mass and lower resistance (e.g., leg [knee] extension, triceps pushdown, biceps curl) (10).

Older adults who are resistance trained and prefer to do more exercises, multiple exercise sets, or both, may split their workouts into lower body and upper body sessions to avoid lengthy training periods. For example, they may perform exercises for the leg and trunk muscles on Mondays and Thursdays, and exercises for the torso and arm muscles on Wednesdays and Saturdays.

Speed

Muscle strength may be best increased by training with relatively heavy resistance at controlled movement speeds (131), whereas muscle power may be best increased by training with moderate resistance at fast movement speeds (183). Older adults training for increased muscle strength may attain better results by lifting loads greater than 60% of maximum at controlled movement speeds, whereas those training for muscle power may attain better results by lifting loads less than 60% of maximum at faster movement speeds.

As a general rule, older adults should begin exercising with a training program to first increase muscular strength and progress to include power training protocols. Power training, which appears to be safe, productive, and well tolerated by older adults, has demonstrated neuromuscular adaptations that may reduce the likelihood of falls and resulting disabilities (26). For example, medicine ball throws are recommended for older adult power training, as such exercises enable both fast movement speeds and resistance release at the end of each throwing action to reduce joint stress (10).

Range of Joint Movement

The National Strength and Conditioning Association advises adults and older adults to perform exercises through the full range of joint movement to enhance muscle strength and joint flexibility (181). Studies with a variety of major muscle groups have demonstrated greater muscle strength gains when the exercises are performed through a full movement range rather than through a partial movement range (65, 125, 145). Although full range of joint movement training is recommended, the actual range of each exercise should be limited to pain-free movements. This is an important consideration for older adults who may have some form of arthritis, a health issue experienced by more than 53 million Americans (9), or other deleterious joint condition.

Breathing

Another important aspect of resistance training technique for older adults is continuous breathing throughout each exercise bout. Regardless of the exercise intensity, older adults should never hold their breath when resistance training. Breath holding, known as the **Valsalva maneuver**, increases internal pressure to levels that can impede venous blood flow, elevate blood pressure, and cause undesirable sensations of light-headedness or blackouts (64). The generally recommended breathing technique for older adults during resistance training is to exhale throughout each concentric muscle action and to inhale throughout each eccentric muscle action (10).

Based on the preponderance of research, older adults are advised to begin resistance training in accordance with the guidelines presented in table 12.1.

Table 12.1   Resistance Training Guidelines for Older Adults

Program variable	Recommendation
Frequency	Train for 2 or 3 nonconsecutive days per week.
Sets	Begin training with 1 set of each exercise and progress to more sets as desired. Multiple-set protocols should allow 2- to 3-min recovery time between successive sets.
Repetitions	Begin training with 10 to 15 repetitions and progress to fewer repetitions with heavier loads as desired (e.g., 8-12 repetitions; 4-8 repetitions).
Resistance	Begin training with 40% to 60% 1RM and progress to 60% to 70% 1RM for 10 to 15 repetitions. If desired, transition to heavier loads and fewer repetitions (e.g., 70% to 80% 1RM for 8 to 12 repetitions; 80% to 90% 1RM for 4 to 8 repetitions).
Progression	When the end range of repetitions can be completed with correct technique, increase the resistance by approximately 5%.
Exercise selection	Perform mostly multiple-joint exercises supplemented with single-joint exercises that cumulatively address all of the major muscle groups.
Movement speed	Perform repetitions at moderate movement speeds with relatively heavy resistance for strength and hypertrophy training, and perform repetitions at fast movement speeds with relatively light resistance for power training.
Range of motion	Perform repetitions through a full range of pain-free movement.
Breathing	Breathe continuously throughout every repetition, generally exhaling during the concentric (lifting) actions and inhaling during the eccentric (lowering) actions.

Aerobic Endurance Training

General recommendations for older adult aerobic endurance training are 20 to 60 minutes of large-muscle aerobic activity, performed most days of the week, at a training intensity of 60% to 90% of maximum (age-predicted) heart rate (181). More specifically, the guidelines for aerobic endurance exercise have two categories according to training intensity (73). The first category is for *moderate intensity training* (40% to <60% $\dot{V}O_2$ or heart rate reserve; e.g., walking), and the second category is for *vigorous intensity training* (≥60-90% $\dot{V}O_2$ or heart rate reserve; e.g., jogging or running). The following section presents the recommendations for both categories of aerobic endurance training with respect to frequency, duration, intensity, and type of exercise activity for older adults (3).

Frequency

The training frequency for aerobic endurance training is actually an individualized decision as to how the recommended weekly exercise time is performed in accordance with one's personal schedule and lifestyle. The recommended amount of aerobic endurance exercise for the moderate intensity training category is between 150 and 300 minutes per week (2.5 to 5.0 hours), and the recommended training frequency is five days per week. As an example, 200 minutes of weekly moderate intensity aerobic activity could be attained by doing 40 minutes of walking on Tuesdays, Wednesdays, Thursdays, Saturdays, and Sundays. The recommended amount of aerobic endurance exercise for the vigorous intensity training category is between 75 and 150 minutes per week (1.25 to 2.5 hours), and the recommended training frequency is three days per week. For example, 90 minutes of weekly vigorous intensity aerobic activity could be attained by doing 30 minutes of jogging on Mondays, Wednesdays, and Fridays.

Duration

The guidelines for aerobic endurance training duration are given in minutes per day but may be divided into smaller segments for moderate intensity exercise in order to accommodate one's daily schedule. For the moderate intensity training category, the recommended daily duration is a minimum of 30 minutes, which may be accumulated in exercise bouts of at least 10 minutes each. For the vigorous intensity training category, the recommended daily duration is a minimum of 20 minutes, which should be attained in a single exercise bout. A combination of moderate intensity and vigorous intensity aerobic endurance training may be performed in accordance with the respective training durations.

Intensity

Although previous guidelines for training intensity have been based on exercise heart rate, older adults have relatively large variations in maximal heart rate and are more likely to take medications that affect their heart rate response to exercise. Consequently, the current guidelines are based on one's perceived physical exertion during the exercise session. On a scale of 0 to 10, it is recommended that people performing moderate intensity training do so at a perceived physical exertion level of 5 to 6, and that people performing vigorous intensity training do so at a perceived physical exertion level of 7 to 8.

Activities

Aerobic endurance may be effectively improved by regularly performing large-muscle, rhythmic-type activities that involve more than 20 minutes of vigorous intensity exercise or more than 30 minutes of moderate intensity exercise. Older adults who have difficulty doing weight-bearing activities may perform recumbent cycling, upright cycling, rowing, swimming, or other weight-supported aerobic endurance exercises. In addition to these aerobic activities, older adults who are capable of doing weight-bearing exercise may also perform walking, jogging, running, stepping, elliptical training, dancing, or other ambulatory activities.

Key Point

Older adults are advised to perform aerobic endurance training at moderate intensity for 150 to 300 minutes per week or at a vigorous intensity for 75 to 150 minutes per week, or a combination of these training intensities and durations.

In accordance with research-based recommendations, older adults are encouraged to follow the aerobic endurance training guidelines presented in table 12.2.

RECOMMENDED STRATEGIES FOR INSTRUCTING OLDER ADULTS

Exercise professionals should be sure to provide a high level of positive reinforcement when implementing an exercise training program with older adults. As previously discussed, most older adults respond favorably to resistance training with progressive increases in muscle mass and strength. Anecdotally, they are often impressed by their relatively rapid improvements in physical fitness, and indebted to their exercise professional for teaching them how to perform resistance training safely and effectively.

However, it can be challenging to initially engage older adults in resistance training and also to keep them committed during the first few training sessions. It is therefore suggested that exercise professionals working with older adults place equal emphasis on education and motivation. Research from the Centers for Disease Control and Prevention (170) reveals that fewer than 5% of adults over age 50 perform moderate intensity physical activity on a regular basis, let alone engage in resistance exercise. Experience indicates that older adults may have health-related concerns about resistance training, such as stressing their joints, injuring their muscles, or harming their heart, as well as personal concerns such as experiencing discomfort, appearing weak, and embarrassing themselves by improper exercise performance. Consequently, a high priority for exercise professionals may be to help older adults develop a positive attitude toward resistance training. First, explain the physiological benefits of regular resistance as presented earlier in this chapter. Second, provide reinforcing training sessions through interactive teaching techniques. Exercise professionals who incorporate specific instructional strategies appear to be more effective in helping older adults gain competence in their exercise performance and confidence in their training program (5-7).

Key Point

Older adult exercise instruction should include clear objectives, concise explanations, precise demonstrations, gradual progression, positive reinforcement, specific feedback, and appropriate assistance.

Older adults like to be acknowledged by name, affirmed, and appreciated for participating in an exercise program (178). In addition to these important interactions, Baechle and Westcott (10) have identified 10 instructional guidelines for educating and motivating older adults.

1. **Understandable performance objectives.** Although this is often ignored, it is essential to begin each exercise session with the

Table 12.2 Aerobic Endurance Training Guidelines for Older Adults

Program variable	Recommendation
Frequency	Perform 5 or more days per week of moderate intensity (40% to <60% $\dot{V}O_2$ or heart rate reserve) aerobic endurance training totaling 150 to 300 min, or 3 or more days per week of vigorous intensity (≥60-90% $\dot{V}O_2$ or heart rate reserve) aerobic endurance training totaling 75 to 150 min, or a combination of these activities.
Duration	Perform moderate intensity aerobic endurance exercise for 30 to 60 min each training day in bouts of at least 10 min, or vigorous intensity aerobic endurance exercise for 20 to 30 min each training day.
Intensity	Perform moderate intensity aerobic endurance training at a perceived physical exertion rating of 5 to 6 on a 10-point scale, or vigorous intensity aerobic endurance training at a perceived physical exertion rating of 7 to 8 on a 10-point scale.
Mode	Perform large-muscle, weight-supported aerobic activities such as cycling, rowing, and swimming, or large-muscle, weight-bearing aerobic activities such as walking, jogging, and stepping.

desired performance objectives. The exercise professional should simply state what he would like the individual to accomplish during the workout. For example, *"Today, our objective is to perform every resistance exercise through a full range of pain-free joint movement."*

2. **Concise instruction with precise demonstration.** Although it is important to speak clearly, concise instructional statements are recommended for older adult communications. Exercise instruction should always be coupled with exercise demonstration, as older adults tend to be visual learners. Model the proper exercise performance as many times as necessary, emphasizing the execution objective. For example, *"Watch me perform the seated row exercise through the full range of joint movement, beginning with my arms fully extended and finishing with my hands at my chest."*

3. **Attentive supervision.** After explaining and demonstrating an exercise, be attentive as the older adult attempts to imitate the demonstration. Actively observing an older adult perform a new exercise enhances her confidence and enables the exercise professional to immediately detect and correct any errors in training technique. As an example, *"I will watch carefully as you perform 10 full-range repetitions of the seated row exercise."*

4. **Appropriate assistance.** With the older adult's approval, it is sometimes helpful to provide some level of manual assistance during the exercise performance. Guiding an older adult through the proper movement pattern may be particularly useful when training with elastic bands and free weights. For example, the exercise professional may help the client pull the seated row handles to the at-chest position so he can experience the feel of full muscle contraction.

5. **One task at a time.** Most resistance training exercises require a sequence of specific tasks for correct completion. Older adults typically master exercise performance more efficiently when instructors present the key exercise components one at a time. For example, the first task in the seated row exercise may be to sit tall with elbows extended and hands gripping the handles. The second task may be to pull the handles to the chest and pause. The third task may be to return the handles to the starting position. The fourth task may be to exhale during the pulling movement. The fifth task may be to inhale during the return movement. The sixth task may be to perform the pulling movement in 2 seconds. The seventh task may be to perform the return movement in 2 seconds.

6. **Gradual progression.** In addition to a gradual progression in exercise resistance, older adults should begin with a few basic exercises and systematically add new exercises only after they have mastered the previous ones. For example, the exercise professional may start an older adult client with just one upper back exercise, such as the seated row. When this exercise is performed properly and consistently, a second upper back exercise (such as the lat pulldown) may be introduced.

7. **Positive reinforcement.** Older adults typically experience some degree of uncertainty about performing resistance training. It is therefore advisable to affirm their exercise efforts with various forms of positive reinforcement, including encouraging comments, performance compliments, and stars on their workout cards. Positive reinforcement is most effective when it is received during or immediately following exercise performance—for example, *"Excellent exercise technique, Tom!"*

8. **Specific feedback.** Positive reinforcement may be enhanced by inclusion of specific information feedback that gives the client a reason for the compliment. The combination of positive reinforcement and specific feedback has value from both a motivational and an educational perspective. For example, *"Excellent exercise technique, Tom; you are pulling the handles all the way to your chest on each repetition."*

9. **Careful questioning.** Older adults may not voluntarily provide information about how they feel when resistance training. Consequently, it may be helpful to ask if they are feeling the exercise effort in the target muscles. For example, while Tom is performing seated rows, the exercise professional can say, *"Tom, please tell me where you feel the most effort while doing seated rows."*

10. **Pre- and postexercise dialogue.** Older adults generally appreciate a brief dialogue with their instructor before beginning and after completing their exercise session. The entry conversation may emphasize encouragement for attaining the workout objectives, and the exit conversation may feature reinforcement for the exercise performance. For example, the exercise professional may initiate a preexercise dialogue by saying, *"Thanks for coming to class today, Tom; what would you like to accomplish during your exercise session, and how can I assist you?"* A sample postexercise dialogue might begin with, *"Great workout Tom; tell me how you felt using the heavier weights."*

These same concepts may be applied to aerobic endurance training, with special emphasis on positive reinforcement. The longer duration required for sustained aerobic endurance exercise and the less visible physiological changes may make aerobic training more challenging for older adults.

Case Study

Older Adults

Mrs. R, a 69-year-old woman, joined an exercise program at the urging of her son, a medical doctor, to address the age-related issues of sarcopenia (muscle loss) and osteopenia (bone loss). Mrs. R's initial body composition readings were as follows: body weight 136.5 pounds (61.9 kg), percent fat 24.6%, lean weight 102.9 pounds (46.7 kg), and fat weight 33.6 pounds (15.2 kg).

During the next eight months, Mrs. R trained Mondays, Wednesdays, and Fridays in a college fitness center. Her resistance training program consisted of the following 12 resistance machines: leg (knee) extension, leg (knee) curl, leg press, hip adduction–hip abduction, chest press, lat pulldown, shoulder press, seated row, abdominal curl, low back extension, torso rotation, and neck flexion–extension. She performed each exercise for one set of 8 to 12 repetitions and increased the resistance by approximately 5% whenever 12 repetitions could be completed. Her aerobic training program progressed from a few minutes on the recumbent cycle to 20 minutes of continuous cycling at about 70% of her age-predicted maximal heart rate and a perceived exertion rating of 14 on the Borg 6- to 20-point scale (17).

After eight months of training, Mrs. R's body composition had improved significantly, to the following readings: body weight 134.4 pounds (61.0 kg), percent fat 20.3%, lean weight 107.2 pounds (48.6 kg), and fat weight 27.2 pounds (12.3 kg). Although her body weight decreased by only 2.1 pounds (1 kg), Mrs. R improved her percent fat reading by 4.3 points (24.6% to 20.3%). She actually added 4.3 pounds (2 kg) of lean (muscle) weight and lost 6.4 pounds (2.9 kg) of fat weight, for a 10.7-pound (4.9 kg) improvement in her body composition and physical appearance.

Over the same time period, Mrs. R increased her leg press 10-repetition load from 100 pounds (45 kg) to 250 pounds (113 kg) for a very impressive strength gain. In addition, her dual x-ray absorptiometry (DXA) scan revealed a small increase in her BMD rather than the 1% to 2% reduction normally experienced by women 70 years of age.

Mrs. R's periodic body composition assessments over the eight-month exercise period are presented in the table.

Mrs. R's Body Composition Changes During an Eight-Month Resistance Training Program

Parameter	Start	2 months	5 months	8 months
Age	69 years	69 years	70 years	70 years
Body weight	136.5 lb (61.9 kg)	136.3 lb (61.8 kg)	132.7 lb (60.2 kg)	134.4 lb (61.0 kg)
Percent fat	24.6%	23.3%	20.3%	20.3%
Lean weight	102.9 lb (46.7 kg)	104.6 lb (47.5 kg)	105.8 lb (48.1 kg)	107.2 lb (48.6 kg)
Fat weight	33.6 lb (15.2 kg)	31.7 lb (14.4 kg)	26.9 lb (12.2 kg)	27.2 lb (12.3 kg)

Recommended Readings

American College of Sports Medicine, Chodzko-Zajko, WJ, Proctor, DN, Fiatarone Singh, MA, Minson, CT, Nigg, CR, Salem, GJ, and Skinner, JS. American College of Sports Medicine position stand. Exercise and physical activity for older adults. *Med Sci Sports Exerc* 41:1510-1530, 2009.

Flack, K, Davy, K, Hulver, M, Winett, R, Frisard, M, and Davy, B. Aging, resistance training, and diabetes prevention. *J Aging Res* 2011:127315, 2011.

Going, S and Laudermilk, M. Osteoporosis and strength training. *Am J Lifestyle Med* 3:310-319, 2009.

Kasch, F, Wallace, J, and VanCamp, S. The effects of physical activity and inactivity on aerobic power in older men: a longitudinal study. *Physician Sportsmed* 18:73-83, 1990.

Lakatta, E. Changes in cardiovascular function with aging. *Eur Heart J* 11:22-29, 1990.

O'Connor, P, Herring, M, and Caravalho, A. Mental health benefits of strength training in adults. *Am J Lifestyle Med* 4: 377-396, 2010.

Singh, M. Exercise and aging. *Clin Geriatr Med* 20:201-221, 2004.

Strasser, B and Schobersberger, W. Evidence of resistance training as a treatment therapy in obesity. *J Obes* 2011:482564, 2011.

Strasser, B, Siebert, U, and Schobersberger, W. Resistance training in the treatment of metabolic syndrome. *Sports Med* 40:397-415, 2010.

Wolfe, R. The unappreciated role of muscle in health and disease. *Am J Clin Nutr* 84:475-482, 2006.

CONCLUSION

The aging process is associated with undesirable but normal changes in the muscular system, cardiovascular system, and nervous system that contribute to reduced physical function and a number of debilitating health issues. Resistance training has been shown to enhance physical function and to reduce the risk of many major medical conditions by increasing muscle mass and strength, increasing resting energy expenditure, decreasing body fat, resisting type 2 diabetes, reducing resting blood pressure, improving blood lipid profiles, improving cardiovascular health, increasing BMD, enhancing mental and emotional health, and reversing specific aging factors. Resistance training recommendations for older adults call for up to 10 basic exercises that address the major muscle groups, performed for one to three sets of 4 to 15 repetitions each, two or three nonconsecutive days a week, using progressively higher resistance, moderate movement speed, and full movement range. Research reveals that resistance training is a safe and effective means for older adults to improve their functional abilities, physical fitness, and personal health.

Aerobic endurance training has been demonstrated to improve cardiorespiratory fitness by increasing aerobic capacity; to benefit general health by reducing resting blood pressure, improving blood lipid profiles, decreasing body fat, and enhancing cognitive function; and to reduce the risk of type 2 diabetes and cardiovascular disease. Aerobic endurance training guidelines for older adults include options of moderate intensity large-muscle activities for 30 to 60 minutes per session, totaling 150 to 300 minutes per week; or vigorous intensity large-muscle activities for 20 to 30 minutes per session, totaling 75 to 150 minutes per week; or a combination of moderate and vigorous training sessions with corresponding durations. Aerobic endurance training may be performed with weight-bearing activities such as walking, jogging, and stepping, or with weight-supporting activities such as cycling, rowing, and swimming.

Key Terms

aerobic capacity
Functional Independence Measure (FIM®)
Golgi tendon organ
intra-abdominal fat
maximal oxygen uptake
microtrauma
mitochondria
multiple-joint exercise
muscle hypertrophy
muscle spindles

myokines
osteopenia
osteoporosis
sarcopenia
single-joint exercise
Type I muscle fibers
Type II muscle fibers
Valsalva maneuver

Study Questions

1. _____ decrease(s) more rapidly than _____ with age.

   a. Bone mass; muscle mass

   b. Type I muscle fibers; Type II muscle fibers

   c. Muscle endurance; muscle strength

   d. Muscle mass; metabolic rate

2. Which of the following is true regarding the effects of resistance training in older adults?

   a. It has little to no effect on managing blood sugar levels.

   b. It can attenuate the loss of muscle mass, but not prevent it completely.

   c. It generally does not improve blood pressure due to the Valsalva maneuver.

   d. It can increase metabolic rate, but only as a consequence of increased muscle mass.

3. One mechanism by which resistance training may affect insulin resistance in older adults is the

   a. increase in resting metabolic rate

   b. reduction in intra-abdominal fat

   c. increase in blood flow as a result of lower blood pressures

   d. increase in release of nitric oxide during higher-intensity resistance training

4. You inherit a 62-year-old client from a departing exercise professional. The client would like to begin exercising again after a long period of inactivity, and he indicated that mobility and lower body strength were his priorities. The departing exercise professional wrote this initial program:

4 sets of:

Bodyweight wall squat	15 repetitions
Machine leg (knee) extension	15 repetitions
Machine leg (knee) curl	15 repetitions

2 sets of:

Machine shoulder press	10 repetitions
Machine lat pulldown	10 repetitions
Machine triceps extension	10 repetitions
Dumbbell biceps curl	10 repetitions
Machine abdominal curl	10 repetitions
Machine low back extension	10 repetitions

All exercises use loads of 50% of his estimated 1RM with 3 minutes of rest between sets and exercises for 2 sessions a week (with 2-3 days between sessions).

Which of the following is the best adjustment to make to the program?

    a. Increase the intensity of the upper body exercises to 75% 1RM.

    b. Reduce all exercises to 1 set and progress to 2 sets as tolerated.

    c. Add an exercise for the calf muscles to the lower body training day.

    d. Perform the lower body exercises twice a week and the upper body exercises twice a week.

Female-Specific Conditions

Jill A. Bush, PhD, CSCS,*D

After completing this chapter, you will be able to

◆ understand the characteristics of the conditions regarding the female athlete triad, pregnancy, postpartum, menopause, and postmenopause;

◆ recognize and identify the major signs or symptoms of women with the female athlete triad, pregnant and postpartum women, and women going through menopause and postmenopause;

◆ identify and administer proper exercise and exercise programming for women with the female athlete triad, pregnant and postpartum women, and women going through menopause and postmenopause; and

◆ understand modifications and precautions for exercise for women with the female athlete triad, pregnant and postpartum women, and women going through menopause and postmenopause.

There are considerations related to women of all ages that an exercise professional needs to be aware of if he is to have clients who are female. These include the female athlete triad, pregnancy and postpartum, and menopause and postmenopause. The female athlete triad consists of three components that are affected by energy availability, menstrual function, and changes to the skeletal system. Pregnant women have exercise-related considerations that can affect both the mother and growing baby. Upon delivery, women going through the postpartum period experience numerous changes in hormones and body shape related to the child-birthing process. Later, as a woman ages, changes in her body and hormonal profile lead to menopause and postmenopause, when she will experience decreases in estrogen and changes in fat and bone metabolism that are linked to risks of osteopenia and osteoporosis.

An exercise professional needs to know how to design and modify a client-specific exercise program based on or in response to the female athlete triad, pregnancy, and menopause. Often, this requires that the exercise professional work closely with her female clients' family physician and other health care professionals such as a registered dietitian or a counselor.

This chapter focuses on exercise-related considerations for the female athlete triad, pregnancy and postpartum, and menopause and postmenopause. Certain clinical conditions and common physician-prescribed medications and over-the-counter remedies that relate to these female concerns are discussed. Recommendations for exercise, precautions, and contraindications are also presented where applicable. Additionally, recommended readings are listed at the end of each section.

FEMALE ATHLETE TRIAD

The **female athlete triad** exists on a continuum involving interrelationships between energy availability, menstrual function, and bone function (figure 13.1) (39, 51, 83, 90), which can be expressed as the clinical manifestations of eating disorders, amenorrhea, and osteoporosis, respectively (90). A woman does not need to exhibit all three components at the same time, as any one

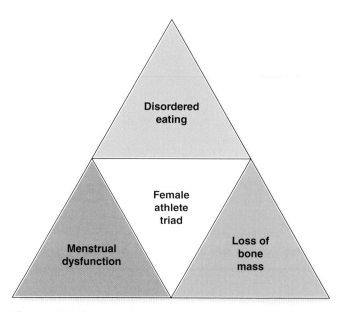

Figure 13.1 Female athlete triad consisting of disordered eating, menstrual dysfunction, and loss of bone mass.

of these components alone can be a risk to her health. Thus, it is important to recognize the signs and symptoms to ensure prevention and treatment. Risk factors for developing the female athlete triad include playing a sport that specifically requires body weight to be monitored, social isolation, exercising more than necessary for a sport, pressure to feel the need to win, punitive consequences for body weight gain, and having parents or coaches who are controlling or overbearing (90). In this section, we explore the pathophysiology of the female athlete triad, common medications given to women with the female athlete triad, effects of exercise, and exercise recommendations for women with the female athlete triad.

Key Point

The female athlete triad is characterized by an interrelationship among eating disorders, menstrual dysfunction, and loss of bone mass.

Pathophysiology of the Female Athlete Triad

Girls and adult women who participate in a sport that favors a lean physique such as gymnastics, figure skating, or long-distance running or a sport that has weight classes such as rowing, as well as female athletes who are required to wear revealing uniforms such as swimsuits or track uniforms, can be at increased risk for insufficient or unhealthy eating habits and subsequently the female athlete triad (90).

Early detection of signs for the female athlete triad is important. Ten risk factors can be assessed: "(1) history of menstrual irregularities and amenorrhea; (2) history of stress fractures; (3) history of critical comments about eating or weight from parent, coach or teammate; (4) a history of depression; (5) a history of dieting; (6) personality factors (such as perfectionism and obsessiveness); (7) pressure to lose weight and/or frequent weight cycling; (8) early start of sport-specific training; (9) overtraining; and (10) recurrent and non-healing injuries" (39).

Other sources (19, 78) provide the exercise professional with a list of common signs and symptoms of the female athlete triad:

- Irregular or absent menstrual cycles
- Constant feelings of tiredness and fatigue
- Sleeping disorders
- Stress fractures and recurrent injuries
- Self-restricted food consumption
- Constant efforts to be thinner
- Eating less food than what's needed in an effort to improve performance or physical appearance
- Cold hands and feet

The interrelatedness of the three conditions that characterize the triad warrants an understanding of the pathophysiology of menstrual dysfunction, bone mass loss, and eating disorders.

Menstrual Dysfunction

Young girls have their first menstrual cycle during puberty, typically at the age of 11 or 12 years (13). Low energy availability (low consumption of foodstuffs) or energy deficiency disrupts the proper functioning of the reproductive system in girls (i.e., ovaries and uterus) (13, 121). This can result in irregular or less frequent menstrual cycles (**oligomenorrhea**) (78). When three or more menstrual cycles are missed consecutively, the condition is considered **amenorrhea**. Not consuming sufficient amounts of calories in order to meet the demands of the body, energy expenditure, body growth, and basal metabolic functions, can delay the onset of menstruation until the age of 15 years (78). When the menstrual cycle becomes disrupted, less estrogen is produced from the ovaries and bone structure can be negatively affected.

Bone Mass Loss

Osteoporosis is a progressive bone disease characterized by a decrease in bone mass or bone mineral density (143). Women with the female athlete triad are at a greater risk for lower levels of bone mass, which leads to osteopenia and possibly osteoporosis (143). Osteopenia and osteoporosis are diagnosed by a medical professional using a bone scan via dual-energy x-ray absorptiometry (DXA). According to the World Health Organization (143), osteoporosis is defined as having a bone mineral density 2.5 or more standard deviations below the mean peak bone mass of an average, healthy 30-year old woman as measured by DXA. **Osteopenia** is a condition in which bone mass or bone mineral density is lower than in an average, healthy 30-year old woman, with a score between –1.0 and –2.5, and is considered a precursor to osteoporosis. It should be noted that not all women who are diagnosed with osteopenia develop osteoporosis (143). Osteopenia occurs more in postmenopausal women due to the loss of estrogen and may worsen with a sedentary lifestyle, consumption of too much alcohol, smoking, or prolonged use of glucocorticoid medications (a class of steroid hormones with anti-inflammatory and metabolic properties; cortisol is the most common) (1, 30, 80).

A diagnosis of osteoporosis, and possibly osteopenia, increases the risk for stress and full fractures because the bones are more brittle (1, 30, 80). There is also an imbalance in the cells that build bones and the cells that break down bone such that the process of bone breakdown occurs at a greater rate than replacement of bone (i.e., there is a net bone loss). This is also related to the decrease in energy availability and decrease in estrogen (14, 68, 71). There is a greater risk for bone-related issues during later years of life, like increased risk of fractures, if women have less bone mass by the third decade of life (e.g., 20-29 years) (51). Loss of bone mass is related to deficiencies in consumption of calcium and vitamin D (18, 56).

Eating Disorders

The *Diagnostic and Statistical Manual of Mental Disorders* (**DSM-5**), published in 2013, provides updated details on feeding and eating disorders, which are both considered mental disorders (9). Feeding and eating disorders include the following conditions: anorexia nervosa, bulimia nervosa, pica, rumination disorders, avoidant/restrictive food intake disorder, and "other specified feeding or eating disorders" (OSFED), which, before 2013, was classified as "eating disorders not otherwise specified" (EDNOS) (9). Binge-eating disorder is a separate category classified in DSM-5, but before 2013 it was included under the classification of feeding and eating disorders. The cause of feeding and eating disorders is not entirely clear. Both biological and environmental variables seem to play a role (9). In general, medical treatments for feeding and eating disorders are effective and can include changes in diet, psychological treatments, and prescription medications. After about five years of treatment, approximately 70% of those with anorexia nervosa and 50% of those with bulimia nervosa recover. Binge-eating disorder recovery occurs in 20% to 60% of those affected. However, both anorexia nervosa and bulimia nervosa increase the risk of death (118). Anorexia nervosa and bulimia nervosa are estimated to affect 0.9% to 4.3% and 2% to 3% of women at one point in their life, respectively (117). Binge-eating disorders affect 1.6% of women per year (9).

Anorexia nervosa is characterized by low body weight, obsessing about body shape and size, including the desire to look thin and fear of gaining any body weight, and restrictive eating behaviors (9, 84). Before 2013, amenorrhea (the absence of the menstrual cycle) was a required component to diagnose anorexia nervosa, but it is no longer required in DSM-5 (9). Many women believe they are overweight even though they physically are not. Various ways of obtaining weight loss include weighing self on a scale frequently, using laxatives, forcing oneself to vomit, exercising excessively, and eating only small amounts of food. Medical complications of anorexia nervosa include osteoporosis, reduction or loss of menses, infertility, and heart damage (9, 88). Anorexia nervosa arises from a complex interaction of psychological, behavioral, biological, and social variables.

Some signs of anorexia nervosa include brittle hair and nails, dry and yellowish skin, constipation, muscle wasting and weakness, low blood pressure, sluggishness, and reduced body temperature making one feel cold (88). There is also a greater risk of heart damage, which can increase the risk of heart attacks, heart-related problems, and death (92). Also, energy consumed and energy expended from exercise are out of balance with this condition (9). When energy availability is low, individuals can experience lower muscle strength and power output and lower aerobic endurance capacity (36, 109). Low energy intake can also lead to a greater risk for illnesses, recurring illnesses, greater levels of fatigue, and slower recovery from bouts of exercise (32, 33, 76). Additionally, if the individual is young, an insufficient energy intake can disrupt normal growth patterns (78).

Medical treatment for anorexia nervosa includes restoring the woman to a healthy body weight, treating any psychological issues, and reducing or eliminating the behaviors or thoughts that can lead to a relapse (88). Treatment solely via medication appears to have a limited benefit, however (102).

Bulimia nervosa is a repeating pattern characterized by binge eating followed by other behaviors to compensate for the overeating, including forced vomiting (purging), excessive use of laxatives or diuretics, fasting, excessive exercise, or a combination of these behaviors (88). Women with this condition consume large amounts of food and then sense that they are out of control after these eating sessions (88). Binge eating is defined as occurring at least one time per week over the past three months (9, 84). Those diagnosed with bulimia nervosa typically have a normal body weight and are sometimes even categorized as overweight. Usually, bulimic behaviors are done in secret and reflect feelings of shame or guilt (88). Symptoms of bulimia nervosa include inflamed and sore throat, swollen glands, worn tooth enamel, acid reflux disorder, gastrointestinal distress from laxative abuse, dehydration from fluid loss, and electrolyte imbalance (levels of sodium, calcium, potassium, or more than one of these minerals that are too low or two high), which can lead to a possible heart attack (88). Medical treatment for anorexia nervosa includes reducing or eliminating the purging or binge-eating behaviors, treating psychological issues, or prescribing medications such as antidepressants (88).

Binge-eating disorders have the five following criteria (9):

1. An episode of binge eating is characterized by eating, in a discrete period of time (e.g., a 1-hour period), a larger than normal amount of food in a similar amount of time and a lack of control over eating during the episode (e.g., a feeling that one cannot stop eating or control what or how much one is eating).

2. Binge-eating episodes that are associated with three or more of the following: eating faster than normal; eating until uncomfortably satiated; eating large amounts of food when not hungry; eating alone due to embarrassment about amount of food consumed; or feeling disgusted with oneself, depressed, or guilty after eating.

3. Feelings of significant emotional or psychological distress or anxiety regarding binge eating.

4. Binge-eating episodes that occur at least once a week for three months.

5. Binge eating is not associated with the repeated use of inappropriate compensatory behavior as is observed in bulimia nervosa (e.g., vomiting, using laxatives, or exercising excessively) and does not occur exclusively during the course of bulimia nervosa or anorexia nervosa.

Medical treatments for binge eating are consistent with those for bulimia nervosa. The only medication approved by the Federal Drug and Food Administration for the treatment of binge eating, as of January 2015, was lisdexamfetamine (44, 48).

The classification of **other specified feeding or eating disorder (OSFED)** includes an eating or feeding disorder not fully meeting the DSM-5 criteria for anorexia nervosa, bulimia nervosa, or binge-eating disorder (124). The OSFED classification includes five conditions: atypical anorexia nervosa, atypical bulimia nervosa and binge-eating disorder (both with low frequency, limited duration, or both), purging disorder, and night eating syndrome (9). Atypical anorexia nervosa includes all the criteria for anorexia nervosa except that body weight remains within normal ranges even though weight loss occurs. Atypical bulimia nervosa and the category of binge-eating disorder include all the criteria for bulimia nervosa and binge-eating disorder, respectively, except that the binge eating occurs less than once per week or for fewer than three months. Purging is a category of self-induced vomiting or misusing laxatives, diuretics, or enemas to control body weight. Night eating syndrome is repeated episodes of eating at night, such as excess calorie intake after dinner or awakening from sleep and then eating (9). Research shows that night eating syndrome should include the consumption of at least 25% of daily caloric intake after dinner, awakenings during the night with intake at least two times per week, or both (4). Symptoms of purging include frequenting the rest room right after a meal, frequent use of laxatives, obsession about body weight, and signs of excessive vomiting including swollen cheeks, popped eye blood vessels, and yellow teeth (86).

Briefly, **pica** is characterized as having an appetite for nonnutritive substances such as paper, chalk, or sand. Complications of the condition arise from issues associated with the consumption of the substances such as gastrointestinal stress and blockages (9). **Rumination disorder** is characterized by "effortless regurgitation following most meals induced by involuntary contraction of the abdominal muscles where there is no retching, nausea, heartburn, odor, or abdominal pain associated with the regurgitation" (9). The cause is unknown. **Avoidant/restrictive food intake disorder**, also known as selective eating disorder, is characterized by prevention of consuming certain types of food. The change in eating can be caused by significant weight loss, nutrition deficiency, use of a feeding tube or dietary supplements, or a significant psychosocial interference (9).

Common Medications Given to Women With the Female Athlete Triad

There are no medications that are prescribed to a woman or girl because she has been diagnosed by her physician or other health care professional with female athlete triad, but there are medications used to treat a condition related to or within the female athlete triad. For example, a woman who has a menstrual dysfunction and is at risk for osteoporosis may benefit from being on estrogen, or, if the physician is concerned about long-term estrogen use, an estrogen agonist–antagonist that targets some tissues (brain and bone) but acts as an antagonist in other tissues (breast or endometrium). For women who have a diagnosed eating disorder, antidepressants may be helpful.

For additional details, including a summary of common side effects and the medications' effects on exercise, see medications tables 13.1 and 13.2 near the end of the chapter.

Effects of Exercise in Women With the Female Athlete Triad

An obvious outcome of exercise, of any type, is caloric expenditure and the potential impact that it has on overall caloric balance. For a woman exhibiting any of the three conditions of the female athlete triad, insufficient energy availability—and its resulting effects—can be exacerbated by even the most minor amount of caloric expenditure. Therefore, exercise can increase risk and severity of the female athlete triad.

Exercise Recommendations for Women With the Female Athlete Triad

Recovery and treatment related to any of the three conditions of the female athlete triad do not progress at the same rate (39). Energy availability in the body can take only days or weeks to

recover and improve. Once energy availability has improved, over a few months, menstrual status will likely be recovered and improved. However, bone mineral density recovery can take up to several years upon improvements in energy status to the body along with adequate estrogen levels (39). With respect to recovery of energy status, the individual should first work on attaining the body weight at which normal menses was last observed.

Exercise recommendations for women with eating disorders include shifting attention from training and competition to treatment (depending on the woman's medical status) and making modifications to exercise type, duration, frequency, and intensity (17, 90, 126, 127) to decrease overall energy expenditure (39). Further, it is recommended that the calculated body mass index be increased to ≥18.5 kg/m^2 (normal-weight body mass index is 19-24.9 kg/m^2). **Body mass index** is derived from a ratio of body weight to body height and categorizes a woman as underweight (≤18.5 kg/m^2), normal weight (19-24.9 kg/m^2), overweight (25-29.9 kg/m^2), or obese (≥30 kg/m^2) based on that calculated value.

If the female athlete triad is exacerbated by low bone mass, the recommendations are to increase energy intake (e.g., to at least 2,000 kcal/day) and vitamin D and calcium consumption (39), as well as adding resistance exercise to improve bone mass and muscle strength (63). However, high-impact movements should be avoided as they could lead to the risk for fractures (72).

Key Point

Women should have preexercise screenings for symptoms associated with the female athlete triad. Exercise professionals should be aware that there is a complex interaction of psychological, behavioral, biological, and social variables related to the female athlete triad.

Prevention of the Female Athlete Triad

The best way to prevent the female athlete triad is through education of the exercise professional, coach, athlete, and parents about components, signs, and symptoms (9, 18, 90). The best care is

Case Study

Female Athlete Triad

Ms. V, 21 years old, is an avid endurance runner and is not consuming the number of calories required to balance and offset the calories expended via her training. Her body mass index is 17 kg/m², which is categorized as under normal weight. She has had a reduction in the frequency of regular menses (i.e., menses not occurring on a regular monthly basis). She has consulted with her physician, who is concerned about her body weight, body mass index, and reduced caloric intake. She has not been diagnosed with an eating disorder, osteopenia, or osteoporosis, although her estrogen levels are on the low end of the normal blood estrogen range. Ms. V has also consulted with a registered dietitian who is working with her to increase caloric consumption as well as increase calcium and vitamin D in her diet, which have been determined to be deficient.

It is not the role of the exercise professional to work on this case alone but rather to work in concert with other allied health professionals in a team approach to assist Ms. V through various treatment options. First, the registered dietitian has recommended an increase in caloric consumption to at least 2,000 kcal/day to improve body weight and body mass index and an increase in vitamin D and calcium-rich foods to maintain or improve bone mass. A psychologist might work with Ms. V on psychological

concerns related to the female athlete triad. The physician would closely monitor her treatment and recovery process in collaboration with the other allied health and exercise professionals.

It is recommended that Ms. V reduce her training volume until caloric consumption can be increased to improve body weight. Once intake levels of calories and protein have been determined by the registered dietitian to be adequate, the exercise professional can design a resistance exercise program (e.g., a two- or three-day per week program composed of 8-10 different exercises targeting all major muscle groups including multijoint exercises [108] using 8-12 repetitions per set). Resistance exercise can be completed using various modes and equipment including free weights, resistance bands, machines, and medicine balls (108). For weeks 1 through 3, three sets of 8 to 12 repetitions of both lower and upper body exercises can be completed on two days per week. The resistance is lighter during this time to accommodate the start of a resistance training program. For weeks 4 through 6, once nutritional intake is maintained, three sets of 8 to 12 repetitions can be completed on three days per week. Since changes in bone remodeling can take at minimum six months (1), resistance exercise training would need to continue at least for this time period.

Recommended Readings

Barrack, MT, Gibbs, JC, de Souza, MJ, Williams, NI, Nichols, JF, Rauh, MJ, and Nattiv, A. Higher incidence of bone stress injuries with increasing female athlete triad-related risk factors: a prospective multisite study of exercising girls and women. *Am J Sports Med* 42:949-958, 2014.

Bonci, CM, Bonci, LJ, Granger, LR, Johnson, CL, Malina, RM, Milne, LW, Ryan, RR, and Vanderbunt, EM. National Athletic Trainers' Association position statement: preventing, detecting, and managing disordered eating in athletes. *J Athl Train* 43(1):80-108, 2008.

de Souza, MJ, Nattiv, A, Joy, E, Misra, M, Williams, NI, Mallinson, RJ, Gibbs, JC, Olmsted, M, Goolsby, M, and Matheson, G. 2014 Female Athlete Triad Coalition Consensus Statement on Treatment and Return to Play of the Female Athlete Triad: 1st international conference held in San Francisco, CA, May 2012, and 2nd international conference held in Indianapolis, IN, May 2013. *Clin J Sport Med* 24(2):96-119, 2014.

(continued)

Recommended Readings *(continued)*

Manore, MM, Kam, LC, and Loucks, AB. The female athlete triad: components, nutrition issues, and health consequences. International Association of Athletics Federations. *J Sports Sci* 25(suppl 1):S61-S71, 2007.

Nattiv A, Loucks, AB, Manore, MM, Sanborn, CF, Sundgot-Borgen, J, and Warren, MP. American College of Sports Medicine position stand. The female athlete triad. *Med Sci Sports Exerc* 39(10):1867-1882, 2007.

Sangenis, P, Drinkwater, BL, Loucks, A, Sherman, RT, Sundgot-Borgen, J, and Thompson, RA. International Olympic Committee Medical Commission Working Group Women in Sport. Position Stand on the Female Athlete Triad. International Olympic Committee. 2005. https://stillmed.olympic.org/media/Document%20 Library/OlympicOrg/IOC/Who-We-Are/Commissions/Medical-and-Scientific-Commission/EN-Position-Stand-on-the-Female-Athlete-Triad.pdf#_ga=1.118851721.1640999716.1482507714. Accessed December 23, 2016.

through an integrated team approach consisting of the coach, exercise professional, medical care, and nutritional and psychological counseling (9, 18, 90). This integrated approach is outside the scope of practice of a single certified exercise professional; thus, the best practice is to refer to a licensed professional (i.e., physician, registered dietitian, psychologist) with consultation with the coach. It is, however, important to have a working knowledge about maintaining healthy body weight, along with activities that expend calories, to provide education and support to the athlete. First and foremost, though, prevention begins with a healthy attitude toward food and exercise and possible preparticipation screenings (61, 82, 132, 139).

The following are five guidelines that can aid in the prevention of the female athlete triad (18, 39, 90, 111, 121).

1. Keep a written record of the monthly menstrual cycle and discuss with a physician or other health care professional if any changes in the menstrual cycle occur.

2. Keep track of daily caloric consumption in order to maintain energy availability to the body and to maintain body weight.

3. Eat every 3 to 4 hours, with three meals a day and at least two snacks to provide energy for exercise and recovery from exercise (77).

4. Consider snacks as a mini-meal with constituents that are nutritious and healthy and that fit into the person's lifestyle (67).

5. Keep a written record of daily exercise including mode, type, time, and intensity.

This record can be used to track the amount, type, and intensity level of the woman or girl and assist the exercise professional and integrative health team in prevention or treatment of symptoms or components of the female athlete triad.

Table 13.1 provides additional suggestions and strategies to help reduce the risk of the female athlete triad.

PREGNANCY AND POSTPARTUM

Many physiological changes occur in the body during pregnancy, and it has been shown that being physically active during pregnancy poses little risk to the mother and baby if there are no pregnancy-related complications (6). During pregnancy, exercise can help to maintain health and fitness levels, assist with weight management, reduce incidence of gestational diabetes, and improve psychological health (6). It has also been shown that being physically active during postpartum can assist in weight loss, in particular with respect to the body fat added during pregnancy, and improve fitness levels and psychological well-being without altering milk production necessary for breastfeeding (6, 42, 74, 75, 104). In this section, we address the pathophysiology of pregnancy and postpartum, common medications and over-the-counter supplements, effects of exercise, and exercise recommendations for pregnant and postpartum women.

Table 13.1 Considerations in the Prevention of the Female Athlete Triad

Consideration	Explanation regarding prevention
Diet	Eat healthfully and appropriately via consultations with a sport dietitian to ensure proper energy intake for success in training and sport performance
Body image	Have a positive body image that does not emphasize body weight too often; seek counseling if focus is on being too thin
Support system	Have a support system every day—family, coaches, and teammates
Professionals	Have dietitians, athletic trainers, counselors, physicians (or a combination of these or other health care professionals) available for any consultations
Menstrual cycle	Monitor the menstrual cycle and consult a physician or other health care professional regarding any irregularities in the menstrual cycle or frequent injuries

Reference: (39)

Pathophysiology of Pregnancy and Postpartum

Pregnancy is marked by increasing weight gain over an approximate 40-week period commensurate with development of the baby and supportive structures, and is divided into trimesters each lasting approximately 12 to 13 weeks (5). The menstrual cycle ceases, the lining of the uterus thickens, and blood vessels and blood volume expand to accommodate an increased blood flow to nourish the baby (5).

Pregnancy hormones include estrogen, progesterone, human chorionic gonadotropin, human placental lactogen, relaxin, and prolactin (5). As pregnancy continues, progesterone prevents the uterus from contracting until the delivery date, and decreased prostaglandin production allows the baby to grow. During pregnancy, estrogen has an anabolic effect on the body to promote breast tissue development and blood vessel enlargement, as well as regulating levels of progesterone. During the third trimester, estrogen and progesterone can be nearly 100-fold and 10- to 15-fold higher, respectively, than nonpregnant levels (5). In combination, estrogen and progesterone control the beginning of breast milk production, which is initiated by the increasing levels of prolactin. During postpartum, estrogen and progesterone decrease, allowing prolactin to stimulate breast milk production. Progesterone can also cause hyperventilation episodes at rest due to progesterone's effect on the brain's respiratory center (16, 60).

Human placental lactogen can function like growth hormone to alter metabolic properties to deliver more energy to the growing baby. It does this by decreasing insulin sensitivity to allow increased levels of glucose in order to ensure adequate nutrition to the baby. Fat breakdown is also increased to deliver more free fatty acids to the growing baby. Adequate amounts of energy through proper nutrition are needed to nourish the growing baby and allow for proper weight gain during pregnancy. If caloric intake is not appropriate, hypoglycemia (e.g., low blood glucose levels) may occur, resulting in nausea, dizziness, and fatigue (79, 130).

The amount of weight gain recommended during pregnancy to support maternal health and baby growth depends on the woman's pre-pregnancy body mass index (table 13.2) (5, 107). During pregnancy and postpartum, women can become less physically active and gain body weight, thus increasing the risk of developing sedentary-based diseases such as obesity and gestational diabetes (41, 54, 95, 99). Given that over 60% of the U.S. population is overweight or obese, there is concern with respect to additional weight gain during pregnancy that might continue during postpartum (52, 62, 91, 110). Starting a pregnancy when one is overweight or obese increases the likelihood of excessive pregnancy weight gain (twofold higher likelihood compared with normal-weight women) (26).

The incidence of lower back pain during pregnancy is common; the cause of its development is unclear but likely is related to increasing body

Table 13.2 Recommendations for Total and Rate of Weight Gain During Pregnancy Based on Prepregnancy Body Mass Index (BMI)

Category	Prepregnancy BMI (kg/m²)	Total weight gain	Weekly weight gain during 2nd and 3rd trimester
Underweight	<18.5	28-40 lb (13-18 kg)	1-1.3 lb (0.5-0.6 kg)
Normal weight	18.5-24.9	25-35 lb (11-16 kg)	0.8-1.1 lb (0.4-0.5 kg)
Overweight	25.0-29.9	15-25 lb (7-11 kg)	0.5-0.7 lb (0.2-0.3 kg)
Obese (including all classes)	≥30.0	11-20 lb (5-9 kg)	0.4-0.6 lb (0.2-0.3 kg)

References: (5, 107)

weight and changes in hormones (74, 104). One such hormone is relaxin, which softens ligaments of the pelvis allowing for passage of the baby during delivery, thus perhaps increasing joint laxity. However, relaxin also affects other joints in the body and may lead to inflammation and pain. Back pain can also extend into the postpartum period.

Postpartum is the period immediately following birth through about six weeks after delivery. The physiological and body changes that occur with the processes of pregnancy can persist from one to two months postpartum. Within four or five days postpartum, estrogen and progesterone levels decrease and there is a rapid drop in progesterone, which allows prolactin and cortisol to bind to receptors on cells to initiate the lactation process. Oxytocin from the pituitary gland in the brain is released upon nipple suckling by the baby and is responsible for the milk ejection reflex (i.e., milk "let-down"). Oxytocin also stimulates uterine contractions, which, postpartum, assist in the uterus returning to prepregnancy size. During breastfeeding, the menstrual cycle and thus menses may not return to normal levels until six to nine months postpartum (136). During the postpartum period, musculoskeletal changes in the pelvic floor muscles and pubic symphysis continue (74, 104). The laxity in the ligaments of the pubic symphysis in the pelvis can cause pain during movement, but performing pelvic floor exercises can reduce the pain and help prevent urinary incontinence (74, 104).

Key Point

Although many physiological and body changes that occur during pregnancy return to normal after delivery, changes persist during the postpartum period that can affect a mother's exercise program.

Common Medications Given to Women During Pregnancy and Postpartum

In consultation with a medical professional, pregnant women might take over-the-counter remedies to alleviate various side effects of being pregnant. These can include headaches, constipation, hemorrhoids, diarrhea, nausea, bloating, and heartburn. Medications table 13.3 near the end of the chapter provides a summary of common over-the-counter remedies and their side effects.

Also, during pregnancy most women take a prenatal vitamin supplement that contains folic acid, calcium, and iron to help prevent brain and spinal cord defects and increase bone growth in the baby, retard the loss of bone mass in the mother, and improve the oxygen-carrying capacity of the mother's and baby's red blood cells. Although folic acid is found in green leafy vegetables, nuts, beans, citrus fruits, and many fortified foods, its critical role in fetal development is the reason for the recommendation that women take a supplement (400 µg/day one month before conception and 600 μg/day during pregnancy). Daily iron and calcium intake should be 27 mg and 1,000 mg, respectively; and because vitamin D helps the body absorb calcium, 600 IU should be taken daily (5).

Effects of Exercise in Women Who Are Pregnant or Postpartum

There are numerous benefits for pregnant women of engaging in moderate intensity exercise for at least 30 minutes per day (38, 103, 105). Benefits include promotion of muscle strength and endurance; increased energy; improvement in body posture; improvement in sleep; improvement in overall mood; decrease in backaches, bloating, swelling, and constipation; improvement in the ability to manage labor; and allowing for an easier return to prepregnancy body shape (6, 7). Aerobic exercise training can also reduce the incidence of gestational diabetes by 55% (116).

Despite these reported benefits, some research does not support strenuous exercise or activity during pregnancy (3, 120). Further, an extensive review of literature by Hinman and colleagues (2015) showed that although exercise is safe for the mother and fetus, research is inconsistent regarding proposed benefits of strenuous exercise during pregnancy such as preventing gestational diabetes, **preeclampsia** (high blood pressure in the pregnant woman), or perinatal depression. However, the authors noted that in a normal pregnancy, the use of moderate- to high-intensity exercise is safe for the developing baby (55). In support of this, women in their first 20 weeks of pregnancy who participated in physical activity including walking and stair climbing showed reductions in preeclampsia compared to women who were not physically active during that same time period (6, 74, 119).

Pregnant women may become overheated during exercise, which can lead to dehydration (6, 7). During pregnancy, blood flow to the skin naturally increases, and exercising in hot, humid environments could put undue stress on the mother's body and developing baby due to increased redirection of blood to the skin for cooling (8).

Pregnant women exercising in a 33°C (91.4°F) swimming pool experienced slight increases in core body temperature but were deemed within safe limits (20).

Another effect of exercise during pregnancy that the exercise professional should be aware of is that while lactic acid production is a normal outcome of exercise, even a small lowering of pH during exercise in the woman can affect the baby and its oxygen levels. However, adequate buffering of this lactate can decrease the chances of a drop in pH in the woman (96).

Women who were lactating and breastfeeding during a 24-week postpartum period showed an improvement in maximal oxygen capacity, lower total body fat, and more energy expended during moderate exercise without any change to the production in breast milk (75). Even women who were not physically active during pregnancy and early postpartum derived significant benefits after starting an exercise program eight weeks postpartum (42). These previously sedentary women lost 3.5 pounds (1.6 kg) and improved their aerobic capacity after 12 weeks of exercise at 60% to 70% of their heart rate reserve with no change in breast milk production.

Exercise Recommendations for Women During Pregnancy and Postpartum

According to the physical activity guidelines published by the U.S. Department of Health and Human Services, it is recommended that pregnant women who are healthy should get at least 150 minutes per week of moderate intensity aerobic activity, such as brisk walking, during and after their pregnancy, distributing the activity throughout the week (135). Healthy women "who already do vigorous intensity aerobic activity, such as running, or large amounts of activity can continue doing so during and after their pregnancy provided they stay healthy and discuss with their health care provider how and when activity should be adjusted over time" (28). However, pregnant women who were previously sedentary or engaged in only moderate intensity exercise should not engage in vigorous intensity exercise during pregnancy (6, 7, 47, 129).

It was recommended in the past that exercise activity during pregnancy be reduced to heart rate levels below 140 beats/min (15). However, there is limited current research to support that recommendation in relation to the developing baby. For example, a study by Szymanski and Satin (128) evaluated the baby's cardiovascular response in active and sedentary women participating in moderate and vigorous aerobic exercise. Neither moderate- nor vigorous-intensity exercise by either group negatively affected heart rate or blood pressure. To guard against a blunted heart rate response to exercise, the American Congress of Obstetricians and Gynecologists recommend that moderate intensity aerobic activity should be assigned and monitored using a rating of perceived exertion (RPE) rather than heart rate (6, 7). On a 6- to 20-point scale, an RPE of 13-14 (corresponding to *somewhat hard*) should be used (6, 7).

Prolonged exercise should occur in a thermoneutral environment or under air conditioning, and maintaining hydration and consuming sufficient calories to maintain energy availability are priorities (6). Some warning signs indicate that women should stop exercising and seek medical attention. These signs include vaginal bleeding, shortness of breath before exercise, dizziness, headache, chest pain, muscle weakness, calf pain or swelling (need to rule out inflammation of the vein caused by blood clots), preterm labor, decreased fetal movements, and amniotic fluid leakage (7).

It should also be noted that several studies have shown that there is an increase in the positive connection between a pregnant woman and her part-ner or spouse during this time (100, 112). Thus one way to engage pregnant women in exercise may be to have their partner exercise with them.

After the first trimester, exercises lying on the back should be avoided as this puts undue pressure on the vena cava in the abdomen, reducing blood flow to the heart and uterus and thus making the woman feel dizzy, short of breath, and nauseated (6, 7). It also increases **orthostatic hypotension** (i.e., low blood pressure when standing up or stretching) (31). Also, holding one's breath should be avoided due to the accompanying increased blood pressure and potentially negative effects on the baby (12, 106, 128).

Involvement in sports and activities that have high contact, such as ice hockey and soccer, could cause trauma to both the woman and developing baby and as such should be avoided. Also, activities involving a high risk of falls, such as skiing and exercising at high altitudes, put the pair at additional bodily risk (7, 10). Other risks for injuries and falls are related to the shift in balance within the body and should be acknowledged in exercise programming. Exercises performed in the water are appropriate as they present a low risk of injury while combining both aerobic and muscle-strengthening exercises (10, 20). Additionally, aquatic exercise causes less stress upon the joints (10, 20).

Resistance exercise training can be performed during pregnancy; however, safety is paramount. In the second and third trimesters, exercises should not be performed in a supine position; and if a pregnant woman will complete more than one set of each exercise, the rest period between the sets should be longer (2-4 minutes) to allow for recovery of energy sources and heart rate (12, 103, 106).

A variety of resistance training exercises can be performed using machines, free weights, elastic bands, elastic tubing, and, in some cases, simply body weight. Note, though, that the use of certain machines can be a limitation as their design may be less accommodating to the pregnant woman's body. Upper and lower back resistance exercises can be done to enhance posture and maintain pelvic alignment since the uterus and breast tissue are enlarging and shifting the center of gravity forward (141), which places

Key Point

Exercise should be stopped and pregnant women should consult their physician or other health care professional immediately if negative signs exist around exercise, including vaginal bleeding, regular painful contractions, amniotic fluid leakage, dyspnea before exertion, dizziness, headache, chest pain, muscle weakness affecting balance, or calf pain or swelling. Pregnant women should avoid exercise in a supine position after the first trimester.

undue stress on the lower back. Abdominal exercises should focus on improving the muscle strength needed during labor and delivery and can include isometric muscle actions (while breathing normally) to reduce risk of **diastasis recti** (a separation of the two sides of the rectus abdominis muscle). Table 13.3 presents a summary of basic exercise program guidelines for women who are pregnant.

During the postpartum period, women should resume exercise gradually due to the detraining effect that may have occurred during pregnancy, as well as physiological and anatomical changes that are still occurring after birth including musculoskeletal changes in the pelvic floor muscles and pubic symphysis (74, 104). Performing

Kegel or **pelvic floor exercises** (i.e., repeatedly contracting and relaxing pelvic floor muscles to improve muscle strength) during pregnancy and postpartum can assist in the restoration of musculoskeletal function in the pelvic floor muscles (87, 104) and alleviate urinary and anal incontinence, pelvic organ prolapse, sexual dysfunction, and chronic pain (21). Further, Pilates exercise that begins 72 hours postdelivery and is performed five days per week has been shown to improve the quality of sleep in postpartum women (11). Brisk walking is also a good mode of exercise after giving birth, and this can prepare the woman for higher-intensity and strenuous types of exercises to be added progressively during the postpartum time period (6, 7).

Table 13.3 Basic Exercise Program Guidelines for Women Who Are Pregnant

Exercise	Frequency	Intensity	Volume
Aerobic exercise			
Lower skill level and balance activities (e.g., walking, stationary cycling, or swimming)	3-5 days per week but not to exceed 5 days per week	Up to an RPE between 13-14 ("somewhat hard") on a 6- to 20-point scale	At least 150 min/week
Resistance exercise			
Machines or free weights in a seated position (no supine exercises after the first trimester)	Two or three sessions per week but not to exceed five sessions per week	60-80% of a 10 repetition maximum[a] 12-15 repetitions per set (not to fatigue) After 28 weeks of pregnancy, perform 12-15 repetitions but begin with a lighter resistance.	Varied based on the time needed to train all major muscle groups with necessary technique and equipment modifications[b]
Flexibility exercise			
Stretches that do not cause discomfort associated with pregnancy-related physical changes (e.g., increased abdominal size)	Daily	Maintain each stretch below discomfort threshold to reduce injury due to increased joint elasticity.	Hold each stretch for 10-30 s
Kegel exercises			
Contract the pelvic floor muscles	Daily	Can be done in sitting or standing position. Squeeze the pelvic floor, moving posterior to anterior. Complete 10 repetitions.	Hold for 3 s, then release

[a]Consider being conservative; higher intensities may reduce blood flow and supply of oxygen to the fetus, thus causing a drop in fetal heart rate (12).

[b]Examples of exercises include seated row, lateral raise, seated machine chest press, dumbbell curl, triceps kickback, dumbbell squat, cable hip extension, standing calf raise, bird dog, and side bridge (115).

References: (6, 7, 38, 103-105, 135, 141)

Case Study

Pregnancy and Postpartum

Mrs. G, 25 years old, is in the first trimester of pregnancy (weeks 1-12). She wishes to begin an exercise program as her obstetrician–gynecologist has told her that exercise could be beneficial both to herself and to the baby. She meets with an exercise professional at four weeks into her pregnancy. She has reported to the exercise professional that she has had no physiological complications during her pregnancy and thus is deemed a low-risk pregnancy. The exercise professional first reviews Mrs. G's exercise history with her. The exercise professional is careful to note the safe exercises that can be performed during pregnancy. The exercise professional begins each exercise session with a proper warm-up consisting of low-impact stretches of all the major muscle groups. Since Mrs. G is at only four weeks of pregnancy, these stretching exercises can be done lying down.

For resistance training, the exercise professional recommends starting with one or two sets of 12 to 15 repetitions for seven or eight primary exercises at an intensity that is challenging but does not result in maximal fatigue. Over the next five to six weeks, one or two more exercises can be added by alternatingly adding an upper body exercise one week followed by a lower body exercise the next week and so on. Aerobic training of up to 30 minutes of moderate intensity (up to an RPE of 12-13) can be performed three days per week. Over the next six weeks, if tolerated, an additional day of exercise can be added.

Beginning in the second trimester, all stretching and resistance training exercises that were performed in a supine position are modified to be side-lying or on all fours.

During the last several weeks leading up to delivery, the exercise professional can consider decreasing the volume of exercise and amount of resistance or intensity. During all of these sessions, the exercise professional needs to make sure that Mrs. G is staying well hydrated and looking for any warning signs to stop the exercise session. During each session, the exercise professional stresses the use of Kegel exercises to strengthen the pelvic floor muscles for delivery and reduce urinary incontinence.

During the postpartum period, if Mrs. G has been medically cleared to continue the exercise program, the exercise professional needs to gradually increase the exercise to moderate intensity to improve weight loss and fitness without affecting breast milk production if Mrs. G decides to breastfeed.

Recommended Readings

American College of Obstetricians and Gynecologists. 2013. Weight Gain During Pregnancy. Committee Opinion. No. 548. www.acog.org/Resources-And-Publications/Committee-Opinions/Committee-on-Obstetric-Practice/Weight-Gain-During-Pregnancy. Accessed December 24, 2016.

American College of Obstetricians and Gynecologists. 2015. Physical Activity and Exercise During Pregnancy and the Postpartum Period. No. 650. www.acog.org/Resources-And-Publications/Committee-Opinions/Committee-on-Obstetric-Practice/Physical-Activity-and-Exercise-During-Pregnancy-and-the-Postpartum-Period. Accessed December 24, 2015.

American College of Obstetricians and Gynecologists. 2016. Exercise During Pregnancy. FAQ 119. www.acog.org/Patients/FAQs/Exercise-During-Pregnancy. Accessed December 24, 2016.

Pruett, MD and Caputo, JL, 2011. Exercise guidelines for pregnant and postpartum women. *Strength Cond J* 33(3):100-103.

MENOPAUSE AND POSTMENOPAUSE

During menopause and postmenopause, a number of hormones in the body undergo changes; the most notable change is decreases in estrogen. Decreases in estrogen are associated with changes in bone and fat metabolism. The changes in estrogen can lead to osteoporosis, which occurs due to an imbalance in the bone remodeling system such that bone becomes more porous and brittle, subsequently leading to increased fractures. Both aerobic and resistance exercise are beneficial for women experiencing menopausal symptoms and psychological issues, as well as for enhancing muscular strength and increasing bone mass and density. Improvements in both the physical and psychological aspects of health thus can improve not only overall health but also quality of life. In this section, we discuss the pathophysiology of menopause; postmenopause and osteoporosis; common medications and over-the-counter supplements; exercise effects; and exercise recommendations for women with menopause, postmenopause, and osteoporosis.

Pathophysiology of Menopause and Postmenopause

Menopause (from the Greek words *men* [month] and *pausis* [cessation]) occurs beginning in the fifth or sixth decade of life (i.e., 40-50 years of age) (34, 50, 101, 114). **Menopause** is characterized by the loss of ovarian follicular function and subsequently cessation of childbearing. There is a transition period between childbearing years and menopause called **perimenopause**, which lasts five to eight years (34, 50, 101, 114). During perimenopause, symptoms include rapid heart rate; vasomotor inability to regulate body temperature (hot and cold flashes); mood changes; depression; irritability; anxiety; sleep disturbances; cognitive issues such as lack of focus or concentration; bladder irritability; and an erratic ovulatory cycle resulting in irregular menses, heavy bleeding, and vaginal dryness (34, 50, 101, 114).

Postmenopause is defined as no menses for a 12-month period during which a woman is not pregnant or lactating. In the case in which the uterus is not present, postmenopause is determined by a very high blood level of follicle-stimulating hormone (34, 50, 101, 114). Women may experience headaches, fatigue, itchiness, night sweats, back and muscle pain, ringing in the ears, dry skin and cracked heels, loss of lean muscle mass, weight gain, increase in visceral abdominal fat, bloating, indigestion, constipation, low libido, hypo- or hyperthyroidism, cravings, increased fungal infections, heavy eyes, loss of memory, thinning hair, heart palpitations, or a combination of any of these (70). Those experiencing menopause also have an increased risk of cancer, type 2 diabetes, osteoporosis, or cardiovascular disease (125).

One concern of menopausal and postmenopausal women is the increased risk of osteoporosis. Osteoporosis affects almost 10 million Americans, most of whom are women (35, 89, 94). Osteoporosis makes bones more porous and thus fragile due to negative changes in estrogen and loss of calcium (35, 89, 94). The bones are placed at an increased risk of fracture, especially in the spine, hip, and wrist (35, 89, 94). The following characteristics are associated with an increased risk of osteoporosis (94):

- Being female
- Being small-boned
- Caucasian or Asian descent
- Age over 55 years
- Family history of osteoporosis or hip fractures
- Physical inactivity
- Diet low in calcium and vitamin D
- Smoking
- High consumption of alcohol

Key Point

Menopausal and postmenopausal women are at a greater risk of experiencing a spine, hip, or wrist fracture and developing osteoporosis than men or younger women.

Bone constantly renews and adapts through a process called **remodeling** that consists of two stages: bone resorption (breakdown or removal) and bone formation (growth). During resorption, cells called osteoclasts on the bone's surface break down bone tissue and create small holes. During formation, other cells called osteoblasts fill in these holes with new bone. Usually, a balance exists between the action of the osteoclasts and osteoblasts; but during menopause, an imbalance results, leading to greater net bone loss and increased risk of fractures.

In addition to changes in bone tissue, there are also changes in several estrogen-related hormones. Estrone is widespread throughout the body and the only one of these hormones present after menopause; estriol is derived from the placenta during pregnancy. Estradiol is the primary sex hormone in women, formed in the ovaries and responsible for female characteristics, and is also important to bone health (23).

Estrogen can have dramatic effects on fat distribution, exercise, and metabolism by increasing activation of the receptors in the lower body and slowing the release of fat, thereby contributing to the "pear" shape of fat distribution in women (98). Additionally, estrogen seems to have an antithyroid effect, which influences metabolic rate (137). An increase in thyroid hormones plus epinephrine can promote fat metabolism, but the use of hormone replacement therapy seems to be ineffective at promoting fat loss; some women even gain body weight while on hormone replacement therapy (137). The interaction of estrogen with other hormones can provide some understanding of why women do not immediately lose weight while on hormone replacement therapy (98, 137).

Common Medications for Menopause-Related Osteoporosis

There are two categories of common osteoporosis medications: antiresorptive medications and anabolic medications (see medications table 13.1 near the end of the chapter; some medications associated with treating osteoporosis within the female athlete triad are also used to treat menopause-related osteoporosis). The goal of antiresorptive medications is to prevent bone loss and lower the risk of breaking bones. When women first take these, they stop losing bone as quickly as before but still make new bone at the same pace; therefore, bone density can increase (48, 133, 142, 144). The goal of anabolic medications is to increase the rate of bone formation and thus bone strength (48, 133, 142, 144).

Common Medications for Menopausal Symptoms

An approach to treating menopause symptoms is with hormone replacement therapy. Such medications can reduce the frequency and severity of hot flashes; improve irritability and sleep disorders related to hormonal changes; increase skin collagen level, which is responsible for the stretch in skin and muscle; and assist in decreasing postmenopausal osteoporosis by slowing bone loss and promoting increase in bone density (48, 133, 142, 144). Side effects of these medications can include headaches, nausea, fluid retention, weight gain, and breast tenderness; but these effects may subside after the first few weeks (48, 133, 142, 144). Other more serious potential side effects include increased risk of breast cancer, heart disease, stroke, and blood clots (144). Various factors have been shown to affect the risk of these side effects, including the specific type of therapy and the timing and duration of treatment (53, 113).

If a woman cannot take hormones or chooses not to, other medications can help reduce some of the symptoms of menopause. Low doses of medications that are commonly used as antidepressants (e.g., escitalopram, fluoxetine, paroxetine, and venlafaxine) may reduce the frequency and severity of hot flashes (22, 49). Also, paroxetine and a conjugated estrogens–bazedoxifene formula have been developed specifically to treat hot flashes (140). For additional details, see medications table 13.4 near the end of the chapter.

Effects of Exercise in Women Who Are Menopausal or Postmenopausal

Reductions in estrogen levels in women are reported to be the main cause of the symptoms associated with menopause (94). Regular exercise can alleviate the more common symptoms in menopausal women by improving the cardiorespiratory system (43, 65, 73), psychological health (46, 134), and overall quality of life (2).

Especially as it relates to menopause-associated osteoporosis, resistance training has been shown to improve bone mass due to mechanical strain, which can stimulate bone growth and thus improve bone strength, thereby reducing the risk of fractures (35). Further, a four-year exercise program with a combination of aerobic endurance, jumping, and resistance training exercises of high intensity and low volume in early postmenopausal women supplemented with calcium and cholecalciferol showed positive benefits on blood lipids, increased muscular strength, and maintenance of bone mass in the spine and femoral head (64). Older adults who varied the intensity of a three times per week resistance training program improved their ability to perform daily activities of living (58, 59).

Key Point

Resistance training that sufficiently loads the body can stimulate net bone growth and reduce the risk of femoral fractures.

There is not enough information to determine any positive benefits in relieving menopause symptoms through yoga (37, 45, 93). However, moderate aerobic exercise has been shown to provide improvements in sleep quality, insomnia, and mood (123). Exercising just 3 hours per week for 12 weeks showed improvements in both physical and psychological health, overall quality of life, and decreased symptoms of menopause (138). Even light-intensity exercises such as walking and dancing led to similar improvements (40).

Exercise Recommendations for Women Who Are Menopausal and Postmenopausal

Much of the attention on exercise recommendations focuses on menopausal and postmenopausal women who are at risk of or who have osteoporosis. See table 13.4 for a sample beginning program and figures 13.2 to 13.6 for exercises that specifically improve spinal flexibility and strength. Of note, resistance training is a priority to increase bone density and muscle strength, assist in the oxidation of body fat, and increase metabolism and body functions that are affected during

Table 13.4 Beginning Resistance Training Program for an Individual Who Has Osteoporosis

Mode	Movement	Intensity, repetitions, and sets
Warm-up	Treadmill, stationary bike, elliptical machine, or stair climber	50% MHR for 5-10 min
Resistance training exercises	Alternate between upper and lower body exercises: Lower body Horizontal leg press, hamstring curl, hip abduction, hip adduction Upper body Bench press, upright row, lat pulldown, shoulder press	40-60% 1RM for 15-20 repetitions for 1-2 sets
Spine-specific exercises*	Prone press-up	15-20 repetitions for 1-2 sets
	Prone press-up and quadruped stabilization	15-20 repetitions for 1-2 sets
	Thoracic extension on a foam roll	8-10 repetitions for 1 set
	Thoracic extension with a pectoral stretch	20-s holds for 5 repetitions
	Thoracic extension in a prone position	10-s holds for 5 repetitions

*See photos of these exercises in the box titled "Spine-Specific Exercises for Osteoporosis."

Adapted, by permission, from E.J. Chaconas et al., 2013, "Exercise Interventions for the Individual with Osteoporosis," *Strength and Conditioning Journal* 35(4): 49-55.

Spine-Specific Exercises for Osteoporosis

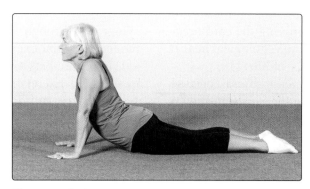

Figure 13.2 Prone press-up.

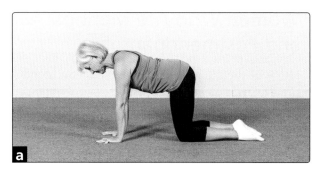

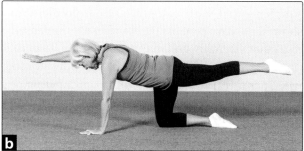

Figure 13.3 Quadruped stabilization: *(a)* starting position, *(b)* ending position.

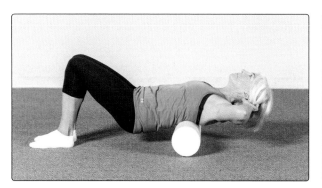

Figure 13.4 Thoracic extension on a foam roll.

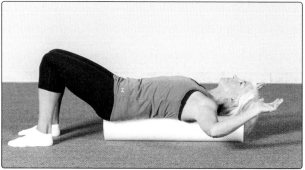

Figure 13.5 Thoracic extension with a pectoral stretch.

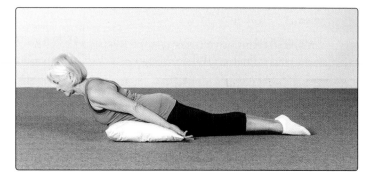

Figure 13.6 Thoracic extension in a prone position.

Menopause and Postmenopause

Ms. B, 65 years old, has been diagnosed with osteoporosis. She wishes to begin an exercise program, mostly because she is interested in being stronger to do activities of daily living. The exercise professional wants to focus on an exercise program that offers a combination of aerobic, resistance, and flexibility exercises to improve overall cardiovascular health, increase bone mass and strength, increase muscle mass and strength, and improve range of motion.

The exercise professional has developed the following exercise program for Ms. B, which can serve as a simple sample program for an older woman with osteoporosis. The goal, over time, is to progress to performing aerobic exercise two or three days per week and resistance training two or three days per week. Aerobic exercise can include walking, cycling, and swimming for 15 to 20 minutes at a light intensity (55% to <65% MHR) with a gradual progression up to 45 minutes at a moderate intensity (65% to <75% MHR). For resistance training, the program should begin with learning proper exercise technique and adjusting to the new program using light loads (40-60% 1RM) and more repetitions (15-20) for one set. Once proper technique has been learned, Ms. B could progress to two sets of 15 to 20 repetitions of, for example, the machine Smith squat (or leg press or leg extension exercise) and leg curl exercises and one set of 15 to 20 repetitions of the abdominal crunch, seated row, bench press, and shoulder press exercises. Then, in two-week phases, she can gradually increase the load, decrease the repetitions, and add sets until she is lifting moderate loads (60-80% 1RM) for fewer repetitions (8 to 15) and more (two or three) sets.

Recommended Readings

Centers for Disease Control and Prevention. CDC recommendation regarding selected conditions affecting women's health. *MMWR* 49(No. RR-2), 2000.

Chaconas, EJ, Olivencia, O, and Russ, BS. Exercise interventions for the individual with osteoporosis. *Strength Cond J* 35(4):49-55, 2013.

Kemmler, K, Engelke, K, Von Stengel, S, Weineck, J, Lauber, D, and Kalender, WA. Long-term four-year exercise has a positive effect on menopausal risk factors: the Erlangen fitness osteoporosis prevention study. *J Strength Cond Res* 21(1):232-239, 2007.

Office of the Surgeon General. 2004. Bone Health and Osteoporosis: A Report of the Surgeon General. www.ncbi.nlm.nih.gov/books/NBK45513/. Accessed December 24, 2016.

Stojanovskaa, L, Apostolopoulosa, V, Polmanb, R, and Borkolesb, E. To exercise, or, not to exercise, during menopause and beyond. *Maturitas* 77:318-323, 2014.

Writing Group for the Women's Health Initiative Investigators. Risks and benefits of estrogen plus progestin in healthy postmenopausal women: principal results from the Women's Health Initiative randomized controlled trial. *JAMA* 288(3):321-333, 2002.

menopause (27, 66). More specifically, Howe and colleagues (57) suggested that exercises to improve bone mass at the femoral neck should be done through progressive resistance training of the lower body. For exercises to improve bone mass at the spine, women should perform a combination of aerobic and resistance training exercises (57).

Although they are beneficial to overall health, walking, jogging, and running do not seem to provide sufficient mechanical loading on bone to adequately promote improvements in bone mass (25, 80, 85). Therefore, performing resistance exercise that applies an additional external load on the body will promote greater bone mass increases in areas prone to fractures, including the wrist, hip, and spine (57, 63). However, a gradual progression needs to be applied; an increase of less than 5% per week is recommended (29).

The exercise intensity should be sufficient to reach a desired threshold resulting in beneficial strength and bone mineral density changes. This is probably in the range of 80% to 85% of one repetition maximum (1RM). Multiple sets (e.g., two or three) in the 8- to 15-repetition range appear to be beneficial for this population (57). Power training might also be incorporated into the program; Stengel and colleagues (122) showed a reduction in the rate of bone loss at the hip and spine with performance of a fast or explosive concentric movement phase compared to a slow (4-second) concentric movement phase. At the beginning of a resistance training program, though, light loads (40-60% 1RM) and more repetitions are recommended (29).

CONCLUSION

Numerous concerns arise with women and girls with the female athlete triad, women who are pregnant and postpartum, and women who are menopausal and postmenopausal. The female athlete triad concerns three areas: menstrual dysfunction; eating disorders, which can limit the amount of energy available to the body; and loss of bone mass. A team approach on the part of professionals is typically used to assist girls and women in treatment and recovery outcomes. Pregnant women have concerns related to a shift of their center of gravity, back pain, joint laxity, and care for the developing baby. Exercise programming needs to be adjusted to accommodate these physiological and physical changes. During postpartum, the body is also changing, and the woman can be actively breastfeeding. Again, programming needs to be altered to start with a slow progression and intensity at first. Concerns during menopause and postmenopause are largely related to changes in estrogen levels. One main issue is osteoporosis, in which bone is more brittle and more susceptible to fractures. Programming can be aimed at improving both muscle and bone strength.

Key Terms

amenorrhea
anorexia nervosa
avoidant/restrictive food intake disorder
binge-eating disorder
body mass index
bulimia nervosa
Diagnostic and Statistical Manual of Mental Disorders (DSM-5)
diastasis recti
female athlete triad
Kegel exercises
menopause
oligomenorrhea
orthostatic hypotension
osteoblasts

osteoclasts
osteopenia
osteoporosis
other specified feeding or eating disorder (OSFED)
pelvic floor exercises
perimenopause
pica
postmenopause
postpartum
preeclampsia
remodeling
rumination disorder

Study Questions

1. Which of the following is a health issue that is a part of the female athlete triad?

    a. sarcopenia

    b. amenorrhea

    c. cardiomyopathy

    d. low body weight

2. Greater than _____ standard deviation(s) below the bone mineral density of an average 30-year-old woman is considered osteoporosis, whereas _____ standard deviation(s) below is considered osteopenia.

    a. 1.0; 0.5

    b. 1.0; 2.5

    c. 2.5; 1.0

    d. 3.0; 2.5

3. Which of the following is a valid safety or health concern for pregnant women or women in the postpartum period?

    a. Moderate exercise can negatively affect breast milk production postpartum.

    b. Exercise causes overheating more easily in pregnant women.

    c. Exercise is likely to result in greater incidence of backaches.

    d. Moderate exercise can reduce blood flow to the baby.

4. Adjustments to exercise practices for pregnant women in the third trimester include

    a. keeping the exercise heart rate below 140 beats/min

    b. performing only dumbbell exercises in the supine position

    c. monitoring exercise intensity using a rating of perceived exertion

    d. limiting total exercise time to 150 minutes per week of moderate-intensity aerobic activity

Medications Table 13.1 Common Medications Used to Treat Menstrual Dysfunction and Osteoporosis Within the Female Athlete Triad

Drug class and names	Mechanism of action	Most common side effects	Effects on exercise
bisphosphonates (Actonel)	Increase bone mineral density by slowing the actions of osteoclasts (bone-absorbing cells)	Nausea; inflammation; bone, joint, or musculoskeletal pain; atrial fibrillation (abnormal heart rhythm) in women related to fluctuations of calcium levels in the blood	No apparent effect on heart rate, blood pressure, muscular strength, or aerobic endurance
Estrogen and estrogen agonists–antagonists	Offer bone health benefits of hormone therapy but without the increased cancer risks; may play a role in suppressing binge eating	Headaches, abdominal pain, nervousness, nausea, back pain, joint pain, vaginal bleeding, loss of menses, breast tenderness, and increase in sexual drive and possibility of skin rash	Systolic blood pressure increases with no change in diastolic blood pressure
teriparatide (Forteo)	Form of parathyroid hormone that increases the rate of bone formation; used to treat osteoporosis in people who have a high risk of fractures	Headache, nausea, dizziness, and limb pain, which could create discomfort during exercise	May experience a drop in blood pressure while standing up from seated or lying position
Calcium and vitamin D coingestion	Prevents or treats low blood calcium levels and conditions affected by low calcium levels including osteoporosis, weak bones, decreased activity of the parathyroid gland, and certain muscle diseases	No common side effects have been reported. Allergic reactions can occur including rash and difficulty breathing, loss of appetite, nausea, vomiting, or constipation.	No apparent effect on heart rate, blood pressure, muscular strength, or aerobic endurance

References: (48, 133, 142, 144)

Medications Table 13.2 Common Medications Used to Treat Eating Disorders Within the Female Athlete Triad

Condition	Drug class and names	Mechanism of action	Most common side effects	Effects on exercise
Binge eating	lisdexamfetamine (Vyvanse)	Central nervous system stimulant	Hypertension or hypotension, decreased blood flow to legs and arms, increased heart rate, abdominal pain, weight loss, loss of appetite, increased alertness, and decreased sense of fatigue	Increased physical strength, acceleration, stamina, and aerobic endurance; reduced reaction time
Bulimia nervosa	Antidepressants including fluoxetine (Prozac) and sertraline (Zoloft)	Actions not entirely clear but believed to be related to increasing serotonin activity in the brain	Trouble sleeping, loss of appetite, dry mouth, rash, excessive sweating, and uncontrolled shaking of body parts	Strength and high-intensity exercise are not affected

References: (69, 97)

Medications Table 13.3 Over-the-Counter Medications Used to Treat Symptoms During Pregnancy

Drug name	Mechanism of action	Most common side effects	Effects on exercise
acetaminophen	Pain relief through the inhibition of cyclooxygenase	Unusual bleeding or bruising, unusual tiredness or weakness, and skin irritations	Aerobic endurance performance seems unaffected (24) or improved (81)
psyllium	Relief from constipation (as a laxative) through the absorption of excess water while normal bowel movements are stimulated	Gastrointestinal distress such as mild diarrhea, nausea, regurgitation, and vomiting, which can be uncomfortable during exercise	None reported
simethicone	An antacid that relieves heartburn	Usually no known side effects when taken as directed. Could experience gastrointestinal symptoms including mild diarrhea, nausea, regurgitation, and vomiting.	None reported

References: (24, 48, 81)

Medications Table 13.4 Common Medications Used to Treat Menopausal Symptoms

Drug class and names	Mechanism of action	Most common side effects	Effects on exercise
escitalopram (Lexapro), fluoxetine (Prozac), paroxetine (Paxil), and venlafaxine (Effexor)	Affect the brain's use of serotonin and norepinephrine, which is linked to the regulation of body heat and reduces the frequency and severity of hot flashes	Drowsiness, dizziness, insomnia, nausea, gas, heartburn, constipation, weight changes, decreased sex drive, and dry mouth	May decrease energy and physical comfort levels (and thereby reduce desire to exercise)
paroxetine (Brisdelle) and conjugated estrogens–bazedoxifene (Duavee)	Specifically formulated to reduce the frequency and severity of hot flashes	Nausea–vomiting, bloating, breast tenderness, headache, muscle spasms, diarrhea, and weight changes	May reduce capacity for higher-intensity aerobic exercise

References: (22, 49, 131, 140)

Answers to Study Questions

Chapter 1
1. a, 2. d, 3. c, 4. d

Chapter 2
1. d, 2. c, 3. c, 4. b

Chapter 3
1. b, 2. c, 3. d, 4. d

Chapter 4
1. a, 2. c, 3. c, 4. a

Chapter 5
1. b, 2. b, 3. a, 4. a

Chapter 6
1. b, 2. b, 3. d, 4. c

Chapter 7
1. d, 2. d, 3. c, 4. d

Chapter 8
1. a, 2. d, 3. d, 4. d

Chapter 9
1. b, 2. d, 3. c, 4. b

Chapter 10
1. d, 2. c, 3. d, 4. c

Chapter 11
1. d, 2. b, 3. b, 4. b

Chapter 12
1. a, 2. b, 3. b, 4. b

Chapter 13
1. b, 2. c, 3. b, 4. c

References

Chapter 1 Rationale and Considerations for Training Special Populations

1. Alexander, NB, Galecki, AT, Grenier, ML, Nyquist, LV, Hofmeyer, MR, Grunawalt, JC, Medell, JL, and Fry-Welch, D. Task-specific resistance training to improve the ability of activities of daily living-impaired older adults to rise from a bed and from a chair. *J Am Geriatr Soc* 49:1418-1427, 2001.

2. Arias, E. United States life tables, 2009. In *National Vital Statistics Reports.* Hyattsville, MD: National Center for Health Statistics, 7, 2009.

3. Armstrong, MJ and Sigal, RJ. Exercise as medicine: key concepts in discussing physical activity with patients who have Type 2 diabetes. *Can J Diabetes* 2671:747-749, 2015.

4. Beaulieu, L, Butterfield, SA, and Mason, CA. Physical activity and U.S. public elementary schools: implications for our profession. *ICHPER-SD Journal of Research* 7:13-16, 2012.

5. Benavent-Caballer, V, Rosado-Calatayud, P, Segura-Orti, E, Amer-Cuenca, JJ, and Lison, JF. Effects of three different low-intensity exercise interventions on physical performance, muscle CSA and activities of daily living: a randomized controlled trial. *Exp Gerontol* 58:159-165, 2014.

6. Booth, FW, Roberts, CK, and Laye, MJ. Lack of exercise is a major cause of chronic diseases. *Compr Physiol* 2:1143-1211, 2014.

7. Brownson, RC, Boehmer, TK, and Luke, DA. Declining rates of physical activity in the United States: what are the contributors? *Annu Rev Public Health* 26:421-443, 2005.

8. Caban-Martinez, AJ, Courtney, TK, Chang, W, Lombardi, DA, Huang, Y, Brennan, MJ, Perry, MJ, Katz, KN, Christiani, DC, and Verma, SK. Leisure-time physical activity, falls, and fall injuries in middle-aged adults. *Am J Prev Med* 49:888-901, 2015.

9. Census Bureau. *Current Population Reports.* Washington, DC: Department of Commerce, 2010.

10. Centers for Disease Control and Prevention. Overcoming Barriers to Physical Activity. 2011. www.cdc.gov/physicalactivity/basics/adding-pa/barriers.html. Accessed January 31, 2017.

11. Centers for Disease Control and Prevention. *National Diabetes Statistics Report: Estimates of Diabetes and Its Burden in the United States, 2014.* Atlanta: U.S. Department of Health and Human Services, 2014.

12. Centers for Disease Control and Prevention. NCHS data on obesity. 2014. www.cdc.gov/nchs/data/factsheets/factsheet_obesity.htm. Accessed May 2014.

13. Department of Health and Human Services. *Physical Activity Guidelines for Americans.* Washington, DC: U.S. Department of Health and Human Services, 2008.

14. Department of Justice. *The 2010 ADA Standards for Accessible Design.* Washington, DC: U.S. Department of Justice, 2010.

15. Diaz, KM and Shimbo, D. Physical activity and the prevention of hypertension. *Curr Hypertens Rep* 15:659-668, 2013.

16. Donnelly, JE, Blair, SN, Jakicic, JM, Manore, MM, Rankin, JW, and Smith, BK. Appropriate physical activity intervention strategies for weight loss and prevention of weight regain for adults. *Med Sci Sports Exerc* 41:459-469, 2009.

17. Finkelstein, EA, Trogdon, JG, Cohen, JW, and Dietz, W. Annual medical spending attributable to obesity: payer- and service-specific estimates. *Health Aff (Millwood)* 28:w822-w831, 2009.

18. Frank, L, Andresen, MA, and Schmid, TL. Obesity relationships with community design, physical activity, and time spent in cars. *Am J Prev Med* 27:87-96, 2004.

19. Frumkin, H. Urban sprawl and public health. *Public Health Rep* 117:201-217, 2002.

20. Heath, GW and Fentem, PH. Physical activity among persons with disabilities--a public health perspective. *Exerc Sport Sci Rev* 26:195-234, 1997.

21. Herman, WH. The economic costs of diabetes: is it time for a new treatment paradigm? *Diabetes Care* 6:775-776, 2013.

22. Hogan, CL, Mata, J, and Carstensen, LL. Exercise holds immediate benefits for affect and cognition in younger and older adults. *Psychol Aging* 28:587-594, 2013.

23. Jacobsen, LA, Kent, M, Lee, M, and Mather, M. America's aging population. *Popul Bull* 66, 2011.

24. Kinsella, KG. Changes in life expectancy 1900–1990. *Am J Clin Nutr* 55:1196S-1202S, 1992.

25. Knight, JA. Physical inactivity: associated diseases and disorders. *Ann Clin Lab Sci* 42:320-337, 2012.

26. Lee, MA and Mather, M. U.S. labor force trends. *Popul Bull* 63, 2008.

27. Levine, MA. Assessing bone health in children and adolescents. *Ind J Endocrin Metab* 16:S205-S212, 2012.

28. Manson, JE, Skerrett, PJ, Greenland, P, and VanItallie, TB. The escalating pandemics of obesity and sedentary lifestyle. A call to action for clinicians. *Arch Intern Med* 164:249-258, 2004.

29. McDonnell, MN, Hillier, SL, Hooker, SP, Le, A, Judd, SE, and Howard, VJ. Physical activity frequency and risk of incident stroke in a national US study of blacks and whites. *Stroke* 44:2519-2524, 2013.

30. McGovern, JN. *Recreation Access Rights Under the ADA*. Bloomington, IN: National Center on Accessibility, 2014.

31. Ogden, CL, Carroll, MD, Kit, BK, and Flegal, KM. Prevalence of childhood and adult obesity in the United States, 2011-2012. *JAMA* 311:806-814, 2014.

32. Okubo, Y, Schoene, D, and Lord, SR. Step training improves reaction time, gait and balance and reduces falls in older people: a systematic review and meta-analysis. *Br J Sports Med*, 2015. [e-pub ahead of print].

33. Rimmer, JH. Promoting inclusive physical activity communities for people with disabilities. *Res Dig Pres Counc Phys Fit Sports* 9:1-8, 2008.

34. Rosenberg, DE, Bombardier, CH, Hoffman, JM, and Belza, B. Physical activity among persons aging with mobility disabilities: shaping a research agenda. *J Aging Res* 2011:708510, 2011.

35. Sarzynski, M, Burton, J, Rankinen, T, Blair, S, Church, T, Despres, J, Hagberg, J, Lander-Ramos, R, Leon, A, Mikus, C, Rao, D, Seip, R, Skinner, J, Slentz, C, Thompson, P, Wilund, K, Kraus, W, and Bouchard, C. The effects of exercise on lipoprotein profile: a meta-analysis of 10 interventions. *Atherosclerosis* 243:364-372, 2015.

36. Takahashi, S. Facility and equipment layout and maintenance. In *NSCA's Essentials of Personal Training*. Coburn, JW, and Malek, MH, eds. Champaign, IL: Human Kinetics, 2012.

37. Thyfault, JP and Booth, FW. Lack of regular physical exercise or too much inactivity. *Curr Opin Clin Nutr Metab Care* 14:374-378, 2011.

38. Vincent, GK and Velcoff, VA. *The Next Four Decades: The Older Population in the United States: 2010 to 2050*. Washington, DC: U.S. Census Bureau, 2010.

39. Warburton, DER, Nicol, CW, and Bredin, SSD. Health benefits of physical activity: the evidence. *CMAJ* 174:801-809, 2006.

40. Ward, B, Schiller, J, and Goodman, R. Multiple chronic conditions among US adults: a 2012 update. *Prev Chronic Dis* 11:130389, 2014.

41. Warren, TY, Barry, V, Hooker, SP, Sui, X, Church, TS, and Blair, SN. Sedentary behaviors increase risk of cardiovascular disease mortality in men. *Med Sci Sports Exerc* 42:879-885, 2010.

42. Zafari, AM and Mackie, BD. Physical activity and the metabolic syndrome. *Hosp Physician* 42:26-38, 2006.

Chapter 2 Health Appraisal and Fitness Assessments

1. Albert, CM, Mittleman, MA, Chae, CU, Lee, IM, Hennekens, CH, and Manson, JE. Triggering of sudden death from cardiac causes by vigorous exertion. *N Engl J Med* 343:1355-1361, 2000.

2. American College of Sports Medicine. *ACSM's Guidelines for Exercise Testing and Prescription*. 9th ed. Baltimore: Lippincott Williams & Wilkins, 40-57, 2014.

3. American Thoracic Society and American College of Chest Physicians. American Thoracic Society/American College of Chest Physicians statement on cardiopulmonary exercise testing. *Am J Respir Crit Care Med* 167:211-277, 2003.

4. Balady, GJ, Weiner, DA, Rose, L, and Ryan, TJ. Physiologic responses to arm ergometry exercise relative to age and gender. *J Am Coll Cardiol* 16:130-135, 1990.

5. Balke, B and Ware, RW. An experimental study of physical fitness of Air Force personnel. *U S Armed Forces Med J* 10:675-688, 1959.

6. Billinger, SA, Loudon, JK, and Gajewski, BJ. Validity of a total body recumbent stepper exercise test to assess cardiorespiratory fitness. *J Strength Cond Res* 22:1556-1562, 2008.

7. Billinger, SA, Swearingen, E, McClain, M, Lentz, AA, and Good, MB. Recumbent stepper submaximal exercise test to predict peak oxygen uptake. *Med Sci Sports Exerc* 44:1539-1544, 2012.

8. Bovend'Eerdt, TJH, Botell, RE, and Wade, DT. Writing SMART rehabilitation goals and achieving goal attainment scaling: a practical guide. *Clin Rehabil* 23:352-361, 2009.

9. Bruce, RA, Kusumi, F, and Hosmer, D. Maximal oxygen intake and nomographic assessment of functional aerobic impairment in cardiovascular disease. *Am Heart J* 85:546-562, 1973.

10. Buchfuhrer, MJ, Hansen, JE, Robinson, TE, Sue, DY, Wasserman, K, and Whipp, BJ. Optimizing the exercise protocol for cardiopulmonary assessment. *J Appl Physiol* 55:1558-1564, 1983.

11. Centers for Disease Control and Prevention. Death and Mortality. National Center for Health Statistics FastStats. www.cdc.gov/nchs/fastats/deaths.htm. Accessed December 22, 2016.

12. U.S. Department of Health and Human Services. The Seventh Report of the Joint National Committee on Prevention, Detection, Evaluation, and Treatment of High Blood Pressure. 2004, p 12.

13. Dahabreh, IJ and Paulus, JK. Association of episodic physical and sexual activity with triggering of acute cardiac events: systemic review and meta-analysis. *JAMA* 305:1225-1233, 2011.

14. Evetovich, TK and Hinnerichs, KR. Client consultation and health appraisal. In *NSCA's Essentials of Personal Training*. 2nd ed. Coburn, JW, and Malek, MH, eds. Champaign, IL: Human Kinetics, 147-163, 178, 2012.

15. Faigenbaum, AD. Age and sex-related differences and their implications for resistance training. In *Essentials of Strength Training and Conditioning*. 3rd ed. Baechle, TR, and Earle, RW, eds. Champaign, IL: Human Kinetics, 141-158, 2008.

16. Franklin, BA and McCullough, PA. Cardiovascular fitness: an independent and additive marker of risk stratification and health outcomes. *Mayo Clin Proc* 84:776-779, 2009.

17. Golding, LA. *YMCA Fitness Testing and Assessment Manual*. Champaign, IL: Human Kinetics, 2000.

18. Gordon, SMBS. Health appraisal in the non-medical setting. In *ACSM's Resource Manual for Guidelines for Exercise Testing and Prescription*. 2nd ed. Durstine JL, ed. Philadelphia: Williams & Wilkins, 219-228, 1993.

19. Hambrecht, RP, Schuler, GC, Muth, T, Grunze, MF, Marburger, CT, Niebauer, J, Methfessel, SM, and Kubler, W. Greater diagnostic sensitivity of treadmill versus cycle exercise testing of asymptomatic men with coronary artery disease. *Am J Cardiol* 70:141-146, 1992.

20. Hatfield, BD and Kaplan, P. Exercise psychology for the personal trainer. In *NSCA's Essentials of Personal Training*. 2nd ed. Coburn, JW, and Malek, MH, eds. Champaign, IL: Human Kinetics, 125-144, 2012.

21. Herbert, DL. Legal aspects of personal training. In *NSCA's Essentials of Personal Training*. 2nd ed. Coburn, JW, and Malek, MH, eds. Champaign, IL: Human Kinetics, 623-633, 2012.

22. Heyward, VH and Gibson, AL. *Advanced Fitness Assessment and Exercise Prescription*. 7th ed. Champaign, IL: Human Kinetics, 23-44, 79-118, 219-265, 305-324, 2014.

23. Hollingsworth, V, Bendick, P, Franklin, B, Seymour, G, and Timmis, GC. Validity of arm ergometer blood pressures immediately after exercise. *Am J Cardiol* 65:1358-1360, 1990.

24. Iverson, GL and Koehle, MS. Normative data for the balance error scoring system in adults. *Rehabil Res Pract* 2013:846418, 2013.

25. Jamnik, VK, Warburton, DE, Makarski, J, McKenzie, DC, Shephard, RJ, Stone, JA, Charlesworth, S, and Gledhill, N. Enhancing the effectiveness of clearance for physical activity participation: background and overall process. *Appl Physiol Nutr Metab* 36(suppl 1):S3-S13, 2011.

26. Kaminsky, LA and Whaley, MH. Evaluation of a new standardized ramp protocol: the BSU/Bruce Ramp Protocol. *J Cardiopulm Rehabil* 18:438-444, 1998.

27. Locke, EA and Latham, GP. Building a practically useful theory of goal setting and task motivation. *Am Psychol* 57:705-717, 2002.

28. McGuigan, M. Administration, scoring, and interpretation of selected tests. In *Essentials of Strength Training and Conditioning*. 4th ed. Haff, GG, and Triplett, NT, eds. Champaign, IL: Human Kinetics, 259-294, 2016.

29. McInnis, KJ and Balady, GJ. Higher cardiovascular risk clients in health clubs: an overview of new guidelines from the AHA and the ACSM on risk screening, emergency procedures, and staffing at health/fitness facilities. *ACSMs Health Fit J* 3(1):19-24, 1999.

30. Moore, GE, Marsh, AP, and Durstine, JL. Approach to exercise and disease. In *ACSM's Exercise Management for Persons with Chronic Diseases and Disabilities*. 3rd ed. Durstine, JL, Moore, GE, Painter, PL, and Roberts, SO, eds. Champaign, IL: Human Kinetics, 12-17, 2013.

31. Morrow Jr, JR, Mood, D, Disch, J, and Kang, M. *Measurement and Evaluation in Human Performance*. 4th ed. Champaign, IL: Human Kinetics, 2011.

32. Myers, J, Buchanon, N, Smith, D, Neutel, J, Bowes, E, Walsh, D, and Froelicher, VF. Individualization ramp treadmill. Observations on a new protocol. *Chest* 101:2365-2415, 1992.

33. Myers, J, Buchanon, N, Walsh, D, Kraemer, M, and McAuley, P. Comparison of the ramp versus standard exercise protocols. *J Am Coll Cardiol* 17:1334-1342, 1991.

34. Pollock, ML, Schmidt, DH, and Jackson, AS. Measurement of cardio-respiratory fitness and body composition in a clinical setting. *Comp Ther* 6:12-27, 1980.

35. Rana, S and White, JB. Fitness assessment selection and administration. In *NSCA's Essentials of Personal Training*. 2nd ed. Coburn, JW, and Malek, MH, eds. Champaign, IL: Human Kinetics, 147-163, 2012.

36. Riebe, D, Franklin, BA, Thompson, PD, Garber, CE, Whitfield, GP, Magal, M, and Pescatello, LS. Updating ACSM's recommendations for exercise preparticipation health screening. *Med Sci Sports Exerc* 47:2473-2479, 2015.

37. Riemann, BL, Guskiewicz, KM, and Shields, EW. Relationship between clinical and forceplate measures of postural stability. *J Sport Rehabil* 8:71-82, 1999.

38. Rikli, RE and Jones, CJ. *Senior Fitness Test Manual*. 2nd ed. Champaign, IL: Human Kinetics, 18, 64-77, 154, 2013.

39. Rodgers, WM and Loitz, CC. The role of motivation in behavior change: how do we encourage our clients to be active? *ACSMs Health Fit J* 13:7-12, 2009.

40. Ryan, ED and Cramer, JT. Fitness testing protocols and norms. In *NSCA's Essentials of Personal Training*. 2nd ed. Coburn, JW, and Malek, MH, eds. Champaign, IL: Human Kinetics, 201-232, 2012.

41. Thompson, PD, Franklin, BA, Balady, GJ, Blair, SN, Corrado, D, Estes, NA, Fulton, JE, Gordon, NF, Haskell, WL, Link, MS, Maron, MA, American Heart Association Council on Nutrition, Physical Activity and Metabolism, American Heart Association Council on Clinical Cardiology, and American College of Sports Medicine. Exercise and acute cardiovascular events placing the risks into perspective: a scientific statement from the American Heart Association Council on Nutrition, Physical Activity, and Metabolism and the Council on Clinical Cardiology. *Circulation* 115:2358-2368, 2007.

42. Warburton, DER, Gledhill, N, Jamnik, VK, Bredin, SSD, Mckenzie, DC, Stone, J, Charlesworth, S, and Shepard, RJ. Evidence-based risk assessment and recommendations for physical activity clearance: consensus document. *Appl Physiol Nutr Metab* 36:S266-S298, 2011.

43. Ward, BW, Schiller, JS, and Goodman, RA. Multiple chronic conditions among US adults: a 2012 update. *Prev Chronic Dis* 11:130389, 2014.

44. Welk, GJ and Meredith, MD. Factors that influence physical fitness in children and adolescents. In *FITNESSGRAM/ACTIVITYGRAM Reference Guide*. Pangrazi, RP, and Corbin, CB, eds. Dallas: The Cooper Institute, 52-60, 2008.

Chapter 3 Musculoskeletal Conditions and Disorders

1. Airaksinen, O, Brox, JI, Cedraschi, C, Hildebrandt, J, Klaber-Moffett, J, Kovacs, F, Mannion, AF, Reis, S, Staal, JB, Ursin, H, and Zanoli, G. Chapter 4. European guidelines for the management of chronic nonspecific low back pain. *Eur Spine J* 15(suppl 2):S192-S300, 2006.

2. Allen, GJ, Hartl, TL, Duffany, S, Smith, SF, VanHeest, JL, Anderson, JM, Hoffman, JR, Kraemer, WJ, and Maresh, CM. Cognitive and motor function after administration of hydrocodone bitartrate plus ibuprofen, ibuprofen alone, or placebo in healthy subjects with exercise-induced muscle damage: a randomized, repeated-dose, placebo-controlled study. *Psychopharmacology (Berl)* 166:228-233, 2003.

3. Altman, RD and Barthel, HR. Topical therapies for osteoarthritis. *Drugs* 71:1259-1279, 2011.

4. American Academy of Orthopaedic Surgeons. Elbow Dislocation. 2007. http://orthoinfo.aaos.org/topic.cfm?topic=A00029. Accessed January 6, 2017.

5. American Academy of Orthopaedic Surgeons. Osteoarthritis. 2007. http://orthoinfo.aaos.org/topic.cfm?topic=a00227. Accessed April 25, 2015.

6. American Academy of Orthopaedic Surgeons. Foot and Ankle Conditioning Program. 2012. http://orthoinfo.aaos.org/topic.cfm?topic=A00667. Accessed January 6, 2017.

7. American Academy of Orthopaedic Surgeons. Rotator Cuff and Shoulder Conditioning Program. 2012. http://orthoinfo.aaos.org/topic.cfm?topic=A00663. Accessed January 6, 2017.

8. American Academy of Orthopaedic Surgeons and American Orthopaedic Foot and Ankle Society. Sprained Ankle. 2012. http://orthoinfo.aaos.org/topic.cfm?topic=a00150. Accessed January 6, 2017.

9. American College of Rheumatology Subcommittee on Osteoarthritis. Recommendations for the medical management of osteoarthritis of the hip and knee: 2000 update. *Arthritis Rheum* 43:1905-1915, 2000.

10. American Geriatrics Society Panel on Exercise and Osteoarthritis. Exercise prescription for older adults with osteoarthritis pain: consensus practice recommendations. A supplement to the AGS Clinical Practice Guidelines on the management of chronic pain in older adults. *J Am Geriatr Soc* 49:808-823, 2001.

11. Anwer, S and Alghadir, A. Effect of isometric quadriceps exercise on muscle strength, pain, and function in patients with knee osteoarthritis: a randomized controlled study. *J Phys Ther Sci* 26:745-748, 2014.

12. Balady, G, Berra, K, Goldling, L, Gordon, N, Mahler, D, Myers, J, and Sheldahl, L. General principles of exercise prescription. In *ACSM's Guidelines for Exercise Testing and Prescription*. Franklin, B, Whaley, M, Howley, E, and Balady, G, eds. Philadelphia: Lippincott Williams & Wilkins, 137-164, 2000.

13. Bansal, S, Katzman, WB, and Giangregorio, LM. Exercise for improving age-related hyperkyphotic posture: a systematic review. *Arch Phys Med Rehabil* 95:129-140, 2014.

14. Bayles, C, Chan, S, and Robare, J. Frailty. In *ACSM's Exercise Management for Persons With Chronic Diseases and Disabilities*. Durstine, J, Moore, G, Painter, P, and Roberts, S, eds. Champaign, IL: Human Kinetics, 201-208, 2009.

15. Bean, JF, Leveille, SG, Kiely, DK, Bandinelli, S, Guralnik, JM, and Ferrucci, L. A comparison of leg power and leg strength within the InCHIANTI study: which influences mobility more? *J Gerontol A Biol Sci Med Sci* 58:728-733, 2003.

16. Beaudart, C, Rizzoli, R, Bruyere, O, Reginster, JY, and Biver, E. Sarcopenia: burden and challenges for public health. *Arch Public Health* 72:45, 2014.

17. Been, E and Kalichman, L. Lumbar lordosis. *Spine J* 14:87-97, 2014.

18. Blume, SW and Curtis, JR. Medical costs of osteoporosis in the elderly Medicare population. *Osteoporos Int* 22:1835-1844, 2011.

19. Boachie-Adjei, O and Lonner, B. Spinal deformity. *Pediatr Clin North Am* 43:883-897, 1996.

20. Bolton, KL, Egerton, T, Wark, J, Wee, E, Matthews, B, Kelly, A, Craven, R, Kantor, S, and Bennell, KL. Effects of exercise on bone density and falls risk factors in post-menopausal women with osteopenia: a randomised controlled trial. *J Sci Med Sport* 15:102-109, 2012.

21. Brandi, ML and Black, D. A drinkable formulation of alendronate: potential to increase compliance and decrease upper GI irritation. *Clin Cases Miner Bone Metab* 10:187-190, 2013.

22. Britnell, SJ, Cole, JV, Isherwood, L, Sran, MM, Britnell, N, Burgi, S, Candido, G, and Watson, L. Postural health in women: the role of physiotherapy. *J Obstet Gynaecol Can* 27:493-510, 2005.

23. Bruce, SA, Newton, D, and Woledge, RC. Effect of age on voluntary force and cross-sectional area of human adductor pollicis muscle. *Q J Exp Physiol* 74:359-362, 1989.

24. Buckinx, F, Rolland, Y, Reginster, JY, Ricour, C, Petermans, J, and Bruyere, O. Burden of frailty in the elderly population: perspectives for a public health challenge. *Arch Public Health* 73:19, 2015.

25. Buckwalter, JA, Saltzman, C, and Brown, T. The impact of osteoarthritis: implications for research. *Clin Orthop Relat Res*:S6-S15, 2004.

26. Burton, LA and Sumukadas, D. Optimal management of sarcopenia. *Clin Interv Aging* 5:217-228, 2010.

27. Cameron, M and Chrubasik, S. Topical herbal therapies for treating osteoarthritis. *Cochrane Database Syst Rev* 5:CD010538, 2013.

28. Carvalho, J, Marques, E, Soares, JM, and Mota, J. Isokinetic strength benefits after 24 weeks of multicomponent exercise training and combined exercise training in older adults. *Aging Clin Exp Res* 22:63-69, 2010.

29. Centers for Disease Control and Prevention. Public health and aging: trends in aging--United States and worldwide. *JAMA* 289:1371-1373, 2003.

30. Chau, DL, Walker, V, Pai, L, and Cho, LM. Opiates and elderly: use and side effects. *Clin Interv Aging* 3:273-278, 2008.

31. Chen, CY, Wu, SC, Chen, LJ, and Lue, BH. The prevalence of subjective frailty and factors associated with frailty in Taiwan. *Arch Gerontol Geriatr* 50(suppl 1):S43-S47, 2010.

32. Chesnut, CH, 3rd, Silverman, S, Andriano, K, Genant, H, Gimona, A, Harris, S, Kiel, D, LeBoff, M, Maricic, M, Miller, P, Moniz, C, Peacock, M, Richardson, P, Watts, N, and Baylink, D. A randomized trial of nasal spray salmon calcitonin in postmenopausal women with established osteoporosis: the prevent recurrence of osteoporotic fractures study. PROOF Study Group. *Am J Med* 109:267-276, 2000.

33. Chin, A, Paw, MJ, van Uffelen, JG, Riphagen, I, and van Mechelen, W. The functional effects of physical exercise training in frail older people: a systematic review. *Sports Med* 38:781-793, 2008.

34. Chou, CH, Hwang, CL, and Wu, YT. Effect of exercise on physical function, daily living activities, and quality of life in the frail older adults: a meta-analysis. *Arch Phys Med Rehabil* 93:237-244, 2012.

35. Clarke, BL and Khosla, S. Physiology of bone loss. *Radiol Clin North Am* 48:483-495, 2010.

36. Clegg, A, Young, J, Iliffe, S, Rikkert, MO, and Rockwood, K. Frailty in elderly people. *Lancet* 381:752-762, 2013.

37. Cooper, R, Naclerio, F, Allgrove, J, and Jimenez, A. Creatine supplementation with specific view to exercise/sports performance: an update. *J Int Soc Sports Nutr* 9:33, 2012.

38. Cosman, F, De Beur, SJ, LeBoff, MS, Lewiecki, EM, Tanner, B, Randall, S, and Lindsay, R. Clinician's guide to prevention and treatment of osteoporosis. *Osteoporos Int* 25:2359-2381, 2014.

39. Culham, EG, Jimenez, HA, and King, CE. Thoracic kyphosis, rib mobility, and lung volumes in normal women and women with osteoporosis. *Spine* 19:1250-1255, 1994.

40. Dagenais, S, Caro, J, and Haldeman, S. A systematic review of low back pain cost of illness studies in the United States and internationally. *Spine J* 8:8-20, 2008.

41. Delmonico, MJ, Kostek, MC, Doldo, NA, Hand, BD, Bailey, JA, Rabon-Stith, KM, Conway, JM, Carignan, CR, Lang, J, and Hurley, BF. Effects of moderate-velocity strength training on peak muscle power and movement velocity: do women respond differently than men? *J Appl Physiol (1985)* 99:1712-1718, 2005.

42. Dent, E, Chapman, I, Howell, S, Piantadosi, C, and Visvanathan, R. Frailty and functional decline indices predict poor outcomes in hospitalised older people. *Age Ageing* 43:477-484, 2014.

43. Di Iorio, A, Abate, M, Di Renzo, D, Russolillo, A, Battaglini, C, Ripari, P, Saggini, R, Paganelli, R, and Abate, G. Sarcopenia: age-related skeletal muscle changes from determinants to physical disability. *Int J Immunopathol Pharmacol* 19:703-719, 2006.

44. Dickinson, JM, Volpi, E, and Rasmussen, BB. Exercise and nutrition to target protein synthesis impairments in aging skeletal muscle. *Exerc Sport Sci Rev* 41:216-223, 2013.

45. Docking, RE, Fleming, J, Brayne, C, Zhao, J, Macfarlane, GJ, and Jones, GT. Epidemiology of back pain in older adults: prevalence and risk factors for back pain onset. *Rheumatology (Oxford)* 50:1645-1653, 2011.

46. Doherty, C, Delahunt, E, Caulfield, B, Hertel, J, Ryan, J, and Bleakley, C. The incidence and prevalence of ankle sprain injury: a systematic review and meta-analysis of prospective epidemiological studies. *Sports Med* 44:123-140, 2014.

47. Edmond, SL, Kiel, DP, Samelson, EJ, Kelly-Hayes, M, and Felson, DT. Vertebral deformity, back symptoms, and functional limitations among older women: the Framingham Study. *Osteoporos Int* 16:1086-1095, 2005.

48. Erickson, JM and Messer, TM. Glucosamine and chondroitin sulfate treatment of hand osteoarthritis. *J Hand Surg Am* 38:1638-1640, 2013.

49. Evans, WJ. Protein nutrition, exercise and aging. *J Am Coll Nutr* 23:601S-609S, 2004.

50. Evans, WJ and Campbell, WW. Sarcopenia and age-related changes in body composition and functional capacity. *J Nutr* 123:465-468, 1993.

51. Fairhall, N, Langron, C, Sherrington, C, Lord, SR, Kurrle, SE, Lockwood, K, Monaghan, N, Aggar, C, Gill, L, and Cameron, ID. Treating frailty--a practical guide. *BMC Med* 9:83, 2011.

52. Fiatarone, MA, Marks, EC, Ryan, ND, Meredith, CN, Lipsitz, LA, and Evans, WJ. High-intensity strength training in nonagenarians. Effects on skeletal muscle. *JAMA* 263:3029-3034, 1990.

53. Fielding, RA, Vellas, B, Evans, WJ, Bhasin, S, Morley, JE, Newman, AB, Abellan van Kan, G, Andrieu, S, Bauer, J, Breuille, D, Cederholm, T, Chandler, J, De Meynard, C, Donini, L, Harris, T, Kannt, A, Keime Guibert, F, Onder, G, Papanicolaou, D, Rolland, Y, Rooks, D, Sieber, C, Souhami, E, Verlaan, S, and Zamboni, M. Sarcopenia: an undiagnosed condition in older adults. Current consensus definition: prevalence, etiology, and consequences. International Working Group on Sarcopenia. *J Am Med Dir Assoc* 12:249-256, 2011.

54. Frankel, JE, Bean, JF, and Frontera, WR. Exercise in the elderly: research and clinical practice. *Clin Geriatr Med* 22:239-256; vii, 2006.

55. Franko, J, Kish, KJ, O'Connell, BG, Subramanian, S, and Yuschak, JV. Advanced age and preinjury warfarin anticoagulation increase the risk of mortality after head trauma. *J Trauma* 61:107-110, 2006.

56. Frontera, WR, Hughes, VA, Fielding, RA, Fiatarone, MA, Evans, WJ, and Roubenoff, R. Aging of skeletal muscle: a 12-yr longitudinal study. *J Appl Physiol (1985)* 88:1321-1326, 2000.

57. Fusco, C, Zaina, F, Atanasio, S, Romano, M, Negrini, A, and Negrini, S. Physical exercises in the treatment of adolescent idiopathic scoliosis: an updated systematic review. *Physiother Theory Pract* 27:80-114, 2011.

58. Garcia-Garcia, FJ, Carcaillon, L, Fernandez-Tresguerres, J, Alfaro, A, Larrion, JL, Castillo, C, and Rodriguez-Manas, L. A new operational definition of frailty: the Frailty Trait Scale. *J Am Med Dir Assoc* 15:e7-e371, 2014.

59. Geerts, WH, Bergqvist, D, Pineo, GF, Heit, JA, Samama, CM, Lassen, MR, and Colwell, CW. Prevention of venous thromboembolism: American College of Chest Physicians Evidence-Based Clinical Practice Guidelines (8th Edition). *Chest* 133:381S-453S, 2008.

60. Griggs, RC, Kingston, W, Jozefowicz, RF, Herr, BE, Forbes, G, and Halliday, D. Effect of testosterone on muscle mass and muscle protein synthesis. *J Appl Physiol (1985)* 66:498-503, 1989.

61. Grinspoon, S, Friedman, A, Miller, K, Lippman, J, Olson, W, and Warren, M. Effects of a triphasic combination oral contraceptive containing norgestimate/ethinyl estradiol on biochemical markers of bone metabolism in young women with osteopenia secondary to hypothalamic amenorrhea. *J Clin Endocrinol Metab* 88:3651-3656, 2003.

62. Harman, SM, Metter, EJ, Tobin, JD, Pearson, J, and Blackman, MR. Longitudinal effects of aging on serum total and free testosterone levels in healthy men. Baltimore Longitudinal Study of Aging. *J Clin Endocrinol Metab* 86:724-731, 2001.

63. Helmick, C and Watkins-Castillo, S. United States Bone and Joint Initiative: The Burden of Musculoskeletal Diseases in the United States (BMUS). 2014. www.boneandjointburden.org. Accessed May 25, 2015.

64. Henrotin, Y, Marty, M, and Mobasheri, A. What is the current status of chondroitin sulfate and glucosamine for the treatment of knee osteoarthritis? *Maturitas* 78:184-187, 2014.

65. Hochberg, MC, Altman, RD, April, KT, Benkhalti, M, Guyatt, G, McGowan, J, Towheed, T, Welch, V, Wells, G, and Tugwell, P. American College of Rheumatology 2012 recommendations for the use of nonpharmacologic and pharmacologic therapies in osteoarthritis of the hand, hip, and knee. *Arthritis Care Res (Hoboken)* 64:465-474, 2012.

66. Hoy, D, Bain, C, Williams, G, March, L, Brooks, P, Blyth, F, Woolf, A, Vos, T, and Buchbinder, R. A systematic review of the global prevalence of low back pain. *Arthritis Rheum* 64:2028-2037, 2012.

67. Hruda, KV, Hicks, AL, and McCartney, N. Training for muscle power in older adults: effects on functional abilities. *Can J Appl Physiol* 28:178-189, 2003.

68. Hubbard, RE, O'Mahony, MS, and Woodhouse, KW. Medication prescribing in frail older people. *Eur J Clin Pharmacol* 69:319-326, 2013.

69. Inouye, SK, Studenski, S, Tinetti, ME, and Kuchel, GA. Geriatric syndromes: clinical, research, and policy implications of a core geriatric concept. *J Am Geriatr Soc* 55:780-791, 2007.

70. Janssen, I, Shepard, DS, Katzmarzyk, PT, and Roubenoff, R. The healthcare costs of sarcopenia in the United States. *J Am Geriatr Soc* 52:80-85, 2004.

71. Jimbo, S, Kobayashi, T, Aono, K, Atsuta, Y, and Matsuno, T. Epidemiology of degenerative lumbar scoliosis: a community-based cohort study. *Spine* 37:1763-1770, 2012.

72. Jordan, JM, Helmick, CG, Renner, JB, Luta, G, Dragomir, AD, Woodard, J, Fang, F, Schwartz, TA, Abbate, LM, Callahan, LF, Kalsbeek, WD, and Hochberg, MC. Prevalence of knee symptoms and radiographic and symptomatic knee osteoarthritis in African Americans and Caucasians: the Johnston County Osteoarthritis Project. *J Rheumatol* 34:172-180, 2007.

73. Kanis, JA and McCloskey, EV. Risk factors in osteoporosis. *Maturitas* 30:229-233, 1998.

74. Kim, Y, Park, J, Lee, J, Kim, J, Yang, S, Jeon, D, Kim, M, Jeong, T, Lee, Y, and Rhee, B. Prevalence and risk factors of the osteoporosis of perimenopausal women in the community population. *Hanguk Uiyak* 62:11-24, 2002.

75. Klibanski, A, Adams-Campbell, L, Bassford, TL, Blair, SN, Boden, SD, Dickersin, K, Gifford, DR, Glasse, L, Goldring, SR, Hruska, K, and Johnson, SR. Osteoporosis prevention, diagnosis, and therapy. *JAMA* 285:785-795, 2001.

76. Knight, JA. Physical inactivity: associated diseases and disorders. *Ann Clin Lab Sci* 42:320-337, 2012.

77. Kralinger, FS, Golser, K, Wischatta, R, Wambacher, M, and Sperner, G. Predicting recurrence after primary anterior shoulder dislocation. *Am J Sports Med* 30:116-120, 2002.

78. Krishnan, GM and Thompson, PD. The effects of statins on skeletal muscle strength and exercise performance. *Curr Opin Lipidol* 21:324-328, 2010.

79. Kritz, M and Cronin, J. Static posture assessment screen of athletes: benefits and considerations. *Strength Cond J* 30:18-27, 2008.

80. Lamberts, SW, van den Beld, AW, and van der Lely, AJ. The endocrinology of aging. *Science* 278:419-424, 1997.

81. Latham, N and Liu, CJ. Strength training in older adults: the benefits for osteoarthritis. *Clin Geriatr Med* 26:445-459, 2010.

82. Lawrence, RC, Felson, DT, Helmick, CG, Arnold, LM, Choi, H, Deyo, RA, Gabriel, S, Hirsch, R, Hochberg, MC, Hunder, GG, Jordan, JM, Katz, JN, Kremers, HM, and Wolfe, F. Estimates of the prevalence of arthritis and other rheumatic conditions in the United States. Part II. *Arthritis Rheum* 58:26-35, 2008.

83. Lexell, J. Human aging, muscle mass, and fiber type composition. *J Gerontol A Biol Sci Med Sci* 50 Spec No:11-16, 1995.

84. Lisse, JR, MacDonald, K, Thurmond-Anderle, ME, and Fuchs, JE, Jr. A double-blind, placebo-controlled study of acetylsalicylic acid (ASA) in trained runners. *J Sports Med Phys Fitness* 31:561-564, 1991.

85. Litwic, A, Edwards, MH, Dennison, EM, and Cooper, C. Epidemiology and burden of osteoarthritis. *Br Med Bull* 105:185-199, 2013.

86. Liu, H, Bravata, DM, Olkin, I, Friedlander, A, Liu, V, Roberts, B, Bendavid, E, Saynina, O, Salpeter, SR, Garber, AM, and Hoffman, AR. Systematic review: the effects of growth hormone on athletic performance. *Ann Intern Med* 148:747-758, 2008.

87. Macaluso, A and De Vito, G. Muscle strength, power and adaptations to resistance training in older people. *Eur J Appl Physiol* 91:450-472, 2004.

88. Macfarlane, GJ, Beasley, M, Jones, EA, Prescott, GJ, Docking, R, Keeley, P, McBeth, J, and Jones, GT. The prevalence and management of low back pain across adulthood: results from a population-based cross-sectional study (the MUSICIAN study). *Pain* 153:27-32, 2012.

89. Maggio, M, Lauretani, F, and Ceda, GP. Sex hormones and sarcopenia in older persons. *Curr Opin Clin Nutr Metab Care* 16:3-13, 2013.

90. Malmstrom, TK, Miller, DK, and Morley, JE. A comparison of four frailty models. *J Am Geriatr Soc* 62:721-726, 2014.

91. Manson, JE, Chlebowski, RT, Stefanick, ML, Aragaki, AK, Rossouw, JE, Prentice, RL, Anderson, G, Howard, BV, Thomson, CA, LaCroix, AZ, Wactawski-Wende, J, Jackson, RD, Limacher, M, Margolis, KL, Wassertheil-Smoller, S, Beresford, SA, Cauley, JA, Eaton, CB, Gass, M, Hsia, J, Johnson, KC, Kooperberg, C, Kuller, LH, Lewis, CE, Liu, S, Martin, LW, Ockene, JK, O'Sullivan, MJ, Powell, LH, Simon, MS, Van Horn, L, Vitolins, MZ, and Wallace, RB. Menopausal hormone therapy and health outcomes during the intervention and extended poststopping phases of the Women's Health Initiative randomized trials. *JAMA* 310:1353-1368, 2013.

92. Marsh, AP, Miller, ME, Saikin, AM, Rejeski, WJ, Hu, N, Lauretani, F, Bandinelli, S, Guralnik, JM, and Ferrucci, L. Lower extremity strength and power are associated with 400-meter walk time in older adults: the InCHIANTI study. *J Gerontol A Biol Sci Med Sci* 61:1186-1193, 2006.

93. Martin, RL, Davenport, TE, Paulseth, S, Wukich, DK, and Godges, JJ. Ankle stability and movement coordination impairments: ankle ligament sprains. *J Orthop Sports Phys Ther* 43:A1-A40, 2013.

94. Mathews, AE, Laditka, SB, Laditka, JN, Wilcox, S, Corwin, SJ, Liu, R, Friedman, DB, Hunter, R, Tseng, W, and Logsdon, RG. Older adults' perceived physical activity enablers and barriers: a multicultural perspective. *J Aging Phys Act* 18:119-140, 2010.

95. Mayer, F and Dickhuth, H. FIMS Position Statement: Physical activity after total joint replacement. *Int SportMed J* 9:39-43, 2008.

96. Mayer, F, Scharhag-Rosenberger, F, Carlsohn, A, Cassel, M, Muller, S, and Scharhag, J. The intensity and effects of strength training in the elderly. *Dtsch Arztebl Int* 108:359-364, 2011.

97. Mentes, J. Oral hydration in older adults: greater awareness is needed in preventing, recognizing, and treating dehydration. *Am J Nurs* 106:40-49; quiz 50, 2006.

98. Metter, EJ, Conwit, R, Tobin, J, and Fozard, JL. Age-associated loss of power and strength in the upper extremities in women and men. *J Gerontol A Biol Sci Med Sci* 52:B267-B276, 1997.

99. Metter, EJ, Talbot, LA, Schrager, M, and Conwit, R. Skeletal muscle strength as a predictor of all-cause mortality in healthy men. *J Gerontol A Biol Sci Med Sci* 57:B359-B365, 2002.

100. Moreira, LD, Oliveira, ML, Lirani-Galvao, AP, Marin-Mio, RV, Santos, RN, and Lazaretti-Castro, M. Physical exercise and osteoporosis: effects of different types of exercises on bone and physical function of postmenopausal women. *Arq Bras Endocrinol Metabol* 58:514-522, 2014.

101. Mosti, MP, Carlsen, T, Aas, E, Hoff, J, Stunes, AK, and Syversen, U. Maximal strength training improves bone mineral density and neuromuscular performance in young adult women. *J Strength Cond Res* 28:2935-2945, 2014.

102. Mosti, MP, Kaehler, N, Stunes, AK, Hoff, J, and Syversen, U. Maximal strength training in postmenopausal women with osteoporosis or osteopenia. *J Strength Cond Res* 27:2879-2886, 2013.

103. Murphy, L and Helmick, CG. The impact of osteoarthritis in the United States: a population-health perspective: a population-based review of the fourth most common cause of hospitalization in U.S. adults. *Orthop Nurs* 31:85-91, 2012.

104. National Scoliosis Foundation. Scoliosis Information and Support. 2007. www.scoliosis.org/info.php. Accessed October 16, 2016.

105. National Strength and Conditioning Association. *Essentials of Strength Training and Conditioning.* 4th ed. Champaign, IL: Human Kinetics, 2016.

106. Neogi, T and Zhang, Y. Epidemiology of osteoarthritis. *Rheum Dis Clin North Am* 39:1-19, 2013.

107. Newman, AB, Lee, JS, Visser, M, Goodpaster, BH, Kritchevsky, SB, Tylavsky, FA, Nevitt, M, and Harris, TB. Weight change and the conservation of lean mass in old age: the Health, Aging and Body Composition Study. *Am J Clin Nutr* 82:872-878, 2005.

108. Nuesch, E, Dieppe, P, Reichenbach, S, Williams, S, Iff, S, and Juni, P. All cause and disease specific mortality in patients with knee or hip osteoarthritis: population based cohort study. *BMJ* 342:d1165, 2011.

109. O'Connell, MD and Wu, FC. Androgen effects on skeletal muscle: implications for the development and management of frailty. *Asian J Androl* 16:203-212, 2014.

110. Pahor, M, Guralnik, JM, Ambrosius, WT, Blair, S, Bonds, DE, Church, TS, Espeland, MA, Fielding, RA, Gill, TM, Groessl, EJ, King, AC, Kritchevsky, SB, Manini, TM, McDermott, MM, Miller, ME, Newman, AB, Rejeski, WJ, Sink, KM, and Williamson, JD. Effect of structured physical activity on prevention of major mobility disability in older adults: the LIFE study randomized clinical trial. *JAMA* 311:2387-2396, 2014.

111. Papageorgiou, AC, Croft, PR, Ferry, S, Jayson, MI, and Silman, AJ. Estimating the prevalence of low back pain in the general population. Evidence from the South Manchester Back Pain Survey. *Spine* 20:1889-1894, 1995.

112. Parise, G, Bosman, MJ, Boecker, DR, Barry, MJ, and Tarnopolsky, MA. Selective serotonin reuptake inhibitors: their effect on high-intensity exercise performance. *Arch Phys Med Rehabil* 82:867-871, 2001.

113. Percope de Andrade, M, Campos, T, and Abreu-E-Silva, G. Supplementary methods in the nonsurgical treatment of osteoarthritis. *Arthroscopy* 31:785-792, 2015.

114. Peterson, MD, Rhea, MR, and Alvar, BA. Applications of the dose-response for muscular strength development: a review of meta-analytic efficacy and reliability for designing training prescription. *J Strength Cond Res* 19:950-958, 2005.

115. Porter, MM. The effects of strength training on sarcopenia. *Can J Appl Physiol* 26:123-141, 2001.

116. Poudel, A, Hubbard, RE, Nissen, L, and Mitchell, C. Frailty: a key indicator to minimize inappropriate medication in older people. *QJM* 106:969-975, 2013.

117. Predel, HG, Rohden, C, Heine, O, Prinz, U, and Rost, RE. ACE inhibition and physical exercise: studies on physical work capacity, energy metabolism, and maximum oxygen uptake in well-trained, healthy subjects. *J Cardiovasc Pharmacol* 23(suppl 1):S25-S28, 1994.

118. Prieto-Alhambra, D, Judge, A, Javaid, MK, Cooper, C, Diez-Perez, A, and Arden, NK. Incidence and risk factors for clinically diagnosed knee, hip and hand osteoarthritis: influences of age, gender and osteoarthritis affecting other joints. *Ann Rheum Dis* 73:1659-1664, 2014.

119. Rahl, R. *Physical Activity and Health Guidelines: Recommendations for Various Ages, Fitness Levels, and Conditions From 57 Authoritative Sources.* Champaign, IL: Human Kinetics, 2010.

120. Rantanen, T, Guralnik, JM, Foley, D, Masaki, K, Leveille, S, Curb, JD, and White, L. Midlife hand grip strength as a predictor of old age disability. *JAMA* 281:558-560, 1999.

121. Riggs, BL. Endocrine causes of age-related bone loss and osteoporosis. *Novartis Found Symp* 242:247-259; discussion 260-264, 2002.

122. Riggs, BL, Khosla, S, and Melton, LJ, 3rd. Primary osteoporosis in men: role of sex steroid deficiency. *Mayo Clin Proc* 75(suppl):S46-S50, 2000.

123. Roddy, E, Zhang, W, Doherty, M, Arden, NK, Barlow, J, Birrell, F, Carr, A, Chakravarty, K, Dickson, J, Hay, E, Hosie, G, Hurley, M, Jordan, KM, McCarthy, C, McMurdo, M, Mockett, S, O'Reilly, S, Peat, G, Pendleton, A, and Richards, S. Evidence-based recommendations for the role of exercise in the management of osteoarthritis of the hip or knee--the MOVE consensus. *Rheumatology (Oxford)* 44:67-73, 2005.

124. Roghani, T, Torkaman, G, Movasseghe, S, Hedayati, M, Goosheh, B, and Bayat, N. Effects of short-term aerobic exercise with and without external loading on bone metabolism and balance in postmenopausal women with osteoporosis. *Rheumatol Int* 33:291-298, 2013.

125. Rosenberg, I. Summary comments. *Am J Clin Nutr* 50:1231-1233, 1989.

126. Rosenberg, IH. Sarcopenia: origins and clinical relevance. *Clin Geriatr Med* 27:337-339, 2011.

127. Roth, SM, Ferrell, RF, and Hurley, BF. Strength training for the prevention and treatment of sarcopenia. *J Nutr Health Aging* 4:143-155, 2000.

128. Roubenoff, R. Origins and clinical relevance of sarcopenia. *Can J Appl Physiol* 26:78-89, 2001.

129. Rudolf, R, Khan, MM, Labeit, S, and Deschenes, MR. Degeneration of neuromuscular junction in age and dystrophy. *Front Aging Neurosci* 6:99, 2014.

130. Sacks, JJ, Helmick, CG, and Langmaid, G. Deaths from arthritis and other rheumatic conditions, United States, 1979-1998. *J Rheumatol* 31:1823-1828, 2004.

131. Sarwark, JF and Kramer, A. Pediatric spinal deformity. *Curr Opin Pediatr* 10:82-86, 1998.

132. Sayer, AA, Robinson, SM, Patel, HP, Shavlakadze, T, Cooper, C, and Grounds, MD. New horizons in the pathogenesis, diagnosis and management of sarcopenia. *Age Ageing* 42:145-150, 2013.

133. Sayers, SP. High-speed power training: a novel approach to resistance training in older men and women. A brief review and pilot study. *J Strength Cond Res* 21:518-526, 2007.

134. Schindel, CS, Hommerding, PX, Melo, DA, Baptista, RR, Marostica, PJ, and Donadio, MV. Physical exercise recommendations improve postural changes found in

children and adolescents with cystic fibrosis: a randomized controlled trial. *J Pediatr* 166:710-716, 2015.

135. Schlosser, TP, Vincken, KL, Rogers, K, Castelein, RM, and Shah, SA. Natural sagittal spino-pelvic alignment in boys and girls before, at and after the adolescent growth spurt. *Eur Spine J* 24:1158-1167, 2015.

136. Schutzer, KA and Graves, BS. Barriers and motivations to exercise in older adults. *Prev Med* 39:1056-1061, 2004.

137. Seguin, R and Nelson, ME. The benefits of strength training for older adults. *Am J Prev Med* 25:141-149, 2003.

138. Seynnes, O, Fiatarone Singh, MA, Hue, O, Pras, P, Legros, P, and Bernard, PL. Physiological and functional responses to low-moderate versus high-intensity progressive resistance training in frail elders. *J Gerontol A Biol Sci Med Sci* 59:503-509, 2004.

139. Sherrington, C, Lord, SR, and Finch, CF. Physical activity interventions to prevent falls among older people: update of the evidence. *J Sci Med Sport* 7:43-51, 2004.

140. Simmonds, MJ. Exercise and activity for individuals with nonspecific back pain. In *ACSM's Resources for Clinical Exercise Physiology: Musculoskeletal, Neuromuscular, Neoplastic, Immunologic and Hematologic Conditions.* American College of Sports Medicine, ed. Philadelphia: Lippincott Williams & Wilkins, 148-161, 2010.

141. Simmonds, MJ and Derghazarian, T. Lower back pain syndrome. In *ACSM's Exercise Management for Persons with Chronic Diseases and Disabilities.* Durstine, JL, Moore, GE, Painter, PL, and Roberts, SO, eds. Champaign, IL: Human Kinetics, 266-269, 2009.

142. Simpson, MR. Benign joint hypermobility syndrome: evaluation, diagnosis, and management. *J Am Osteopath Assoc* 106:531-536, 2006.

143. Skelton, DA, Greig, CA, Davies, JM, and Young, A. Strength, power and related functional ability of healthy people aged 65-89 years. *Age Ageing* 23:371-377, 1994.

144. Skovron, ML, Szpalski, M, Nordin, M, Melot, C, and Cukier, D. Sociocultural factors and back pain. A population-based study in Belgian adults. *Spine* 19:129-137, 1994.

145. Smit, E, Winters-Stone, KM, Loprinzi, PD, Tang, AM, and Crespo, CJ. Lower nutritional status and higher food insufficiency in frail older US adults. *Br J Nutr* 110:172-178, 2013.

146. Smith, SS, Wang, CE, and Bloomfield, SA. Osteoporosis. In *ACSM's Exercise Management for Persons with Chronic Diseases and Disabilities.* Durstine, JL, Moore, GE, Painter, PL, and Roberts, SO, eds. Champaign, IL: Human Kinetics, 270-279, 2009.

147. Spector, TD and MacGregor, AJ. Risk factors for osteoarthritis: genetics. *Osteoarthritis Cartilage* 12(suppl A):S39-S44, 2004.

148. Stanos, SP and Galluzzi, KE. Topical therapies in the management of chronic pain. *Postgrad Med* 125:25-33, 2013.

149. Strand, V, McIntyre, LF, Beach, WR, Miller, LE, and Block, JE. Safety and efficacy of US-approved viscosupplements for knee osteoarthritis: a systematic review and meta-analysis of randomized, saline-controlled trials. *J Pain Res* 8:217-228, 2015.

150. Tesch, PA. Exercise performance and beta-blockade. *Sports Med* 2:389-412, 1985.

151. Thompson, BJ, Conchola, EC, Palmer, TB, and Stock, MS. Effects of aging on maximal and rapid velocity capacities of the leg extensors. *Exp Gerontol* 58:128-131, 2014.

152. Tocchi, C. Frailty in older adults: an evolutionary concept analysis. *Res Theory Nurs Pract* 29:66-84, 2015.

153. Trappe, TA, White, F, Lambert, CP, Cesar, D, Hellerstein, M, and Evans, WJ. Effect of ibuprofen and acetaminophen on postexercise muscle protein synthesis. *Am J Physiol Endocrinol Metab* 282:E551-E556, 2002.

154. Tsutsumi, T, Don, BM, Zaichkowsky, LD, and Delizonna, LL. Physical fitness and psychological benefits of strength training in community dwelling older adults. *Appl Human Sci* 16:257-266, 1997.

155. United States Surgeon General. In *Bone Health and Osteoporosis: A Report of the Surgeon General.* Rockville, MD: U.S. Department of Health and Human Services, Office of the Surgeon General, 2004.

156. U.S. Department of Health and Human Services. Physical Activity Guidelines for Americans. 2008. www.health.gov/paguidelines/guidelines. Accessed January 7, 2017.

157. van Tulder, M, Becker, A, Bekkering, T, Breen, A, del Real, MT, Hutchinson, A, Koes, B, Laerum, E, and Malmivaara, A. Chapter 3. European guidelines for the management of acute nonspecific low back pain in primary care. *Eur Spine J* 15(suppl 2):S169-S191, 2006.

158. Vandervoot, AA and Symons, TB. Functional and metabolic consequences of sarcopenia. *Can J Appl Physiol* 26:90-101, 2001.

159. Vincent, KR, Conrad, BP, Fregly, BJ, and Vincent, HK. The pathophysiology of osteoarthritis: a mechanical perspective on the knee joint. *PM R* 4:S3-S9, 2012.

160. Vogel, LA, Carotenuto, G, Basti, JJ, and Levine, WN. Physical activity after total joint arthroplasty. *Sports Health* 3:441-450, 2011.

161. Walsh, K, Cruddas, M, and Coggon, D. Low back pain in eight areas of Britain. *J Epidemiol Community Health* 46:227-230, 1992.

162. Waterman, BR, Owens, BD, Davey, S, Zacchilli, MA, and Belmont, PJ, Jr. The epidemiology of ankle sprains in the United States. *J Bone Joint Surg Am* 92:2279-2284, 2010.

163. Waters, DL, Baumgartner, RN, and Garry, PJ. Sarcopenia: current perspectives. *J Nutr Health Aging* 4:133-139, 2000.

164. Watts, NB, Lewiecki, EM, Miller, PD, and Baim, S. National Osteoporosis Foundation 2008 Clinician's Guide to Prevention and Treatment of Osteoporosis and the World Health Organization Fracture Risk Assessment Tool (FRAX): what they mean to the bone densitometrist and bone technologist. *J Clin Densitom* 11:473-477, 2008.

165. Weinstein, AM, Rome, BN, Reichmann, WM, Collins, JE, Burbine, SA, Thornhill, TS, Wright, J, Katz, JN, and Losina, E. Estimating the burden of total knee replacement in the United States. *J Bone Joint Surg Am* 95:385-392, 2013.

166. Weinstein, SL, Dolan, LA, Cheng, JC, Danielsson, A, and Morcuende, JA. Adolescent idiopathic scoliosis. *Lancet* 371:1527-1537, 2008.

167. Wilson, NA, Schneller, ES, Montgomery, K, and Bozic, KJ. Hip and knee implants: current trends and policy considerations. *Health Aff (Millwood)* 27:1587-1598, 2008.

168. Woo, J. Relationships among diet, physical activity and other lifestyle factors and debilitating diseases in the elderly. *Eur J Clin Nutr* 54(suppl 3):S143-S147, 2000.

169. Wright, NC, Looker, AC, Saag, KG, Curtis, JR, Delzell, ES, Randall, S, and Dawson-Hughes, B. The recent prevalence of osteoporosis and low bone mass in the United States based on bone mineral density at the femoral neck or lumbar spine. *J Bone Miner Res* 29:2520-2526, 2014.

170. Zacchilli, MA and Owens, BD. Epidemiology of shoulder dislocations presenting to emergency departments in the United States. *J Bone Joint Surg Am* 92:542-549, 2010.

171. Zaina, F, Donzelli, S, Lusini, M, Minnella, S, and Negrini, S. Swimming and spinal deformities: a cross-sectional study. *J Pediatr* 166:163-167, 2015.

172. Zhang, Y and Jordan, JM. Epidemiology of osteoarthritis. *Clin Geriatr Med* 26:355-369, 2010.

Chapter 4 Metabolic Conditions and Disorders

1. Akesson, A, Weismayer, P, Newby, P, and Wolk, A. Combined effect of low-risk dietary and lifestyle behaviors in primary prevention of myocardial infarction in women. *Arch Intern Med* 167:2122-2127, 2007.

2. Albuquerque, D, Stice, E, Rodríguez-López, R, Manco, L, and Nóbrega, C. Current review of genetics of human obesity: from molecular mechanisms to an evolutionary perspective. *Mol Genet Genomics* 290:1191-1221, 2015.

3. Altena, T, Michaelson, J, Ball, S, Guilford, B, and Thomas, T. Lipoprotein subfraction changes after continuous or intermittent exercise training. *Med Sci Sports Exerc* 38:367-372, 2006.

4. American College of Cardiology and American Heart Association Task Force on Practice Guidelines. Expert panel report: guidelines (2013) for the management of overweight and obesity in adults. *Obesity* 22:S41, 2014.

5. American College of Sports Medicine. *ACSM's Guidelines for Exercise Testing and Prescription*. 9th ed. Baltimore: Wolters Kluwer/Lippincott Williams & Wilkins, 2014.

6. American Diabetes Association. Insulin Basics. www.diabetes.org/living-with-diabetes/treatment-and-care/medication/insulin/insulin-basics.html. Accessed December 21, 2016.

7. American Diabetes Association. Diagnosis and classification of diabetes mellitus. *Diabetes Care* 35:S64-S71, 2012.

8. American Diabetes Association. Standards of medical care in diabetes—2016. *Diabetes Care* 35:S1-S112, 2016.

9. Anderson, J, Konz, E, Frederich, R, and Wood, C. Long-term weight-loss maintenance: a meta-analysis of U.S. studies. *Am J Clin Nutr* 74:579-584, 2001.

10. Arabshahi, S, Ibiebele, T, Hughes, M, Lahmann, P, Williams, G, and van der Pols, J. Dietary patterns and weight change: 15-year longitudinal study in Australian adults. *Eur J Nutr* 55:1-11, 2016.

11. Arnarson, A, Ramel, A, Geirsdottir, O, Jonsson, P, and Thorsdottir, I. Changes in body composition and use of blood cholesterol lowering drugs predict changes in blood lipids during 12 weeks of resistance exercise training in older adults. *Aging Clin Exp Res* 26:287-292, 2014.

12. Bacchi, E, Negri, C, Zanolin, M, Milanese, C, Faccioli, N, Trombetta, M, Zoppini, G, Ceyese, A, Bonadonna, R, Schena, F, Bonora, E, Lanza, M, and Meghetti, P. Metabolic effects of aerobic and resistance training in type 2 diabetic subjects. *Diabetes Care* 25:1729-1736, 2012.

13. Bally, L, Zueger, T, Buehler, T, Dokumaci, A, Speck, C, Pasi, N, Ciller, C, Paganini, D, Feller, K, Loher, H, and Rosset, R. Metabolic and hormonal response to intermittent high-intensity and continuous moderate intensity exercise in individuals with type 1 diabetes: a randomised crossover study. *Diabetologia* 59:776-784, 2016.

14. Bambs, C, Kip, K, Dinga, A, Mulukutla, S, Aiyer, A, and Reis, S. Low prevalence of "ideal cardiovascular health" in a community-based population. *Circulation* 2011:850-857, 2011.

15. Bansal, N. Prediabetes diagnosis and treatment: a review. *World J Diabetes* 6:296-303, 2015.

16. Bansal, S, Buring, J, Rifai, N, Mora, S, Sacks, F, and Ridker, R. Fasting compared with nonfasting triglycerides and risk of cardiovascular events. *JAMA* 298:309-316, 2007.

17. Barnard, R, Lattimore, L, Holly, R, Cherry, S, and Pritikin, N. Response of non-insulin dependent diabetes patients to an intensive program of diet and exercise. *Diabetes Care* 5:370-374, 1982.

18. Baskin, H, Cobin, R, Duick, D, Gharib, H, Guttler, R, Kaplan, M, and Segal, R. American Association

of Clinical Endocrinologists medical guidelines for clinical practice for the evaluation and treatment of hyperthyroidism and hypothyroidism. *Endocr Pract* 8:457-469, 2001.

19. Bellenir, K. *Basic Consumer Health Information About Type 1 Diabetes (Insulin-Dependent or Juvenile-Onset Diabetes), Type 2 Diabetes (Noninsulin-Dependent or Adult-Onset Diabetes), and Related Disorders (Health Reference Series)*. Omnigraphics, 1999.

20. Botero, J, Shiguemoto, G, Prestes, J, Marin, C, Do Prado, W, Pontes, C, Guerra, R, Ferreia, F, Baldissera, V, and Perez, S. Effects of long-term periodized resistance training on body composition, leptin, resistin and muscle strength in elderly post-menopausal women. *J Sports Med Phys Fitness* 53:289-294, 2013.

21. Bousquet-Santos, K, Vaisman, M, Barreto, N, Cruz-Filho, R, Salvador, B, Frontera, W, and Nobrega, A. Resistance training improves muscle function and body composition in patients with hyperthyroidism. *Arch Phys Med Rehabil* 87:1123-1130, 2006.

22. Brown, P. Why Did Afrezza Flop? www.medpageto-day.com/cardiology/type1diabetes/55663. Accessed December 21, 2016.

23. Budal, K, Mirzahosseini, A, Bela, N, and Toth, G. The pharmacotherapy of obesity. *Acta Pharm Hung* 85:3-17, 2015.

24. Buysschaert, M, Medina, J, Bergman, M, Shah, A, and Lonier, J. Prediabetes and associated disorders. *Endocrine* 48:371-393, 2015.

25. Calabro, P, Limongelli, G, Pacileo, G, Di Salvo, G, Golino, P, and Calabro, R. The role of adiposity as a determinant of an inflammatory milieu. *J Cardiovasc Med* 9:450-460, 2008.

26. Campaigne, B, Landt, K, Mellies, M, James, F, Glueck, C, and Sperling, M. The effects of physical training on blood lipid profiles in adolescents with insulin-dependent diabetes mellitus. *Phys Sportsmed* 13:83-89, 1985.

27. Carroll, M, Kit, B, Lacher, D, and Sung, S. Total and High-Density Lipoprotein Cholesterol in Adults: NHANES, 2011-2012. NCHS Data Brief No. 132, 2013.

28. Centers for Disease Control and Prevention. *National Diabetes Statistics Report: Estimates of Diabetes and Its Burden in the United States*. Atlanta: U.S. Department of Health and Human Services, 2014.

29. Chakera, A, Pearce, S, and Vaidya, B. Treatment for primary hypothyroidism: current approaches and future possibilities. *Drug Des Devel Ther* 6:1-11, 2012.

30. Chetty, V, Almulla, A, Odueyungbo, A, and Thabane, L. The effect of continuous subcutaneous glucose monitoring (CGMS) versus intermittent whole blood finger-stick glucose monitoring (SBGM) on hemoglobin A1c (HbA1c) levels in Type I diabetic patients: a systematic review. *Diabetes Res Clin Pract* 81:79-87, 2008.

31. Chiang, J, Kirkman, M, Laffel, L, and Peters, A. Type 1 diabetes through the life span: a position statement of the American Diabetes Association. *Diabetes Care* 37:2034-2054, 2014.

32. Chiuve, S, Rexrode, K, Speigelman, D, Logroscino, G, Manson, J, and Rimm, E. Primary prevention of stroke by healthy lifestyle. *Circulation* 118:947-954, 2008.

32a. Choquet, H and Meyre, D. Genetics of obesity: what have we learned? *Curr Genomics* 12:169-179, 2011.

33. Church, T, Blair, S, Cocreham, S, Johannsen, N, Johnson, W, Kramer, K, Mikus, C, Myers, V, Nauta, M, Rodarte, R, Sparks, L, Thompson, A, and Earnest, C. Effects of aerobic and resistance training on hemoglobin A1c levels in patients with type 2 diabetes. *JAMA* 304:2253-2262, 2010.

34. Clarke, T, Ward, B, Freeman, G, and Schiller, J. Early release of selected estimates based on data from the January-September 2015 National Health Interview Survey. National Center for Health Statistics. 2016. www.cdc.gov/nchs/nhis.htm. Accessed January 8, 2017.

35. Colberg, S. Diabetic Medications and Exercise, Part 2: Use of Symlin and Byetta. www.diabetesincontrol.com/diabetic-medications-and-exercise-part-2-use-of-symlin-and-byetta. Accessed December 7, 2016.

36. Colberg, S, Sigal, R, Fernhall, B, Regensteiner, J, Blissmer, B, Rubin, R, Chasan-Taber, L, Albright, A, and Braun, B. Exercise and type 2 diabetes: the American College of Sports Medicine and the American Diabetes Association joint position statement. *Diabetes Care* 33:e147-e167, 2010.

37. Colberg, S, Sigal, R, Yardley, J, Riddell, M, Dunstan, D, Dempsey, P, Horton, E, Castorino, K, and Tate, D. Physical activity/exercise and diabetes: a position statement of the American Diabetes Association. *Diabetes Care* 39:2065-2079, 2016.

38. Colditz, G, Willett, W, Rotnitzky, A, and Manson, J. Weight gain as a risk factor for clinical diabetes mellitus in women. *Ann Intern Med* 122:481-486, 1995.

39. Cuff, D, Menelly, G, Martin, A, Ignaszewski, A, Tildesley, H, and Frohlich, J. Effective exercise modality to reduce insulin resistance in women with type 2 diabetes. *Diabetes Care* 26:2977-2982, 2003.

40. Dabelea, D, Mayer-Davis, E, Saydah, S, Imperatore, G, Linder, B, Divers, J, Bell, R, Badaru, A, Talton, J, Crume, T, and Liese, A. Prevalence of type 1 and type 2 diabetes among children and adolescents from 2001 to 2009. *JAMA* 311:1778-1786, 2014.

41. Davidson, L, Hudson, R, Kilpatrick, K, Kuk, J, McMillan, K, Janiszewski, P, Lee, S, Lam, M, and Ross, R. Effects of exercise modality on insulin resistance and functional limitation in older adults: a randomized controlled study. *Arch Intern Med* 169:122-131, 2009.

42. Delbridge, E and Proietto, J. State of the science: VLED (very low energy diet) for obesity. *Asia Pac J Clin Nutr* 15:49-54, 2006.

43. Demers, L and Spencer, C. Laboratory medicine practice guidelines: laboratory support for the diagnosis and monitoring of thyroid disease. *Thyroid* 13:3-126, 2003.

44. Denke, M. Dietary prescriptions to control dyslipidemias. *Circulation* 105:132-135, 2002.

45. Despres, J, Lemieux, I, Bergeron, J, Pibarot, P, Mathieu, P, Larose, E, Rodés-Cabau, J, Bertrand, O, and Poirier, P. Abdominal obesity and the metabolic syndrome and contribution to global cardiometabolic risk. *Arterioscler Thromb Vasc Biol* 28:1039-1049, 2008.

46. Diabetes Prevention Program Research Group. 10-year follow-up of diabetes incidence and weight loss in the Diabetes Prevention Program Outcomes Study. *Lancet* 374:1677-1686, 2009.

47. Dimitropoulos, G, Tahrani, A, and Stevens, M. Cardiac autonomic neuropathy in patients with diabetes mellitus. *World J Diabetes* 5:17-39, 2014.

48. Donnelly, JE, Blair, SN, Jakicic, JM, Manore, MM, Rankin, JW, and Smith, BK. Appropriate physical activity intervention strategies for weight loss and prevention of weight regain for adults. *Med Sci Sports Exerc* 41:459-471, 2009.

49. Drugs.com. Medications for Diabetes, Type 1. www.drugs.com/condition/diabetes-mellitus-type-i.html. Accessed December 7, 2016.

50. Drugs.com. Medications for Diabetes, Type 2. www.drugs.com/condition/diabetes-mellitus-type-ii.html. Accessed December 1, 2016.

51. Drugs.com. Medications for High Cholesterol. www.drugs.com/condition/hyperlipidemia.html. Accessed December 1, 2016.

52. Drugs.com. Medications for Hyperthyroidism. www.drugs.com/condition/hyperthyroidism.html. Accessed December 1, 2016.

53. Drugs.com. Medications for Obesity. www.drugs.com/condition/obesity.html. Accessed December 1, 2016.

54. Drugs.com. Medications for Underactive Thyroid (Hypothyroidism). www.drugs.com/condition/hypothyroidism.html. Accessed December 1, 2016.

55. Dubé, M, Lavoie, C, and Weisnagel, S. Glucose or intermittent high-intensity exercise in glargine/glulisine users with T1DM. *Med Sci Sports Exerc* 45:3-7, 2013.

56. Durstine, J, Moore, G, and Polk, D. Hyperlipidemia. In *ACSM's Exercise Management for Persons with Chronic Diseases and Disabilities*. 3rd ed. Durstine, J, Moore, G, Painter, P, and Roberts, S, eds. Champaign, IL: Human Kinetics, 167-174, 2009.

57. Dyck, D. Leptin sensitivity in skeletal muscle is modulated by diet and exercise. *Exerc Sport Sci Rev* 33:189-194, 2005.

58. Ebbeling, C, Swain, J, Feldman, H, Wong, W, Hachey, D, Garcia-Lago, E, and Ludwig, D. Effects of dietary composition on energy expenditure during weight-loss maintenance. *JAMA* 307:2627-2634, 2012.

59. Eberhardt, M, Ogden, C, Engelgau, M, Cadwell, B, Hedley, A, and Saydah, S. Prevalence of overweight and obesity among adults with diagnosed diabetes—United States, 1988-1994 and 1999-2002. *MMWR* 53:1066-1068, 2004.

60. Eckel, R, Jakicic, J, Ard, J, De Jesus, J, Miller, N, Hubbard, V, I-Min, L, Lichtenstein, A, Loria, C, Millen, B, Nonas, C, Sacks, F, Smith, S, Jr, Svetkey, L, Wadden, T, and Yanovski, S. 2013 AHA/ACC guideline on lifestyle management to reduce cardiovascular risk: a report of the American College of Cardiology/American Heart Association Task Force on Practice Guidelines. *J Am Coll Cardiol* 63, 3027-3028, 2014.

61. Ekblom-Bak, E, Ekblom, B, Vikström, M, de Faire, U, and Hellénius, M. The importance of non-exercise physical activity for cardiovascular health and longevity. *Br J Sports Med* 48:233-238, 2014.

62. Ertek, S and Cicero, A. Hyperthyroidism and cardiovascular complications: a narrative review on the basis of pathophysiology. *Arch Med Sci* 9:944-952, 2013.

63. Feingold, K and Grunfeld, C. Diabetes and dyslipidemia. In Endotext [Internet]. De Groot, LJ, Chrousos, G, Dungan, K, Grossman, A, Hershman, JM, McLachlan, R, New, M, Rebar, R, Singer, F, Vinik, A, and Weickart, MO, eds. South Dartmouth, MA: MDTextcom, 2015. www.ncbi.nlm.nih.gov/books/NBK305900.

64. Fock, K and Khoo, J. Diet and exercise in the management of obesity and overweight. *J Gastroenterol Hepatol* 28:59-63, 2013.

65. Ford, E, Bergmann, M, Kroger, J, Schienkiewitz, A, Weikert, C, and Boeing, H. Healthy living is the best revenge: findings from the European Prospective Investigation Into Cancer and Nutrition-Potsdam Study. *Arch Intern Med* 169:1355-1362, 2009.

66. Ford, E, Li, C, Zhao, G, Pearson, W, and Capewell, S. Trends in the prevalence of low risk factor burden for cardiovascular disease among United States adults. *Circulation* 120:1181-1188, 2009.

67. Ford, E, Li, C, Zhao, G, Pearson, W, and Mokdad, A. Hypertriglyceridemia and its pharmacologic treatment among U.S. adults. *Arch Intern Med* 169:572-578, 2009.

68. Foster-Schubert, K, Alfano, C, Duggan, C, Xiao, L, Campbell, K, Kong, A, Bain, C, Wang, C, Blacburn, G, and McTiernan, A. Effect of diet and exercise, alone or combined, on weight and body composition in overweight-to-obese postmenopausal women. *Obesity* 20:1628-1638, 2012.

69. Frigolet, M, Ramos Barragán, V, and Tamez Gonzalez, M. Low-carbohydrate diets: a matter of love or hate. *Ann Nutr Metab* 58:320-334, 2011.

70. Ganga, H, Sim, H, and Thompson, P. A systematic review of statin-induced muscle problems in clinical trials. *Am Heart J* 168:6-15, 2014.

71. Gardner, C. Glimmers of light: new clues to weight gain and loss. *Nutrition Action Health Letter* December:1-6, 2013.

72. Garg, S, Zisser, H, Schwartz, S, Bailey, T, Kaplan, R, Ellis, S, and Jovanovic, L. Improvement in glycemic excursions with a transcutaneous, real-time continuous glucose sensor: a randomized controlled trial. *Diabetes Care* 29:44-50, 2006.

73. George, E, Rosenkranz, R, and Kolt, G. Chronic disease and sitting time in middle-aged Australian males: findings from the 45 and Up Study. *Int J Behav Nutr Phys Act* 10:10-20, 2013.

74. Ghandehari, H, Kamai-Bahi, K, and Wong, N. Prevalence and extent of dyslipidemia and recommended lipid levels in U.S. adults with and without cardiovascular comorbidities: the National Health and Nutrition Examination Survey 2003-2004. *Am Heart J* 156:112-119, 2008.

75. Go, A, Mozaffarian, D, Roger, V, Benjamin, E, Berry, J, Blaha, M, Dai, S, Ford, E, Fox, C, Franco, S, and Fullerton, H. AHA statistical update. *Circulation* 127:e62-e245, 2013.

76. Goodman, C and Helgeson, K. *Exercise Prescription for Medical Conditions: Handbook for Physical Therapists.* Philadelphia: Davis, 2010.

77. Grøntved, A, Pan, A, Mekary, R, Stampfer, M, Willett, W, Manson, J, and Hu, F. Muscle-strengthening and conditioning activities and risk of type 2 diabetes: a prospective study in two cohorts of U.S. women. *PLoS Med* 11:e1001587, 2014.

78. Grundy, S, Smith, H, Eckel, R, Redberg, R, and Bonow, R. Prevention Conference VI: Diabetes and cardiovascular disease: executive summary. *Circulation* 105:2231-2239, 2002.

79. Guelfi, K, Jones, T, and Fournier, P. The decline in blood glucose levels is less with intermittent high-intensity compared with moderate exercise in individuals with type 1 diabetes. *Diabetes Care* 28:1289-1294, 2005.

80. Guelfi, K, Jones, T, and Fournier, P. New insights into managing the risk of hypoglycaemia associated with intermittent high-intensity exercise in individuals with type 1 diabetes mellitus. *Sports Med* 37:937-946, 2007.

81. Gustafson, B, Hammarstedt, A, Andersson, C, and Smith, U. Inflamed adipose tissue: a culprit underlying the metabolic syndrome and atherosclerosis. *Arterioscler Thromb Vasc Biol* 27:2276-2283, 2007.

82. Hall, K, Bemis, T, Brychta, R, Chen, K, Courville, A, Crayner, E, Goodwin, S, Gu, J, Howard, L, Knuth, N, Miller III, B, Prado, C, Siervo, M, Skarulis, M, Walter, M, Walter, P, and Yannai, L. Calorie for calorie, dietary fat restriction results in more body fat loss than carbohydrate restriction in people with obesity. *Cell Metab* 22:1-10, 2015.

83. Hall, K, Sacks, G, Chandramohan, D, Chow, C, Yang, Y, Gortmaker, S, and Swinburn, B. Quantification of the effect of energy imbalance on bodyweight. *Lancet* 378:826-836, 2011.

84. Heyman, E, Delamarche, P, Berthon, P, Meeusen, R, Briard, D, Vincent, S, DeKerdanet, M, and Delamarche, A. Alteration in sympathoadrenergic activity at rest and during intense exercise despite normal aerobic fitness in late pubertal adolescent girls with type 1 diabetes. *Diabetes Metab* 33:422-429, 2007.

85. Hill, J, Galloway, J, Goley, A, Marrero, D, Minners, R, Montgomery, B, Peterson, G, Ratner, R, Sanchez, E, and Aroda, V. Scientific statement: socioecological determinants of prediabetes and type 2 diabetes. *Diabetes Care* 36:2430-2439, 2013.

86. Hill, J, Wyatt, H, and Peters, J. Energy balance and obesity. *Circulation* 126:126-132, 2012.

87. Hollowell, J, Staehling, N, Flanders, W, Hannon, W, Gunter, E, Spencer, C, and Braverman, L. Serum TSH, T(4), and thyroid antibodies in the United States population (1988 to 1994): National Health and Nutrition Examination Survey (NHANES III). *J Clin Endocrinol Metab* 87:489-498, 2002.

88. Hu, F, Manson, J, Stampfer, M, Colditz, G, and Liu, S. Diet, lifestyle, and the risk of type 2 diabetes mellitus in women. *N Engl J Med* 345:790-797, 2001.

89. Ingelsson, E, Massaro, J, Sutherland, P, Jacques, P, Levy, D, D'Agostino, R, Vasan, R, and Robins, S. Contemporary trends in dyslipidemia in the Framingham Heart Study. *Arch Intern Med* 169:279-286, 2009.

90. Iscoe, K and Riddell, M. Continuous moderate-intensity exercise with or without intermittent high-intensity work: effects on acute and late glycaemia in athletes with Type 1 diabetes mellitus. *Diabet Med* 28:824-832, 2011.

91. Ismail, I, Keating, S, Baker, M, and Johnson, N. A systematic review and meta-analysis of the effect of aerobic vs. resistance exercise training on visceral fat. *Obes Rev* 13:68-91, 2012.

92. Jaggers, J, Hynes, K, and Wintergerst, K. Exercise and sport participation for individuals with type 1 diabetes: safety considerations and the unknown. *ACSMs Health Fit J* 20:40-44, 2016.

93. Jellinger, P, Smith, D, Mehta, A, Ganda, O, Handelsman, Y, Rodbard, H, Shepherd, M, and Seibel, J. American Association of Clinical Endocrinologists' guidelines for management of dyslipidemia and prevention of atherosclerosis. *Endocr Pract* 18:1-78, 2012.

94. Johansen, K. Exercise and chronic kidney disease: current recommendations. *Sports Med* 35:485-499, 2005.

95. Johansen, K. Exercise in the end-stage renal disease population. *J Am Soc Nephrol* 18:1845-1854, 2007.

96. Johansen, K. Exercise and dialysis. *Hemodial Int* 12:290-300, 2008.

97. Johansen, K, Chertow, G, Kutner, N, Dalrymple, L, Grimes, B, and Kaysen, G. Low level of self-reported physical activity in ambulatory patients new to dialysis. *Kidney Int* 78:1164-1170, 2010.

98. Johansen, K, Finkelstein, F, Revicki, D, Gitlin, M, Evans, C, and Mayne, T. Systematic review and meta-analysis of exercise tolerance and physical functioning in dialysis patients treated with erythropoiesis-stimulating agents. *Am J Kidney Dis* 55:535-548, 2010.

99. Johansen, K and Painter, P. Exercise in individuals with chronic kidney disease. *Am J Kidney Dis* 59:128-134, 2012.

100. Johansen, K, Painter, P, Sakkas, G, Gordon, P, Doyle, J, and Shubert, T. Effects of resistance exercise training and nandrolone deconate on body composition and muscle function among patients who receive hemodialysis: a randomized, controlled trial. *J Am Soc Nephrol* 17:2307-2314, 2006.

101. Johnson, C, Levey, A, Coresh, J, Levin, A, Lau, J, and Eknoyan, G. Clinical practice guidelines for chronic kidney disease in adults: part I. definition, disease stages, evaluation, treatment, and risk factors. *Am Fam Physician* 70:869-876, 2004.

101a. Jou, C. The biology and genetics of obesity: a century of inquiries. *N Engl J Med* 320:1874-1877, 2014.

102. Kahaly, G, Hellermann, J, Mohr-Kahaly, S, and Treese, N. Impaired cardiopulmonary exercise capacity in patients with hyperthyroidism. *Chest* 109:57-61, 1996.

103. Kahaly, G, Kampmann, C, and Mohr-Kahaly, S. Cardiovascular hemodynamics and exercise tolerance in thyroid disease. *Thyroid* 12:473-481, 2002.

104. Karfopoulou, E, Brikou, D, Mamalaki, E, Bersimis, F, Anastasiou, C, Hill, J, and Yannakouilia, M. Dietary patterns in weight loss maintenance: results from the medweight study. *Eur J Nutr* 55:1-12, 2016.

105. Katzmarzyk, P, Church, T, Craig, C, and Bouchard, C. Sitting time and mortality from all causes, cardiovascular disease, and cancer. *Med Sci Sports Exerc* 41:998-1005, 2009.

106. Kaufman, F. *Diabesity: A Doctor and Her Patients on the Front Lines of the Obesity-Diabetes Epidemic.* New York: Random House, 2006.

107. Klecha, A, Barreiro Arcos, M, and Frick, L. Immune-endocrine interactions in autoimmune thyroid disease. *Neuroimmunomodulation* 15:68-75, 2008.

108. Klein, E and Danzi, S. Thyroid disease and the heart. *Circulation* 116:1725-1755, 2007.

109. Knowler, W, Barrett-Connor, E, Fowler, S, Hamman, R, Lachin, J, Walker, E, and Nathan, D. Reduction in the incidence of type 2 diabetes with lifestyle intervention or metformin. *N Engl J Med* 346:393-403, 2002.

110. Kraemer, R, Chu, H, and Castracane, V. Leptin and exercise. *Exp Biol Med* 227:701-708, 2002.

111. Krishnan, C and Thompson, P. The effects of statins on skeletal muscle strength and exercise performance. *Curr Clin Lipidol* 21:124-128, 2010.

112. Kujala, U, Kaprio, J, Sarna, S, and Koskenvuo, M. Relationship of leisure-time physical activity and mortality. *JAMA* 279:440-444, 1998.

113. Kurihara, O, Takano, M, Seino, Y, Shimizu, W, and Mizuno, K. Coronary atherosclerosis is already ongoing in pre-diabetic status: insight from intravascular imaging modalities. *World J Diabetes* 15:184-191, 2015.

114. Laaksonen, D, Atalay, M, Niskanen, L, Mustonen, T, Sen, C, Lakka, T, and Uusitupa, M. Aerobic exercise and the lipid profile in type 1 diabetic men: a randomized controlled trial. *Med Sci Sports Exerc* 32:1541-1548, 2000.

115. Larsen, P, Kronenberg, H, Melmed, S, and Polonsky, K. *Williams' Textbook of Endocrinology.* 10th ed. Philadelphia: Saunders, 2002.

116. Lee, Y and Pratley, R. Abdominal obesity and cardiovascular disease risk: the emerging role of the adipocyte. *J Cardiopulm Rehabil Prev* 27:2-10, 2007.

117. Lenz, O and Fornoni, A. Renin–angiotensin system blockade and diabetes: moving the adipose organ from the periphery to the center. *Kidney Int* 74:851-853, 2008.

118. Levine, J, Vander Weg, M, Hill, J, and Klesges, R. Non-exercise activity thermogenesis: the crouching tiger hidden dragon of societal weight gain. *Arterioscler Thromb Vasc Biol* 26:729-736, 2006.

119. Li, C, Ford, E, Zhao, G, and Mokdad, A. Prevalence of pre-diabetes and its association with clustering of cardiometabolic risk factors and hyperinsulinemia among U.S. adolescents. *Diabetes Care* 32:342-347, 2009.

120. Libby, P, Ridker, P, and Hannson, GK. Progress and challenges in translating the biology of atherosclerosis. *Nature* 473:317-324, 2011.

121. Liese, A, Schulz, M, Moore, C, and Mayer-Davis, E. Dietary patterns, insulin sensitivity and adiposity in the multi-ethnic insulin resistance atherosclerosis study population. *Br J Nutr* 92:973-984, 2004.

122. Lim, J, Iyer, A, Liu, L, Suen, J, and Lohman, R. Diet-induced obesity, adipose inflammation, and metabolic dysfunction correlating with PAR2 expression are attenuated by PAR2 antagonism. *FASEB J* 27:4757-4767, 2013.

123. Ling, C, Holme, B, Cotillard, A, Habii-Rachedi, F, Brazeilles, R, Gougis, S, Gausseres, N, Cani, P, Fellahi, S, Bastard, J, Kennedy, S, Dure, J, Erlich, S, Zucker, J, Rizkalia, S, and Clement, K. Dietary patterns differentially associate with inflammation and gut microbiota in overweight and obese subjects. *PLoS One* 9:e109434, 2014.

124. Loprinzi, P, Branscum, A, Hanks, J, and Smit, E. Healthy lifestyle characteristics and their joint association with cardiovascular disease biomarkers in U.S. adults. *Mayo Clin Proc* 91:432-442, 2016.

125. MacDonald, M. Postexercise late-onset hypoglycemia in insulin-dependent diabetic patients. *Diabetes Care* 10:584-588, 1987.

126. Maran, A, Pavan, P, Bonsembiante, B, Brugin, E, Ermolao, A, Avogaro, A, and Zaccaria, M. Continuous glucose monitoring reveals delayed nocturnal hypoglycemia after intermittent high-intensity exercise in nontrained patients with type 1 diabetes. *Diabetes Technol Ther* 12:763-768, 2010.

127. Martin, M, Heymsfeld, S, Haft, C, Kahn, B, Laughlin, M, Leibel, R, Tschop, M, and Yanovski, J. Defining leptin resistance: challenges and opportunities. *Cell Metab* 15:150-156, 2012.

128. Marwick, T, Hordern, M, Miller, T, Chyun, D, Bertoni, A, Blumenthal, R, Philippides, G, and Rocchini, A. Exercise training for type 2 diabetes mellitus and impact on cardiovascular risk: a scientific statement from the American Heart Association. *Circulation* 119:3244-3262, 2009.

129. Mayer, J, Purnima, R, and Mitra, K. Relation between caloric intake, body weight, and physical work studies in an industrial male population in West Bengal. *Am J Clin Nutr* 4:169-175, 1956.

130. Mayo Clinic. Diseases and Conditions: High cholesterol: Treatment. www.mayoclinic.org/diseases-conditions/high-blood-cholesterol/diagnosis-treatment/treatment/txc-20181958. Accessed December 1, 2016.

131. Mayo Clinic. Diseases and Conditions: Hyperthyroidism (overactive thyroid): Treatment and drugs. www.mayoclinic.org/diseases-conditions/hyperthyroidism/basics/treatment/con-20020986. Accessed December 1, 2016.

132. Mayo Clinic. Diseases and Conditions: Obesity: Treatment and drugs. www.mayoclinic.org/diseases-conditions/obesity/basics/treatment/con-20014834. Accessed December 1, 2016.

133. Mayo Clinic. Diseases and Conditions: Type 1 diabetes. www.mayoclinic.org/diseases-conditions/type-1-diabetes/basics/tests-diagnosis/con-20019573. Accessed December 1, 2016.

134. Mayo Clinic. Diseases and Conditions: Type 1 diabetes: Treatment and drugs. www.mayoclinic.org/diseases-conditions/type-1-diabetes/basics/treatment/con-20019573. Accessed December 1, 2016.

135. Mayo Clinic. Diseases and Conditions: Type 2 diabetes: Treatment. www.mayoclinic.org/diseases-conditions/type-2-diabetes/diagnosis-treatment/treatment/txc-20169988. Accessed December 1, 2016.

136. McAllister, R, Delp, M, and Laughlin, M. Thyroid status and exercise tolerance: cardiovascular and metabolic considerations. *Sports Med* 20:189-198, 1995.

137. McQueen, M. Exercise aspects of obesity treatment. *Ochsner J* 9:140-143, 2009.

138. Mikus, C, Boyle, L, Borengasser, S, Oberlin, D, Naples, S, Fletcher, J, Meers, G, Ruebel, M, Laughlin, M, Dellsperger, K, Fadel, P, and Thyfault, J. Simvastatin impairs exercise training adaptations. *J Am Coll Cardiol* 62:709-714, 2013.

139. Mistry, N, Wass, J, and Turner, M. When to consider thyroid dysfunction in the neurology clinic. *Pract Neurol* 9:145-156, 2009.

140. Miyashita, M, Burns, S, and Stensel, D. An update on accumulating exercise and postprandial lipemia: translating theory into practice. *J Prev Med Public Health* 46:S3-S11, 2013.

141. Moore, G, Painter, P, Brinker, K, Stray-Gundersen, J, and Mitchell, J. Cardiovascular response to submaximal stationary cycling during hemodialysis. *Am J Kidney Dis* 31:613-617, 1998.

142. Moore, G, Parsons, D, Stray-Gundersen, J, Painter, P, Brinker, K, and Mitchell, J. Uremic myopathy limits aerobic capacity in hemodialysis patients. *Am J Kidney Dis* 22:277-287, 1993.

143. Moy, C, Songer, T, LaPorte, R, Dorman, J, Kriska, A, Orchard, T, Becker, D, and Drash, A. Insulin-dependent diabetes mellitus, physical activity, and death. *Am J Epidemiol* 137:74-81, 1993.

144. Murphy, M, Blair, S, and Murtagh, E. Accumulated versus continuous exercise for health benefit: a review of empirical studies. *Sports Med* 39:29-43, 2009.

145. Mustafa, K, DeFronzo, R, and Abdul-Ghani, M. Treatment of prediabetes. *World J Diabetes* 2015:1207-1222, 2015.

146. National Cholesterol Education Program. Third report of the National Cholesterol Education Program (NCEP) Expert Panel on Detection, Evaluation, and Treatment of High Blood Cholesterol in Adults (Adult Treatment Panel III) Final Report. *Circulation* 106:3143-3421, 2002.

147. National Heart Lung and Blood Institute. *The Practical Guide: Identification, Evaluation, and Treatment of Overweight and Obesity in Adults.* NIH Publication No. DO-4084. Bethesda, MD: National Institutes of Health, 2000.

148. National Institute of Diabetes and Digestive and Kidney Diseases. Anemia in CKD. 2014. www.niddk.nih.gov/health-information/health-topics/kidney-disease/anemia-in-kidney-disease-and-dialysis/Pages/facts.aspx. Accessed December 23, 2016.

149. National Kidney Foundation. K/DOQU clinical practice guidelines for chronic kidney disease: evaluation, classification, and stratification. *Am J Kidney Dis* 39:S1-S266, 2002.

150. Nichols, G, Gullion, C, Koro, C, Ephross, S, and Brown, J. The incidence of congestive heart failure in type 2 diabetes: an update. *Diabetes Care* 27:1879-1884, 2004.

151. Nordestgaard, B, Benn, M, Schnohr, P, and Tybjaerg-Hansen, A. Nonfasting triglycerides and risk of myocardial infarction, ischemic heart disease, and death in men and women. *JAMA* 298:299-308, 2007.

152. Norris, R, Carroll, D, and Cochrane, R. The effects of aerobic and anaerobic training on fitness, blood pressure, and psychological stress and well-being. *J Psychosom Res* 34:367-375, 1990.

153. Nuffer, W, Trujillo, J, and Meqveri, J. A comparison of new pharmacological agents for the treatment of obesity. *Ann Pharmacother* 50:376-388, 2016.

154. O'Donnell, M, Xavier, D, Liu, L, Zhang, H, and Chen, S. Risk factors for ischemic and intracerebral haemorrhagic stroke in 22 countries (the INTERSTROKE study): a case-control study. *Lancet* 376:112-123, 2010.

155. O'Gorman, D, Karlson, H, McQuaid, S, Yousif, O, Rahman, Y, Gasparro, D, Glund, S, Chibalin, A, Zierath, J, and Nolan, J. Exercise training increases insulin stimulated glucose disposal and Glut-4 (SCL2A4) protein content in patients with type 2 diabetes. *Diabetologia* 49:2983-2992, 2006.

156. Ogden, C, Carroll, M, Kit, B, and Flegal, K. Prevalence of obesity and trends in body mass index among U.S. children and adolescents, 1999-2010. *JAMA* 307:483-490, 2012.

157. Ogden, C, Carroll, M, Kit, B, and Flegal, K. *Prevalence of Obesity in the United States, 2009-2010.* NCHS Data Brief No. 82. Hyattsville, MD: National Center for Health Statistics, 2012.

158. Painter, P. Physical functioning in end-stage renal disease: update 2005. *Hemodial Int* 9:218-235, 2005.

159. Painter, P. Chronic kidney and liver disease. In *ACSM's Exercise Management for Persons with Chronic Diseases and Disabilities.* 4th ed. Moore, G, Durstine, J, and Painter, P, eds. Champaign, IL: Human Kinetics, 201-207, 2016.

160. Painter, P, Hector, L, Ray, K, Lynes, L, Dibble, S, Paul, S, Tomlanovich, S, and Ascher, N. A randomized trial of exercise training after renal transplantation. *Transplantation* 74:42-48, 2002.

161. Painter, P, Hector, L, Ray, K, Lynes, L, Paul, S, Dodd, M, Tomlanovich, S, and Ascher, N. Effects of exercise training on coronary heart disease risk factors in renal transplant recipients. *Am J Kidney Dis* 42:363-369, 2003.

162. Painter, P, Nelson-Worel, J, Hill, M, Thornbery, D, Shelp, W, Harrington, A, and Weinstein, A. Effects of exercise training during hemodialysis. *Nephron* 43:87-92, 1986.

163. Paoli, A, Pacelli, Q, Moro, T, Marcolin, G, Neri, M, Battaglia, G, Sergi, G, Bolzetta, F, and Bianco, A. Effects of high-intensity circuit training, low-intensity circuit training and endurance training on blood pressure and lipoproteins in middle-aged overweight men. *Lipids Health Dis* 12:131, 2013.

164. Parker, B and Thompson, P. Effect of statins on skeletal muscle: exercise, myopathy, and muscle outcomes. *Exerc Sport Sci Rev* 40:188-194, 2012.

165. Persinger, R, Foster, C, Gibson, M, Fater, D, and Porcari, J. Consistency of the talk test for exercise prescription. *Med Sci Sports Exerc* 36:1632-1636, 2004.

166. Pollock, M, Franklin, B, Balady, G, Chaitman, B, Fleg, J, Fletcher, B, Limacher, M, Piña, I, Stein, R, Williams, M, and Bazzarre, T. Resistance exercise in individuals with and without cardiovascular disease: benefits, rationale, safety, and prescription. An advisory from the Committee on Exercise, Rehabilitation, and Prevention, Council on Clinical Cardiology, American Heart Association. *Circulation* 101:828-833, 2000.

167. Pontzer, H. Constrained total energy expenditure and the evolutionary biology of energy balance. *Exerc Sport Sci Rev* 43:110-116, 2015.

168. Rabasa-Lhoret, R, Bourque, J, Ducros, F, and Chiasson, J. Guidelines for premeal insulin dose reduction for postprandial exercise of different intensities and durations in type 1 diabetic subjects treated intensively with a basal-bolus insulin regimen (ultralente-lispro). *Diabetes Care* 24:625-630, 2001.

169. Ramalho, A, de Lourdes Lima, M, Nunes, F, Cambuí, Z, Barbosa, C, Andrade, A, Viana, A, Martins, M, Abrantes, V, Aragão, C, and Temístocles, M. The effect of resistance versus aerobic training on metabolic control in patients with type-1 diabetes mellitus. *Diabetes Res Clin Pract* 72:271-276, 2006.

170. Rivera, J, O'Hare, A, and Harper, G. Update on the management of chronic kidney disease. *Am Fam Physician* 86:749-754, 2012.

171. Roberts, C and Barnard, R. Effects of diet and exercise on chronic disease. *J Appl Physiol* 98:3-30, 2005.

172. Rodgers, R, Tschop, M, and Wilding, J. Anti-obesity drugs: past, present, and future. *Dis Model Mech* 5:621-626, 2012.

173. Roitman, J and LaFontaine, T. *The Exercise Professional's Guide to Optimizing Health.* Baltimore: Wolters Kluwer/Lippincott Williams & Wilkins, 2012.

174. Rosenkranz, R, Duncan, M, Rosenkranz, S, and Kolt, G. Active lifestyles related to excellent self-rated health and quality of life: cross sectional findings from 194,545 participants in the 45 and up study. *BMC Public Health* 13:1071, 2013.

175. Saran, R, Li, Y, Robinson, B, Abbott, K, Agodoa, L, Ayanian, J, Bragg-Gresham, J, Balkrishnan, R, Chen, J, Cope, E, and Eggers, P. U.S. renal data system 2015: annual data report: epidemiology of kidney disease in the United States. *Am J Kidney Dis* 67:A7, 2016.

176. Schwingshackl, L, Dias, S, Strasser, B, and Hoffmann, G. Impact of different training modalities on anthropometric and metabolic characteristics in overweight/obese subjects: a systematic review and network meta-analysis. *PLoS Med* 8:e82853, 2013.

177. Segura-Orti, E and Johansen, K. Exercise in end-stage renal disease. *Semin Dial* 23:422-430, 2010.

178. Sideravičiūtė, S, Gailiūniene, A, Visagurskiene, K, and Vizbaraite, D. The effect of long-term swimming program on body composition, aerobic capacity and blood lipids in 14-19-year aged healthy girls and girls with type 1 diabetes mellitus. *Medicina (Kaunas)* 42:661-666, 2006.

179. Sigal, R, Kenny, G, Boulé, N, Wells, G, Prud'homme, D, Fortier, M, Reid, R, Tulloch, H, Coyle, D, Phillips,

P, Jennings, A, and Jaffey, J. Effects of aerobic training, resistance training, or both on glycemic control in type 2 diabetes: a randomized trial. *Ann Intern Med* 147:357-369, 2007.

180. Sigal, R, Kenny, G, Wasserman, D, and Castaneda-Sceppa, C. Physical activity/exercise and type 2 diabetes. *Diabetes Care* 27:2518-2539, 2004.

181. Sigal, R, Kenny, G, Wasserman, D, Castaneda-Sceppa, C, and White, R. Physical activity/exercise and Type 2 diabetes: a consensus statement from the American Diabetes Association. *Diabetes Care* 29:1433-1438, 2006.

182. Skugor, M. Hypothyroidism and Hyperthyroidism. 2014. www.clevelandclinicmeded.com/medicalpubs/diseasemanagement/endocrinology/hypothyroidism-and-hyperthyroidism. Accessed January 8, 2017.

183. Slentz, C, Houmard, J, Johnson, J, Bateman, L, Tanner, C, McCartney, J, Duscha, B, and Kraus, W. Inactivity, exercise training and detraining, and plasma lipoproteins: STRRIDE: a randomized, controlled study of exercise intensity and amount. *J Appl Physiol* 103:432-442, 2007.

184. Smart, N, Williams, A, Levinger, I, Selig, S, Howden, E, Coombes, J, and Fassett, R. Exercise and Sports Science Australia (ESSA) position statement on exercise and chronic kidney disease. *J Sci Med Sport* 16:406-411, 2013.

185. Smith-Marsh, D. Type 1 Diabetes Risk Factors. www.endocrineweb.com/conditions/type-1-diabetes/type-1-diabetes-risk-factors. Accessed December 6, 2016.

186. Sorace, P, LaFontaine, T, and Thomas, T. Know the risks: lifestyle management of dyslipidemia. *ACSMs Health Fit J* 10:18-25, 2006.

187. Sparling, P, Franklin, B, and Hill, J. Energy balance: the key to a unified message on diet and physical activity. *J Cardiopulm Rehabil Prev* 33:12-15, 2013.

188. Spring, B, Ockene, J, Gidding, S, Mozaffarian, D, and Moore, S. Better population health through behavior change in adults: a call to action. *Circulation* 128:2169-2176, 2013.

189. Steven, S, Hollingsworth, K, Al-Mrabeh, A, Avery, L, Aribisala, B, Caslake, M, and Taylor, R. Very-low-calorie diet and 6 months of weight stability in type 2 diabetes: pathophysiologic changes in responders and nonresponders. *Diabetes Care* 39:808-815, 2016.

190. Stone, N, Robinson, J, Lichtenstein, A, Merz, C, Blum, C, Eckel, R, Goldberg, A, Gordon, D, Levy, D, Lloyd-Jones, D, and McBride, P. ACC/AHA guideline on the treatment of blood cholesterol to reduce atherosclerotic cardiovascular risk in adults: a report of the American College of Cardiology/American Heart Association task force on practice guidelines. *J Am Coll Cardiol* 63:2889-2934, 2013.

191. Stöppler, M. HbA1c Test. www.emedicinehealth.com/hemoglobin_a1c_hba1c/article_em.htm. Accessed December 21, 2016.

192. Strasser, B, Arvandi, M, and Siebert, U. Resistance training, visceral obesity, and inflammatory response: a review of the evidence. *Obes Rev* 13:578-591, 2012.

193. Stuckey, M and Petrella, R. Heart rate variability in type 2 diabetes mellitus. *Crit Rev Biomed Eng* 41:137-147, 2013.

194. Tansey, M, Tsalikian, E, Beck, R, Mauras, N, Buckingham, B, Weinzimer, S, Janz, K, Kollman, C, Xing, D, Ruedy, K, and Steffes, M. The effects of aerobic exercise on glucose and counterregulatory hormone concentrations in children with type 1 diabetes. *Diabetes Care* 29:20-25, 2006.

195. Taplin, C, Cobry, E, Messer, L, McFann, K, Chase, H, and Fiallo-Scharer, R. Preventing post-exercise nocturnal hypoglycemia in children with type 1 diabetes. *J Pediatr* 157:784-788, 2010.

196. Thomas, T and LaFontaine, T. Exercise, nutritional strategies and lipoproteins. In *ACSM's Resource Manual for the Guidelines for Exercise Testing and Prescription*. 4th ed. Roitman, J, ed. Baltimore: Wolters Kluwer/Lippincott Williams & Wilkins, 2001.

197. Tonoli, C, Heyman, E, Roelands, B, Buyse, L, Cheung, S, Berthoin, S, and Meeusen, R. Effects of different types of acute and chronic (training) exercise on glycaemic control in type 1 diabetes mellitus. *Sports Med* 42:1059-1080, 2012.

198. Torre, D, Lamb, G, and Van Ruiswyck, J. *Koshar's Clinical Medicine for Students*. 5th ed. Baltimore: Wolters Kluwer/Lippincott Williams & Wilkins, 2008.

199. Trombold, J, Christmas, K, Machin, D, Kim, I, and Coyle, E. Acute high-intensity exercise is more effective than moderate-intensity exercise for attenuation of postprandial triglyceride elevation. *J Appl Physiol* 114:792-800, 2013.

200. Tsalikian, E, Mauras, N, Beck, R, Tamborlane, W, Janz, K, Chase, H, Wysocki, T, Weinzimer, S, Buckingham, B, Kollman, C, and Xing, D. Impact of exercise on overnight glycemic control in children with type 1 diabetes mellitus. *J Pediatr* 147:528-534, 2005.

201. Tuominen, J, Karonen, S, Melamies, L, Bolli, G, and Koivisto, V. Exercise-induced hypoglycaemia in IDDM patients treated with a short-acting insulin analogue. *Diabetologia* 38:106-111, 1995.

202. U.S. Department of Health and Human Services and U.S. Department of Agriculture. 2015-2020 Dietary Guidelines for Americans, Eighth Edition. 2015. http://health.gov/dietaryguidelines/2015/guidelines/. Accessed January 7, 2017.

203. U.S. National Library of Medicine. ACE inhibitors. https://medlineplus.gov/ency/patientinstructions/000087.htm. Accessed January 31, 2017.

204. U.S. National Library of Medicine. Pramlintide Injection. https://medlineplus.gov/druginfo/meds/a605031.html. Accessed December 7, 2016.

205. U.S. News and World Report. 2016. Diet rankings. www.usnews.com/info/blogs/pressroom/2016/01/05/us-news-reveals-the-2016-best-diets-rankings. Accessed March 25, 2016.

206. Vehik, K, Hamman, R, Lezotte, D, Norris, J, Klingensmith, G, Bloch, C, Rewers, M, and Dabelea, D. Increasing incidence of type 1 diabetes in 0-to 17-year-old Colorado youth. *Diabetes Care* 30:503-509, 2007.

207. Vinik, A and Erbas, T. Neuropathy. In *Handbook of Exercise in Diabetes*. 2nd ed. Ruderman, N, ed. Alexandria, VA: American Diabetes Association, 463-496, 2002.

208. Vinik, A and Erbas, T. Diabetic autonomic neuropathy. *Handb Clin Neurol* 117:279-294, 2013.

209. Wang, Y, Simar, D, and Fiatarone Singh, M. Adaptations to exercise training within skeletal muscle in adults with type 2 diabetes or impaired glucose tolerance: a systematic review. *Diabetes Metab Res Rev* 25:13-40, 2009.

210. WebMD Medical Reference. Inhaled Insulin. www.webmd.com/diabetes/inhaled-insulin. Accessed December 21, 2016.

211. WebMD Medical Reference. Types of Insulin for Diabetes Treatment. www.webmd.com/diabetes/guide/diabetes-types-insulin#1. Accessed December 21, 2016.

212. Westman, E, Feinman, R, Mavropoulos, J, Vernon, M, Volek, J, Wortman, J, Yancy, W, and Phinney, S. Low-carbohydrate nutrition and metabolism. *Am J Clin Nutr* 86:276-284, 2007.

213. Willett, W and Stampfer, M. Current evidence on healthy eating. *Annu Rev Public Health* 34:77-95, 2013.

214. Williams, P. High density lipoprotein cholesterol and other risk factors for coronary artery disease in female runners. *N Engl J Med* 334:1298-1303, 1996.

215. Williams, P. Incident hypercholesterolemia in relation to changes in vigorous physical activity. *Med Sci Sports Exerc* 41:73-80, 2009.

216. Williams, P, Blanche, P, and Kraus, R. Behavioral versus genetic correlates of lipoproteins and adiposity in identical twins discordant for exercise. *Circulation* 112:350-356, 2005.

217. Williams, P, Stefanick, M, Vranizan, K, and Wood, P. The effects of weight loss by exercise or dieting on high-density lipoprotein (HDL) levels in men with low, intermediate, and normal-to-high HDL at baseline. *Metabolism* 43:917-924, 1994.

218. Willis, L, Slentz, C, Bateman, L, Shields, A, Piner, L, Bales, C, Houmard, J, and Kraus, W. Effects of aerobic and/or resistance training on body mass and fat mass in overweight or obese adults. *J Appl Physiol* 113:1831-1837, 2012.

219. Wing, R. Physical activity in the treatment of the adulthood overweight and obesity: current evidence and research issues. *Med Sci Sports Exerc* 31:S547-S552, 1999.

220. Wing, R and Hill, J. National Weight Control Registry Research Findings. http://nwcr.ws/Research/published%20research.htm. Accessed February 5, 2014.

221. Wong, C, Chiang, Y, Wai, J, Lo, F, Yeh, C, Chung, S, and Chang, C. Effects of a home-based aerobic exercise programme in children with type 1 diabetes mellitus. *J Clin Nurs* 20:681-691, 2011.

222. World Cancer Research Fund and American Institute for Cancer Research. Food, Nutrition, Physical Activity, and the Prevention of Cancer: A Global Perspective. 2007. www.aicr.org/assets/docs/pdf/reports/Second_Expert_Report.pdf. Accessed May 7, 2016.

223. Yang, Z, Scott, C, Mao, C, Tang, J, and Farmer, A. Resistance exercise versus aerobic exercise for type 2 diabetes: a systematic review and meta-analysis. *Sports Med* 44:487-499, 2014.

224. Yardley, J, Kenny, G, Perkins, B, Riddell, M, Balaa, N, Malcolm, J, Boulay, P, Khandwala, F, and Sigal, R. Resistance versus aerobic exercise acute effects on glycemia in type 1 diabetes. *Diabetes Care* 36:537-542, 2013.

225. Zaharieva, D and Riddell, M. Prevention of exercise-associated dysglycemia: a case study-based approach. *Diabetes Spectr* 28:55-62, 2015.

226. Zhang, J, Thomas, T, and Ball, S. Effect of exercise timing on postprandial lipemia and HDL cholesterol subfractions. *J Appl Physiol* 85:1516-1522, 1998.

Chapter 5 Pulmonary Disorders and Conditions

1. Adde, F, Rodrigues, J, and Cardoso, A. Nutritional follow-up of cystic fibrosis patients: the role of nutrition education. *J Pediatr (Rio J)* 80:475-482, 2004.

2. Aguilaniu, B. Impact of bronchodilator therapy on exercise tolerance in COPD. *Int J Chron Obstruct Pulmon Dis* 5:57-71, 2010.

3. Ahidjo, B, Maiga, M, Ihms, E, Maiga, M, Ordonez, A, Cheung, L, Beck, S, Andrade, B, Jain, S, and Bishai, W. The antifibrotic drug pirfenidone promotes pulmonary cavitation and drug resistance in a mouse model of chronic tuberculosis. *JCI Insight* 1:e86017, 2016.

4. Allen, D. Effects of inhaled steroids on growth, bone metabolism, and adrenal function. *Adv Pediatr* 53:101-110, 2006.

5. Allen, D, Bielory, L, Derendorf, H, Dluhy, R, Colice, G, and Szefler, S. Inhaled corticosteroids: past lessons and future issues. *J Allergy Clin Immunol* 112:S1-S40, 2003.

6. Allen, D, Mullen, M, and Mullen, B. A meta-analysis of the effect of oral and inhaled corticosteroids on growth. *J Allergy Clin Immunol* 93:967-976, 1994.

7. American Academy of Allergy Asthma & Immunology. Asthma results in missed sleep, school days for children. 2012. http://acaai.org/news/asthma-results-missed-sleep-school-days-children?f5tp=1. Accessed January 27, 2017.

8. American Academy of Allergy Asthma & Immunology. Asthma Statistics. 2017. www.aaaai.org/conditions-and-treatments/asthma/Asthma-Statistics. Accessed January 27, 2017.

9. American College of Chest Physicians. CDC reports annual financial cost of COPD to be $36 billion in the United States. 2014. www.chestnet.org/News/Press-Releases/2014/07/CDC-reports-36-billion-in-annual-financial-cost-of-COPD-in-US. Accessed January 27, 2017.

10. American Lung Association. Trends in COPD (chronic bronchitis and emphysema): morbidity and mortality. 2013. www.lung.org/assets/documents/research/copd-trend-report.pdf. Accessed January 27, 2017.

11. American Lung Association. How serious is COPD. 2016. www.lung.org/lung-health-and-diseases/lung-disease-lookup/copd/learn-about-copd/how-serious-is-copd.html. Accessed January 27, 2017.

12. American Lung Association. What causes COPD. 2016. www.lung.org/lung-health-and-diseases/lung-disease-lookup/copd/symptoms-causes-risk-factors/what-causes-copd.html. Accessed January 27, 2017.

13. Anderson, S. Airway drying and exercise-induced asthma. In *Exercise-Induced Asthma*. McFadden, E, ed. New York: Marcel Dekker, 77-114, 1999.

14. Anderson, S, Connolly, N, and Godfrey, S. Comparison of bronchoconstriction induced by cycling and running. *Thorax* 26:396-401, 1971.

15. Anderson, S and Daviskas, E. Pathophysiology of exercise-induced asthma: the role of respiratory water loss. In *Allergic and Respiratory Disease in Sports Medicine*. Weiler, J, ed. New York: Marcel Dekker, 87-114, 1997.

16. Anderson, S and Daviskas, E. The mechanism of exercise-induced asthma is . . . *J Allergy Clin Immunol* 106:453-459, 2000.

17. Anderson, S, Schoeffel, R, Follet, R, Perry, C, Daviskas, E, and Kendall, M. Sensitivity to heat and water loss at rest and during exercise in asthmatic patients. *Eur J Respir Dis* 63:459-471, 1982.

18. Anderson, S, Seale, J, Ferris, L, Schoeffel, R, and Lindsay, D. An evaluation of pharmacotherapy for exercise-induced asthma. *J Allergy Clin Immunol* 64:612-624, 1979.

19. Andrianopoulos, V, Klijn, P, Franssen, F, and Spruit, M. Exercise training in pulmonary rehabilitation. *Clin Chest Med* 35:313-322, 2014.

20. Arena, R. Exercise testing and training in chronic lung disease and pulmonary arterial hypertension. *Prog Cardiovasc Dis* 53:454-463, 2011.

21. Arena, R, Cahalin, L, Borghi-Silva, A, and Myers, J. The effect of exercise training on the pulmonary arterial system in patients with pulmonary hypertension. *Prog Cardiovasc Dis* 57:480-488, 2015.

22. Aris, R, Renner, J, Winders, A, Buell, H, Riggs, D, Lester, G, and Ontjes, D. Increased rate of fractures and severe kyphosis: sequelae of living into adulthood with cystic fibrosis. *Ann Intern Med* 128:186-193, 1998.

23. Asher, M, Pardy, R, Coates, A, Thomas, E, and Macklem, P. The effects of inspiratory muscle training in patients with cystic fibrosis 1-4. *Am Rev Respir Dis* 126:855-859, 1982.

24. Babu, A, Padmakumar, R, Maiya, A, Mohapatra, A, and Kamath, R. Effects of exercise training on exercise capacity in pulmonary arterial hypertension: a systematic review of clinical trials. *Heart Lung Circ* 25:333-341, 2016.

25. Backer, V and Ulrik, C. Bronchial responsiveness to exercise in a random sample of 494 children and adolescents from Copenhagen. *Clin Exp Allergy* 22:741-747, 1992.

26. Baker, S. Delayed release pancrelipase for the treatment of pancreatic exocrine insufficiency associated with cystic fibrosis. *Ther Clin Risk Manag* 4:1079-1084, 2008.

27. Balfour-Lynn, I. Anti-inflammatory approaches to cystic fibrosis airways disease. *Curr Opin Pulm Med* 13:522-528, 2007.

28. Barnes, N, Marone, G, Di Maria, G, Visser, S, Utama, I, and Payne, S. A comparison of fluticasone propionate, 1 mg daily, with beclomethasone dipropionate, 2 mg daily, in the treatment of severe asthma. International Study Group. *Eur Respir J* 6:877-885, 1993.

29. Barnes, N, Sharma, R, Lettis, S, and Calverley, P. Blood eosinophils as a marker of response to inhaled corticosteroids in COPD. *Eur Respir J* 47:1374-1382, 2016.

30. Bastos, H, Neves, I, Redondo, M, Cunha, R, Pereira, J, Magalhães, A, and Fernandes, G. Influence of emphysema distribution on pulmonary function parameters in COPD patients. *J Bras Pneumol* 41:489-495, 2015.

31. Beasley, R, Semprini, A, and Mitchell, E. Risk factors for asthma: is prevention possible? *Lancet* 386:1075-1085, 2015.

32. Beck, K, Offord, K, and Scanlon, P. Bronchoconstriction occurring during exercise in asthmatic subjects. *Am J Respir Crit Care Med* 149:352-357, 1994.

33. Becker, A and Simons, F. Formoterol, a new long-acting selective beta-2-agonist, decreases airway responsiveness in children with asthma. *Lung* 168:99-102, 1990.

34. Becker, J, Rogers, J, Rossini, G, Mirchandani, H, and D'Alonzo, G. Asthma deaths during sports: report of a 7-year experience. *J Allergy Clin Immunol* 113:264-267, 2004.

35. Bel, E, Wenzel, S, Thompson, P, Prazma, C, Keene, O, Yancey, S, Ortega, H, Pavord, I, and SIRIUS Investigators. Oral glucocorticoid-sparing effect of mepolizumab in eosinophilic asthma. *N Engl J Med* 371:1189-1197, 2014.

36. Belkin, R, Henig, N, Singer, L, Chaparro, C, Rubenstein, R, Xie, S, Yee, J, Kotloff, R, Lipson, D, and Bunin, G. Risk factors for death of patients with cystic fibrosis awaiting lung transplantation. *Am J Respir Crit Care Med* 173:659-666, 2006.

37. Bernard, S, Whittom, F, Leblanc, P, Jobin, J, Belleau, R, Bérubé, C, Carrier, G, and Maltais, F. Aerobic and strength training in patients with chronic obstructive pulmonary disease. *Am J Respir Crit Care Med* 159:896-901, 1999.

38. Berstad, A and Brandtzaeg, P. Does reduced microbial exposure contribute to increased prevalence of allergy? *Tidsskr Nor Laegeforen* 120:915-919, 2000.

39. Bertolaso, C, Groleau, V, Schall, J, Maqbool, A, Mascarenhas, M, Latham, N, Dougherty, K, and Stallings, V. Fat-soluble vitamins in cystic fibrosis and pancreatic insufficiency: efficacy of a nutrition intervention. *J Pediatr Gastroenterol Nutr* 58:443-448, 2014.

40. Bollmeier, S and Prosser, T. Combination of fluticasone furoate and vilanterol for the treatment of chronic obstructive pulmonary disease. *Ann Pharmacother* 48:250-257, 2014.

41. Boulet, L, Becker, A, Bérubé, A, Beveridge, R, and Ernst, P. Canadian asthma consensus report. *CMAJ* 161:S1-S62, 1999.

42. Bourbeau, J and Johnson, M. New and controversial therapies for chronic obstructive pulmonary disease. *Proc Am Thorac Soc* 6:553-554, 2009.

43. Bradley, J and Moran, F. Physical training for cystic fibrosis. *Cochrane Database Syst Rev* 5:1-59, 2011.

44. Briggs, E, Nguyen, T, Wall, M, and MacDonald, K. Oral antimicrobial use in outpatient cystic fibrosis pulmonary exacerbation management: a single-center experience. *Clin Respir J* 6:56-64, 2012.

45. Buntain, H, Schluter, P, Bell, S, Greer, R, Wong, J, Batch, J, Lewindon, P, and Wainwright, C. Controlled longitudinal study of bone mass accrual in children and adolescents with cystic fibrosis. *Thorax* 61:146-154, 2006.

46. Burte, E, Nadif, R, and Jacquemin, B. Susceptibility factors relevant for the association between long-term air pollution exposure and incident asthma. *Curr Environ Health Rep* 3:23-39, 2016.

47. Camargo, CJ, Weiss, S, Zhang, S, Willett, W, and Speizer, F. Prospective study of body mass index, weight change, and risk of adult-onset asthma in women. *Arch Intern Med* 159:2582-2588, 1999.

48. Carlin, B. Asthma. In *ACSM's Clinical Exercise Physiology*. 3rd ed. Ehrman, J, Gordon, P, Visich, P, and Keteyian, S, eds. Champaign, IL: Human Kinetics, 342, 2013.

49. Caronia, J. Restrictive lung disease. 2016. http://emedicine.medscape.com/article/301760-overview. Accessed January 29, 2017.

50. Carson, K, Chandratilleke, M, Picot, J, Brinn, M, Esterman, A, and Smith, B. Physical training for asthma. *Cochrane Database Syst Rev* 9:CD001116-001172, 2013.

51. Castricum, A, Holzer, K, Brukner, P, and Irving, L. The role of the bronchial provocation challenge tests in the diagnosis of exercise-induced bronchoconstriction in elite swimmers. *Br J Sports Med* 44:736-740, 2010.

52. Castro-Rodriguez, J, Holberg, C, Morgan, W, Wright, A, and Martinez, F. Increased incidence of asthmalike symptoms in girls who become overweight or obese during the school years. *Am J Respir Crit Care Med* 163:1344-1349, 2001.

53. Centers for Disease Control and Prevention. Asthma in the US. 2011. www.cdc.gov/VitalSigns/Asthma/index.html. Accessed January 27, 2017.

54. Centers for Disease Control and Prevention. Asthma. 2017. www.cdc.gov/nchs/fastats/asthma.htm. Accessed January 27, 2017.

55. Cerny, F. Relative effects of bronchial drainage and exercise for in-hospital care of patients with cystic fibrosis. *Phys Ther* 69:633-639, 1989.

56. Cerny, F, Armitage, L, Hirsch, J, and Bishop, B. Respiratory and abdominal muscle responses to expiratory threshold loading in cystic fibrosis. *J Appl Physiol* 72:842-850, 1992.

57. Chan, L, Chin, L, Kennedy, M, Woolstenhulme, J, Nathan, S, Weinstein, A, Connors, G, Weir, N, Drinkard, B, Lamberti, J, and Keyser, R. Benefits of intensive treadmill exercise training on cardiorespiratory function and quality of life in patients with pulmonary hypertension. *Chest* 143:333-343, 2013.

58. Chang, P, Bhavsar, P, Michaeloudes, C, Khorasani, N, and Chung, K. Corticosteroid insensitivity of chemokine expression in airway smooth muscle of patients with severe asthma. *J Allergy Clin Immunol* 130:877-885, 2012.

59. Chaouat, A, Sitbon, O, Mercy, M, Ponçot-Mongars, R, Provencher, S, Guillaumot, A, Gomez, E, Selton-Suty, C, Malvestio, P, Regent, D, and Paris, C. Prognostic value of exercise pulmonary haemodynamics in pulmonary arterial hypertension. *Eur Respir J* 44:704-713, 2014.

60. Chen, W and Horton, D. Heat and water loss from the airways and exercise-induced asthma. *Respiration* 34:305-313, 1977.

61. Chia, E, Lau, E, Xuan, W, Celermajer, D, and Thomas, L. Exercise testing can unmask right ventricular dysfunction in systemic sclerosis patients with normal resting pulmonary artery pressure. *Int J Cardiol* 204:179-186, 2016.

62. Choby, G and Lee, S. Pharmacotherapy for the treatment of asthma: current treatment options and future directions. *Int Forum Allergy Rhinol* 5(suppl 1):S35-S40, 2015.

63. Chung, K, Wenzel, S, Brozek, J, Bush, A, Castro, M, Sterk, P, Adcock, I, Bateman, E, Bel, E, Bleecker, E, Boulet, L, Brightling, C, Chanez, P, Dahlen, S,

Djukanovic, R, Frey, U, Gaga, M, Gibson, P, Hamid, Q, Jajour, N, Mauad, T, Sorkness, R, and Teague, W. International ERS/ATS guidelines on definition, evaluation and treatment of severe asthma. *Eur Respir J* 43:343-373, 2014.

64. Coates, A, Boyce, P, Muller, D, Mearns, M, and Godfrey, S. The role of nutritional status, airway obstruction, hypoxia, and abnormalities in serum lipid composition in limiting exercise tolerance in children with cystic fibrosis. *Acta Paediatr* 69:353-358, 1980.

65. Collie, D, Glendinning, L, Govan, J, Wright, S, Thornton, E, Tennant, P, Doherty, C, and McLachlan, G. Lung microbiota changes associated with chronic pseudomonas aeruginosa lung infection and the impact of intravenous colistimethate sodium. *PLoS One* 10:e0142097, 2015.

66. Coreno, A, Skowronski, M, Kotaru, C, and McFadden Jr, E. Comparative effects of long-acting β2-agonists, leukotriene receptor antagonists, and 5-lipoxygenase inhibitor on exercise-induced asthma. *J Allergy Clin Immunol* 106:500-506, 2000.

67. Crapo, R, Casaburi, R, Coates, A, Enright, P, Hankinson, J, Irvin, C, MacIntyre, N, McKay, R, Wanger, J, Anderson, S, Cockcroft, D, Fish, J, and Sterk, P. Guidelines for methacholine and exercise challenge testing. *Am J Respir Crit Care Med* 161:309-329, 2000.

68. Cropp, G, Pullano, T, Cerny, F, and Nathanson, I. Exercise tolerance and cardiorespiratory adjustments at peak work capacity in cystic fibrosis. *Am Rev Respir Dis* 126:211-216, 1982.

69. Cystic Fibrosis Foundation. Patient registry annual data report. 2015. www.cff.org/Our-Research/CF-Patient-Registry/2015-Patient-Registry-Annual-Data-Report.pdf. Accessed January 27, 2017.

70. D'Alonzo, G, Nathan, R, Henochowicz, S, Morris, R, Ratner, P, and Rennard, S. Salmeterol xinafoate as maintenance therapy compared with albuterol in patients with asthma. *JAMA* 271:1412-1416, 1994.

71. D'Andrea, A, La Gerche, A, Golia, E, Padalino, R, Calabrò, R, Russo, M, and Bossone, E. Physiologic and pathophysiologic changes in the right heart in highly trained athletes. *Herz* 40:369-378, 2015.

72. D'Urzo, A, Donohue, J, Kardos, P, Miravitlles, M, and Price, D. A re-evaluation of the role of inhaled corticosteroids in the management of patients with chronic obstructive pulmonary disease. *Expert Opin Pharmacother* 16:1845-1860, 2015.

73. Darbee, J, Ohtake, P, Grant, B, and Cerny, F. Physiologic evidence for the efficacy of positive expiratory pressure as an airway clearance technique in patients with cystic fibrosis. *Phys Ther* 84:524-537, 2004.

74. Davidson, T, Murphy, C, Mitchell, M, Smith, C, and Light, M. Management of chronic sinusitis in cystic fibrosis. *Laryngoscope* 105:354-358, 1995.

75. De Brandt, J, Spruit, M, Derave, W, Hansen, D, Vanfleteren, L, and Burtin, C. Changes in structural and metabolic muscle characteristics following exercise-based interventions in patients with COPD: a systematic review. *Expert Rev Respir Med* 10:521-545, 2016.

76. de Man, F, van Hees, H, Handoko, M, Niessen, H, Schalij, I, Humbert, M, Dorfmüller, P, Mercier, O, Bogaard, H, Postmus, P, and Westerhof, N. Diaphragm muscle fiber weakness in pulmonary hypertension. *Am J Respir Crit Care Med* 183:1411-1418, 2011.

77. De Simone, G, Aquino, G, Di Gioia, C, Mazzarella, G, Bianco, A, and Calcagno, G. Efficacy of aerobic physical retraining in a case of combined pulmonary fibrosis and emphysema syndrome: a case report. *J Med Case Rep* 9:85, 2015.

78. Decramer, M, de Bock, V, and Dom, R. Functional and histologic picture of steroid-induced myopathy in chronic obstructive pulmonary disease. *Am J Respir Crit Care Med* 153:1958-1964, 1996.

79. Del Giacco, S, Firinu, D, Bjermer, L, and Carlsen, K. Exercise and asthma: an overview. *Eur Clin Respir J* 2:27984, 2014.

80. Del Giacco, S and Garcia-Larsen, V. Aerobic exercise training reduces bronchial hyper-responsiveness and serum pro-inflammatory cytokines in patients with asthma. *Evid Based Med* 21:70, 2016.

81. Dentice, R, Elkins, M, Middleton, P, Bishop, J, Wark, P, Dorahy, D, Harmer, C, Hu, H, and Bye, P. A randomised trial of hypertonic saline during hospitalisation for exacerbation of cystic fibrosis. *Thorax* 71:141-147, 2016.

82. Di Stefano, A, Capelli, A, Lusuardi, M, Balbo, P, Vecchio, C, Maestrelli, P, Mapp, C, Fabbri, L, Donner, C, and Saetta, M. Severity of airflow limitation is associated with severity of airway inflammation in smokers. *Am J Respir Crit Care Med* 158:1277-1285, 1998.

83. Dodge, J and Turck, D. Cystic fibrosis: nutritional consequences and management. *Best Pract Res Clin Gastroenterol* 20:531-546, 2006.

84. Dogra, S, Kuk, J, Baker, J, and Jamnik, V. Exercise is associated with improved asthma control in adults. *Eur Respir J* 37:318-323, 2011.

85. Domínguez-Muñoz, J. Pancreatic enzyme replacement therapy for pancreatic exocrine insufficiency: when is it indicated, what is the goal and how to do it? *Adv Med Sci* 56:1-5, 2011.

86. Dong, F, Zhang, Y, Chi, F, Song, Q, Zhang, L, Wang, Y, and Che, C. Clinical efficacy and safety of ICS/LABA in patients with combined idiopathic pulmonary fibrosis and emphysema. *Int J Clin Exp Med* 8:8617-8625, 2015.

87. Doull, I. What and when to collect from infants with cystic fibrosis. *Arch Dis Child* 92:831-832, 2007.

88. Dowman, L, Hill, C, and Holland, A. Pulmonary rehabilitation for interstitial lung disease. *Cochrane Database Syst Rev* 10:CD006322, 2014.

89. Drazen, J, Israel, E, and O'Byrne, P. Treatment of asthma with drugs modifying the leukotriene pathway. *N Eng J Med* 340:197-206, 1999.

90. Drugs.com. Azathioprine. www.drugs.com/cdi/azathioprine.html. Accessed February 1, 2017.

91. Drugs.com. Aztreonam inhalation. www.drugs.com/cdi/aztreonam-inhalation.html. Accessed February 1, 2017.

92. Drugs.com. Cyclophosphamide side effects. www.drugs.com/sfx/cyclophosphamide-side-effects.html. Accessed February 1, 2017.

93. Drugs.com. Dornase alfa (inhalation). www.drugs.com/mtm/dornase-alfa-inhalation.html. Accessed February 1, 2017.

94. Drugs.com. Ivacaftor side effects. www.drugs.com/sfx/ivacaftor-side-effects.html. Accessed February 1, 2017.

95. Drugs.com. Medications for asthma. www.drugs.com/condition/asthma.html. Accessed January 30, 2017.

96. Drugs.com. Medications for pulmonary hypertension. www.drugs.com/condition/pulmonary-hypertension.html. Accessed February 1, 2017.

97. Drugs.com. Pancrelipase side effects. www.drugs.com/sfx/pancrelipase-side-effects.html. Accessed February 1, 2017.

98. Drugs.com. Tobramycin. www.drugs.com/cdi/tobramycin.htm. Accessed February 1, 2017.

99. Drzymala-Czyz, S, Jonczyk-Potoczna, K, Lisowska, A, Stajgis, M, and Walkowiak, J. Supplementation of ursodeoxycholic acid improves fat digestion and absorption in cystic fibrosis patients with mild liver involvement. *Eur J Gastroenterol Hepatol* 28:645-649, 2016.

100. Ehsan, Z and Clancy, J. Management of Pseudomonas aeruginosa infection in cystic fibrosis patients using inhaled antibiotics with a focus on nebulized liposomal amikacin. *Future Microbiol* 10:1901-1912, 2015.

101. Eichenberger, P, Diener, S, Kofmehl, R, and Spengler, C. Effects of exercise training on airway hyperreactivity in asthma: a systematic review and meta-analysis. *Sports Med* 43:1157-1170, 2013.

102. Ejiofor, S and Turner, A. Pharmacotherapies for COPD. *Clin Med Insights Circ Respir Pulm Med* 7:17, 2013.

103. Elborn, J, Bell, S, Madge, S, Burgel, P, Castellani, C, Conway, S, De Rijcke, K, Dembski, B, Drevinek, P, Heijerman, H, Innes, J, Lindblad, A, Marshall, B, Olesen, H, Reimann, A, Solé, A, Viviani, L, Wagner, T, Welte, T, and Blasi, F. Report of the European Respiratory Society/European Cystic Fibrosis Society task force on the care of adults with cystic fibrosis. *Eur Respir J* 47:420-428, 2016.

104. Elphick, H and Mallory, G. Oxygen therapy for cystic fibrosis. *Cochrane Database Syst Rev* 7:CD003884, 2013.

105. Equi, A, Balfour-Lynn, I, Bush, A, and Rosenthal, M. Long term azithromycin in children with cystic fibrosis: a randomised, placebo-controlled crossover trial. *Lancet* 360:978-984, 2002.

106. Evans, A, Lewis, S, Ogunbayo, O, and Moral-Sanz, J. Modulation of the LKB1-AMPK signalling pathway underpins hypoxic pulmonary vasoconstriction and pulmonary hypertension. In *Arterial Chemoreceptors in Physiology and Pathophysiology*. Springer International, 89-99, 2015.

107. Eves, N and Davidson, W. Evidence-based risk assessment and recommendations for physical activity clearance: respiratory disease. *Appl Physiol Nutr Metab* 36:S80-S100, 2011.

108. Fabbri, L, Burge, P, Croonenborgh, L, Warlies, F, Weeke, B, Ciaccia, A, and Parker, C. Comparison of fluticasone propionate with beclomethasone dipropionate in moderate to severe asthma treated for one year. *Thorax* 48:817-823, 1993.

109. Fagan, J, Scheff, P, Hryhorczuk, D, Ramakrishan, V, Ross, M, and Persk, V. Prevalence of asthma and other allergic diseases in an adolescent population: association with gender and race. *Ann Allergy Asthma Immunol* 86:177-184, 2001.

110. Fisk, M, Steigerwald, M, Smoliga, J, and Rundell, K. Asthma in swimmers: a review of the current literature. *Phys Sportsmed* 38:28-34, 2010.

111. Flume, P, Mogayzel Jr, P, Robinson, K, Goss, C, Rosenblatt, R, Kuhn, R, Marshall, B, and Clinical Practice Guidelines for Pulmonary Therapies Committee. Cystic fibrosis pulmonary guidelines: treatment of pulmonary exacerbations. *Am J Respir Crit Care Med* 180:802-808, 2009.

112. Flume, P, Robinson, K, O'Sullivan, B, Finder, J, Vender, R, Willey-Courand, D, White, T, Marshall, B, and Clinical Practice Guidelines for Pulmonary Therapies Committee. Cystic fibrosis pulmonary guidelines: airway clearance therapies. *Respir Care* 54:522-537, 2009.

113. Fox, B, Kassirer, M, Weiss, I, Raviv, Y, Peled, N, Shitrit, D, and Kramer, M. Ambulatory rehabilitation improves exercise capacity in patients with pulmonary hypertension. *J Card Fail* 17:196-200, 2011.

114. França-Pinto, A, Mendes, F, de Carvalho-Pinto, R, Agondi, R, Cukier, A, Stelmach, R, Saraiva-Romanholo, B, Kalil, J, Martins, M, Giavina-Bianchi, P, and Carvalho, C. Aerobic training decreases bronchial hyperresponsiveness and systemic inflammation in patients with moderate or severe asthma: a randomised controlled trial. *Thorax* 70:732-739, 2015.

115. Frostell, C, Blomqvist, H, Hedenstierna, G, Lundberg, J, and Zapol, W. Inhaled nitric oxide selectively reverses human hypoxic pulmonary vasoconstriction without causing systemic vasodilation. *Anesthesiology* 78:427-435, 1993.

116. Gaddy, J, Margolskee, D, Bush, R, Williams, V, and Busse, W. Bronchodilation with a potent and selective leukotriene D4 (LTD4) receptor antagonist (MK-571)

in patients with asthma. *Am Rev Respir Dis* 146:358-363, 1992.

117. Galiè, N, Corris, P, Frost, A, Girgis, R, Granton, J, Jing, Z, Klepetko, W, McGoon, M, McLaughlin, V, Preston, I, and Rubin, L. Updated treatment algorithm of pulmonary arterial hypertension. *J Am Coll Cardiol* 25:D60-D72, 2013.

118. Galiè, N, Hoeper, M, Humbert, M, Torbicki, A, Vachiery, J, Barbera, J, Beghetti, M, Corris, P, Gaine, S, Gibbs, J, and Gomez-Sanchez, M. Guidelines for the diagnosis and treatment of pulmonary hypertension. *Eur Heart J* 30:2493-2537, 2009.

119. Galiè, N, Humbert, M, Vachiery, J, Gibbs, S, Lang, I, Torbicki, A, Simonneau, G, Peacock, A, Noordegraaf, A, Beghetti, M, and Ghofrani, A. 2015 ESC/ERS Guidelines for the diagnosis and treatment of pulmonary hypertension. *Eur Heart J* 37:67-119, 2016.

120. Garvey, C, Bayles, M, Hamm, L, Hill, K, Holland, A, Limberg, T, and Spruit, M. Pulmonary rehabilitation exercise prescription in chronic obstructive pulmonary disease: review of selected guidelines: an official statement from the American Association of Cardiovascular and Pulmonary Rehabilitation. *J Cardiopulm Rehabil Prev* 36:75-83, 2016.

121. Gauderman, W, Avol, E, Gilliland, F, Vora, H, Thomas, D, Berhane, K, McConnell, R, Kuenzli, N, Lurmann, F, Rappaport, E, Margolis, H, Bates, D, and Peters, J. The effect of air pollution on lung development from 10 to 18 years of age. *N Engl J Med* 351:1057-1067, 2004.

122. Gaunaurd, I, Gómez-Marín, O, Ramos, C, Sol, C, Cohen, M, Cahalin, L, Cardenas, D, and Jackson, R. Physical activity and quality of life improvements of patients with idiopathic pulmonary fibrosis completing a pulmonary rehabilitation program. *Respir Care* 59:1872-1879, 2014.

123. Gibson, P and Simpson, J. The overlap syndrome of asthma and COPD: what are its features and how important is it? *Thorax* 64:728-735, 2009.

124. Global Initiative for Chronic Obstructive Lung Disease. Global strategy for diagnosis, management, and prevention of COPD. 2016. http://goldcopd.org/global-strategy-diagnosis-management-prevention-copd-2016/. Accessed January 26, 2017.

125. Godfrey, S. Exercise-induced asthma. In *Allergic Diseases from Infancy to Adulthood*. Bierman, C, and Pearlman, D, eds. Philadelphia: Saunders, 597, 1988.

126. Gordon, S, Bruce, N, Grigg, J, Hibberd, P, Kurmi, O, Lam, K, Mortimer, K, Asante, K, Balakrishnan, K, Balmes, J, and Bar-Zeev, N. Respiratory risks from household air pollution in low and middle income countries. *Lancet Respir Med* 2:823-860, 2014.

127. Gosman, M, Willemse, B, Jansen, D, Lapperre, T, van Schadewijk, A, Hiemstra, P, Postma, D, Timens, W, and Kerstjens, H. Increased number of B-cells in bronchial biopsies in COPD. *Eur Respir J* 27:60-64, 2006.

128. Grashoff, W, Sont, J, Sterk, P, Hiemstra, P, de Boer, W, Stolk, J, Han, J, and Van Krieken, J. Chronic obstructive pulmonary disease: role of bronchiolar mast cells and macrophages. *Am J Pathol* 151:1785-1790, 1997.

129. Grassi, V, Carminati, L, Cossi, S, Marengoni, A, and Tantucci, C. Chronic obstructive lung disease. Systemic manifestations. *Recenti Prog Med* 94:217-226, 2003.

130. Greulich, T and Vogelmeier, C. Alpha-1-antitrypsin deficiency: increasing awareness and improving diagnosis. *Ther Adv Respir Dis* 10:72-84, 2016.

131. Gries, C, Bhadriraju, S, Edelman, J, Goss, C, Raghu, G, and Mulligan, M. Obese patients with idiopathic pulmonary fibrosis have a higher 90-day mortality risk with bilateral lung transplantation. *J Heart Lung Transplant* 34:241-246, 2015.

132. Griese, M, App, E, Duroux, A, Burkert, A, and Schams, A. Recombinant human DNase (rhDNase) influences phospholipid composition, surface activity, rheology and consecutively clearance indices of cystic fibrosis sputum. *Pulm Pharmacol Ther* 10:21-27, 1997.

133. Gruber, W, Orenstein, D, Braumann, K, and Hüls, G. Health-related fitness and trainability in children with cystic fibrosis. *Pediatr Pulmonol* 43:953-964, 2008.

134. Grünig, E, Lichtblau, M, Ehlken, N, Ghofrani, H, Reichenberger, F, Staehler, G, Halank, M, Fischer, C, Seyfarth, H, Klose, H, and Meyer, A. Safety and efficacy of exercise training in various forms of pulmonary hypertension. *Eur Respir J* 40:84-92, 2012.

135. Gu, S, Hu, H, and Dong, H. Systematic review of the economic burden of pulmonary arterial hypertension. *PharmacoEconomics* 34:533-550, 2016.

136. Haahtela, T, Järvinen, M, Kava, T, Kiviranta, K, Koskinen, S, Lehtonen, K, Nikander, K, Persson, T, Reinikainen, K, Selroos, O, and Sovijärvi, A. Comparisons of a beta 2-agonist, terbutaline, with an inhaled corticosteroid, budesonide, in newly detected asthma. *N Engl J Med* 325:388-392, 1991.

137. Halank, M, Einsle, F, Lehman, S, Bremer, H, Ewert, R, Wilkens, H, Meyer, F, Grünig, E, Seyfarth, H, Kolditz, M, and Wieder, G. Exercise capacity affects quality of life in patients with pulmonary hypertension. *Lung* 191:337-343, 2013.

138. Hallstrand, T and Henderson Jr, W. An update on the role of leukotrienes in asthma. *Curr Opin Allergy Clin Immunol* 10:60-66, 2010.

139. Hanada, M, Sakamoto, N, Ishimatsu, Y, Kakugawa, T, Obase, Y, Kozu, R, Senjyu, H, Izumikawa, K, Mukae, H, and Kohno, S. Effect of long-term treatment with corticosteroids on skeletal muscle strength, functional exercise capacity and health status in patients with interstitial lung disease. *Respirology* 21:1088-1093, 2016.

140. Haque, R, Hakim, A, Moodley, T, Torrego, A, Essilfie-Quaye, S, Jazrawi, E, Johnson, M, Barnes, P, Adcock, I, and Usmani, O. Inhaled long-acting β2 agonists enhance glucocorticoid receptor nuclear translocation and efficacy in sputum macrophages in COPD. *J Allergy Clin Immunol* 132:1166-1173, 2013.

141. Hasler, E, Müller-Mottet, S, Furian, M, Saxer, S, Huber, L, Maggiorini, M, Speich, R, Bloch, K, and Ulrich, S. Pressure-flow during exercise catheterization predicts survival in pulmonary hypertension. *Chest* 150:57-67, 2016.

142. Health Research Funding. 43 incredible lung transplant survival rate statistics. 2015. http://healthresearchfunding.org/43-incredible-lung-transplant-survival-rate-statistics/. Accessed January 27, 2017.

143. Hebestreit, A, Kersting, U, Basler, B, Jeschke, R, and Hebestreit, H. Exercise inhibits epithelial sodium channels in patients with cystic fibrosis. *Am J Respir Crit Care Med* 164:443-446, 2001.

144. Hebestreit, H, Arets, H, Aurora, P, Boas, S, Cerny, F, Hulzebos, E, Karila, C, Lands, L, Lowman, J, Swisher, A, and Urquhart, D. Statement on exercise testing in cystic fibrosis. *Respiration* 90:332-351, 2015.

145. Hebestreit, H, Kieser, S, Junge, S, Ballmann, M, Hebestreit, A, Schindler, C, Schenk, T, Posselt, H, and Kriemler, S. Long-term effects of a partially supervised conditioning programme in cystic fibrosis. *Eur Respir J* 35:578-583, 2010.

146. Heck, S, Nguyen, J, Le, D, Bals, R, and Dinh, Q. Pharmacological therapy of bronchial asthma: the role of biologicals. *Int Arch Allergy Immunol* 168:241-252, 2016.

147. Herve, P, Lau, E, Sitbon, O, Savale, L, Montani, D, Godinas, L, Lador, F, Jaïs, X, Parent, F, Günther, S, and Humbert, M. Criteria for diagnosis of exercise pulmonary hypertension. *Eur Respir J* 46:728-737, 2015.

148. Higenbottam, T. Pulmonary hypertension and chronic obstructive pulmonary disease: a case for treatment. *Proc Am Thorac Soc* 2:12-19, 2005.

149. Higgins, L, Robertson, R, Kelsey, S, Olson, M, Hoffman, L, Rebovich, P, Haile, L, and Orenstein, D. Exercise intensity self-regulation using the OMNI scale in children with cystic fibrosis. *Pediatr Pulmonol* 48:497-505, 2013.

150. Hoeper, M, Humbert, M, Souza, R, Idrees, M, Kawut, S, Sliwa-Hahnle, K, Jing, Z, and Gibbs, J. A global view of pulmonary hypertension. *Lancet Respir Med* 4:306-322, 2016.

151. Hogg, J, Chu, F, Utokaparch, S, Woods, R, Elliott, W, Buzatu, L, Cherniack, R, Rogers, R, Sciurba, F, Coxson, H, and Paré, P. The nature of small-airway obstruction in chronic obstructive pulmonary disease. *N Engl J Med* 350:2645-2653, 2004.

152. Holland, A. Exercise limitation in interstitial lung disease - mechanisms, significance and therapeutic options. *Chron Respir Dis* 7:101-111, 2010.

153. Holland, A, Dowman, L, and Hill, C. Principles of rehabilitation and reactivation: interstitial lung disease, sarcoidosis and rheumatoid disease with respiratory involvement. *Respiration* 89:89-99, 2015.

154. Holt, P. Infections and the development of allergy. *Toxicol Lett* 86:205-210, 1996.

155. Holt, P, Sly, P, and Bjorksten, B. Atopic versus infectious diseases in childhood: a quesiton of balance? *Pediatr Allergy Immunol* 8:53-58, 1997.

156. Horiguchi, M, Oiso, Y, Sakai, H, Motomura, T, and Yamashita, C. Pulmonary administration of phosphoinositide 3-kinase inhibitor is a curative treatment for chronic obstructive pulmonary disease by alveolar regeneration. *J Control Release* 213:112-119, 2015.

157. Hospers, J, Postma, D, Jijcken, B, Weiss, S, and Schouten, J. Histamine airway hyperresponsiveness and mortality from chronic obstructive pulmonary disease: a cohort study. *Lancet* 356:1313-1317, 2000.

158. Howarth, P. Is allergy increasing?—early life influences. *Clin Exp Allergy* (suppl 6):2-7, 1998.

159. Humbert, M, Sitbon, O, Chaouat, A, Bertocchi, M, Habib, G, Gressin, V, Yaici, A, Weitzenblum, E, Cordier, J, Chabot, F, and Dromer, C. Pulmonary arterial hypertension in France: results from a national registry. *Am J Respir Crit Care Med* 173:1023-1030, 2006.

160. Iepsen, U, Jørgensen, K, Ringbaek, T, Hansen, H, Skrubbeltrang, C, and Lange, P. A systematic review of resistance training versus endurance training in COPD. *J Cardiopulm Rehabil Prev* 35:163-172, 2015.

161. Iheagwara, N and Thomas, T. Pharmacologic treatment of pulmonary hypertension. www.medscape.com/viewarticle/728503_6. Accessed February 1, 2017.

162. Islam, T, Berhane, K, McConnell, R, Gauderman, W, Avol, E, Peters, J, and Gilliland, F. Glutathione-S-transferase (GST) P1, GSTM1, exercise, ozone and asthma incidence in school children. *Thorax* 64:197-202, 2009.

163. Islam, T, Gauderman, W, Berhane, K, McConnell, R, Avol, E, Peters, J, and Gilliland, F. Relationship between air pollution, lung function and asthma in adolescents. *Thorax* 62:957-963, 2007.

164. Israel, E, Cohn, J, Dube, L, and Drazen, J. Effect of treatment with zileuton, a 5-lipoxygenase inhibitor, in patients with asthma. A randomized controlled trial. *JAMA* 275:931-936, 1996.

165. Jiang, Z and Zhu, L. Update on molecular mechanisms of corticosteroid resistance in chronic obstructive pulmonary disease. *Pulm Pharmacol Ther* 37:1-8, 2016.

166. Jones, R and Nzekwu, M. The effects of body mass index on lung volumes. *Chest* 130:827-833, 2006.

167. Joseph, C, Ownby, D, Peterson, E, and Johnson, C. Racial differences in physiologic parameters related to asthma among middle-class children. *Chest* 117:1336-1344, 2000.

168. Kabitz, H, Bremer, H, Schwoerer, A, Sonntag, F, Walterspacher, S, Walker, D, Ehlken, N, Staehler, G, Windisch, W, and Grünig, E. The combination of exercise and respiratory training improves respira-

tory muscle function in pulmonary hypertension. *Lung* 192:321-328, 2014.

169. Karjalainen, E, Laitinen, A, Sue-Chu, M, Altraja, A, Bjermer, L, and Laitinen, L. Evidence of airway inflammation and remodeling in ski athletes with and without bronchial hyperresponsiveness to methacholine. *Am J Respir Crit Care Med* 161:2086-2091, 2000.

170. Kauppi, P, Kupiainen, H, Lindqvist, A, Tammilehto, L, Kilpeläinen, M, Kinnula, V, Haahtela, T, and Laitinen, T. Overlap syndrome of asthma and COPD predicts low quality of life. *Asthma* 48:279-285, 2011.

171. Kholdani, C, Fares, W, and Mohsenin, V. Pulmonary hypertension in obstructive sleep apnea: is it clinically significant? A critical analysis of the association and pathophysiology. *Pulm Circ* 5:220-227, 2015.

172. Kioumis, I, Zarogoulidis, K, Huang, H, Li, Q, Dryllis, G, Pitsiou, G, Machairiotis, N, Katsikogiannis, N, Papaiwannou, A, Lampaki, S, Porpodis, K, Zaric, B, Branislav, P, Mpoukovinas, I, Lazaridis, G, and Zarogoulidis, P. Pneumothorax in cystic fibrosis. *J Thorac Dis* 6:S480-S487, 2014.

173. Klijn, P, Oudshoorn, A, van der Ent, C, van der Net, J, Kimpen, J, and Helders, P. Effects of anaerobic training in children with cystic fibrosis: a randomized controlled study. *Chest* 125:1299-1305, 2004.

174. Kobelska-Dubiel, N, Klincewicz, B, and Cichy, W. Liver disease in cystic fibrosis. *Prz Gastroenterol* 9:136-141, 2014.

175. Koenig, J. Air pollution and asthma. *J Allergy Clin Immunol* 104:717-722, 1999.

176. Krafczyk, M and Asplund, C. Exercise-induced bronchoconstriction: diagnosis and management. *Am Fam Physician* 84:427, 2011.

177. Kriemler, S, Wilk, B, Schurer, W, Wilson, W, and Bar-Or, O. Preventing dehydration in children with cystic fibrosis who exercise in the heat. *Med Sci Sports Exerc* 31:774-779, 1999.

178. Kuk, K and Taylor-Cousar, J. Lumacaftor and ivacaftor in the management of patients with cystic fibrosis: current evidence and future prospects. *Ther Adv Respir Dis* 9:313-326, 2015.

179. Laitinen, L, Laitinen, A, and Haahtela, T. Airway mucosal inflammation even in patients with newly diagnosed asthma. *Am Rev Respir Dis* 147:697-704, 1993.

180. Lama, V and Martinez, F. Resting and exercise physiology in interstitial lung diseases. *Clin Chest Med* 25:435-453, 2004.

181. Lange, P, Parner, J, Vestbo, J, Schnohr, P, and Jensen, G. A 15-year follow-up study of ventilatory function in adults with asthma. *N Engl J Med* 339:1194-1200, 1998.

182. Lannefors, L and Wollmer, P. Mucus clearance with three chest physiotherapy regimes in cystic fibrosis: a comparison between postural drainage, PEP and physical exercise. *Eur Respir J* 5:748-753, 1992.

183. Larsson, L, Hemmingsson, P, and Boethius, G. Self-reported obstructive airway symptoms are common in young cross-country skiers. *Scand J Med Sci Sports* 4:124-127, 1994.

184. Leite, M, Ramos, E, Kalva-Filho, C, Freire, A, de Alencar Silva, B, Nicolino, J, de Toledo-Arruda, A, Papoti, M, Vanderlei, L, and Ramos, D. Effects of 12 weeks of aerobic training on autonomic modulation, mucociliary clearance, and aerobic parameters in patients with COPD. *Int J Chron Obstruct Pulmon Dis* 10:2549-2557, 2015.

185. Leuchte, H, Neurohr, C, Baumgartner, R, Holzapfel, M, Giehrl, W, Vogeser, M, and Behr, J. Brain natriuretic peptide and exercise capacity in lung fibrosis and pulmonary hypertension. *Am J Respir Crit Care Med* 170:360-365, 2004.

186. Leuppi, J, Tandjung, R, Anderson, S, Stolz, D, Brutsche, M, Bingisser, R, Perruchoud, A, Surber, C, Knoblauch, A, Andersson, M, Greiff, L, Chan, H, and Tamm, M. Prediction of treatment-response to inhaled corticosteroids by mannitol-challenge test in COPD. A proof of concept. *Pulm Pharmacol Ther* 18:83-88, 2005.

187. Lima, T, Guimarães, F, Sá Ferreira, A, Penafortes, J, Almeida, V, and Lopes, A. Correlation between posture, balance control, and peripheral muscle function in adults with cystic fibrosis. *Physiother Theory Pract* 30:79-84, 2014.

188. Litonjua, A, Carey, V, Weiss, S, and Gold, D. Race, socioeconomic factors, and area of residence are associated with asthma prevalence. *Pediatr Pulmonol* 28:394-401, 1999.

189. Louie, S, Zeki, A, Schivo, M, Chan, A, Yoneda, K, Avdalovic, M, Morrissey, B, and Albertson, T. The asthma-chronic obstructive pulmonary disease overlap syndrome: pharmacotherapeutic considerations. *Expert Rev Clin Pharmacol* 6:197-219, 2013.

190. Luks, V, Vandemheen, K, and Aaron, S. Confirmation of asthma in an era of overdiagnosis. *Eur Respir J* 36:255-260, 2010.

191. Macchia, A, Marchioli, R, Marfisi, R, Scarano, M, Levantesi, G, Tavazzi, L, and Tognoni, G. A meta-analysis of trials of pulmonary hypertension: a clinical condition looking for drugs and research methodology. *Am Heart J* 153:1037-1047, 2007.

192. Mannino, D, Gagnon, R, Petty, T, and Lydick, E. Obstructive lung disease and low lung function in adults in the United States: data from the National Health and Nutrition Examination Survey, 1988-1994. *Arch Intern Med* 160:1683-1689, 2000.

193. Mannix, E, Farber, M, Palange, P, Galassetti, P, and Manfredi, F. Exercise-induced asthma in figure skaters. *Chest* 109:312-315, 1996.

194. Margaritopoulos, G, Vasarmidi, E, and Antoniou, K. Pirfenidone in the treatment of idiopathic pulmonary fibrosis: an evidence-based review of its place in therapy. *Core Evid* 11:11, 2016.

195. Martiniano, S, Hoppe, J, Sagel, S, and Zemanick, E. Advances in the diagnosis and treatment of cystic fibrosis. *Adv Pediatr* 61:225-243, 2014.

196. Marwick, J, Ito, K, Adcock, I, and Kirkham, P. Oxidative stress and steroid resistance in asthma and COPD: pharmacological manipulation of HDAC-2 as a therapeutic strategy. *Expert Opin Ther Targets* 11:745-755, 2007.

197. Massery, M. Musculoskeletal and neuromuscular interventions: a physical approach to cystic fibrosis. *J R Soc Med* 98(suppl 45):55-66, 2005.

198. Mayo Clinic. Diseases and conditions: asthma. www.mayoclinic.org/diseases-conditions/asthma/in-depth/asthma-medications/art-20045557. Accessed January 30, 2017.

199. McCreanor, J, Cullinan, P, Nieuwenhuijsen, M, Stewart-Evans, J, Malliarou, E, Jarup, L, Harrington, R, Svartengren, M, Han, I, Ohman-Strickland, P, Chung, K, and Zhang, J. Respiratory effects of exposure to diesel traffic in persons with asthma. *N Engl J Med* 357:2348-2358, 2007.

200. McDonald, V, Simpson, J, Higgins, I, and Gibson, P. Multidimensional assessment of older people with asthma and COPD: clinical management and health status. *Age Ageing* 40:42-49, 2011.

201. McGoon, M, Benza, R, Escribano-Subias, P, Jiang, X, Miller, D, Peacock, A, Pepke-Zaba, J, Pulido, T, Rich, S, Rosenkranz, S, and Suissa, S. Pulmonary arterial hypertension: epidemiology and registries. *J Am Coll Cardiol* 62:D51-D59, 2013.

202. McGowan, E, Matsui, E, McCormack, M, Pollack, C, Peng, R, and Keet, C. Effect of poverty, urbanization, and race/ethnicity on perceived food allergy in the United States. *Ann Allergy Asthma Immunol* 115:85-86, 2015.

203. McKenzie, D, McLuckie, S, and Stirling, D. The protective effects of continuous and interval exercise in athletes with exercise-induced asthma. *Med Sci Sports Exerc* 26:951-956, 1994.

204. Medicherla, S, Fitzgerald, M, Spicer, D, Woodman, P, Ma, J, Kapoun, A, Chakravarty, S, Dugar, S, Protter, A, and Higgins, L. P38alpha-selective mitogen-activated protein kinase inhibitor SD-282 reduces inflammation in a subchronic model of tobacco smoke-induced airway inflammation. *J Pharmacol Exp Ther* 324:921-929, 2008.

205. Meltzer, E and Noble, P. Idiopathic pulmonary fibrosis. *Orphanet J Rare Dis* 3:1, 2008.

206. Mereles, D, Ehlken, N, Kreuscher, S, Ghofrani, S, Hoeper, M, Halank, M, Meyer, F, Karger, G, Buss, J, Juenger, J, and Holzapfel, N. Exercise and respiratory training improve exercise capacity and quality of life in patients with severe chronic pulmonary hypertension. *Circulation* 114:1482-1489, 2006.

207. Meyer, F, Lossnitzer, D, Kristen, A, Schoene, A, Kübler, W, Katus, H, and Borst, M. Respiratory muscle dysfunction in idiopathic pulmonary arterial hypertension. *Eur Respir J* 25:125-130, 2005.

208. Mocumbi, A, Thienemann, F, and Sliwa, K. A global perspective on the epidemiology of pulmonary hypertension. *Can J Cardiol* 31:375-381, 2015.

209. Mogayzel, P, Naureckas, E, Robinson, K, Mueller, G, Hadjiliadis, D, Hoag, J, Lubsch, L, Hazle, L, Sabadosa, K, Marshall, B, and Pulmonary Clinical Practice Guidelines Committee. Cystic fibrosis pulmonary guidelines: chronic medications for maintenance of lung health. *Am J Respir Crit Care Med* 187:680-689, 2013.

210. Molis, M and Molis, W. Exercise-induced bronchospasm. *Sports Health* 2:311-317, 2010.

211. Moorcroft, A, Dodd, M, and Webb, A. Exercise testing and prognosis in adult cystic fibrosis. *Thorax* 52:291-293, 1997.

212. Moran, F and Bradley, J. Incorporating exercise into the routine care of individuals with cystic fibrosis: is the time right? *Expert Rev Respir Med* 4:139-142, 2010.

213. Morton, A and Fitch, K. Australian association for exercise and sports science position statement on exercise and asthma. *J Sci Med Sport* 14:312-316, 2011.

214. Naeije, R. Breathing more with weaker respiratory muscles in pulmonary arterial hypertension. *Eur Respir J* 25:6-8, 2005.

215. Nannini, L, Poole, P, Milan, S, Holmes, R, and Normansell, R. Combined corticosteroid and long-acting β2-agonist in one inhaler versus placebo for chronic obstructive pulmonary disease. *Cochrane Database Syst Rev* 11:CD003794, 2013.

216. Nathan, S, du Bois, R, Albera, C, Bradford, W, Costabel, U, Kartashov, A, Noble, P, Sahn, S, Valeyre, D, Weycker, D, and King Jr, T. Validation of test performance characteristics and minimal clinically important difference of the 6-minute walk test in patients with idiopathic pulmonary fibrosis. *Respir Med* 109:914-922, 2015.

217. National Heart, Lung, and Blood Institute. How is COPD treated? 2013. www.nhlbi.nih.gov/health/health-topics/topics/copd/treatment. Accessed January 27, 2017.

218. National Heart, Lung, and Blood Institute. What is COPD? 2014. www.nhlbi.nih.gov/health/health-topics/topics/copd/. Accessed January 27, 2017.

219. Nelson, H, Weiss, S, Bleecker, E, Yancey, S, and Dorinsky, P. The Salmeterol Multicenter Asthma Research Trial: a comparison of usual pharmacotherapy for asthma or usual pharmacotherapy plus salmeterol. *Chest* 129:15-26, 2006.

220. Nici, L, Donner, C, Wouters, E, Zuwallack, R, Ambrosino, N, Bourbeau, J, Carone, M, Celli, B, Engelen, M, Fahy, B, Garvey, C, Goldstein, R, Gosselink, R, Lareau, S, MacIntyre, N, Maltais, F, Morgan, M, O'Donnell, D, Prefault, C, Reardon, J, Rochester, C, Schols, A, Singh, S, and Troosters, T. ATS statement: pulmonary rehabilitation-1999. *Am J Respir Crit Care Med* 159:1666-1682, 1999.

221. Nixon, P, Orenstein, D, and Kelsey, S. Habitual physical activity in children and adolescents with cystic fibrosis. *Med Sci Sports Exerc* 33:30-35, 2001.

222. O'Byrne, P, Bleecker, E, Bateman, E, Busse, W, Woodcock, A, Forth, R, Toler, W, Jacques, L, and Lötvall, J. Once-daily fluticasone furoate alone or combined with vilanterol in persistent asthma. *Eur Respir J* 43:773-782, 2014.

223. O'Donnell, D, Flüge, T, Gerken, F, Hamilton, A, Webb, K, Aguilaniu, B, Make, B, and Magnussen, H. Effects of tiotropium on lung hyperinflation, dyspnoea and exercise tolerance in COPD. *Eur Respir J* 23:832-840, 2004.

224. O'Sullivan, B and Flume, P. The clinical approach to lung disease in patients with cystic fibrosis. *Semin Respir Crit Care Med* 30:505-513, 2009.

225. Oba, Y and Lone, N. Comparative efficacy of inhaled corticosteroid and long-acting beta agonist combinations in preventing COPD exacerbations: a Bayesian network meta-analysis. *Int J Chron Obstruct Pulmon Dis* 9:469-479, 2014.

226. Oda, K, Yatera, K, Fujino, Y, Ishimoto, H, Nakao, H, Hanaka, T, Ogoshi, T, Kido, T, Fushimi, K, Matsuda, S, and Mukae, H. Efficacy of concurrent treatments in idiopathic pulmonary fibrosis patients with a rapid progression of respiratory failure: an analysis of a national administrative database in Japan. *BMC Pulm Med* 16:91, 2016.

227. Orenstein, D, Hovell, M, Mulvihill, M, Keating, K, Hofstetter, C, Kelsey, S, Morris, K, and Nixon, P. Strength vs aerobic training in children with cystic fibrosis: a randomized controlled trial. *Chest* 126:1204-1214, 2004.

228. Panagiotou, M, Peacock, A, and Johnson, M. Respiratory and limb muscle dysfunction in pulmonary arterial hypertension: a role for exercise training? *Pulm Circ* 5:424-434, 2015.

229. Papathanasiou, A and Nakos, G. Why there is a need to discuss pulmonary hypertension other than pulmonary arterial hypertension? *World J Crit Care Med* 4:274-277, 2015.

230. Parasa, R and Maffulli, N. Musculoskeletal involvement in cystic fibrosis. *Bull Hosp Jt Dis* 58:37-44, 1999.

231. Parsons, J, Hallstrand, T, Mastronarde, J, Kaminsky, D, Rundell, K, Hull, J, Storms, W, Weiler, J, Cheek, F, Wilson, K, and Anderson, S. American Thoracic Society subcommittee on exercise-induced bronchoconstriction. *Am J Respir Crit Care Med* 187:1016-1027, 2013.

232. Pastré, J, Prévotat, A, Tardif, C, Langlois, C, Duhamel, A, and Wallaert, B. Determinants of exercise capacity in cystic fibrosis patients with mild-to-moderate lung disease. *BMC Pulm Med* 14:74, 2014.

233. Pedersen, B and Saltin, B. Exercise as medicine—evidence for prescribing exercise as therapy in 26 different chronic diseases. *Scand J Med Sci Sports* 25:1-72, 2015.

234. Pérez, E, Daniels, C, Schroeder, D, St Sauver, J, Hartman, T, Bartholmai, B, Yi, E, and Ryu, J. Incidence, prevalence, and clinical course of idiopathic pulmonary fibrosis: a population-based study. *Chest* 137:129-137, 2010.

235. Pesci, A, Rossi, G, Bertorelli, G, Aufiero, A, Zanon, P, and Olivieri, D. Mast cells in the airway lumen and bronchial mucosa of patients with chronic bronchitis. *Am J Respir Crit Care Med* 149:1311-1316, 1994.

236. Pianosi, P, Leblanc, J, and Almudevar, A. Peak oxygen uptake and mortality in children with cystic fibrosis. *Thorax* 60:50-54, 2005.

237. Porteous, M, Rivera-Lebron, B, Kreider, M, Lee, J, and Kawut, S. Determinants of 6-minute walk distance in patients with idiopathic pulmonary fibrosis undergoing lung transplant evaluation. *Pulm Circ* 6:30-36, 2016.

238. Provost-Craig, M, Arbour, K, Sestilli, D, Chabalko, J, and Ekinol, E. The incidence of exercise-induced bronchospasm in competitive figure skaters. *J Asthma* 33:67-71, 1996.

239. Putman, M, Greenblatt, L, Sicilian, L, Uluer, A, Lapey, A, Sawicki, G, Gordon, C, Bouxsein, M, and Finkelstein, J. Young adults with cystic fibrosis have altered trabecular microstructure by TS-based morphological analysis. *Osteoporos Int* 27:2497-2505, 2016.

240. Radtke, T, Nolan, S, Hebestreit, H, and Kriemler, S. Physical exercise training for cystic fibrosis. *Paediatr Respir Rev* 19:42-45, 2016.

241. Raghu, G, Collard, H, Egan, J, Martinez, F, Behr, J, Brown, K, Colby, T, Cordier, J, Flaherty, K, Lasky, J, and Lynch, D. An official ATS/ERS/JRS/ALAT statement: idiopathic pulmonary fibrosis: evidence-based guidelines for diagnosis and management. *Am J Respir Crit Care Med* 183:788-824, 2011.

242. Ratjen, F and Tullis, E. Cystic fibrosis. In *Clinical Respiratory Medicine: Expert Consult*. 4th ed. Spiro, S, Silvestri, G, and Agusti, A, eds. Philadelphia: Elsevier, 568-579, 2012.

243. Reeves, E, McCarthy, C, McElvaney, O, Vijayan, M, White, M, Dunlea, D, Pohl, K, Lacey, N, and McElvaney, N. Inhaled hypertonic saline for cystic fibrosis: reviewing the potential evidence for modulation of neutrophil signaling and function. *World J Crit Care Med* 4:179-191, 2015.

244. Reix, P, Aubert, F, Werck-Gallois, M, Toutain, A, Mazzocchi, C, Moreux, N, Bellon, G, Rabilloud, M, and Kassai, B. Exercise with incorporated expiratory manoeuvres was as effective as breathing techniques for airway clearance in children with cystic fibrosis: a randomised crossover trial. *J Physiother* 58:241-247, 2012.

245. Richeldi, L, Cottin, V, du Bois, R, Selman, M, Kimura, T, Bailes, Z, Schlenker-Herceg, R, Stowasser, S, and Brown, K. Nintedanib in patients with idiopathic pulmonary fibrosis: combined evidence from the TOMORROW and INPULSIS® trials. *Respir Med* 113:74-79, 2016.

246. Rijcken, B, Schouten, J, Xu, X, Rosner, B, and Weiss, S. Airway hyperresponsiveness to histamine associated with accelerated decline in FEV1. *Am J Respir Crit Care Med* 151:1377-1382, 1995.

247. Rowan, S, Keane, M, Gaine, S, and McLoughlin, P. Hypoxic pulmonary hypertension in chronic lung diseases: novel vasoconstrictor pathways. *Lancet Respir Med* 4:225-236, 2016.

248. Rundell, K, Anderson, S, Sue-Chu, M, Bougault, V, and Boulet, L. Air quality and temperature effects on exercise-induced bronchoconstriction. *Compr Physiol* 5:579-610, 2015.

249. Rundell, K and Slee, J. Exercise and other indirect challenges to demonstrate asthma or exercise-induced bronchoconstriction in athletes. *J Allergy Clin Immunol* 122:238-246, 2008.

250. Rundell, K, Spiering, B, Baumann, J, and Evans, T. Effects of montelukast on airway narrowing from eucapnic voluntary hyperventilation and cold air exercise. *Br J Sports Med* 39:232-236, 2005.

251. Rundell, K and Sue-Chu, M. Air quality and exercise-induced bronchoconstriction in elite athletes. *Immunol Allergy Clin North Am* 33:409-421, 2013.

252. Rundell, K, Wilber, R, Szmedra, L, Jenkinson, D, Mayers, L, and Im, J. Exercise-induced asthma screening of elite athletes: field versus laboratory exercise challenge. *Med Sci Sports Exerc* 32:309-316, 2000.

253. Saglam, M, Arikan, H, Vardar-Yagli, N, Calik-Kutukcu, E, Inal-Ince, D, Savci, S, Akdogan, A, Yokusoglu, M, Kaya, E, and Tokgozoglu, L. Inspiratory muscle training in pulmonary arterial hypertension. *J Cardiopulm Rehabil Prev* 35:198-206, 2015.

254. Sahin, H, Naz, I, Varol, Y, Aksel, N, Tuksavul, F, and Ozsoz, A. Is a pulmonary rehabilitation program effective in COPD patients with chronic hypercapnic failure? *Expert Rev Respir Med* 10:593-598, 2016.

255. Sahlberg, M, Svantesson, U, Thomas, E, and Strandvik, B. Muscular strength and function in patients with cystic fibrosis. *Chest* 127:1587-1592, 2005.

256. Saiman, L, Mayer-Hamblett, N, Anstead, M, Lands, L, Kloster, M, Goss, C, Rose, L, Burns, J, Marshall, B, and Ratjen, F. Open-label, follow-on study of azithromycin in pediatric patients with CF uninfected with Pseudomonas aeruginosa. *Pediatr Pulmonol* 47:641-648, 2012.

257. Salvi, S and Barnes, P. Chronic obstructive pulmonary disease in non-smokers. *Lancet* 374:733-743, 2009.

258. Scherr, A, Schafroth Török, S, Jochmann, A, Miedinger, D, Maier, S, Taegtmeyer, A, Chhajed, P, Tamm, M, and Leuppi, J. Response to add-on inhaled corticosteroids in COPD based on airway hyperresponsiveness to mannitol. *Chest* 42:919-926, 2012.

259. Schneiderman-Walker, J, Pollock, S, Corey, M, Wilkes, D, Canny, G, Pedder, L, and Reisman, J. A randomized controlled trial of a 3-year home exercise program in cystic fibrosis. *J Pediatr* 136:304-310, 2000.

260. Schupp, J, Köhler, T, and Müller-Quernheim, J. Usefulness of cyclophosphamide pulse therapy in interstitial lung diseases. *Respiration* 91:296-301, 2016.

261. Selvadurai, H, Blimkie, C, Meyers, N, Mellis, C, Cooper, P, and Van Asperen, P. Randomized controlled study of in-hospital exercise training programs in children with cystic fibrosis. *Pediatr Pulmonol* 33:194-200, 2002.

262. Selvaggio, A and Noble, P. Pirfenidone initiates a new era in the treatment of idiopathic pulmonary fibrosis. *Annu Rev Med* 67:487-495, 2016.

263. Seys, S, Hox, V, Van Gerven, L, Dilissen, E, Marijsse, G, Peeters, E, Dekimpe, E, Kasran, A, Aertgeerts, S, Troosters, T, Vanbelle, V, Peers, K, Ceuppens, J, Hellings, P, Dupont, L, and Bullens, D. Damage-associated molecular pattern and innate cytokine release in the airways of competitive swimmers. *Allergy* 70:187-194, 2015.

264. Shoemaker, M, Hurt, H, and Arndt, L. The evidence regarding exercise training in the management of cystic fibrosis: a systematic review. *Cardiopulm Phys Ther J* 19:75-83, 2008.

265. Sin, D, Johnson, M, Gan, W, and Man, S. Combination therapy of inhaled corticosteroids and long-acting beta2-adrenergics in management of patients with chronic obstructive pulmonary disease. *Curr Pharm Des* 10:3547-3560, 2004.

266. Sin, D and Man, S. Chronic obstructive pulmonary disease as a risk factor for cardiovascular morbidity and mortality. *Proc Am Thorac Soc* 2:8-11, 2005.

267. Singh, P, Schaefer, A, Parsek, M, Moninger, T, Welsh, M, and Greenberg, E. Quorum-sensing signals indicate that cystic fibrosis lungs are infected with bacterial biofilms. *Nature* 407:762-764, 2000.

268. Solomon, M, Bozic, M, and Mascarenhas, M. Nutritional issues in cystic fibrosis. *Clin Chest Med* 37:97-107, 2016.

269. Sood, A, Petersen, H, Blanchette, C, Meek, P, Belinsky, S, Picchi, M, and Tesfaigzi, Y. Wood smoke-associated chronic obstructive pulmonary disease (COPD)—underappreciated in the United States? *Am J Respir Crit Care Med* 179:A4742, 2009.

270. Soriano, J, Davis, K, Coleman, B, Visick, G, Mannino, D, and Pride, N. The proportional Venn diagram of obstructive lung disease: two approximations from the United States and the United Kingdom. *Chest* 124:474-481, 2003.

271. Soriano, J, Visick, G, Muellerova, H, Payvandi, N, and Hansell, A. Patterns of comorbidities in newly diagnosed COPD and asthma in primary care. *Chest* 128:2099-2107, 2005.

272. Spruit, M, Singh, S, Garvey, C, ZuWallack, R, Nici, L, Rochester, C, Hill, K, Holland, A, Lareau, S, Man, W, and Pitta, F. An official American Thoracic Society/European Respiratory Society statement: key concepts and advances in pulmonary rehabilitation. *Am J Respir Crit Care Med* 188:e13-e64, 2013.

273. Staggenborg, A. Restrictive pulmonary disorders: an overview. 2009. www.westernschools.com/Portals/0/html/H8377/bwVJFC_files/OEBPS/Text/Section0003.html. Accessed January 27, 2017.

274. Stanbury, R and Graham, E. Systemic corticosteroid therapy—side effects and their management. *Br J Ophthalmol* 82:704-708, 1998.

275. Steiner, M and Preston, I. Optimizing endothelin receptor antagonist use in the management of pulmonary arterial hypertension. *Vasc Health Risk Manag* 4:943-952, 2008.

276. Stickland, M, Rowe, B, Spooner, C, Vandermeer, B, and Dryden, D. Effect of warm-up exercise on exercise-induced bronchoconstriction. *Med Sci Sports Exerc* 44:389-391, 2012.

277. Stirling, D, Cotton, D, Graham, B, Hodgson, W, Cockcroft, D, and Dosman, J. Characteristics of airway tone during exercise in patients with asthma. *J Appl Physiol* 54:934-942, 1983.

278. Strannegard, O and Strannegard, I. Why is the prevalence of allergy increasing? Changed microbial load is probably the cause. *Lakartidningen* 96:4306-4312, 1999.

279. Strookappe, B, Elfferich, M, Swigris, J, Verschoof, A, Veschakelen, J, Knevel, T, and Drent, M. Benefits of physical training in patients with idiopathic or end-stage sarcoidosis-related pulmonary fibrosis: a pilot study. *Sarcoidosis Vasc Diffuse Lung Dis* 32:43-52, 2015.

280. Sue-Chu, M, Karjalainen, E, Laitinen, A, Larsson, L, Laitinen, L, and Bjermer, L. Placebo-controlled study of inhaled budesonide on indices of airway inflammation in bronchoalveolar lavage fluid and bronchial biopsies in cross-country skiers. *Respiration* 67:417-425, 2000.

281. Sue-Chu, M, Larsson, L, Moen, T, Rennard, S, and Bjermer, L. Bronchoscopy and bronchoalveolar lavage findings in cross-country skiers with and without "ski-asthma." *Eur Respir J* 13:626-632, 1999.

282. Tan, C, Xuan, L, Cao, S, Yu, G, Hou, Q, and Wang, H. Decreased histone deacetylase 2 (HDAC2) in peripheral blood monocytes (PBMCs) of COPD patients. *PloS One* 11:e0147380, 2016.

283. Tarran, R, Donaldson, S, and Boucher, R. Rationale for hypertonic saline therapy for cystic fibrosis lung disease. *Semin Respir Crit Care Med* 28:295-302, 2007.

284. Tashkin, D, Altose, M, Connett, J, Kanner, R, Lee, W, and Wise, R. Methacholine reactivity predicts changes in lung function over time in smokers with early chronic obstructive pulmonary disease. The Lung Health Study Research Group. *Am J Respir Crit Care Med* 153:1802-1811, 1996.

285. Tashkin, D and Fabbri, L. Long-acting beta-agonists in the management of chronic obstructive pulmonary disease: current and future agents. *Respir Res* 11:149, 2010.

286. Tashkin, D and Murray, R. Smoking cessation in chronic obstructive pulmonary disease. *Respir Med* 103:963-974, 2009.

287. Turchetta, A, Salerno, T, Lucidi, V, Libera, F, Cutrera, R, and Bush, A. Usefulness of a program of hospital-supervised physical training in patients with cystic fibrosis. *Pediatr Pulmonol* 38:115-118, 2004.

288. Urquhart, D and Vendrusculo, F. Clinical interpretation of cardiopulmonary exercise testing in cystic fibrosis and implications for exercise counselling. *Paediatr Respir Rev*, 2015. [e-pub ahead of print].

289. Vainshelboim, B, Fox, B, Kramer, M, Izhakian, S, Gershman, E, and Oliveira, J. Short-term improvement in physical activity and body composition after supervised exercise training program in idiopathic pulmonary fibrosis. *Arch Phys Med Rehabil* 97:788-797, 2016.

290. Vainshelboim, B, Fox, B, Oliveira, J, and Kramer, M. Exercise training in idiopathic pulmonary fibrosis. *Expert Rev Respir Med* 10:69-77, 2016.

291. Vainshelboim, B, Oliveira, J, Fox, B, Adir, Y, Ollech, J, and Kramer, M. Physiological profile and limitations in exercise in idiopathic pulmonary fibrosis. *J Cardiopulm Rehabil Prev* 36:270-278, 2016.

292. Vainshelboim, B, Oliveira, J, Fox, B, and Kramer, M. The prognostic role of ventilatory inefficiency and exercise capacity in idiopathic pulmonary fibrosis. *Respir Care* 61:1100-1109, 2016.

293. Vainshelboim, B, Oliveira, J, Fox, B, Soreck, Y, Fruchter, O, and Kramer, M. Long-term effects of a 12-week exercise training program on clinical outcomes in idiopathic pulmonary fibrosis. *Lung* 193:345-354, 2015.

294. Vainshelboim, B, Oliveira, J, Yehoshua, L, Weiss, I, Fox, B, Fruchter, O, and Kramer, M. Exercise training-based pulmonary rehabilitation program is clinically beneficial for idiopathic pulmonary fibrosis. *Respiration* 88:378-388, 2014.

295. van Doorn, N. Exercise programs for children with cystic fibrosis: a systematic review of randomized controlled trials. *Disabil Rehabil* 32:41-49, 2010.

296. van Essen-Zandvliet, E, Hughes, M, Waalkens, H, Duiverman, E, Pocock, S, and Kerrebijn, K. Effects of 22 months of treatment with inhaled corticosteroids and/or beta-2-agonists on lung function, airway responsiveness, and symptoms in children with asthma. *Am Rev Respir Dis* 146:547-554, 1992.

297. van Staa, T, Cooper, C, Leufkens, H, and Bishop, N. Children and the risk of fractures caused by oral corticosteroids. *J Bone Miner Res* 18:913-918, 2003.

298. Vazquez-Levin, M, Kupchik, G, Torres, Y, Chaparro, C, Shtainer, A, Bonforte, R, and Nagler, H. Cystic fibrosis and congenital agenesis of the vas deferens, antisperm antibodies and CF-genotype. *J Reprod Immunol* 27:199-212, 1994.

299. Vignaud, H, Cullin, C, and Bouchecareilh, M. Alpha-1 antitrypsin deficiency: a model of alteration of protein homeostasis or proteostasis. *Rev Mal Respir* 32:1059-1071, 2015.

300. Villaça, D, Lerario, M, Dal Corso, S, and Neder, J. New treatments for chronic obstructive pulmonary disease using ergogenic aids. *J Bras Pneumol* 32:66-74, 2006.

301. Volmer, T. The socio-economics of asthma. *Pulm Pharmacol Ther* 14:55-60, 2001.

302. Von Kries, R, Hermann, M, Grunert, V, and Von Mutius, E. Is obesity a risk factor for childhood asthma? *Allergy* 56:318-322, 2001.

303. Wang, C, Chou, P, Joa, W, Chen, L, Sheng, T, Ho, S, Lin, H, Huang, C, Chung, F, Chung, K, and Kuo, H. Mobile-phone-based home exercise training program decreases systemic inflammation in COPD: a pilot study. *BMC Pulm Med* 14:142, 2014.

304. Wark, P, McDonald, V, and Jones, A. Nebulised hypertonic saline for cystic fibrosis. *Cochrane Database Syst Rev* 3:CD001506, 2005.

305. WebMD. Anticholinergics for chronic obstructive pulmonary disease (COPD). www.webmd.com/lung/copd/anticholinergics-for-chronic-obstructive-pulmonary-disease-copd. Accessed January 30, 2017.

306. WebMD. Beta2-agonists for chronic obstructive pulmonary disease (COPD). www.webmd.com/lung/copd/beta2-agonists-for-chronic-obstructive-pulmonary-disease-copd. Accessed February 1, 2017.

307. WebMD. COPD (chronic obstructive pulmonary disease) - medications. www.webmd.com/lung/copd/tc/chronic-obstructive-pulmonary-disease-copd-medications. Accessed January 30, 2017.

308. WebMD. Corticosteroids for chronic obstructive pulmonary disease (COPD). www.webmd.com/lung/copd/corticosteroids-for-chronic-obstructive-pulmonary-disease-copd. Accessed February 1, 2017.

309. Weiler, J, Anderson, S, Randolph, C, Bonini, S, Craig, T, Pearlman, D, Rundell, K, Silvers, W, Storms, W, Bernstein, D, Blessing-Moore, J, Cox, L, Khan, D, Lang, D, Nicklas, R, Oppenheimer, J, Portnoy, J, Schuller, D, Spector, S, Tilles, S, Wallace, D, Henderson, W, Schwartz, L, Kaufman, D, Nsouli, T, Shieken, L, and Rosario, N. Pathogenesis, prevalence, diagnosis, and management of exercise-induced bronchoconstriction: a practice parameter. *Ann Allergy Asthma Immunol* 105:S1-S47, 2010.

310. Weiler, J, Layton, T, and Hunt, M. Asthma in United States Olympic athletes who participated in the 1996 summer games. *J Allergy Clin Immunol* 102:722-726, 1998.

311. Weinstein, A, Chin, L, Keyser, R, Kennedy, M, Nathan, S, Woolstenhulme, J, Connors, G, and Chan, L. Effect of aerobic exercise training on fatigue and physical activity in patients with pulmonary arterial hypertension. *Respir Med* 107:778-784, 2013.

312. Wensel, R, Francis, D, Meyer, F, Opitz, C, Bruch, L, Halank, M, Winkler, J, Seyfarth, H, Gläser, S, Blumberg, F, and Obst, A. Incremental prognostic value of cardiopulmonary exercise testing and resting haemodynamics in pulmonary arterial hypertension. *Int J Cardiol* 167:1193-1198, 2013.

313. Wilber, R, Rundell, K, Szmedra, L, Jenkinson, D, Im, J, and Drake, S. Incidence of exercise-induced bronchospasm in Olympic winter sport athletes. *Med Sci Sports Exerc* 32:732-737, 2000.

314. Williams, P and Shapiro, G. Asthma in children. In *Conn's Current Therapy 1995*. Rakel, R, ed. Philadelphia: Saunders, 682-691, 1995.

315. Wilschanski, M and Durie, P. Patterns of GI disease in adulthood associated with mutations in the CFTR gene. *Gut* 56:1153-1163, 2007.

316. Wollin, L, Wex, E, Pautsch, A, Schnapp, G, Hostettler, K, Stowasser, S, and Kolb, M. Mode of action of nintedanib in the treatment of idiopathic pulmonary fibrosis. *Eur Respir J* 45:1434-1445, 2015.

317. Wood-Baker, R, Walters, J, and Walters, E. Systemic corticosteroids in chronic obstructive pulmonary disease: an overview of Cochrane systematic reviews. *Respir Med* 101:371-377, 2007.

318. Yakubovich, A, Cluver, L, and Gie, R. Socioeconomic factors associated with asthma prevalence and severity among children living in low-income South African communities. *S Afr Med J* 106:404-412, 2016.

319. Yuan, P, Yuan, X, Sun, X, Pudasaini, B, Liu, J, and Hu, Q. Exercise training for pulmonary hypertension: a systematic review and meta-analysis. *Int J Cardiol* 178:142-146, 2015.

320. Yusen, R, Edwards, L, Kucheryavaya, A, Benden, C, Dipchand, A, Goldfarb, S, Levvey, B, Lund, L, Meiser, B, Rossano, J, and Stehlik, J. The registry of the International Society for Heart and Lung Transplantation: thirty-second official adult lung and heart-lung transplantation report—2015; focus theme: early graft failure. *J Heart Lung Transplant* 34:1264-1277, 2015.

321. Zach, M, Oberwaldner, B, and Hausler, F. Cystic fibrosis: physical exercise versus chest physiotherapy. *Arch Dis Child* 57:587-589, 1982.

322. Zach, M, Purrer, B, and Oberwaldner, B. Effect of swimming on forced expiration and sputum clearance in cystic fibrosis. *Lancet* 2:1201-1203, 1981.

323. Zambom-Ferraresi, F, Cebollero, P, Gorostiaga, E, Hernández, M, Hueto, J, Cascante, J, Rezusta, L, Val, L, and Anton, M. Effects of combined resistance and endurance training versus resistance training alone on strength, exercise capacity, and quality of life in patients with COPD. *J Cardiopulm Rehabil Prev* 35:446-453, 2015.

Chapter 6 Cardiovascular Conditions and Disorders

1. Adams, V, Doring, C, and Schuler, G. Impact of physical exercise on alterations in the skeletal muscle in patients with chronic heart failure. *Front Biosci* 13:302-311, 2008.

2. American College of Sports Medicine. American College of Sports Medicine position stand. Progression models in resistance training for healthy adults. *Med Sci Sports Exerc* 41:687-708, 2009.

3. American College of Sports Medicine. *ACSM's Guidelines for Exercise Testing and Prescription.* 9th ed. Baltimore: Lippincott Williams & Wilkins, 2013.

4. American Heart Association. Types of Blood Pressure Medications. www.heart.org/HEARTORG/Conditions/HighBloodPressure/PreventionTreatmentof-HighBloodPressure/Types-of-Blood-Pressure-Medications_UCM_303247_Article.jsp#.VsX7Mk32YdU. Accessed January 7, 2017.

5. American Heart Association. High Blood Pressure. Statistical Fact Sheet 2013 Update. 2013. www.heart.org/idc/groups/heart-public/@wcm/@sop/@smd/documents/downloadable/ucm_319587.pdf. Accessed March 7, 2015.

6. Anderson, JL, Halperin, JL, Albert, NM, Bozkurt, B, Brindis, RG, Curtis, LH, DeMets, D, Guyton, RA, Hochman, JS, and Kovacs, RJ. Management of patients with peripheral artery disease (compilation of 2005 and 2011 ACCF/AHA guideline recommendations). *Circulation* 127:1425-1443, 2013.

7. Ben-Dor, I and Battler, A. Treatment of stable angina. *Heart* 93:868-874, 2007.

8. Bittner, V. Angina pectoris: reversal of the gender gap. *Circulation* 117:1505-1507, 2008.

9. Blumenthal, JA, Sherwood, A, Gullette, EC, Babyak, M, Waugh, R, Georgiades, A, Craighead, LW, Tweedy, D, Feinglos, M, Appelbaum, M, Hayano, J, and Hinderliter, A. Exercise and weight loss reduce blood pressure in men and women with mild hypertension: effects on cardiovascular, metabolic, and hemodynamic functioning. *Arch Intern Med* 160:1947-1958, 2000.

10. Bolooki, HM and Askari, A. Acute Myocardial Infarction. 2010. www.clevelandclinicmeded.com/medical-pubs/diseasemanagement/cardiology/acute-myocardial-infarction/. Accessed January 8, 2017.

11. Brawner, C and Lewis, B. Pacemakers and implantable cardioverter defibrillators. In *ACSM's Exercise Management for Persons with Chronic Diseases and Disabilities.* 4th ed. Durstine, JL, Moore, GE, Painter, PL, and Roberts, SO, eds. Champaign, IL: Human Kinetics, 149-154, 2016.

12. Brubaker, PH and Myers, JN. Chronic heart failure. In *ACSM's Exercise Management for Persons With Chronic Diseases and Disabilities.* 4th ed. Moore, G, Durstine, J, and Painter, P, eds. Champaign, IL: Human Kinetics, 135-142, 2009.

13. Camm, AJ, Kirchhof, P, Lip, GY, Schotten, U, Savelieva, I, Ernst, S, Van Gelder, IC, Al-Attar, N, Hindricks, G, and Prendergast, B. Guidelines for the management of atrial fibrillation: the Task Force for the Management of Atrial Fibrillation of the European Society of Cardiology (ESC). *Eur Heart J* 31:2369-2429, 2010.

14. Carretero, OA and Oparil, S. Essential hypertension. Part I: definition and etiology. *Circulation* 101:329-335, 2000.

15. Colilla, S, Crow, A, Petkun, W, Singer, DE, Simon, T, and Liu, X. Estimates of current and future incidence and prevalence of atrial fibrillation in the U.S. adult population. *Am J Cardiol* 112:1142-1147, 2013.

16. Contractor, AS, Gordon, TL, and Gordon, NF. Hypertension. In *Clinical Exercise Physiology.* 3rd ed. Ehrman, JK, Gordon, PM, Visich, PS, and Keteyian, SJ, eds. Champaign, IL: Human Kinetics, 137-154, 2013.

17. Cook, C, Cole, G, Asaria, P, Jabbour, R, and Francis, DP. The annual global economic burden of heart failure. *Int J Cardiol* 171:368-376, 2014.

18. Cooper, C, Dolezal, B, Durstine, J, Gordon, B, Pinkstaff, S, Babu, A, and Phillips, S. Chronic conditions very strongly associated with tobacco. In *ACSM's Exercise Management for Persons With Chronic Diseases and Disabilities.* 4th ed. Moore, G, Durstine, J, and Painter, P, eds. Champaign, IL: Human Kinetics, 95-114, 2016.

19. Durstine, J, Moore, G, Painter, P, Macko, R, Gordon, B, and Kraus, W. Chronic conditions strongly associated with physical inactivity. In *ACSM's Exercise Management for Persons with Chronic Diseases and Disabilities.* 4th ed. Moore, G, Durstine, J, and Painter, P, eds. Champaign, IL: Human Kinetics, 71-94, 2016.

20. Esler, M. The sympathetic system and hypertension. *Am J Hypertens* 13:99S-105S, 2000.

21. Franklin, B. Myocardial infarction. In *ACSM's Exercise Management for Persons with Chronic Diseases and Disabilities.* Durstine, JL, Moore, GE, Painter, PL, and Roberts, SO, eds. Champaign, IL: Human Kinetics, 49-57, 2009.

22. Franklin, B. Revascularization: CABGS and PTCA or PCI. In *ACSM's Exercise Management for Persons with Chronic Diseases and Disabilities.* Durstine, JL, Moore, GE, Painter, PL, and Roberts, SO, eds. Champaign, IL: Human Kinetics, 58-65, 2009.

23. Graham, TE and Spriet, LL. Metabolic, catecholamine, and exercise performance responses to various doses of caffeine. *J Appl Physiol (1985)* 78:867-874, 1995.

24. Hamer, M, Taylor, A, and Steptoe, A. The effect of acute aerobic exercise on stress related blood pressure responses: a systematic review and meta-analysis. *Biol Psychol* 71:183-190, 2006.

25. James, PA, Oparil, S, Carter, BL, Cushman, WC, Dennison-Himmelfarb, C, Handler, J, Lackland, DT, LeFevre, ML, MacKenzie, TD, Ogedegbe, O, Smith, SC, Jr, Svetkey, LP, Taler, SJ, Townsend, RR, Wright, JT, Jr, Narva, AS, and Ortiz, E. 2014 evidence-based guideline for the management of high blood pressure in adults: report from the panel members appointed to the Eighth Joint National Committee (JNC 8). *JAMA* 311:507-520, 2014.

26. Jones, DW and Hall, JE. Seventh report of the Joint National Committee on Prevention, Detection, Evaluation, and Treatment of High Blood Pressure and evidence from new hypertension trials. *Hypertension* 43:1-3, 2004.

27. Kawano, H, Tanaka, H, and Miyachi, M. Resistance training and arterial compliance: keeping the benefits while minimizing the stiffening. *J Hypertens* 24:1753-1759, 2006.

28. Keteyian, S. General principles of pharmacology. In *Clinical Exercise Physiology.* 3rd ed. Ehrman, JK, Gordon, PM, Visich, PS, and Keteyian, SJ, eds. Champaign, IL: Human Kinetics, 33-44, 2013.

29. Keteyian, S. High intensity interval training in patients with cardiovascular disease: a brief review of physiologic adaptations and suggestions for future research. *Clin Exerc Physiol* 2:12-19, 2013.

30. Keteyian, SJ. Chronic heart failure. In *Clinical Exercise Physiology.* 3rd ed. Ehrman, JK, Gordon, PM, Visich, PS, and Keteyian, SJ, eds. Champaign, IL: Human Kinetics, 259-276, 2013.

31. Keteyian, SJ, Hibner, BA, Bronsteen, K, Kerrigan, D, Aldred, HA, Reasons, LM, Saval, MA, Brawner, CA, Schairer, JR, Thompson, TM, Hill, J, McCulloch, D, and Ehrman, JK. Greater improvement in cardiorespiratory fitness using higher-intensity interval training in the standard cardiac rehabilitation setting. *J Cardiopulm Rehabil Prev* 34:98-105, 2014.

32. Lesho, EP, Manngold, J, and Gey, DC. Management of peripheral arterial disease. *Am Fam Physician* 69, 525-532, 2004.

33. Mampuya, WM. Cardiac rehabilitation past, present and future: an overview. *Cardiovasc Diagn Ther* 2:38-49, 2012.

34. Manire, J, Kipp, R, and Hagerman, P. Compendium of resistance training exercise. In *Resistance Training for Special Populations.* Swank, AM, and Hagerman, P, eds. New York: Delmar Cengage, 2010.

35. Mays, RJ, Casserly, IP, and Regensteiner, JG. Peripheral artery disease. In *Clinical Exercise Physiology.* 3rd ed. Ehrman, JK, Gordon, PM, Visich, PS, and Keteyian, SJ, eds. Champaign, IL: Human Kinetics, 277-296, 2013.

36. Moholdt, T, Aamot, IL, Granoien, I, Gjerde, L, Myklebust, G, Walderhaug, L, Brattbakk, L, Hole, T, Graven, T, Stolen, TO, Amundsen, BH, Molmen-Hansen, HE, Stoylen, A, Wisloff, U, and Slordahl, SA. Aerobic interval training increases peak oxygen uptake more than usual care exercise training in myocardial infarction patients: a randomized controlled study. *Clin Rehabil* 26:33-44, 2012.

37. Montalescot, G, Andersen, HR, Antoniucci, D, Betriu, A, de Boer, MJ, Grip, L, Neumann, FJ, and Rothman, MT. Recommendations on percutaneous coronary intervention for the reperfusion of acute ST elevation myocardial infarction. *Heart* 90:e37, 2004.

38. Moore, GE, Painter, PL, Lyerly, GW, and Durstine, JL. Managing exercise in persons with multiple chronic conditions. In *ACSM's Exercise Management for Persons with Chronic Diseases and Disabilities.* Durstine, JL, Moore, GE, Painter, PL, and Roberts, SO, eds. Champaign, IL: Human Kinetics, 31-37, 2009.

39. Mozaffarian, D, Benjamin, EJ, Go, AS, Arnett, DK, Blaha, MJ, Cushman, M, de Ferranti, S, Despres, JP, Fullerton, HJ, Howard, VJ, Huffman, MD, Judd, SE, Kissela, BM, Lackland, DT, Lichtman, JH, Lisabeth, LD, Liu, S, Mackey, RH, Matchar, DB, McGuire, DK, Mohler, ER, 3rd, Moy, CS, Muntner, P, Mussolino, ME, Nasir, K, Neumar, RW, Nichol, G, Palaniappan, L, Pandey, DK, Reeves, MJ, Rodriguez, CJ, Sorlie, PD, Stein, J, Towfighi, A, Turan, TN, Virani, SS, Willey, JZ, Woo, D, Yeh, RW, and Turner, MB. Heart disease and stroke statistics--2015 update: a report from the American Heart Association. *Circulation* 131:e29-e322, 2015.

40. Murphy, S, Xu, J, and Kochanek, K. Deaths: final data for 2010. *Natl Vital Stat Rep* 61:1-117, 2013.

41. Myers, J and Atwood, J. Atrial fibrillation. In *ACSM's Exercise Management for Persons with Chronic Diseases and Disabilities.* 4th ed. Durstine, JL, Moore, GE, Painter, PL, and Roberts, SO, eds. Champaign, IL: Human Kinetics, 143-148, 2016.

42. National Health Services. Treating atrial fibrillation. 2015. www.nhs.uk/Conditions/Atrial-fibrillation/Pages/Treatment.aspx. Accessed November 11, 2016.

43. Parker, M. Valvular heart disease. In *ACSM's Exercise Management for Persons With Chronic Diseases and Disabilities.* 4th ed. Moore, G, Durstine, J, and Painter, P, eds. Champaign, IL: Human Kinetics, 155-162, 2016.

44. Patterson, MA. Revascularization of the heart. In *Clinical Exercise Physiology.* 3rd ed. Ehrman, JK, Gordon, PM, Visich, PS, and Keteyian, SJ, eds. Champaign, IL: Human Kinetics, 239-258, 2013.

45. Pescatello, LS, Franklin, BA, Fagard, R, Farquhar, WB, Kelley, GA, and Ray, CA. American College of Sports Medicine position stand. Exercise and hypertension. *Med Sci Sports Exerc* 36:533-553, 2004.

46. Pina, IL, Apstein, CS, Balady, GJ, Belardinelli, R, Chaitman, BR, Duscha, BD, Fletcher, BJ, Fleg, JL, Myers, JN, and Sullivan, MJ. Exercise and heart failure: a statement from the American Heart Association Committee on exercise, rehabilitation, and prevention. *Circulation* 107:1210-1225, 2003.

47. Reininger, AJ, Bernlochner, I, Penz, SM, Ravanat, C, Smethurst, P, Farndale, RW, Gachet, C, Brandl, R, and Siess, W. A 2-step mechanism of arterial thrombus formation induced by human atherosclerotic plaques. *J Am Coll Cardiol* 55:1147-1158, 2010.

48. Sacks, FM, Svetkey, LP, Vollmer, WM, Appel, LJ, Bray, GA, Harsha, D, Obarzanek, E, Conlin, PR, Miller, ER, 3rd, Simons-Morton, DG, Karanja, N, and Lin, PH. Effects on blood pressure of reduced dietary sodium and the Dietary Approaches to Stop Hypertension (DASH) diet. DASH-Sodium Collaborative Research Group. *N Engl J Med* 344:3-10, 2001.

49. Squires, RW. Acute coronary syndromes: unstable angina and acute myocardial infarction. In *Clinical Exercise Physiology*. 3rd ed. Ehrman, JK, Gordon, PM, Visich, PS, and Keteyian, S, eds. Champaign, IL: Human Kinetics, 215-234, 2013.

50. Stewart, K and Spragg, DD. Cardiac electrical pathophysiology. In *Clinical Exercise Physiology*. 3rd ed. Ehrman, JK, Gordon, PM, Visich, PS, and Keteyian, SJ, eds. Champaign, IL: Human Kinetics, 297-313, 2013.

51. Swank, AM. Resistance training strategies for individuals with chronic heart failure. In *Resistance Training for Special Populations*. Swank, AM, and Hagerman, P, eds. New York: Delmar Cengage, 169-184, 2009.

52. Talbot, S and Smith, AJ. Factors predisposing to postural hypotensive symptoms in the treatment of high blood pressure. *Br Heart J* 37:1059-1063, 1975.

53. Thomas, S, Gokhale, R, Boden, WE, and Devereaux, PJ. A meta-analysis of randomized controlled trials comparing percutaneous coronary intervention with medical therapy in stable angina pectoris. *Can J Cardiol* 29:472-482, 2013.

54. Triposkiadis, F, Karayannis, G, Giamouzis, G, Skoularigis, J, Louridas, G, and Butler, J. The sympathetic nervous system in heart failure physiology, pathophysiology, and clinical implications. *J Am Coll Cardiol* 54:1747-1762, 2009.

55. Unger, T and Li, J. The role of the renin-angiotensin-aldosterone system in heart failure. *J Renin Angiotensin Aldosterone Syst* 5(suppl 1):S7-S10, 2004.

56. Vahanian, A, Alfieri, O, Andreotti, F, Antunes, MJ, Baron-Esquivias, G, Baumgartner, H, Borger, MA, Carrel, TP, De Bonis, M, Evangelista, A, Falk, V, Lung, B, Lancellotti, P, Pierard, L, Price, S, Schafers, HJ, Schuler, G, Stepinska, J, Swedberg, K, Takkenberg, J, Von Oppell, UO, Windecker, S, Zamorano, JL, and Zembala, M. Guidelines on the management of valvular heart disease (version 2012): the Joint Task Force on the Management of Valvular Heart Disease of the European Society of Cardiology (ESC) and the European Association for Cardio-Thoracic Surgery (EACTS). *Eur J Cardiothorac Surg* 42:S1-S44, 2012.

57. Whelton, SP, Chin, A, Xin, X, and He, J. Effect of aerobic exercise on blood pressure: a meta-analysis of randomized, controlled trials. *Ann Intern Med* 136:493-503, 2002.

58. Wyndham, CR. Atrial fibrillation: the most common arrhythmia. *Tex Heart Inst J* 27:257-267, 2000.

59. Yancy, CW, Jessup, M, Bozkurt, B, Butler, J, Casey, DE, Jr, Drazner, MH, Fonarow, GC, Geraci, SA, Horwich, T, Januzzi, JL, Johnson, MR, Kasper, EK, Levy, WC, Masoudi, FA, McBride, PE, McMurray, JJ, Mitchell, JE, Peterson, PN, Riegel, B, Sam, F, Stevenson, LW, Tang, WH, Tsai, EJ, and Wilkoff, BL. 2013 ACCF/AHA guideline for the management of heart failure: a report of the American College of Cardiology Foundation/American Heart Association Task Force on practice guidelines. *Circulation* 128:e240-e327, 2013.

60. Zucker, IH, Xiao, L, and Haack, KK. The central renin-angiotensin system and sympathetic nerve activity in chronic heart failure. *Clin Sci (Lond)* 126:695-706, 2014.

Chapter 7 Immunologic and Hematologic Disorders

1. Centers for Disease Control and Prevention. Blood-borne Infectious Diseases. www.cdc.gov/niosh/topics/bbp/universal.html. Accessed December 8, 2016.

2. Work group recommendations: 2002 Exercise and Physical Activity Conference, St. Louis, Missouri. Session VI: population approaches to health promotion and disability prevention through physical activity. *Arthritis Rheum* 49:477, 2003.

3. Acquired immunodeficiency syndrome. In *Professional Guide to Diseases*. Harold, C, ed. Philadelphia: Lippincott Williams & Wilkins, 2009.

4. Etiology and pathogenesis of rheumatoid arthritis. In *Kelley's Textbook of Rheumatology*. Firestein, GS, and Kelley, WN, eds. Philadelphia: Saunders/Elsevier, 1035-1086, 2009.

5. Human immunodeficiency virus. In *Mosby's Medical Dictionary*. 8th ed. Myers, T, ed. St. Louis: Elsevier, 893-894, 2009.

6. Abrahão, MI, Gomiero, AB, Peccin, MS, Grande, AJ, and Trevisani, V. Cardiovascular training vs. resistance training for improving quality of life and physical function in patients with system lupus erythematosus: a randomized controlled trial. *Scand J Rheumatol* 45:197-201, 2016.

7. Adis Medical Writers. Both prevention and treatment are important when managing sickle cell disease. *Drugs Ther Perspect* 30:411-416, 2014.

8. Adler, M. *ABC of AIDS*. 5th ed. London: BMJ Books, 2001.

9. Aerenhouts, D, Ickmans, K, Clarys, P, Zinzen, E, Meersdom, G, Lambrecht, L, and Nijs, J. Sleep characteristics, exercise capacity and physical activity in patients with chronic fatigue syndrome. *Disabil Rehabil* 37:2044-2050, 2015.

10. Afari, N and Buchwald, D. Chronic fatigue syndrome: a review. *Am J Psychiatry* 160:221-236, 2003.

11. AIDS Info. FDA-Approved HIV Medicines. www.aidsinfo.nih.gov/education-materials/fact-sheets/21/58/fda-approved-HIV-medicines. Accessed December 1, 2015.

12. Al Kitani, M, Thompson, D, and Stokes, D. Responses to exercise in Omani children with sickle cell disease or sickle cell trait, compared with healthy controls. *Int J Sports Sci Fit* 4:39-52, 2014.

13. Alcorn, R, Bowser, B, Henley, E, and Holloway, V. Fluidotherapy and exercise in the management of sickle cell anemia. A clinical report. *Phys Ther* 64:1520-1522, 1984.

14. Aletaha, D, Neogi, T, Silman, AJ, Funovits, J, Felson, DT, Bingham, CO 3rd, Birnbaum, NS, Burmester, GR, Bykerk, VP, Cohen, MD, Combe, B, Costenbader, KH, Dougados, M, Emery, P, Ferraccioli, G, Hazes, JM, Hobbs, K, Huizinga, TW, Kavanaugh, A, Kay, J, Kvien, TK, Laing, T, Mease, P, Ménard, HA, Moreland, LW, Naden, RL, Pincus, T, Smolen, JS, Stanislawska-Biernat, E, Symmons, D, Tak, PP, Upchurch, KS, Vencovsky, J, Wolfe, F, and Hawker, G. Rheumatoid arthritis classification criteria: an American College of Rheumatology/European League Against Rheumatism collaborative initiative [published correction appears in *Ann Rheum Dis* 69(10):1892, 2010]. *Ann Rheum Dis* 69:1580-1588, 2010.

15. Alexy, T, Sangkatumvong, S, Connes, P, Pais, E, Tripette, J, Barthelemy, J, and Coates, T. Sickle cell disease: selected aspects of pathophysiology. *Clin Hemorheol Microcirc* 44:155-166, 2010.

16. Alvarado, A, Ward, K, Muntz, D, Thompson, A, Rodeghier, M, Fernhall, B, and Liem, R. Heart rate recovery is impaired after maximal exercise testing in children with sickle cell anemia. *J Pediatr* 166:389-393, 2015.

17. American Society of Hematology. State of sickle cell disease: 2016 report. 2016. www.scdcoalition.org/report.html. Accessed December 8, 2016.

18. Anderson, A and Forsyth, A. Playing it Safe: Bleeding Disorders, Sports, and Exercise. 2005. www.hemophilia.org/Community-Resources/NHF-Publications/Playing-it-Safe-Bleeding-Disorders-Sports-and-Exercise. Accessed December 8, 2016.

19. Arthritis Foundation. Drug Types. www.arthritis.org/living-with-arthritis/treatments/medication/drug-types. Accessed December 8, 2016.

20. National Fibromyalgia & Chronic Pain Association. Fibromyalgia treatment. 2014. www.fmcpaware.org/fibromyalgia/treatment.html. Accessed December 8, 2016.

21. Avellaneda, FA, Pérez, MA, Izquierdo, MM, Arruti, BM, Barbado, HF, de la Cruz, LJ, Díaz-Delgado, PR, Gutiérrez, RE, Palacín, DC, Rivera, RJ, and Ramón, GJ. Chronic fatigue syndrome: aetiology, diagnosis, and treatment. *BMC Psychiatry* 9(suppl 1):S1, 2009.

22. Aviña-Zubieta, JA, Choi, HK, Sadatsafavi, M, Etminan, M, Esdaile, JM, and Lacaille, D. Risk of cardiovascular mortality in patients with rheumatoid arthritis: a meta-analysis of observational studies. *Arthritis Rheum* 59:1690-1697, 2008.

23. Ayán, C and Martín, V. Systemic lupus erythematosus and exercise. *Lupus* 16:5-9, 2007.

24. Bailey, S and Nieman, D. Chronic fatigue syndrome. In *ACSM's Exercise Management for Persons with Chronic Disease and Disability*. Moore, GE, Durstine, JL, and Painter, PL, eds. Champaign, IL: Human Kinetics, 215-220, 2016.

25. Beltrame, LG, Abreu, L, Almeida, J, and Boullosa, DA. The acute effect of moderate intensity aquatic exercise on coagulation factors in haemophiliacs. *Clin Physiol Funct Imaging* 35:191-196, 2015.

26. Bested, AC and Marshall, LM. Review of myalgic encephalomyelitis/chronic fatigue syndrome: an evidence-based approach to diagnosis and management by clinicians. *Rev Environ Health* 30:223-249, 2015.

27. Bidonde, J, Busch, AJ, Webber, SC, Schachter, CL, Danyliw, A, Overend, TJ, Richards, RS, and Rader, T. Aquatic exercise training for fibromyalgia. *Cochrane Database Syst Rev* 10:CD011336, 2014.

28. Bircan, C, Karasel, SA, Akgun, B, El, O, and Alper, S. Effects of muscle strengthening versus aerobic exercise program in fibromyalgia. *Rheumatol Int* 28:527-532, 2008.

29. Bostrom, C, Elfving, B, Dupre, B, Opava, CH, Lundberg, IE, and Jansson, E. Effects of a one-year physical activity programme for women with systemic lupus erythematosus - a randomized controlled study. *Lupus* 25:602-616, 2016.

30. Breedland, I, van Scheppingen, C, Leijsma, M, Verheij-Jansen, NP, and van Weert, E. Effects of a group-based exercise and educational program on physical performance and disease self-management in rheumatoid arthritis: a randomized controlled study. *Phys Ther* 91:879-893, 2011.

31. Burckhardt, CS, Mannerkorpi, K, Hedenberg, L, and Bjelle, A. A randomized, controlled clinical trial of education and physical training for women with fibromyalgia. *J Rheumatol* 21:714-720, 1994.

32. Buskilla, D. Neuroendocrine mechanisms in fibromyalgia-chronic fatigue: the best practice and research. *Clin Rheumatol* 15:747-758, 2001.

33. Calandre, EP, Rico-Villademoros, F, and Slim, M. An update on pharmacotherapy for the treatment of fibromyalgia. *Expert Opin Pharmacother* 16:1347-1368, 2015.

34. Carr, A and Cooper, DA. Adverse effects of antiretroviral therapy. *Lancet* 356:1423-1430, 2000.

35. Carruthers, B, van de Sande, M, De Meirleir, K, Klimas, N, Broderick, G, Mitchell, T, Staines, D, Powles, A, Speight, N, Vallings, R, and Bateman, L. Myalgic encephalomyelitis: international consensus criteria. *J Intern Med* 270:327-338, 2011.

36. Cash, E, Salmon, P, Weissbecker, I, Rebholz, WN, Bayley-Veloso, R, Zimmaro, LA, Floyd, A, Dedert, E, and Sephton, SE. Mindfulness meditation alleviates fibromyalgia symptoms in women: results of a randomized clinical trial. *Ann Behav Med* 49:319-330, 2015.

37. Centers for Disease Control and Prevention. *HIV/AIDS Surveillance Report, 2007*. Atlanta: CDC, 2009.

38. Centers for Disease Control and Prevention. CDC Fact Sheet. New HIV Infections in the United States. 2012. www.cdc.gov/std/hiv/stdfact-std-hiv.html.

39. Centers for Disease Control and Prevention. About HIV/AIDS. 2015. www.cdc.gov/hiv/basics/whatIshiv.html. Accessed December 8, 2016.

40. Centers for Disease Control and Prevention. Sickle Cell Disease. 2016. www.cdc.gov/ncbddd/sicklecell/treatments.html. Accessed December 8, 2016.

41. Centers for Disease Control and Prevention. Lupus. 2016. www.cdc.gov/lupus/index.htm. Accessed February 5, 2016.

42. Chambers, D, Bagnall, A, Hempel, S, and Forbes, C. Interventions for the treatment, management and rehabilitation of patients with chronic fatigue syndrome/myalgic encephalomyelitis: an updated systematic review. *J R Soc Med* 99:506-520, 2006.

43. Chan, JS, Ho, RT, Chung, KF, Wang, CW, Yao, TJ, Ng, SM, and Chan, CL. Qigong exercise alleviates fatigue, anxiety, and depressive symptoms, improves sleep quality, and shortens sleep latency in persons with chronic fatigue syndrome-like illness. *Evid Based Complement Alternat Med* 2014:106048, 2014.

44. Chapplain, J, Beillot, J, Begue, J, Souala, F, Bouvier, C, Arvieux, C, Tattevin, P, Dupont, M, Chapon, F, Duvauferrier, R, and Hespel, J. Mitochondrial abnormalities in HIV-infected lipoatrophic patients treated with antiretroviral agents. *J Acquir Immune Defic Syndr* 37:1477-1488, 2004.

45. Cheungpasitporn, W, Thongprayoon, C, Ungprasert, P, and Erickson, SB. Outcomes of living kidney donors with rheumatoid arthritis. *Prog Transplant* 25:307-310, 2015.

46. Ciccone, CD. *Davis's Drug Guide for Rehabilitation Professionals*. Philadelphia: Davis, 2013.

47. Clarke-Jennssen, AC, Fredriksen, PM, Lilleby, V, and Mengshoel, AM. Effects of supervised aerobic exercise in patients with systemic lupus erythematosus: a pilot study. *Arthritis Rheum* 53:308-312, 2005.

48. Clauw, DJ. Fibromyalgia: update on mechanisms and management. *J Clin Rheumatol* 13:102-109, 2007.

49. Cleare, AJ, Reid, S, Chalder, T, Hotopf, M, and Wessely, S. Chronic fatigue syndrome. *BMJ Clin Evid* pii:1101, 2015.

50. Connes, P, Machado, R, Hue, O, and Reid, H. Exercise limitation, exercise testing and exercise recommendations in sickle cell anemia. *Clin Hemorheol Microcirc* 49:151-163, 2011.

51. Connes, P, Machado, R, Hue, O, and Reid, H. Exercise limitation, exercise testing and exercise recommendations in sickle cell disease. *Clin Hemorheol Microcirc* 49:151-163, 2011.

52. Cooney, JK, Law, RJ, Matschke, V, Lemmey, AB, Moore, JP, Ahmad, Y, Jones, JG, Maddison, P, and Thom, JM. Benefits of exercise in rheumatoid arthritis. *J Aging Res* 2011:681640, 2011.

53. Cramer, CR. Fibromyalgia and chronic fatigue syndrome: an update for athletic trainers. *J Athl Train* 33:359-361, 1998.

54. Creamer, P. Effective management of fibromyalgia. *J Musculoskelet Med* 16:622-637, 1999.

55. Crofford, L. Fibromyalgia. 2015. www.rheumatology.org/I-Am-A/Patient-Caregiver/Diseases-Conditions/Fibromyalgia. Accessed December 8, 2016.

56. Crowson, C, Matteson, E, Myasoedova, E, Michet, C, Ernste, F, Warrington, K, Davis, J, Hunder, G, Therneau, T, and Gabriel, S. The lifetime risk of adult-onset rheumatoid arthritis and other inflammatory autoimmune rheumatic diseases. *Arthritis Rheum* 63:633-639, 2011.

57. Curtis, R, Baker, J, Riske, B, Ullman, M, Niu, X, Norton, K, Lou, M, and Nichol, MB. Young adults with hemophilia in the U.S.: demographics, comorbidities, and health status. *Am J Hematol* 90(suppl 2):S11-S16, 2015.

58. Da Silva, E, Pinto, RS, Cadore, E, and Kruel, LF. Nonsteroidal anti-inflammatory drug use and endurance during running in male long-distance runners. *J Athl Train* 50:295-302, 2015.

59. Davis, J and Matteson, E. My treatment approach to rheumatoid arthritis. *Mayo Clin Proc* 87:659-673, 2012.

60. Dawes, J. One on one: guidelines for fibromyalgia. *Strength Cond J* 24:16-17, 2001.

61. Dawes, J and Stephenson, MD. One on one: training those with chronic fatigue. *Strength Cond J* 30:55-57, 2008.

62. De Carvalho, MRP, Sato, EI, Tebexreni, AS, Heidecher, RTC, Schenkman, S, and Neto, TLB. Effects of supervised cardiovascular training program on exercise tolerance, aerobic capacity, and quality of life in patients with systemic lupus erythematosus. *Arthritis Rheum* 53:838-844, 2005.

63. de Jong, Z and Vliet Vlieland, TP. Safety of exercise in patients with rheumatoid arthritis. *Curr Opin Rheumatol* 17:177-182, 2005.

64. de Medeiros Fernandes, T, de Medeiros, T, Alves, J, Bezerra, C, Fernandes, J, Serafim, É, Fernandes, M, and de Fatima Sonati, M. Socioeconomic and demographic characteristics of sickle cell disease patients from a low-income region of northeastern Brazil. *Rev Bras Hematol Hemoter* 37:172-177, 2015.

65. Dedeken, L, Chapusette, R, Lê, PQ, Heijmans, C, Devalck, C, Huybrechts, S, Ziereisen, F, Hanssens, L, Rozen, L, Noubouossie, D, Mujinga, MN, and Ferster, A. Reduction of the six-minute walk distance in children with sickle cell disease is correlated with silent infarct: results from a cross-sectional evaluation in a single center in Belgium. *PLoS One* 9:e108922, 2014.

66. Dishman, RK, Washburn, RA, and Heath, GW. *Physical Activity Epidemiology*. Champaign, IL: Human Kinetics, 2004.

67. Drawz, P, Ayyappan, S, Nouraie, M, Saraf, S, Gordeuk, V, Hostetter, T, Gladwin, M, and Little, J. Kidney disease among patients with sickle cell disease, hemoglobin SS and SC. *Clin J Am Soc Nephrol* 11:207-215, 2016.

68. Dudgeon, WD, Phillips, KD, Carson, JA, Brewer, RB, Durstine, JL, and Hand, GA. Counteracting muscle wasting in HIV-infected individuals. *HIV Med* 7:299-310, 2006.

69. Duncan, HV and Achara, G. A rare initial manifestation of systemic lupus erythematosus—acute pancreatitis: case report and review of the literature. *J Am Board Fam Med* 16:334-338, 2003.

70. Duncan, MJ, Thake, CD, and Downs, PJ. Effect of caffeine ingestion on torque and muscle activity during resistance exercise in men. *Muscle Nerve* 50:523-527, 2014.

71. Dunkin, M. What you need to know about DMARDs. *Arthritis Today* 26:58-62, 2012.

72. Eichner, ER. Sickle cell trait in sports. *Curr Sports Med Rep* 9:347-351, 2010.

73. Eichner, ER. Exertional sickling deaths in Army recruits with sickle cell trait. *Mil Med* 177:56-59, 2012.

74. Erdman, KM. A review of treatment options for chronic fatigue syndrome. *Physician Assist* 27:16-25, 2003.

75. Evans, S, Cousins, L, Tsao, JC, Subramanian, S, Sternlieb, B, and Zeltzer, LK. A randomized controlled trial examining Iyengar yoga for young adults with rheumatoid arthritis: a study protocol. *Trials* 12:19, 2011.

76. Fahey, JL and Fleming, DS. *AIDS/HIV Reference Guide for Medical Professionals.* 4th ed. (Center for Interdisciplinary Research in Immunology and Disease at UCLA). Williams & Wilkins, 1997.

77. Fenton, KA. Changing epidemiology of HIV/AIDS in the United States: implications for enhancing and promoting HIV testing strategies. *Clin Infect Dis* 45(suppl 4):S213-S220, 2007.

78. Ferreira, MP and Norwood, JM. Strength training for the athlete with HIV/AIDS: practical implications for the performance team. *Strength Cond J* 19:50-57, 1997.

79. Fisher, SD, Kanda, BS, Miller, TL, and Lipshultz, SE. Cardiovascular disease and therapeutic drug-related cardiovascular consequences in HIV-infected patients. *Am J Cardiovasc Drugs* 11:383-394, 2011.

80. Fleischman, A, Johnsen, S, Systrom, D, Hrovat, M, Farrar, C, Frontera, W, Fitch, K, Thomas, B, Torriani, M, Côte, H, and Grinspoon, S. Effects of nucleoside reverse transcriptase inhibitor, stavudine, on glucose disposal and mitochondrial function in muscle of healthy adults. *Am J Physiol Endocrinol Metab* 292:666-673, 2007.

81. Forsyth, A, Quon, D, and Konkle, B. Role of exercise and physical activity on hemophilic arthropathy, fall prevention and osteoporosis. *Haemophilia* 17:e870-e876, 2011.

82. Forsyth, AL, Gregory, M, Nugent, D, Garrido, C, Pilgaard, T, Cooper, DL, and Iorio, A. Haemophilia experiences, results and opportunities (HERO) study: methodology and population demographics. *Haemophilia* 20:44-51, 2014.

83. Friis-Møller, N, Thiébaut, R, Reiss, P, Weber, R, Monforte, AD, De Wit, S, El-Sadr, W, Fontas, E, Worm, S, Kirk, O, Phillips, A, Sabin, CA, Lundgren, JD, and Law, MG. Predicting the risk of cardiovascular disease in HIV-infected patients: the data collection on adverse effects of anti-HIV drugs study. *Eur J Cardiovasc Prev Rehabil* 17:491-501, 2010.

84. Furst, DE and Emery, P. Rheumatoid arthritis pathophysiology: update on emerging cytokine and cytokine-associated cell targets. *Rheumatology* 53:1560-1569, 2014.

85. Gavi, M, Vassalo, D, Amaral, F, Macedo, D, Gava, P, Dantas, E, and Valim, V. Strengthening exercises improve symptoms and quality of life, but do not change autonomic modulation in fibromyalgia: a randomized clinical trial. *PLoS One* 9:e90767, 2014.

86. Gettings, L. Psychological well-being in rheumatoid arthritis: a review of the literature. *Musculoskeletal Care* 8:99-106, 2010.

87. Goel, R and Krishnamurti, L. Mortality, health care utilization and associated diagnoses in hospitalized patients with haemophilia in the United States: first reported nationwide estimates. *Haemophilia* 18:688-692, 2012.

88. Goldenberg, DL, Simms, RW, Geiger, A, and Komaroff, AL. High frequency of fibromyalgia in patients with chronic fatigue seen in primary care practice. *Arthritis Rheum* 33:381, 1990.

89. Gomes-Neto, M, Conceição, CS, Carvalho, VO, and Brites, C. A systematic review of the effects of different types of therapeutic exercise on physiologic and functional measurements in patients with HIV/AIDS. *Clinics* 68:1157-1167, 2013.

90. Gordon, B and Lubitz, L. Promising outcomes of an adolescent chronic fatigue syndrome inpatient programme. *J Paediatr Child Health* 45:286-290, 2009.

91. Gordon, BA, Knapman, LM, and Lubitz, L. Graduated exercise training and progressive resistance training in adolescents with chronic fatigue syndrome: a randomized controlled pilot study. *Clin Rehabil* 24:1072-1079, 2010.

92. Graham, T. Caffeine and exercise: metabolism, endurance and performance. *Sports Med* 31:785-807, 2001.

93. Grimbacher, B, Warnatz, K, Yong, PF, Korganow, AS, and Peter, HH. The crossroads of autoimmunity and immunodeficiency: lessons from polygenic traits and monogenic defects. *J Allergy Clin Immunol* 137:3-17, 2016.

94. Groen, WG, Den Uijl, IEM, Van Der Net, J, Grobbee, DE, De Groots, G, and Fischer, K. Protected by nature? Effects of strenuous physical exercise in FVIII activity in moderate and mild haemophilia. *Haemophilia* 19:519-523, 2013.

95. Guymer, E and Clauw, D. Treatment of fatigue in fibromyalgia. *Rheum Dis Clin North Am* 28:367-378, 2002.

96. Häkkinen, A, Häkkinen, K, Hannonen, P, and Allen, M. Strength training induced adaptations in neuromuscular function in pre-menopausal women with fibromyalgia: comparison with healthy women. *Ann Rheum Dis* 60:21-26, 2001.

97. Hallowell, RW and Horton, MR. Interstitial lung disease in patients with rheumatoid arthritis: spontaneous and drug induced. *Drugs* 74:443-450, 2014.

98. Han, A, Robinson, V, Judd, M, Taixiang, W, Wells, G, and Tugwell, P. Tai chi for treating rheumatoid arthritis. *Cochrane Database Syst Rev* CD004849, 2004.

99. Hanly, JG, Fisk, JD, Sherwood, G, Jones, E, Jones, JV, and Eastwood, B. Cognitive impairment in patients with systemic lupus erythematosus. *J Rheumatol* 19:562-567, 1992.

100. Harris, E. The rationale for combination therapy of rheumatoid arthritis based on pathophysiology. *J Rheumatol* 23:2-4, 1996.

101. Hashimoto, T, Yoshiuchi, K, Inada, S, Shirakura, K, Wada, N, Takeuchi, K, and Matsushita, M. Physical activity of elderly patients with rheumatoid arthritis and healthy individuals: an actigraphy study. *Biopsychosoc Med* 9:1-8, 2015.

102. Häuser, W, Klose, P, Langhorst, J, Moradi, B, Steinbach, M, Schiltenwolf, M, and Busch, A. Efficacy of different types of aerobic exercise in fibromyalgia syndrome: a systematic review and meta-analysis of randomized controlled trials. *Arthritis Res Ther* 12:R79, 2010.

103. Helmick, C, Felson, D, Lawrence, R, Gabriel, S, Hirsch, R, Kwoh, C, Liang, M, Kremers, H, Mayes, M, Merkel, P, Pillemer, S, Reveille, J, and Stone, J. Estimates of the prevalence of arthritis and other rheumatic conditions in the United States. Part I. *Arthritis Rheum* 58:15-25, 2008.

104. Hilberg, T, Herbsleb, M, Puta, C, Gabriel, H, and Schramm, W. Physical training increases isometric muscular strength and proprioceptive performance in hemophilic subjects. *Haemophilia* 9:86-93, 2003.

105. Hopkinson, ND, Doherty, M, and Powell, RJ. Clinical features and race-specific incidence/prevalence rates of systemic lupus erythematosus in a geographically complete cohort of patients. *Ann Rheum Dis* 53:675-680, 1994.

106. Howard, J, Inusa, B, Liossi, C, Jacob, E, Murphy, PB, Hart, N, Gavlak, J, Sahota, S, Chorozoglou, M, Nwosu, C, Gwam, M, Gupta, A, Rees, DC, Thein, SL, Reading, IC, Kirkham, FJ, and Cheng, MY. Prevention of morbidity in sickle cell disease—qualitative outcomes, pain and quality of life in a randomised cross-over pilot trial of overnight supplementary oxygen and auto-adjusting continuous positive airways pressure (POMS2a): study protocol for a randomised controlled trial. *Trials* 16:1-11, 2015.

107. Huerta, MDR, Tujillo-Martin, MM, Rua-Figueroa, I, Cuellar-Pompas, L, Quiros-Lopez, R, Serrano-Aguilar, P, and Spanish SLE CPG Development Group. Healthy lifestyle habits for patients with systemic lupus erythematosus: a systemic review. *Semin Arthritis Rheum* 45:463-470, 2016.

108. Hyatt, G. *Exercise and Fibromyalgia*. Tucson: Desert Southwest Fitness, Inc., 1998.

109. Isomeri, R, Mikkelson, M, Latikka, P, and Kammonen, K. Effects of amitriptyline and cardiovascular fitness training on pain in patients with primary fibromyalgia. *J Musculoskelet Pain* 1:253-260, 1993.

110. Jahanbin, I, Moghadam, H, Nazarinia, MA, Ghodsbin, F, Bagheri, Z, and Ashraf, AR. The effect of conditioning exercise on the health status and pain in patients with rheumatoid arthritis: a randomized controlled clinical trial. *Int J Community Based Nurs Midwifery* 2:169-176, 2014.

111. Jama, AH, Salem, AH, and Dabbous, IA. Massive splenic infarction in Saudi patients with sickle cell anemia: a unique manifestation. *Am J Hematol* 69:205-209, 2002.

112. James, JA, Neas, BN, Moser, KL, Hall, T, Bruner, GR, Sestak, AL, and Harley, JB. Systemic lupus erythematosus in adults is associated with previous Epstein-Barr virus exposure. *Arthritis Rheum* 44:1122-1126, 1998.

113. Jason, LA, Richman, JA, Rademaker, AW, Jordan, KM, Plioplys, AV, Raylor, RR, McCready, W, Huang, CF, and Plioplys, S. Community-based study of chronic fatigue syndrome. *Arch Intern Med* 159:2129-2137, 1999.

114. Jay, GW and Barkin, RL. Fibromyalgia. *Dis Mon* 61:66-111, 2015.

115. Jiao, J, Vincent, A, Cha, S, Luedtke, C, and Oh, T. Relation of age with symptom severity and quality of life in patients with fibromyalgia. *Mayo Clin Proc* 89:199-206, 2014.

116. Jones, G, Atzeni, F, Beasley, M, Flüβ, E, Sarzi-Puttini, P, and MacFarlane, G. The prevalence of fibromyalgia in the general population. *Arthritis Rheum* 67:568-575, 2015.

117. Jones, KD, Adams, DG, Winters, K, and Burckhardt, CS. Exercise in fibromyalgia: a comprehensive review of 47 intervention studies: 1988-2005. *Health Qual Life Outcomes* 4:67-89, 2006.

118. Jones, KD and Clark, SR. Individualizing the exercise prescription for persons with fibromyalgia. *Rheum Dis Clin North Am* 28:419-436, 2002.

119. Jones, KD, Clark, SR, and Bennett, RM. Prescribing exercise for people with fibromyalgia. *AACN Clin Issues* 13:277-293, 2002.

120. Kaaja, RJ and Greer, IA. Manifestations of chronic disease during pregnancy. *JAMA* 294:2751-2757, 2008.

121. Kaleth, A, Slaven, J, and Ang, D. Increasing steps/day predicts improvements in physical function and pain interference in adults with fibromyalgia. *Arthritis Care Res* 66:1887-1894, 2014.

122. Khair, K, Collier, C, Meerabeau, L, and Gibson, F. Multimethodology research with boys with severe haemophilia. *Nurse Res* 20:40-44, 2013.

123. Kibar, S, Yildiz, H, Ay, S, Evcik, D, and Ergin, E. New approach in fibromyalgia exercise program: a preliminary study regarding the effectiveness of balance training. *Arch Phys Med Rehabil* 96:1576-1582, 2015.

124. Kimberly, RP. Research advances in systemic lupus erythematosus. *JAMA* 285:650-652, 2001.

125. Kitahata, M, Gange, S, Abraham, A, Merriman, B, Saag, M, Justice, A, Hogg, R, Deeks, S, Eron, J, Brooks, J, Rourke, S, Gill, M, Bosch, R, Martin, J, Klein, M, Jacobson, L, Rodriguez, B, Sterling, T, Kirk, G, Napravnik, S, Rachlis, A, Calzavara, L, Horberg, M, Silverberg, M, Gebo, K, Goedert, J, Benson, C, Collier, A, Van Rompaey, S, Crane, H, McKaig, R, Lau, B, Freeman, A, and Moore, R. Effect of early versus deferred antiretroviral therapy for HIV on survival. *N Engl J Med* 360:18, 2009.

126. Komaroff, AL and Buchwald, D. Symptoms and signs of chronic fatigue syndrome. *Rev Infect Dis* 13(suppl 1):S8-S11, 1991.

127. LaFontaine, T. Special populations: strength and conditioning in fibromyalgia patients. *Strength Cond J* 22:42-44, 2000.

128. Lampe, FC, Duprez, DA, Kuller, LH, Tracy, R, Otvos, J, Stroes, E, Cooper, DA, Hoy, J, Paton, NI, Friis-Møller, N, Neuhaus, J, Liappis, AP, and Phillips, AN. Changes in lipids and lipoprotein particle concentrations after interruption of antiretroviral therapy. *J Acquir Immune Defic Syndr* 54:275-284, 2010.

129. Lawrence, RH and Shah, GH. Athletes' perceptions of National Collegiate Athletic Association–mandated sickle cell trait screening: insight for academic institutions and college health professionals. *J Am Coll Health* 62:343-350, 2014.

130. Learnmonth, YC, Paul, L, McFadyen, AK, Marshall-McKenna, R, Mattison, P, Miller, L, and McFarlane, NG. Short-term effect of aerobic exercise on symptoms in multiple sclerosis and chronic fatigue syndrome. *Int J MS Care* 16:76-82, 2014.

131. Lemmey, A, Williams, S, Marcora, S, Jones, J, and Maddison, P. Are the benefits of a high-intensity progressive resistance training program sustained in rheumatoid arthritis patients? A 3-year follow-up study. *Arthritis Care Res* 64:71-75, 2012.

132. Liem, RI, Reddy, M, Pelligra, SA, Savant, AP, Fernhall, B, Rodeghier, M, and Thompson, AA. Reduced fitness and abnormal cardiopulmonary responses to maximal exercise testing in children and young adults with sickle cell anemia. *Physiol Rep* 3:e12338, 2015.

133. Lima, FD, Stamm, DN, Della Pace, ID, Ribeiro, LR, Rambo, LM, Bresciani, G, Ferreira, J, Rossato, MF, Silva, MA, Pereira, ME, Ineu, RP, Santos, AR, Bobinski, F, Fighera, MR, and Royes, LF. Ibuprofen intake increases exercise time to exhaustion: a possible role for preventing exercise-induced fatigue. *Scand J Med Sci Sports* 26:1160-1170, 2015.

134. Liu, W, Zahner, L, Cornell, M, Le, T, Ratner, J, Wang, Y, Pasnoor, M, Dimachkie, M, and Barohn, R. Benefit of Qigong exercise in patients with fibromyalgia: a pilot study. *Int J Neurosci* 122:657-664, 2012.

135. Lupus Foundation of America. What are common triggers for lupus flare? 2013. www.lupus.org/answers/entry/what-are-common-triggers-for-a-lupus-flare. Accessed July 8, 2013.

136. Lynch, GS, Schertzer, JD, and Ryall, JG. Therapeutic approaches for muscle wasting disorders. *Pharmacol Ther* 113:461-487, 2007.

137. Machado, R. Sickle cell anemia-associated pulmonary arterial hypertension. *J Bras Pneumol* 33:583-591, 2007.

138. Makani, J, Soka, D, Rwezaula, S, Krag, M, Mghamba, J, Ramaiya, K, Cox, SE, and Grosse, SD. Health policy for sickle cell disease in Africa: experience from Tanzania on interventions to reduce under-five mortality. *Trop Med Int Health* 20:184-187, 2015.

139. Malita, F, Karelis, A, Toma, E, and Rabasa-Lhoret, R. Effects of different types of exercise on body composition and fat distribution in HIV infected patients: a brief review. *Can J Appl Physiol* 30:233-245, 2005.

140. Manco-Johnson, MJ, Abshire, TC, Shapiro, AD, Riske, B, Hacker, MR, Kilcoyne, R, Ingram, JD, Manco-Johnson, ML, Funk, S, Jacobson, L, and Valentino, LA. Prophylaxis versus episodic treatment to prevent joint disease in boys with severe hemophilia. *N Engl J Med* 357:535-544, 2007.

141. Mannerkorpi, K, Nyberg, B, Ahlme'n, M, and Ekdahl, C. Pool exercise combined with an education program for patients with fibromyalgia syndrome. A prospective, randomized study. *J Rheumatol* 27:2473-2481, 2000.

142. Mannucci, PM and Tuddenham, EG. The hemophilias--from royal genes to gene therapy. *N Engl J Med* 345:384, 2001.

143. Markworth, J, Vella, J, Figueiredo, V, and Cameron-Smith, D. Ibuprofen treatment blunts early translational signaling responses in human skeletal muscle following resistance exercise. *J Appl Physiol* 117:20-28, 2014.

144. Martin, L, Nutting, A, Macintosh, B, Edworthy, S, Butterwick, D, and Cook, J. An exercise program in the treatment of fibromyalgia. *J Rheumatol* 23:1050-1053, 1996.

145. Mayo Clinic. Diseases and Conditions: Hemophilia. www.mayoclinic.org/diseases-conditions/hemophilia/basics/causes/con-20029824. Accessed September 26, 2014.

146. McCain, GA, Bell, DA, Mai, FM, and Halliday, PD. A controlled study of effects of a supervised cardiovascular fitness training program on the manifestations of primary fibromyalgia. *Arthritis Rheum* 31:1135-1141, 1998.

147. McKay, D, Ostring, G, Broderick, C, Chaitow, J, and Singh-Grewal, D. A feasibility study of the effect of intra-articular corticosteroid injection isokinetic muscle strength in children with juvenile idiopathic arthritis. *Pediatr Exerc Sci* 25:221-237, 2013.

148. Meeus, M, Nijs, J, and Meirleir, KD. Chronic musculoskeletal pain in patients with the chronic fatigue syndrome: a systematic review. *Eur J Pain* 11:377-386, 2007.

149. Meremikwu, M and Okomo, U. Sickle cell disease. www.clinicalevidence.bmj.com/x/systematic-review/2402/overview.html. 2016. Accessed December 8, 2016.

150. Merrill, JT, Buyon, JP, and Utset, T. A 2014 update on the management of patients with systemic lupus erythematosus. *Semin Arthritis Rheum* 44:e1-e2, 2014.

151. Merson, MH. The HIV/Aids pandemic at 25–the global response. *N Engl J Med* 354:2414, 2006.

152. Miossi, R, Benatti, FB, Lúciade de Sá Pinto, A, Lima, FR, Borba, EF, Prodo, DM, Perandini, LA, Gualano, B, Bonfá, E, and Roschel, H. Using exercise training to counterbalance chronotropic incompetence and delayed heart rate recover in systemic lupus erythematosus: a randomized trial. *Arthritis Care Res* 64:1159-1166, 2012.

153. Mocroft, A, Kirk, O, Reiss, P, De Wit, S, Sedlacek, D, Beniowski, M, Gatell, J, Phillips, AN, Ledergerber, B, and Lundgren, JD. Estimated glomerular filtration rate, chronic kidney disease and antiretroviral drug use in HIV-positive patients. *AIDS* 24:1667-1678, 2010.

154. Mulvany, R, Zucker-Levin, A, Jeng, M, Joyce, C, Tuller, J, Rose, J, and Dugdale, M. Effects of a 6-week, individualized, supervised exercise program for people with bleeding disorders and hemophilic arthritis. *Phys Ther* 90:509-526, 2010.

155. Mutimura, E, Crowther, N, Cade, T, Yarashesk, K, and Stewart, A. Exercise training reduces central adiposity and improves metabolic indices in HAART-treated HIV-positive subjects in Rwanda: a randomized controlled trial. *AIDS Res Hum Retroviruses* 24:15-23, 2008.

156. Naik, RP, Streiff, MB, Haywood, C, Nelson, JA, and Lanzkron, S. Venous thromboembolism in adults with sickle cell disease: a serious and under-recognized complication. *Am J Med* 126:443-449, 2013.

157. National Hemophila Foundation. Hemophilia A. www.hemophilia.org/Bleeding-Disorders/Types-of-Bleeding-Disorders/Hemophilia-A. 2016. Accessed December 8, 2016.

158. National Institute of Arthritis and Musculoskeletal and Skin Diseases. *Systemic Lupus Erythematosus.* Bethesda, MD: National Institutes of Health, 2003.

159. National Institutes of Health. How is hemophilia treated? www.nhlbi.nih.gov/health/health-topics/topics/hemophilia/treatment. Accessed July 13, 2013.

160. Naz, S and Symmons, D. Mortality in established rheumatoid arthritis. *Best Pract Res Clin Rheumatol* 21:871-883, 2007.

161. Negrei, C, Bojinca, V, Balanescu, A, Bojinca, M, Baconi, D, Spandidos, DA, Tsatsakis, AM, and Stan, M. Management of rheumatoid arthritis: impact and risks of various therapeutic approaches (review). *Exp Ther Med* 11:1177-1183, 2016.

162. Negrier, C, Seuser, A, Forsyth, A, Lobet, S, Llinas, A, Rosas, M, and Heijnen, L. The benefits of exercise for patients with haemophilia and recommendations for safe and effective physical activity. *Haemophilia* 19:487-498, 2013.

163. Neill, J, Belan, I, and Ried, K. Effectiveness of non-pharmacological interventions for fatigue in adults with multiple sclerosis, rheumatoid arthritis, or systemic lupus erythematosus: a systematic review. *J Adv Nurs* 56:617-635, 2006.

164. Neto, MG, Conceico, CS, Carvalho, VO, and Brites, C. Effects of combined aerobic and resistance exercise on exercise capacity, muscle strength and quality of life in HIV patients: a systematic review and meta-analysis. *PLoS One* 10:1-14, 2015.

165. Nieman, D. Fibromyalgia. In *ACSM's Exercise Management for Persons with Chronic Disease and Disability.* Moore, GE, Durstine, JL, and Painter, PL, eds. Champaign, IL: Human Kinetics, 221-226, 2016.

166. Nieman, D, Hand, G, Lyerly, G, and Dudgeon, W. Acquired immune deficiency syndrome. In *ACSM's Exercise Management for Persons with Chronic Disease and Disability.* Moore, GE, Durstine, JL, and Painter, PL, ed. Champaign, IL: Human Kinetics, 209-214, 2016.

167. Nijs, J, Vaherberghen, K, Duquet, W, and Meirlier, KD. Chronic fatigue syndrome: lack of association between pain-related fear of movement and exercise capacity disability. *Phys Ther* 84:696-705, 2004.

168. Nijs, J and Van Parijs, M. Long-term effectiveness of pool exercise therapy and education in patients with fibromyalgia. *J Chron Fat Syndr* 12:73-79, 2004.

169. Oka, T, Tanahashi, T, Chijiwa, T, Lkhagvasuren, B, Sudo, N, and Oka, K. Isometric yoga improves the fatigue and pain of patients with chronic fatigue syndrome who are resistant to conventional therapy: a randomized, controlled trial. *Biopsychosoc Med* 8:27, 2014.

170. Okon, LG and Werth, V. Cutaneous lupus erythematosus: diagnosis and treatment. Best practice and research. *Clin Rheumatol* 27:391-404, 2013.

171. Ovayolu, N, Ovayolu, O, and Karadag, G. Health-related quality of life in ankylosing spondylitis, fibromyalgia syndrome, and rheumatoid arthritis: a comparison with a selected sample of healthy individuals. *Clin Rheumatol* 30:655-664, 2011.

172. Panjwani, S. Early diagnosis and treatment of discoid lupus erythematosus. *J Am Board Fam Med* 22:206-213, 2009.

173. Rahnama, N and Mazloum, V. Effects of strengthening and aerobic exercises on pain severity and function in patients with knee rheumatoid arthritis. *Int J Prev Med* 3:493-498, 2012.

174. Ramsey-Goldman, R, Schilling, EM, Dunlop, D, Langman, C, Greenland, P, Thomas, RJ, and Chang, RW. A pilot study on the effects of exercise in patients with systemic lupus erythematosus. *Arthritis Care Res* 13:262-269, 2000.

175. Reiffenberger, DH and Amundson, LH. Fibromyalgia syndrome: a review. *Am Fam Physician* 53:1698-1712, 1996.

176. Reuter, B and Hagerman, P. Aerobic endurance exercise training. In *Essentials of Strength Training and Conditioning*. 3rd ed. Baechle, T, and Earle, R, eds. Champaign, IL: Human Kinetics, 495, 2008.

177. Robinson, F, Quinn, L, and Rimmer, J. Effects of high-intensity endurance and resistance exercise on HIV metabolic abnormalities: a pilot study. *Biol Res Nurs* 8:177-185, 2007.

178. Rodgers, SE, Duncan, EM, Barbulescu, DM, Quinn, DM, and Lloyd, JV. In vitro kinetics of factor VIII activity in patients with mild haemophilia A and a discrepancy between one-stage and two-stage factor VIII assay results. *Br J Haematol* 136:138-145, 2007.

179. Roozen, M. Training individuals with fibromyalgia. *Strength Cond J* 20:64-66, 1998.

180. Rossi, A, DiLollo, A, Guzzo, M, Giacomelli, C, Atzeni, F, Bazzichi, L, and DiFranco, M. Fibromyalgia and nutrition: what news? *Clin Exp Rheumatol* 33:S117-S125, 2015.

181. Rusu, C, Gee, M, Lagace, C, and Parlor, M. Chronic fatigue syndrome and fibromyalgia in Canada: prevalence and association with six health status indicators. *Health Promot Chronic Dis Prev Can* 35:3-11, 2015.

182. Buckelew, SP, Conway, R, Parker, J, Deuser, WE, Read, J, Witty, TE, Hewett, JE, Minor, M, Johnson, JC, Van Male, L, McIntosh, MJ, Nigh, M, and Kay, DR. Biofeedback/relaxation training and exercise interventions for fibromyalgia: a prospective trial. *Arthritis Care Res* 111:196-209, 1998.

183. Schneider, M, Vernon, H, Gordon, K, Lawson, G, and Penera, J. Chiropractic management of fibromyalgia syndrome: a systematic review of the literature. *J Manipulative Physiol Ther* 32:25-40, 2009.

184. Sevmili, D, Kozanoglu, E, Guzel, R, and Doganay, A. The effects of aquatic, isometric strength-stretching and aerobic exercise on physical and psychological parameters of female patients with fibromyalgia syndrome. *J Phys Ther Sci* 27:1781-1786, 2015.

185. Sheng, L and Wu-kui, CAO. HIV/AIDS epidemiology and prevention in China. *Chin Med J* 121:1230-1236, 2008.

186. Shi, Y and Rui, X. Procalcitonin kinetics: a reliable tool for diagnosis and monitoring of the course of bacterial infection in critically ill patients with autoimmune diseases. *Intensive Care Med* 39:2233-2234, 2013.

187. Siegel, J, Rhinehart, E, Jackson, M, Chiarello, L, and Healthcare Infection Control Practices Advisory Committee. *Guideline for Isolation Precautions: Preventing Transmission of Infectious Agents in Healthcare Settings*, 2007.

188. Souza, JC, Simoes, HG, Campbell, CG, Pontes, FL, Boullosa, DA, and Prestes, JJ. Haemophilia and exercise. *Int J Sports Med* 33:83-88, 2012.

189. Spierer, DK, DeMeersman, RE, Kleinfeld, J, McPherson, E, Fullilove, RE, Alba, A, and Zion, AS. Exercise training improves cardiovascular and autonomic profiles in HIV. *Clin Auton Res* 17:341-348, 2007.

190. Strasser, B, Leeb, G, Strehblow, C, Schobersberger, W, Haber, P, and Cauza, E. The effects of strength and endurance training in patients with rheumatoid arthritis. *Clin Rheumatol* 30:623-632, 2011.

191. Stringer, WW. Mechanisms of exercise limitations in HIV+ individuals. *Med Sci Sports Exerc* 32:S412-S421, 2000.

192. Tan, EM, Sugura, K, and Gupta, S. The case definition of chronic fatigue syndrome. *J Clin Immunol* 22:8-12, 2002.

193. Tebbe, B and Orfanos, CE. Epidemiology and socio-economic impact of skin disease in lupus erythematosus. *Lupus* 6:96-104, 1997.

194. Tench, CM, McCarthy, J, McCurdie, I, White, PD, and D'Cruz, DP. Fatigue in systemic lupus erythematosus: a randomized controlled trial of exercise. *Rheumatology* 42:1050-1054, 2003.

195. The Johns Hopkins Lupus Center. Lupus Medications. 2016. www.hopkinslupus.org/lupus-treatment/lupus-medications/. Accessed December 8, 2016.

196. Tiktinsky, R, Falk, B, Heim, M, and Martinovitz, U. The effect of resistance training on the frequency of bleeding in haemophilia patients: a pilot study. *Haemophilia* 8:22-27, 2002.

197. Tinti, G, Somera, R, Valente, F, and Domingos, C. Benefits of kinesiotherapy and aquatic rehabilitation on sickle cell anemia. A case report. *Genet Mol Res* 9:360-364, 2010.

198. Triant, V, Lee, H, Hadigan, C, and Grinspoon, S. Increased acute myocardial infarction rates and cardiovascular risk factors among patients with human immunodeficiency virus disease. *J Clin Endocrinol Metab* 92:2506-2512, 2007.

199. Tuna, Z, Duger, T, Atalay-Guzel, N, Aral, A, Basturk, B, Haznedaroglu, S, and Goker, B. Aerobic exercise improves oxidant-antioxidant balance in patients with rheumatoid arthritis. *J Phys Ther Sci* 27:1239-1242, 2015.

200. University of Maryland Medical Center. Chronic fatigue syndrome. 2012. www.umm.edu/health/medical/reports/articles/chronic-fatigue-syndrome. Accessed December 8, 2016.

201. van Breukelen-van der Stoep, DF, van Zeben, D, Klop, B, van de Geijn, GJ, Janssen, HJ, Hazes, MJ, Birnie, E, van der Meulen, N, De Vries, MA, and Castro Cabezas, M. Association of cardiovascular risk factors with carotid intima media thickness in patients with rheumatoid arthritis with low disease activity compared to controls: a cross-sectional study. *PLoS One* 10:e0140844, 2015.

202. van Cauwenbergh, D, DeKooning, M, Ickmans, K, and Nijs, J. How to exercise people with chronic fatigue syndrome: evidence-based practice guidelines. *Eur J Clin Invest* 42:1136-1142, 2012.

203. van den Ende, C, Breedveld, F, Cessie, S, Dijkmans, B, de Mug, A, and Hazes, J. Effect of intensive exercise on patients with active rheumatoid arthritis: a randomized clinical trial. *Ann Rheum Dis* 59:615-621, 2000.

204. van Vilsteren, M, Boot, CR, Knol, DR, van Schaardenburg, D, Voskuyl, AE, Steenbeek, R, and Anema, JR. Productivity at work and quality of life in patients with rheumatoid arthritis. *BMC Musculoskelet Disord* 16:107, 2015.

205. Vanness, MJ, Snell, CR, Stayer, DR, Dempsey, L IV, and Stevens, SR. Subclassifying chronic fatigue syndrome through exercise testing. *Med Sci Sports Exerc* 35:908-913, 2003.

206. Verhoeven, F, Tordi, N, Prati, C, Demougeot, C, Mougin, F, and Wendling, D. Physical activity in patients with rheumatoid arthritis. *Joint Bone Spine* 83:265-270, 2016.

207. Vervloesem, N, Van Gils, N, Ovaere, L, Westhovens, R, and Van Assche, D. Are personal characteristics associated with exercise participation in patients with rheumatoid arthritis? A cross-sectional exploratory survey. *Musculoskeletal Care* 10:90-100, 2012.

208. Villareal, DT and Holloszy, JO. DHEA enhances effects of weight training on muscle mass and strength in elderly women and men. *Am J Physiol Endocrinol Metab* 291:E1003-E1008, 2006.

209. Waltz, X and Connes, P. Pathophysiology and physical activity in patients with sickle cell anemia. *Mov Sport Sci* 83:41-47, 2014.

210. Waltz, X, Hedreville, M, Sinnapah, S, Lamarre, Y, Soter, V, Lemonne, N, and Connes, P. Delayed beneficial effect of acute exercise on red blood cell aggregate strength in patients with sickle cell anemia. *Clin Hemorheol Microcirc* 52:15-26, 2012.

211. Wasserman, A. Diagnosis and management of rheumatoid arthritis. *Am Fam Physician* 84:1245-1252, 2011.

212. Westover, AN, Nakonezny, PA, Barlow, CE, Vongpatanasin, W, Adinoff, B, Brown, ES, Mortensen, EM, Halm, EA, and DeFina, LF. Exercise outcomes in prevalent users of stimulant medications. *J Psychiatr Res* 64:32-39, 2015.

213. White, KP and Harth, M. Classification, epidemiology, and natural history of fibromyalgia. *Curr Pain Headache Rep* 5:320-329, 2001.

214. White, PD, Goldsmith, KA, Johnson, AL, Potts, L, Walwyn, R, DeCesare, JC, Baber, HL, Burgess, M, Clark, LV, Cox, DL, Bavinton, J, Angus, BJ, Murphy, G, Murphy, M, O'Dowd, H, Wilks, D, McCrone, P, Chalder, T, Sharpe, M, and PACE Trial Management Group. Comparison of adaptive pacing therapy, cognitive behavior therapy, graded exercise therapy, and specialist medical care for chronic fatigue syndrome (PACE): a randomized trial. *Lancet* 377:823-836, 2011.

215. Whitehill, WR and Wright, KE. Weightroom safety: AIDS: guidelines for the athletic community. *Strength Cond J* 12:64-67, 1990.

216. Williams, C and Dawes, J. One-on-one: guidelines for training individuals with lupus. *Strength Cond J* 29:56-58, 2007.

217. Wilson, B, Spencer, H, and Kortebein, P. Exercise recommendations in patients with newly diagnosed fibromyalgia. *PM R* 4:252-255, 2012.

218. Wong, T and Recht, M. Current options and new developments in the treatment of haemophilia. *Drugs* 71:305-320, 2011.

219. World Health Organization. HIV/AIDS. www.who.int/mediacentre/factsheets/fs360/en/. Accessed December 8, 2016.

220. Yancey, JR and Thomas, SM. Chronic fatigue syndrome: diagnosis and treatment. *Am Fam Physician* 86:741-746, 2012.

221. Young, G. From boy to man: recommendations for the transition process in haemophilia. *Haemophilia* 18(suppl 5):527-532, 2012.

222. Yunus, MB. Gender differences in fibromyalgia and other related syndromes. *J Gend Specif Med* 5:42-47, 2002.

223. Zhang, L, Xia, Y, Zhang, Q, Fu, T, Yin, R, Guo, G, Li, L, and Gu, Z. The correlations of socioeconomic status, disease activity, quality of life, and depression/anxiety in Chinese patients with rheumatoid arthritis. *Psychol Health Med* 22:28-36, 2017.

224. Zippenfening, H and Sirbu, E. Benefits of exercise on physical and mental health in rheumatoid arthritis patients. *Timisoara Med* 7:58-63, 2014.

Chapter 8 Neuromuscular Conditions and Disorders

1. Agarwal, A and Verma, I. Cerebral palsy in children: an overview. *J Clin Orthop Trauma* 3:77-81, 2012.

2. Alemdaroglu, I, Karaduman, A, and Yilmaz, O. Acute effects of different exercises on hemodynamic responses and fatigue in Duchenne muscle dystrophy. *Fizyoter Rehabil* 23:10-16, 2012.

3. Alix, J. The pathophysiology of ischemic injury to developing white matter. *McGill J Med* 9:134-140, 2006.

4. Allam, M, Del Castillo, A, and Navajas, R. Parkinson's disease risk factors: genetic, environmental, or both? *Neurol Res* 27:206-208, 2005.

5. Alter, M, Kahana, E, and Loewenson, R. Migration and risk of multiple sclerosis. *Neurology* 28:1089-1093, 1978.

6. Antonini, A, Abbruzzese, G, Barone, P, Bonuccelli, U, Lopiano, L, Onofrj, M, Zappia, M, and Quattrone, A. COMT inhibition with tolcapone in the treatment algorithm of patients with Parkinson's disease (PD): relevance for motor and non-motor features. *Neuropsychiatr Dis Treat* 4:1-9, 2008.

7. Argenta, L, Zheng, Z, Bryant, A, Tatter, S, and Morykwas, M. A new method for modulating traumatic brain injury with mechanical tissue resuscitation. *Neurosurgery* 70:1281-1295, 2012.

8. Arida, R, Cavalheiro, E, da Silva, A, and Scorza, F. Physical activity and epilepsy: proven and predicted benefits. *Sports Med* 38:607-615, 2008.

9. Ascherio, A. Environmental factors in multiple sclerosis. *Expert Rev Neurother* 13:3-9, 2013.

10. Ascherio, A and Munger, K. Environmental risk factors for multiple sclerosis. Part I: the role of infection. *Ann Neurol* 61:288-299, 2007.

11. Bagnato, F, Centonze, D, Galgani, S, Grasso, M, Haggiag, S, and Strano, S. Painful and involuntary multiple sclerosis. *Expert Opin Pharmacother* 12:763-777, 2011.

12. Balcer, L, Miller, D, Reingold, S, and Cohen, J. Vision and vision-related outcome measures in multiple sclerosis. *Brain* 138:11-27, 2015.

13. Bar-On, L, Molenaers, G, Aertbeliën, E, Van Campenhout, A, Feys, H, Nuttin, B, and Desloovere, K. Spasticity and its contribution to hypertonia in cerebral palsy. *Biomed Res Int* 2015:317047, 2015.

14. Barfield, J, Cobler, D, Pratt, D, and Malone, L. Resistance training recommendations for individuals with neuromuscular disabilities. *Palaestra* 27, 2013.

15. Ben-Menachem, E. Vagus-nerve stimulation for the treatment of epilepsy. *Lancet Neurol* 1:477-482, 2002.

16. Berg, AT, Berkovic, S, Brodie, MJ, Buchhalter, J, Cross, JH, van Emde Boas, W, Engel, J, French, J, Glauser, TA, Mathern, GW, Moshé, SL, Nordli, D, Plouin, P, and Scheffer, IE. Revised terminology and concepts for organization of seizures and epilepsies: report of the ILAE Commission on Classification and Terminology, 2005-2009. *Epilepsia* 51:676-685, 2010.

17. Bhambhani, Y, Rowland, G, and Faraq, M. Effects of circuit training on body composition and peak cardiorespiratory responses in patients with moderate to severe traumatic brain injury. *Arch Phys Med Rehabil* 86:268-276, 2005.

18. Bhutani, V, Zipursky, A, Blencowe, H, Khanna, R, Sgro, M, Ebbesen, F, Bell, J, Mori, R, Slusher, T, Fahmy, N, Paul, V, Du, L, Okolo, A, de Almeida, M, Olusanya, B, Kumar, P, Cousens, S, and Lawn, J. Neonatal hyperbilirubinemia and Rhesus disease of the newborn: incidence and impairment estimates for 2010 at regional and global levels. *Pediatr Res* 74:86-100, 2013.

19. Bonita, R and Beaglehole, R. Recovery of motor function after stroke. *Stroke* 19:1497-1500, 1988.

20. Briellmann, R, Hopwood, M, and Jackson, G. Major depression in temporal lobe epilepsy with hippocampal sclerosis: clinical and imaging correlates. *J Neurol Neurosurg Psychiatr* 78:1226-1230, 2007.

21. Brienesse, L and Emerson, M. Effects of resistance training for people with Parkinson's disease: a systematic review. *J Am Med Dir Assoc* 14:236-241, 2013.

22. Brooks, D. Optimizing levodopa therapy for Parkinson's disease with levodopa/carbidopa/entacapone: implications from a clinical and patient perspective. *Neuropsychiatr Dis Treat* 4:39-47, 2008.

23. Bushby, K, Finkel, R, Birnkrant, D, Case, L, Clemens, P, Cripe, L, Kaul, A, Kinnett, K, McDonald, C, Pandya, S, Poysky, J, Shapiro, F, Tomezsko, J, Constantin, C, and DMD Care Considerations Working Group. Diagnosis and management of Duchenne muscular dystrophy, part 1: diagnosis, and pharmocological and psychosocial management. *Lancet Neurol* 9:77-93, 2010.

24. Calabresi, P. Diagnosis and management of multiple sclerosis. *Am Fam Physician* 70:1935-1944, 2004.

25. Camerota, F, Galli, M, Celletti, C, Vimercati, S, Cimolin, V, Tenore, N, Filippi, G, and Albertini, G. Quantitative effects of repeated muscle vibrations on gait pattern in a 5-year-old child with cerebral palsy. *Case Rep Med* 2011:359126, 2011.

26. Canadian Agency for Drugs and Technology in Health. Management of Relapsing-Remitting Multiple Sclerosis. CADTH Therapeutic Review. 2013. www.cadth.ca/management-relapsing-remitting-multiple-sclerosis. Accessed December 21, 2016.

27. Casa, D, Guskiewicz, K, Anderson, S, Courson, R, Heck, J, Jimenez, C, McDermott, B, Miller, M, Stearns, R, Swartz, E, and Walsh, K. National Athletic Trainers' Association position statement: preventing sudden death in sports. *J Athl Train* 47:96-118, 2012.

28. Center for Excellence for Medical Multimedia. Moderate to Severe TBI: TBI Medication Chart. www.traumaticbraininjuryatoz.org/Moderate-to-Severe-TBI/Treatment-Stages-of-Moderate-to-Severe-TBI/TBI-Medication-Chart. Accessed May 27, 2016.

29. Centers for Disease Control and Prevention. *Report to Congress on Traumatic Brain Injury in the United States: Epidemiology and Rehabilitation.* Atlanta: National Center for Injury Prevention and Control; Division of Unintentional Injury Prevention, 2015.

30. Chahine, L, Stern, M, and Chen-Plotkin, A. Blood-based biomarkers for Parkinson's disease. *Parkinsonism Relat Disord* 20:S99-S103, 2014.

31. Chang, R and Mubarak, S. Pathomechanics of Gowers' sign: a video analysis of a spectrum of Gowers' maneuvers. *Clin Orthop Relat Res* 470:1987-1991, 2012.

32. Cherian, A and Thomas, S. Status epilepticus. *Ann Indian Acad Neurol* 12:140-153, 2009.

33. Chin, L. Spinal cord injuries medication. 2016. www.emedicine.medscape.com/article/793582-medication. Accessed May 27, 2016.

34. Chong, J, Hesdorffer, D, Thurman, D, Lopez, D, Harris, R, Hauser, W, Labiner, E, Velarde, A, and Labiner, D. The prevalence of epilepsy along the Arizona–Mexico border. *Epilepsy Res* 105:206-215, 2013.

35. Claflin, E, Krishnan, C, and Khot, S. Emerging treatments for motor rehabilitation after stroke. *Neurohospitalist* 5:77-88, 2015.

36. Crenshaw, S, Royer, T, Richards, J, and Hudson, D. Gait variability in people with multiple sclerosis. *Mult Scler* 12:613-619, 2006.

37. Cussler, E, Lohman, T, Going, S, Houtkooper, L, Metcalfe, L, Flint-Wagner, H, Harris, R, and Teixeira, P. Weight lifted in strength training predicts bone change in postmenopausal women. *Med Sci Sports Exerc* 35:10-17, 2003.

38. Dalgas, U, Ingemann-Hansen, T, and Stenager, E. Physical exercise and MS recommendations. *Int MS J* 16:5-11, 2009.

39. Dalgas, U, Stenager, E, and Ingemann-Hansen, T. Multiple sclerosis and physical exercise: recommendations for the application of resistance-, endurance- and combined training. *Mult Scler* 14:35-53, 2008.

40. Damiano, D and Abel, M. Functional outcomes of strength training in spastic cerebral palsy. *Arch Phy Med Rehabil* 79:119-125, 1998.

41. Darras, B, Miller, D, and Urion, D. Dystrophinopathies. In *GeneReviews*. Pagon, R, Adam, M, and Ardinger, H, eds. Seattle: University of Washington, 2000.

42. DasGupta, R and Fowler, C. Bladder, bowel and sexual dysfunction in multiple sclerosis: management strategies. *Drugs* 63:153-166, 2003.

43. Davies, D. *Textbook of Adverse Drug Reactions*. Oxford: Oxford University Press, 1977.

44. Davis, G, Plyley, M, and Shepard, R. Gains in cardiorespiratory fitness with arm-crank training in spinally disabled men. *Can J Sport Sci* 16:64-72, 1991.

45. Davis, S, Wilson, T, White, A, and Frohman, E. Thermoregulation in multiple sclerosis. *J Appl Physiol* 109:1531-1537, 1985.

46. de Lima, C, Vancini, R, Arida, R, Guilhoto, L, Mello, M, Barreto, A, Guaranha, M, Yacubian, E, and Tufik, S. Physiological and electroencephalographic responses to acute exhaustive physical exercise in people with juvenile myoclonic epilepsy. *Epilepsy Behav* 22:718-722, 2011.

47. De Silva, D, Woon, F, Moe, K, Chen, C, Chang, H, and Wong, M. Concomitant coronary artery disease among Asian ischaemic stroke patients. *Ann Acad Med Singapore* 37:573-575, 2008.

48. de Souza-Teixeira, F, Costilla, S, Ayán, C, García-López, D, González-Gallego, J, and de Paz, J. Effects of resistance training in multiple sclerosis. *Int J Sports Med* 30:245-250, 2009.

49. Delateur, B and Giaconi, R. Effect on maximal strength of submaximal exercise in Duchenne muscular dystrophy. *Am J Phys Med* 58:26-36, 1979.

50. Deon, L and Gaebler-Spira, D. Assessment and treatment of movement disorders in children with cerebral palsy. *Orthop Clin North Am* 41:507-517, 2010.

51. Dhalla, Z, Bruni, J, and Sutton, J. A comparison of the efficacy and tolerability of controlled-release carbamazepine with conventional carbamazepine. *Can J Neurol Sci* 18:66-68, 1991.

52. Dibble, L, Addison, O, and Papa, E. The effects of exercise on balance in persons with Parkinson's disease: a systematic review across the disability spectrum. *J Neurol Phys Ther* 33:14-26, 2009.

53. Dibble, L, Hale, T, Marcus, RL, Gerber, J, and Lastayo, P. The safety and feasibility of high-force eccentric resistance exercise in persons with Parkinson's disease. *Arch Phys Med Rehabil* 87:1280-1282, 2006.

54. Dobkin, B. Strategies for stroke rehabilitation. *Lancet Neurol* 3:528-536, 2004.

55. Dodd, L, Taylor, N, Shields, N, Presad, D, McDonald, E, and Gillon, A. Progressive resistance training did not improve walking but can improve muscle performance, quality of life and fatigue in adults with multiple sclerosis: a randomized controlled trial. *Mult Scler* 17:1362-1374, 2011.

56. Dupuis, F, Johnston, K, Lavoie, M, Lepore, F, and Lassonde, M. Concussions in athletes produce brain dysfunction as revealed by event-related potentials. *Neuroreport* 11:4087-4092, 2000.

57. Emery, A. The muscular dystrophies. *Lancet* 359:687-695, 2002.

58. Englot, D and Blumenfeld, H. Consciousness and epilepsy: why are complex-partial seizures complex? *Prog Brain Res* 177:147-170, 2009.

59. Epilepsy Foundation. International League Against Epilepsy announces Epilepsy: A New Definition. 2014. www.epilepsy.com/article/2014/4/revised-definition-epilepsy. Accessed November 9, 2016.

60. Espir, M and Millac, P. Treatment of paroxysmal disorders in multiple sclerosis with carbamazepine (Tegretol). *J Neurol Neurosurg Psychiatry* 33:528-531, 1970.

61. Falvo, M, Schilling, B, and Earhart, G. Parkinson's disease and resistive exercise: rationale, review, and recommendations. *Mov Disord* 23:1-11, 2008.

62. Fatemi, A, Wilson, M, and Johnston, M. Hypoxic ischemic encephalopathy in the term infant. *Clin Perinatol* 36:835-vii, 2009.

63. Fernandez, J and Pitetti, K. Training of ambulatory individuals with cerebral palsy. *Arch Phys Med Rehabil* 74:468-472, 1993.

64. Ferrari, A, Sghedoni, A, Alboresi, S, Pedroni, E, and Lombardi, F. New definitions of 6 clinical signs of perceptual disorder in children with cerebral palsy: an observational study through reliability measures. *Eur J Phys Rehabil Med* 50:709-716, 2014.

65. Filipi, M, Kucera, D, Fillipi, E, Ridpath, A, and Leuschen, M. Improvement in strength following resistance training in MS patients despite varied disability levels. *Neurorehabilitation* 28:373-382, 2011.

66. Fink, J. Hereditary spastic paraplegia overview. In *GeneReviews*. Pagon, R, Adam, M, and Ardinger, H, eds. Seattle: University of Washington, 2000.

67. Flanagan, S, Cantor, J, and Ashman, T. Traumatic brain injury: future assessment tools and treatment prospects. *Neuropsychiatr Dis Treat* 4:877-892, 2008.

68. Flanigan, K. Duchenne and Becker muscular dystrophies. *Neurol Clin* 32:671-688, 2014.

69. Fong, AJ, Roy, RR, Ichiyama, RM, Lavrov, I, Courtine, G, Gerasimenko, Y, Tai, YC, Burdick, J, and Edgerton, VR. Recovery of control of posture and locomotion after a spinal cord injury: solutions staring us in the face. *Prog Brain Res* 175:393-418, 2009.

70. Fowler, C. The cause and management of bladder, sexual and bowel symptoms in multiple sclerosis. *Baillieres Clin Neurol* 6:447-466, 1997.

71. Friedman, D, Fahlstrom, R, and EPGP Investigators. Racial and ethnic differences in epilepsy classification among probands in the Epilepsy Phenome/Genome Project (EPGP). *Epilepsy Res* 107:306-310, 2013.

72. Frohman, E. Multiple sclerosis. *Med Clin North Am* 87:867-897, 2003.

73. Frohman, E and Castro, W. Symptomatic therapy in multiple sclerosis. *Ther Adv Neurol Disord* 4:83-98, 2011.

74. Gajewska, E, Sobieska, M, and Samborski, W. Associations between manual abilities, gross motor function, epilepsy, and mental capacity in children with cerebral palsy. *Iran J Child Neurol* 8:45-52, 2014.

75. Garcia-Zozaya, I. Adrenal insufficiency in acute spinal cord injury. *J Spinal Cord Med* 29:67-69, 2006.

76. Gélisse, P, Genton, P, Coubes, P, Tang, N, and Crespel, A. Can emotional stress trigger the onset of epilepsy? *Epilepsy Behav* 48:15-20, 2015.

77. Gianola, S, Pecoraro, V, Lambiase, S, Gatti, R, Banfi, G, and Moja, L. Efficacy of muscle exercise in patients with muscular dystrophy: a systematic review showing a missed opportunity to improve outcomes. *PLoS One* 8:e65414, 2013.

78. Goldenberg, M. Overview of drugs used for epilepsy and seizures: etiology, diagnosis, and treatment. *P T* 35:392-415, 2010.

79. Gourraud, P, Harbo, H, Hauser, S, and Baranzini, S. The genetics of multiple sclerosis: an up-to-date review. *Immunol Rev* 248:87-103, 2012.

80. Gray, E, Hogwood, J, and Mulloy, B. The anticoagulant and antithrombotic mechanisms of heparin. *Handb Exp Pharmacol* 207:43-61, 2012.

81. Grigorean, V, Sandu, A, Popescu, M, Iacobini, MA, Stoian, R, Neascu, C, Strambu, V, and Popa, F. Cardiac dysfunctions following spinal cord injury. *J Med Life* 2:133-145, 2009.

82. Hass, C, Collins, M, and Juncos, J. Resistance training with creatine monohydrate improves upper-body strength in patients with Parkinson's disease: a randomized trial. *Neurorehabil Neural Repair* 21:107-115, 2007.

83. Hassett, L, Moseley, A, Tate, R, and Harmer, A. Fitness training for cardiorespiratory conditioning after traumatic brain injury. *Cochrane Database Syst Rev* 2:CD006123, 2009.

84. Haussleiter, I, Brüne, M, and Juckel, G. Psychopathology in multiple sclerosis. *Ther Adv Neurol Disord* 2:13-29, 2009.

85. Heath, GW and Fentem, PH. Physical activity among persons with disabilities--a public health perspective. *Exerc Sport Sci Rev* 26:195-234, 1997.

86. Helmstaedter, C, Van Roost, D, Clusmann, H, Urbach, H, Elger, C, and Schramm, J. Collateral brain damage, a potential source of cognitive impairment after selective surgery for control of mesial temporal lobe epilepsy. *J Neurol Neurosurg Psychiatry* 75:323-326, 2004.

87. Henry, J, Lalloo, C, and Yashpal, K. Central poststroke pain: an abstruse outcome. *Pain Res Manag* 13:41-49, 2008.

88. Himpens, E, Van den Broeck, C, Oostra, A, Calders, P, and Vanhaesebrouck, P. Prevalence, type, distribution, and severity of cerebral palsy in relation to gestational age: a meta-analytic review. *Dev Med Child Neurol* 50:334-340, 2008.

89. Hirsch, M, Toole, T, Maitland, C, and Rider, R. The effects of balance training and high-intensity resistance training on persons with idiopathic Parkinson's disease. *Arch Phys Med Rehabil* 84:1109-1117, 2003.

90. Hoshide, S, Eguchi, K, Ishikawa, J, Murata, M, Katsuki, T, Mitsuhashi, T, Shimada, K, and Kario, K. Can ischemic stroke be caused by acute reduction of blood pressure in the acute phase of cardiovascular disease? *J Clin Hypertens (Greenwich)* 10:195-200, 2008.

91. Howard, G, Labarthe, D, Hu, J, Yoon, S, and Howard, V. Regional differences in African Americans' high risk for stroke: the remarkable burden of stroke for southern African Americans. *Ann Epidemiol* 17:689-696, 2007.

92. Hylek, E. Complications of oral anticoagulant therapy: bleeding and nonbleeding, rates and risk factors. *Semin Vasc Med* 3:271-278, 2003.

93. Jacobs, P. Effects of resistance and endurance training in persons with paraplegia. *Med Sci Sports Exerc* 41:992-997, 2009.

94. Jacobs, P, Mahoney, E, Robbins, A, and Nash, M. Hypokinetic circulation in persons with paraplegia. *Med Sci Sports Exerc* 34:1401-1407, 2002.

95. Jacobs, P and Nash, M. Exercise recommendations for individuals with spinal cord injury. *Sports Med* 34:727-751, 2004.

96. Jacobs, P, Nash, M, and Rusinowski, J. Circuit training provides cardiorespiratory and strength benefits in persons with paraplegia. *Med Sci Sports Exerc* 33:711-717, 2001.

97. Jankovic, J. Parkinson's disease: clinical features and diagnosis. *J Neurol Neurosurg Psychiatry* 79:369-376, 2008.

98. Jankovic, J and Poewe, W. Therapies in Parkinson's disease. *Curr Opin Neurol* 25:433-447, 2012.

99. Jensen, M, Hoffman, A, Stoelb, B, Abresch, R, Carter, G, and McDonald, C. Chronic pain in persons with myotonic dystrophy and facioscapulohumeral dystrophy. *Arch Phys Med Rehabil* 89:320-328, 2008.

100. Johnson, R. Demyelinating diseases. In *Institute of Medicine (US) Forum on Microbial Threats.* Knobler, S, O'Connor, S, and Lemon, S, eds. Washington, DC: National Academies Press (US), 2004.

101. Jorgensen, H, Nakayama, H, Raaschou, H, and Olsen, T. Recovery of walking function in stroke patients: the Copenhagen stroke study. *Arch Phys Med Rehabil* 76:27-32, 1995.

102. Jorgensen, J, Bech-Perdersen, D, Zeeman, P, Sorensen, J, Anderson, L, and Schonberger, M. Effect of intensive outpatient physical training on gait performance and cardiovascular health in people with hemiparesis after stroke. *Phys Ther* 90:527-537, 2010.

103. Kaakkola, S. Clinical pharmacology, therapeutic use and potential of COMT inhibitors in Parkinson's disease. *Drugs* 59:1233-1250, 2000.

104. Kabadi, S and Faden, A. Neuroprotective strategies for traumatic brain injury: improving clinical translation. *Int J Mol Sci* 15:1216-1236, 2014.

105. Kaiboriboon, K, Bakaki, P, Lhatoo, S, and Koroukian, S. Incidence and prevalence of treated epilepsy among poor health and low-income Americans. *Neurology* 80:1942-1949, 2013.

106. Kanner, A. Depression in epilepsy: prevalence, clinical semiology, pathogenic mechanisms, and treatment. *Biol Psychiatry* 54:388-398, 2003.

107. Káradóttir, R and Attwell, D. Neurotransmitter receptors in the life and death of oligodendrocytes. *Neuroscience* 145:1426-1438, 2007.

108. Kargarfard, M, Etemadifar, M, Baker, P, Mehrabi, M, and Hayatbakhsh, R. Effect of aquatic exercise training on fatigue and health-related quality of life in patients with multiple sclerosis. *Arch Phys Med Rehabil* 93:1701-1708, 2012.

109. Kaspar, R, Allen, H, and Montanaro, F. Current understanding and management of dilated cardiomyopathy in Duchenne and Becker muscular dystrophy. *J Am Acad Pract* 21:241-249, 2009.

110. Katz, D, Cohen, S, and Alexander, M. Mild traumatic brain injury. *Handb Clin Neurol* 127:131-156, 2015.

111. Kelly, J, Kilbreath, S, Davis, G, Zeman, B, and Raymond, J. Cardiorespiratory fitness and walking ability in subacute stroke patients. *Arch Phys Med Rehabil* 84:1780-1785, 2003.

112. Kessler, T, Fowler, C, and Panicker, J. Sexual dysfunction in multiple sclerosis. *Expert Rev Neurother* 9:341-350, 2009.

113. Khaw, A and Kessler, C. Stroke: epidemiology, risk factors, and genetics [in German]. *Hamostaseologie* 26:287-297, 2006.

114. Kieburtz, K and Wunderle, K. Parkinson's disease: evidence for environmental risk factors. *Mov Disord* 28:8-13, 2013.

115. Kim, J and Gean, A. Imaging for the diagnosis and management of traumatic brain injury. *Neurotherapeutics* 8:39-53, 2011.

116. Kjølhede, T, Vissing, K, and Dalgas, U. Multiple sclerosis and progressive resistance training: a systematic review. *Mult Scler* 18:1215-1228, 2012.

117. Kleinman, J, Newhart, M, Davis, C, Heidler-Gary, J, Gottesman, R, and Hillis, A. Right hemispatial neglect: frequency and characterization following acute left hemisphere stroke. *Brain Cogn* 64:50-59, 2007.

118. Knezević-Pogancev, M. Cerebral palsy and epilepsy [in Serbian]. *Med Pregl* 63:527-530, 2010.

119. Knottnerus, I, Gielen, M, Lodder, J, Rouhl, R, Staals, J, Vlietinck, R, and van Oostenbrugge, R. Family history of stroke is an independent risk factor for lacunar stroke subtype with asymptomatic lacunar infarcts at younger ages. *Stroke* 42:1196-2000, 2011.

120. Krassioukov, A and West, C. The role of autonomic function on sport performance in athletes with spinal cord injury. *PM R* 6:S58-S65, 2014.

121. Krupp, L, Serafin, D, and Christodoulou, C. Multiple sclerosis-associated fatigue. *Expert Rev Neurother* 10:1437-1447, 2010.

122. Leddy, J, Kozlowski, K, Donnelly, J, Pendergast, D, Epstein, L, and Willer, B. A preliminary study of subsymptom threshold exercise training for refractory post-concussion syndrome. *Clin J Sports Med* 21:89-94, 2010.

123. Leddy, J and Willer, B. Use of graded exercise testing in concussion and return-to-activity management. *Curr Sports Med Rep* 12:370-376, 2013.

124. Lee, M, Kilbreath, S, Singh, M, Zeman, B, and Davis, G. Effect of progressive resistance training on muscle performance after chronic stroke. *Med Sci Sports Exerc* 42:23-34, 2010.

125. Levy, R, Cooper, P, and Giri, P. Ketogenic diet and other dietary treatments for epilepsy. *Cochrane Database Syst Rev* 14:CD001903, 2012.

126. Liao, H, Liu, Y, Liu, W, and Lin, Y. Effectiveness of loaded sit-to-stand resistance exercise for children with mild spastic diplegia: a randomized clinical trial. *Arch Phys Med Rehabil* 88:25-31, 2007.

127. Lieberman, A. Depression in Parkinson's disease – a review. *Acta Neurol Scand* 113:1-8, 2006.

128. Liew, W and Kang, P. Recent developments in the treatment of Duchenne muscular dystrophy and spinal muscular atrophy. *Ther Adv Neurol Disord* 6:147-160, 2013.

129. Long, A and Dagogo-Jack, S. The comorbidities of diabetes and hypertension: mechanisms and approach to target organ protection. *J Clin Hypertens (Greenwich)* 13:244-251, 2011.

130. Losy, J, Michalowska-Wender, G, and Wende, M. The effect of large-dose prednisone therapy on IgG subclasses in multiple sclerosis. *Acta Neurol Scand* 89:69-71, 1994.

131. Lundberg, A, Ovenfors, C, and Saltin, B. Effect of physical training on school-children with cerebral palsy. *Acta Paediatr Scand* 56:182-188, 1967.

132. MacKay-Lyons, M and Makrides, L. Exercise capacity early after stroke. *Arch Phys Med Rehabil* 83:1697-1702, 2002.

133. Macko, R, Ivey, F, Forrester, L, Hanley, D, Sorkin, JD, Katzel, L, Silver, K, and Goldberg, A. Treadmill exercise rehabilitation improves ambulatory function and cardiovascular fitness in patients with chronic stroke: a randomized controlled trial. *Stroke* 36:2206-2211, 2005.

134. Malmqvist, L, Biering-Sørensen, T, Bartholdy, K, Krassioukov, A, Welling, K, Svendsen, J, Kruse, A, Hansen, B, and Biering-Sørensen, F. Assessment of autonomic function after acute spinal cord injury using heart rate variability analyses. *Spinal Cord* 53:54-58, 2015.

135. Malow, B. Sleep deprivation and epilepsy. *Epilepsy Curr* 4:193-195, 2004.

136. Markert, C, Ambrosio, F, Call, J, and Grange, R. Exercise and Duchenne muscular dystrophy: toward evidence-based exercise prescription. *Muscle Nerve* 43:464-478, 2011.

137. Markert, C, Case, L, Carter, G, Furlong, P, and Grange, R. Exercise and Duchenne muscular dystrophy: where we have been and where we need to go. *Muscle Nerve* 45:746-751, 2012.

138. Markowitz, C. Multiple sclerosis update. *Am J Manag Care* 19:294-300, 2013.

139. Matthews, K, Cunniff, C, Kantamneni, J, Ciafaloni, E, Miller, T, Matthews, D, Cwik, V, Druschel, C, Miller, L, Meaney, F, Sladky, J, and Romitti, P. Muscular dystrophy surveillance tracking and research network (MD STARnet): case definition in surveillance for childhood-onset Duchenne/Becker muscular dystrophy. *J Child Neurol* 25:1098-1102, 2010.

140. Mayo Clinic. Diseases and Conditions: Cerebral palsy: Treatment, Medications. www.mayoclinic. org/diseases-conditions/cerebral-palsy/basics/treatment/con-20030502. Accessed May 27, 2015.

141. Mayo Clinic. Diseases and Conditions: Muscular dystrophy: Treatments and drugs. www.mayoclinic. org/diseases-conditions/muscular-dystrophy/basics/treatment/con-20021240. Accessed May 27, 2016.

142. Mayo Clinic. Diseases and Conditions: Spinal cord injury: Treatments and drugs. 2014. www.mayoclinic. org/diseases-conditions/spinal-cord-injury/basics/treatment/con-20023837. Accessed May 27, 2016.

143. Mayo Clinic. Diseases and Conditions: Traumatic brain injury: Treatments and drugs. 2014. www.mayoclinic.org/diseases-conditions/traumatic-brain-injury/basics/treatment/con-20029302. Accessed May 27, 2016.

144. Mayo Clinic. Diseases and Conditions: Stroke: Treatment. 2016. www.mayoclinic.org/diseases-conditions/stroke/diagnosis-treatment/treatment/txc-20117296. Accessed May 27, 2016.

145. McAuley, J, Long, L, Heise, J, Kirby, T, Buckworth, J, Pitt, C, Lehman, K, Moore, J, and Reeves, A. A prospective evaluation of the effects of a 12-week outpatient exercise program on clinical and behavioral outcomes in patients with epilepsy. *Epilepsy Behav* 2:592-600, 2001.

146. McDonald, C. Clinical approach to the diagnostic evaluation of hereditary and acquired neuromuscular diseases. *Phys Med Rehabil Clin N Am* 23:495-563, 2013.

147. McGreevy, J, Hakim, C, McIntosh, M, and Duan, D. Animal models of Duchenne muscular dystrophy: from basic mechanisms to gene therapy. *Dis Model Mech* 8:195-213, 2015.

148. McKinley, W, Santos, K, Meade, M, and Brooke, K. Incidence and outcomes of spinal cord injury clinical syndromes. *J Spinal Cord Med* 30:215-224, 2007.

149. McNee, A, Gough, M, Morrissey, M, and Shortland, A. Increases in muscle volume after plantarflexor strength training in children with spastic cerebral palsy. *Dev Med Child Neurol* 51:429-435, 2009.

150. Medori, R, Brooke, M, and Waterston, R. Genetic abnormalities in Duchenne and Becker dystrophies: clinical correlations. *Neurology* 39:461-465, 1989.

151. Molik, B, Kosmol, A, Laskin, J, Morgulec-Adamowicz, N, Skucas, K, Dabrowska, A, and Ergun, N. Wheelchair basketball skill tests: differences between athletes' functional classification level and disability type. *Fizyoter Rehabil* 21:11-19, 2010.

152. Moradi, M, Sahraian, M, Aghsaie, A, Kordi, M, Meysamie, A, Abolhasani, M, and Sobhani, V. Effects of eight-week resistance training program in men with multiple sclerosis. *Sports Med* 6:e22838, 2015.

153. Moreau, N, Simpson, K, Teefey, S, and Damiano, D. Muscle architecture predicts maximum strength and is related to activity levels in cerebral palsy. *Phys Ther* 90:1619-1630, 2010.

154. Morris, C, Bowers, R, Ross, K, Stevens, P, and Phillips, D. Orthotic management of cerebral palsy:

recommendations from a consensus conference. *NeuroRehabilitation* 28:37-46, 2011.

155. Mossberg, K, Amonette, W, and Masel, B. Endurance training and cardiorespiratory conditioning after traumatic brain injury. *J Head Trauma Rehabil* 25:173-183, 2010.

156. Mula, M and Hesdorffer, D. Suicidal behavior and antiepileptic drugs in epilepsy: analysis of the emerging evidence. *Drug Healthc Patient Saf* 3:15-20, 2011.

157. Murugan, S, Arthi, C, Thilothammal, N, and Lakshmi, B. Carrier detection in Duchenne muscular dystrophy using molecular methods. *Indian J Med Res* 137:1102-1110, 2013.

158. Muscular Dystrophy Association. Duchenne Muscular Dystrophy: Diagnosis. 2016. www.mda.org/disease/duchenne-muscular-dystrophy/diagnosis. Accessed November 28, 2016.

159. National Center for Health, Physical Activity and Disability. Exercise Programming for Clients with Cerebral Palsy. www.nchpad.org/869/4965/Exercise~Programming~for~Clients~with~Cerebral~Palsy. Accessed May 24, 2016.

160. National Center for Health, Physical Activity and Disability. Fitness Training for Clients with Muscular Dystrophy. 2006. www.nchpad.org/896/5019/Fitness~Training~for~Clients~with~Muscular~Dystrophy. Accessed November 28, 2016.

161. National Institute of Neurological Disorders and Stroke. Stroke: Hope through research. www.ninds.nih.gov/disorders/stroke/detail_stroke.htm. Accessed May 27, 2016.

162. National Institutes of Health. FY 2008 Annual Performance Report. 2008. www.dpcpsi.nih.gov/sites/default/files/opep/document/FY_2008_NIH_Annual_Performance_Report.pdf. Accessed January 19, 2016.

163. National Multiple Sclerosis Society. Medications. www.nationalmssociety.org/Treating-MS/Medications. Accessed May 27, 2016.

164. National Multiple Sclerosis Society. Pediatric MS. www.nationalmssociety.org/What-is-MS/Who-Gets-MS/Pediatric-MS. Accessed January 12, 2016.

165. National Multiple Sclerosis Society. Who Gets MS? (Epidemiology). www.nationalmssociety.org/What-is-MS/Who-Gets-MS. Accessed December 17, 2016.

166. National Multiple Sclerosis Society. Multiple Sclerosis FAQs. 2014. www.nationalmssociety.org/What-is-MS/MS-FAQ-s. Accessed November 28, 2016.

167. National Multiple Sclerosis Society. Stretching for People with MS: An illustrated manual. 2016. www.nationalmssociety.org/NationalMSSociety/media/MSNationalFiles/Brochures/Brochure-Stretching-for-People-with-MS-An-Illustrated-Manual.pdf. Accessed November 28, 2016.

168. National Spinal Cord Injury Statistical Center. Spinal cord injury facts and figures at a glance. 2012. www.nscisc.uab.edu/PublicDocuments/fact_figures_docs/Facts%202012%20Feb%20Final.pdf. Accessed November 28, 2016.

169. Nelson, K and Grether, J. Causes of cerebral palsy. *Curr Opin Pediatr* 11:487-491, 1999.

170. Nersesyan, H and Slavin, K. Current approach to cancer pain management: availability and implications of different treatment options. *Ther Clin Risk Manag* 3:381-400, 2007.

171. Nijboer, T, van de Port, I, Schepers, V, Post, M, and Visser-Meily, A. Predicting functional outcome after stroke: the influence of neglect on basic activities in daily living. *Front Hum Neurosci* 7:182, 2013.

172. Nilsson, S, Staff, P, and Pruett, E. Physical work capacity and the effect of training on subjects with long-standing paraplegia. *Scand J Rehabil Med* 7:51-56, 1975.

173. Novitzke, J. Privation of memory: what can be done to help stroke patients remember? *J Vasc Interv Neurol* 1:122-123, 2008.

174. Nowak, K and Davies, K. Duchenne muscular dystrophy and dystrophin: pathogenesis and opportunities for treatment. *EMBO Rep* 5:872-876, 2004.

175. O'Callaghan, M and MacLennan, A. Cesarean delivery and cerebral palsy: a systematic review and meta-analysis. *Obstet Gynecol* 122:1169-1175, 2013.

176. O'Connell, J and Gray, C. Treatment of post-stroke hypertension. A practical guide. *Drugs Aging* 8:408-415, 1998.

177. O'Shea, T. Diagnosis, treatment, and prevention of cerebral palsy. *Clin Obstet Gynecol* 51:816-828, 2008.

178. Oaklander, A. Neuropathic itch. In *Itch: Mechanisms and Treatment*. Carstens, E, and Akiyama, T, eds. Boca Raton, FL: CRC Press/Taylor & Francis, 2014.

179. Ostwald, S, Davis, S, Hersch, G, Kelley, C, and Godwin, K. Evidence-based educational guidelines for stroke survivors after discharge home. *J Neurosci Nurs* 40:173-191, 2008.

180. Pak, S and Patten, C. Strengthening to promote functional recovery poststroke: an evidence-based review. *Top Stroke Rehabil* 15:177-199, 2008.

181. Pakpoor, J, Handel, A, Giovannoni, G, Dobson, R, and Ramagopalan, S. Meta-analysis of the relationship between multiple sclerosis and migraine. *PLoS One* 7:e45295, 2012.

182. Panayiotopoulos, C. Symptomatic and probably symptomatic focal epilepsies: topographical symptomatology and classification. In *The Epilepsies: Seizures, Syndromes and Management*. Oxfordshire (UK): Bladon Medical, 2005.

183. Paneth, N. Birth and the origins of cerebral palsy. *N Engl J Med* 315:124-126, 1986.

184. Park, E and Kim, W. Meta-analysis of the effect of strengthening interventions in individuals with cerebral palsy. *Res Dev Disabil* 35:239-249, 2014.

185. Parkinson's Disease Foundation. What Causes Parkinon's? www.pdf.org/en/causes. Accessed January 18, 2016.

186. Parkinson's Disease Foundation. Medications & Treatments. www.pdf.org/parkinson_prescription_meds. Accessed May 27, 2016.

187. Parkinson's Disease Foundation. What Is Parkinson's? 2016. www.parkinson.org/understanding-parkinsons/what-is-parkinsons. Accessed November 28, 2016.

188. Passamano, L, Taglia, A, Palladino, A, Viggiano, E, D'Ambrosio, P, and Scutifero, M. Improvement of survival in Duchenne Muscular Dystrophy: retrospective analysis of 835 patients. *Acta Myol* 31:121-125, 2012.

189. Patten, C, Lexell, J, and Brown, H. Weakness and strength training in persons with poststroke hemiplegia: rationale, method, and efficacy. *J Rehabil Res Dev* 41:293-312, 2004.

190. Pavićević, D, Miladinović, J, and Brkušanin, M. Molecular genetics and genetic testing in myotonic dystrophy type 1. *Biomed Res Int* 2013:1-13, 2013.

191. Pennell, P. Hormonal aspects of epilepsy. *Neurol Clin* 27:941, 2009.

192. Pimentel, J, Tojal, R, and Morgado, J. Epilepsy and physical exercise. *Seizure* 25:87-94, 2015.

193. Polman, C and Uitdehagg, B. Drug treatment of multiple sclerosis. *West J Med* 173:398-402, 2000.

194. Potempa, K, Lopez, M, Braun, L, Szidon, J, Fogg, L, and Tincknell, T. Physiological outcomes of aerobic exercise training in hemiparetic stroke patients. *Stroke* 26:101-105, 1995.

195. Pula, J, Newman-Toker, D, and Kattah, J. Multiple sclerosis as a cause of the acute vestibular syndrome. *J Neurol* 260:1649-1654, 2013.

196. Qureshi, A, Suri, M, Kirmani, J, and Divani, A. The relative impact of inadequate primary and secondary prevention on cardiovascular mortality in the United States. *Stroke* 35:2346-2350, 2004.

197. Rafeeyan, Z, Azarbarzin, M, Moosa, F, and Hasanzadeh, A. Effect of aquatic exercise on the multiple sclerosis patients' quality of life. *Iran J Nurs Midwifery Res* 15:43-47, 2010.

198. Rajab, A, Yoo, S, and Abdulgalil, A. An autosomal recessive form of spastic cerebral palsy (CP) with microcephaly and mental retardation. *Am J Med Genet A* 140:1504-1510, 2006.

199. Raminsky, M. The effects of temperature on conduction in demyelinated single nerve fibers. *Arch Neurol* 52:358-363, 1973.

200. Reid, S, Hamer, P, Alderson, J, and Lloyd, D. Neuromuscular adaptations to eccentric strength training in children and adolescents with cerebral palsy. *Dev Med Child Neurol* 52:358-363, 2009.

201. Rodby-Bousquet, E and Hägglund, G. Better walking performance in older children with cerebral palsy. *Clin Orthop Relat Res* 470:1286-1293, 2012.

202. Rolak, L. Multiple sclerosis. *Clin Med Res* 1:57-82, 2003.

203. Rossetti, A, Jeckelmann, S, Novy, J, Roth, P, Weller, M, and Stupp, R. Levetiracetam and pregabalin for antiepileptic monotherapy in patients with primary brain tumors. A phase II randomized study. *Neuro Oncol* 16:584-588, 2014.

204. RxList. Seizure Medications. 2016. www.rxlist.com/seizure_medications/drugs-condition.htm. Accessed May 27, 2016.

205. Sahoo, SK and Fountain, N. Epilepsy in football players and other land-based contact or collision sport athletes: when can they participate and is there an increased risk? *Curr Sports Med Rep* 3:284-288, 2004.

206. Salgado, S, Williams, N, Kotian, R, and Salgado, M. An evidence-based exercise regimen for patients with mild to moderate Parkinson's disease. *Brain Sci* 3:87-100, 2013.

207. Saltz, B, Robinson, D, and Woerner, M. Recognizing and managing antipsychotic drug treatment side effects in the elderly. *Prim Care Companion J Clin Psychiatry* 6:14-19, 2004.

208. Sander, J. Infectious agents and epilepsy. In *Institute of Medicine (US) Forum on Microbial Threats*. Knobler, S, O'Connor, S, and Lemon, S, eds. Washington, DC: National Academies Press (US), 2004.

209. Sawka, M. Physiology of upper-body exercise. In *Exercise and Sport Sciences Reviews*. Pandolf, K, ed. New York: Macmillan, 175-211, 1986.

210. Scandalis, T, Bosak, A, Berliner, JC, Hellman, LL, and Wells, M. Resistance training and gait function in patients with Parkinson's disease. *Am J Phys Med Rehabil* 80:38-43, 2001.

211. Schapiro, R. The symptomatic management of multiple sclerosis. *Ann Indian Acad Neurol* 12:291-295, 2009.

212. Schendel, D. Infection in pregnancy and cerebral palsy. *J Am Med Womens Assoc* 56:105-108, 2001.

213. Schilling, B, Pfeiffer, R, Le Doux, MS, Karlage, RE, Bloomer, RJ, and Falvo, M. Effects of moderate-volume, high-load lower-body resistance training on strength and function in persons with Parkinson's disease: a pilot study. *Parkinsons Dis* 2010:824734, 2010.

214. Scholten, A, Haagsma, J, Andriessen, T, Vos, P, Steyerberg, E, van Beeck, E, and Polinder, S. Health-related quality of life after mild, moderate and severe traumatic brain injury: patterns and predictors of suboptimal functioning during the first year after injury. *Injury* 46:616-624, 2015.

215. Scholtes, V, Becher, J, Comuth, A, Dekkers, H, Van Dijk, L, and Dallmeijer, A. Effectiveness of functional progressive resistance exercise strength training on muscle strength and mobility in children with cerebral palsy: a randomized controlled trial. *Dev Med Child Neurol* 52:e107-e113, 2010.

216. Scholtes, V, Dallmeijer, A, Rameckers, E, Verschuren, O, Tempelaars, E, Hensen, M, and Becher, JG. Lower limb strength training in children with cerebral palsy – a randomized controlled trial protocol for functional strength training based on progressive resistance exercise principles. *BMC Pediatr* 8:41, 2008.

217. Schoser, B and Timchenko, L. Myotonic dystrophies 1 and 2: complex diseases with complex mechanisms. *Curr Genomics* 11:77-90, 2010.

218. Schwarzbold, M, Diaz, A, Martins, E, Rufino, A, Amante, LN, Thais, ME, Quevedo, J, Hohl, A, Linhares, MN, and Walz, R. Psychiatric disorders and traumatic brain injury. *Neuropsychiatr Dis Treat* 4:797-816, 2008.

219. Sharpe, R. The low incidence of multiple sclerosis in areas near the equator may be due to ultraviolet light induced suppressor cells to melanocyte antigens. *Med Hypotheses* 19:319-323, 1986.

220. Showkathali, R and Antonios, T. Autonomic dysreflexia; a medical emergency. *J R Soc Med* 100:382-383, 2007.

221. Siciliano, G, Simoncini, C, Giannotti, S, Zampa, V, Angelini, C, and Ricci, G. Muscle exercise in limb girdle muscular dystrophies: pitfall and advantages. *Acta Myol* 34:3-8, 2015.

222. Sinanović, O, Mrkonjić, Z, Zukić, S, Vidović, M, and Imamović, K. Post-stroke language disorders. *Acta Clin Croat* 50:79-94, 2011.

223. Singleton, A, Farrer, M, and Bonifati, V. The genetics of Parkinson's disease: progress and therapeutic implications. *Mov Disord* 28:14-23, 2013.

224. Smith, B, Carson, S, Fu, R, McDonagh, M, Dana, T, Chan, B, Thakurta, S, and Gibler, A. *Drug class review: disease-modifying drugs for multiple sclerosis: final update 1 report.* Portland, OR: Oregon Health & Science University, 2010.

225. Smith, S and Eskey, C. Hemorrhagic stroke. *Radiol Clin North Am* 49:27-45, 2011.

226. Soler, E and Ruiz, V. Epidemiology and risk factors of cerebral ischemia and ischemic heart diseases: similarities and differences. *Curr Cardiol Rev* 6:138-149, 2010.

227. Sorace, P, Ronai, P, and LaFontaine, T. Clients with spinal cord injury, multiple sclerosis, epilepsy, and cerebral palsy. In *NSCA's Essentials of Personal Training.* 2nd ed. Coburn, J, and Malek, M, eds. Champaign, IL: Human Kinetics, 577-579, 2012.

228. Sospedra, M and Martin, R. Immunology of multiple sclerosis. *Annu Rev Immunol* 23:683-747, 2005.

229. Stafstrom, C. Dietary approaches to epilepsy treatment: old and new options on the menu. *Epilepsy Curr* 4:215-222, 2004.

230. Staskin, D and Zoltan, E. Anticholinergics and central nervous system effects: are we confused? *Rev Urol* 9:191-196, 2008.

231. Stoller, O, de Bruin, E, Schindelholz, M, Schuster-Amft, C, de Bie, R, and Hunt, K. Cardiopulmonary exercise testing early after stroke using feedback-controlled robotics-assisted treadmill exercise: test-retest reliability and repeatability. *J Neuroeng Rehabil* 11:145, 2014.

232. Surmeier, D, Guzman, J, Sanchez-Padilla, J, and Goldberg, J. What causes the death of dopaminergic neurons in Parkinson's disease? *Prog Brain Res* 183:59-77, 2010.

233. Sveen, M, Jeppesen, T, Hauerslev, S, Kober, L, Kraj, T, and Vissing, J. Endurance training improves fitness and strength in patients with Becker muscular dystrophy. *Brain* 131:2824-2831, 2008.

234. Taglia, A, Petillo, R, D'Ambrosio, P, Picillo, E, Torella, A, Orsini, C, Ergoli, M, Scutifero, M, Passamano, L, Palladino, A, Nigro, G, and Politano, L. Clinical features of patients with dystrophinopathy sharing the 45-55 exon deletion of DMD gene. *Acta Myol* 34:9-13, 2015.

235. Taylor, N, Dodd, K, Baker, R, Willoughby, K, Thomason, P, and Graham, H. Progressive resistance training and mobility-related function in young people with cerebral palsy: a randomized controlled trial. *Dev Med Child Neurol* 55:806-812, 2013.

236. Thompson, H, McCormick, W, and Kagan, S. Traumatic brain injury in older adults: epidemiology, outcomes, and future implications. *J Am Geriatr Soc* 54:1590-1595, 2006.

237. Tollback, A, Eriksson, S, Wredenberg, A, Jenner, G, Vargas, R, Borg, K, and Ansved, T. Effects of high resistance training in patients with myotonic dystrophy. *Scand J Rehabil Med* 31:9-16, 1999.

238. Torretti, J and Sengupta, D. Cervical spine trauma. *Indian J Orthop* 41:255-267, 2007.

239. Treadwell, S and Robinson, T. Cocaine use and stroke. *Postgrad Med J* 83:389-394, 2007.

240. Trojano, M, Paolicelli, D, Bellacosa, A, and Cataldo, S. The transition from relapsing-remitting MS to irreversible disability: clinical evaluation. *Neurol Sci* 24(suppl 5):S268-S270, 2003.

241. Tugui, R and Antonescu, D. Cerebral palsy gait, clinical importance. *Maedica (Buchar)* 8:388-393, 2013.

242. Turbanski, S and Schmidbleicher, D. Effects of heavy resistance training on strength and power in upper extremities in wheelchair athletes. *J Strength Cond Res* 24:8-16, 2010.

243. Turner, C and Hilton-Jones, D. The myotonic dystrophies: diagnosis and management. *J Neurol Neurosurg Psychiatr* 81:358-367, 2010.

244. United States Department of Health and Human Services. *Physical Activity Guidelines for Americans.* Washington, DC: U.S. Department of Health and Human Services, 2008.

245. Urbano, L and Bogousslavsky, J. Antiplatelet drugs in ischemic stroke prevention: from monotherapy to combined treatment. *Cerebrovasc Dis* 17(suppl 1):74-80, 2004.

246. Ustrell, X and Pellisé, A. Cardiac workup of ischemic stroke. *Curr Cardiol Rev* 6:175-183, 2010.

247. van der Scheer, J, de Groot, S, Vegter, R, Hartog, J, Tepper, M, Slootman, H, ALLRISC Group, Veeger, D, and van der Woude, L. Low-intensity wheelchair training in inactive people with long-term spinal cord injury: a randomized controlled trial on propulsion technique. *Am J Phys Med Rehabil* 94:975-986, 2015.

248. Vancini, R, Barbosa de Lira, C, Scorza, F, de Albuquerque, M, Sousa, B, de Lima, C, Cavalheiro, E, Carlos da Silva, A, and Arida, R. Cardiorespiratory and electroencephalographic responses to exhaustive acute physical exercise in people with temporal lobe epilepsy. *Epilepsy Behav* 19:504-505, 2010.

249. Varanese, S, Birnbaum, Z, Rossi, R, and Di Rocco, A. Treatment of advanced Parkinson's disease. *Parkinsons Dis* 2010:480260, 2011.

250. Verrotti, A, Trotta, D, Salladini, C, di Corcia, G, Latini, G, Cutarella, R, and Chiarelli, F. Photosensitivity and epilepsy: a follow-up study. *Dev Med Child Neurol* 46:347-351, 2004.

251. Verschuren, O, Ketelaar, M, Gorter, J, Helders, P, Uiterwaal, C, and Takken, T. Exercise training program in children and adolescents with cerebral palsy: a randomized controlled trial. *Arch Pediatr Adolesc Med* 161:1075-1081, 2007.

252. von Sarnowski, B, Putaala, J, Grittner, U, Gaertner, B, Schminke, U, Curtze, S, Huber, R, Tanislav, C, Lichy, C, Demarin, V, Basic-Kes, V, Ringelstein, E, Neumann-Haefelin, T, Enzinger, C, Fazekas, F, Rothwell, P, Dichgans, M, Jungehulsing, GJ, Heuschmann, PU, Kaps, M, Norrving, B, Rolfs, A, Kessler, C, Tatlisumak, T, and sifap1 Investigators. Lifestyle risk factors for ischemic stroke and transient ischemic attack in young adults in the Stroke in Young Fabry Patients study. *Stroke* 44:119-125, 2013.

252a. Vyas, A, Kori, V, Rajagopala, S, and Patel, K. Etiopathological study on cerebral palsy and its management by Shashtika Shali Pinda Sweda and Samvardhana Ghrita. *Ayu* 34:56-62, 2013.

253. Wagle Shukla, A and Okun, M. Surgical treatment of Parkinson's disease: patients, targets, devices, and approaches. *Neurotherapeutics* 11:47-59, 2014.

254. Walberer, M and Rueger, M. The macrosphere model—an embolic stroke model for studying the pathophysiology of focal cerebral ischemia in a translational approach. *Ann Transl Med* 3:123, 2015.

255. Wang, X, Dong, Y, Qi, X, Huang, C, and Hou, L. Cholesterol levels and risk of hemorrhagic stroke: a systematic review and meta-analysis. *Stroke* 44:1833-1839, 2013.

256. WebMD. Drug Treatment for Parkinson's Disease. www.webmd.com/parkinsons-disease/guide/drug-treatments. Accessed May 27, 2016.

257. WebMD. Drugs & Medications Search. www.webmd.com/drugs/condition-1078-Multiple+Sclerosis.aspx?diseaseid=1078&diseasename=Multiple+Sclerosis. Accessed May 17, 2016.

258. WebMD. Cerebral Palsy – Medications. 2014. www.webmd.com/children/tc/cerebral-palsy-medications. Accessed May 27, 2016.

259. WebMD. Stroke Health Center: Medications. 2014. www.webmd.com/stroke/guide/stroke-medications. Accessed May 27, 2016.

260. WebMD. Epilepsy Health Center: Epilepsy drugs to treat seizures. 2015. www.webmd.com/epilepsy/medications-treat-seizures. Accessed May 27, 2016.

261. WebMD. Understanding Muscular Dystrophy – Diagnosis and Treatment. 2015. www.webmd.com/children/understanding-muscular-dystrophy-treatment. Accessed May 27, 2016.

262. Wise, E, Hoffman, J, Powell, J, Bombardier, C, and Bell, K. Benefits of exercise maintenance after traumatic brain injury. *Arch Phys Med Rehabil* 93:1319-1323, 2012.

263. Witenko, C, Moorman-Li, R, Motycka, C, Duane, K, Hincapie-Castillo, J, Leonard, P, and Valaer, C. Considerations for the appropriate use of skeletal muscle relaxants for the management of acute low back pain. *P T* 39:427-435, 2014.

264. Wolf, S, Winstein, C, Miller, J, Taub, E, Uswatte, G, Morris, D, Giuliani, C, Light, K, Nichols-Larsen, D, and EXCITE Investigators. Effect of constraint-induced movement therapy on upper extremity function 3 to 9 months after stroke: the EXCITE randomized clinical trial. *JAMA* 296:2095-2104, 2006.

265. Worth, P. How to treat Parkinson's disease in 2013. *Clin Med (Lond)* 13:93-96, 2013.

266. Xiong, Y, Mahmood, A, and Chopp, M. Emerging treatments for traumatic brain injury. *Expert Opin Emerg Drugs* 14:67-84, 2009.

267. Young, H, Barton, B, Waisbren, S, Portales, D, Ryan, M, Webster, R, and North, K. Cognitive and psychological profile of males with Becker muscular dystrophy. *J Child Neurol* 23:155-162, 2007.

268. Zafeiriou, D, Kontopoulos, E, and Tsikoulas, I. Characteristics and prognosis of epilepsy in children with cerebral palsy. *J Child Neurol* 14:289-294, 1999.

269. Ziemssen, T and Reichmann, H. Cardiovascular autonomic dysfunction in Parkinson's disease. *J Neurol Sci* 289:74-80, 2010.

Chapter 9 Cognitive Conditions and Disorders

1. Alzheimer's Association. Medications for Memory Loss. www.alz.org/alzheimers_disease_standard_prescriptions.asp. Accessed September 21, 2016.

2. Alzheimer's Association. 2015 Alzheimer's disease facts and figures. *Alzheimers Dement* 11:332-384, 2015.

3. Alzheimer's Society. Risk factors. www.alzheimers.org.uk/site/scripts/documents_info.php?documentID. Accessed September 22, 2016.

4. American Psychiatric Association. Task force on DSM-IV. In *Diagnostic and Statistical Manual of Mental Disorders: DSM-IV.* Washington, DC: American Psychiatric Association, 1994.

5. American Psychiatric Association. *Diagnostic and Statistical Manual of Mental Disorders: DSM-IV-TR.* Washington, DC: American Psychiatric Association, 2000.

6. American Psychiatric Association. DSM-5 task force. In *Diagnostic and Statistical Manual of Mental Disorders: DSM-5.* Washington, DC: American Psychiatric Association, 2013.

7. American Psychiatric Association and Task Force on Nomenclature and Statistics. Committee on nomenclature and statistics. In *Diagnostic and Statistical Manual of Mental Disorders.* Washington, DC: American Psychiatric Association, 1980.

8. Autism Speaks. Sports, exercise, and the benefits of physical activity for individuals with autism. 2009. www.autismspeaks.org/science/science-news/sports-exercise-and-benefits-physical-activity-individuals-autism. Accessed November 29, 2016.

9. Bandini, L, Curtin, C, Hamad, C, Tybor, D, and Must, A. Prevalence of overweight in children with developmental disorders in the continuous national health and nutrition examination survey (NHANES) 1999–2002. *J Pediatr* 146:738-743, 2005.

10. Bandini, L, Gleason, J, Curtin, C, Lividini, K, Anderson, S, Cermak, S, Maslin, M, and Must, A. Comparison of physical activity between children with autism spectrum disorders and typically developing children. *Autism* 17:44-54, 2013.

11. Barnes, J. Exercise, cognitive function, and aging. *Adv Physiol Educ* 39:55-62, 2015.

12. Bherer, L, Erickson, KI, and Liu-Ambrose, T. A review of the effects of physical activity and exercise on cognitive and brain functions in older adults. *J Aging Res* 2013:657508, 2013.

13. Canfield, M, Honein, M, Yuskiv, N, Xing, J, Mai, C, Collins, J, Devine, O, Petrini, J, Ramadhani, T, Hobbs, C, and Kirby, R. National estimates and race/ethnic-specific variation of selected birth defects in the United States, 1999-2001. *Birth Defects Res Part A Clin Mol Teratol* 76:747-756, 2006.

14. Carmeli, E, Barchad, S, Masharawi, Y, and Coleman, R. Impact of a walking program in people with Down syndrome. *J Strength Cond Res* 18:180-184, 2004.

15. Carmichael, S, Saper, C, and Schlaug, G. Emergent properties of neural repair: elemental biology to therapeutic concepts. *Ann Neurol* 79:895-906, 2016.

16. Centers for Disease Control and Prevention. Autism spectrum disorder: Data and statistics. 2016. www.cdc.gov/ncbddd/autism/data.html. Accessed September 26, 2016.

17. Centers for Disease Control and Prevention. Facts about Down Syndrome. 2016. www.cdc.gov/ncbddd/birthdefects/downsyndrome.html. Accessed October 16, 2016.

18. Chapman, DP, Williams, S, Strine, T, Anda, R, and Moore, M. Dementia and its implications for public health. *Prev Chronic Dis* 3:A34, 2006.

19. Chen, A, Kim, S, Houtrow, A, and Newacheck, P. Prevalence of obesity among children with chronic conditions. *Obesity* 18:210-213, 2010.

20. Cheng, S. Cognitive reserve and the prevention of dementia: the role of physical and cognitive activities. *Curr Psychiatry Rep* 18:85, 2016.

21. Christensen, D, Baio, J, and Braun, K. Prevalence and characteristics of autism spectrum disorder among children aged 8 years. *MMWR Surveill Summ* 65:1-23, 2012.

22. Climstein, M, Pitetti, K, Barrett, P, and Campbell, K. The accuracy of predicting treadmill VO2max for adults with mental retardation, with and without Down's syndrome, using ACSM gender- and activity-specific regression equations. *J Intellect Disabil Res* 37:521-531, 1993.

23. Corrada, MM, Brookmeyer, R, Paganini-Hill, A, Berlau, D, and Kawas, C. Dementia incidence continues to increase with age in the oldest old: the 90+ study. *Ann Neurol* 67:114-121, 2010.

24. Cotman, C and Berchtold, N. Exercise: a behavioral intervention to enhance brain health and plasticity. *Trends Neurosci* 25:295-301, 2002.

25. Cowley, P, Ploutz-Snyder, L, Baynard, T, Heffernan, K, Jae, S, Hsu, S, Lee, M, Pitetti, K, Reiman, M, and Fernhall, B. The effect of progressive resistance training on leg strength, aerobic capacity and functional tasks of daily living in persons with Down syndrome. *Disabil Rehabil* 33:2229-2236, 2011.

26. Curtin, C, Bandini, L, Perrin, E, Tybor, D, and Must, A. Prevalence of overweight in children and adolescents with attention deficit hyperactivity disorder and autism spectrum disorders: a chart review. *BMC Pediatr* 5:48, 2005.

27. Division of Birth Defects and Developmental Disabilities of the Centers for Disease Control and Prevention. Facts about Down syndrome. 2016. www.cdc.gov/ncbddd/birthdefects/downsyndrome.html#ref. Accessed October 16, 2016.

28. Dodd, KJ and Shields, N. A systematic review of the outcomes of cardiovascular exercise programs for people with Down syndrome. *Arch Phys Med Rehabil* 86:2051-2058, 2005.

29. Ellis, L, Lang, R, Shield, J, Wilkinson, J, Lidstone, J, Coulton, S, and Summerbell, C. Obesity and disability—a short review. *Obes Rev* 7:341-345, 2006.

30. Eshkoor, S, Hamid, T, Mun, C, and Ng, C. Mild cognitive impairment and its management in older people. *Clin Interv Aging* 10:687-693, 2015.

31. Fleck, S and Kraemer, W. *Strength Training for Young Athletes.* 2nd ed. Champaign, IL: Human Kinetics, 2005.

32. Fleck, S and Kraemer, W. *Designing Resistance Training Programs.* 4th ed. Champaign, IL: Human Kinetics, 2014.

33. Gadia, CA, Tuchman, R, and Rotta, NT. Autism and pervasive developmental disorders [in Portuguese]. *J Pediatr (Rio J)* 80:S83-S94, 2004.

34. Geschwind, D. Advances in autism. *Annu Rev Med* 60:367-380, 2009.

35. Global Down Syndrome Foundation. Facts and FAQ About Down Syndrome. 2015. www.globaldownsyndrome.org/about-down-syndrome/facts-about-down-syndrome/. Accessed September 16, 2016.

36. Heller, T, Hsieh, K, and Rimmer, J. Attitudinal and psychosocial outcomes of a fitness and health education program on adults with down syndrome. *Am J Ment Retard* 109:175-185, 2004.

37. Heller, T, McCubbin, J, Drum, C, and Peterson, J. Physical activity and nutrition health promotion interventions: what is working for people with intellectual disabilities? *Intellect Dev Disabil* 49:26-36, 2011.

38. Hielkema, T and Hadders-Algra, M. Motor and cognitive outcome after specific early lesions of the brain - a systematic review. *Dev Med Child Neurol* 58(suppl 4):46-52, 2016.

39. Houston-Wilson, C and Lieberman, L. Strategies for teaching students with autism in physical education. *JOPERD* 74:40-44, 2003.

40. Kern, L, Koegel, R, and Dunlap, G. The influence of vigorous versus mild exercise on autistic stereotyped behaviors. *J Autism Dev Disord* 14:57-67, 1984.

41. Kramer, A and Erickson, K. Capitalizing on cortical plasticity: influence of physical activity on cognition and brain function. *Trends Cogn Sci* 11:138-147, 2007.

42. Landa, R. Diagnosis of autism spectrum disorders in the first 3 years of life. *Nat Clin Pract Neurol* 4:138-147, 2008.

43. Lochbaum, M and Crews, D. Exercise prescription for autistic populations. *J Autism Dev Disord* 25:335-336, 1995.

44. Lourenço, C, Esteves, M, Corredeira, R, and Seabra, A. Assessment of the effects of intervention programs of physical activity in individuals with autism spectrum disorder. *Revista Brasileira de Educação Especial* 21:319-328, 2015.

45. Mendonca, G, Pereira, F, and Fernhall, B. Effects of combined aerobic and resistance exercise training in adults with and without Down syndrome. *Arch Phys Med Rehabil* 92:37-45, 2011.

46. Mohan, M, Bennett, C, and Carpenter, P. Memantine for dementia in people with Down syndrome. *Cochrane Database Syst Rev*:CD007657, 2009.

47. Morley, J, Morris, J, Berg-Weger, M, Borson, S, Carpenter, B, del Campo, N, Dubois, B, Fargo, K, Fitten, LJ, Flaherty, JH, Ganguli, M, Grossberg, GT, Malmstrom, TK, Petersen, RD, Rodriguez, C, Saykin, AJ, Scheltens, P, Tangalos, EG, Verghese, J, Wilcock, G, Winblad, B, Woo, J, and Vellas, B. Brain health: the importance of recognizing cognitive impairment: an IAGG consensus conference. *J Am Med Dir Assoc* 16:731-739, 2015.

48. Murphy, C, Boyle, C, Schendel, D, Decouflé, P, and Yeargin-Allsopp, M. Epidemiology of mental retardation in children. *Ment Retard Dev Disabil Res Rev* 4:6-13, 1998.

49. National Institute on Aging. *Alzmeimer's Disease Medications Fact Sheet*. Bethesda, MD: U.S. Department of Health and Human Services, 2016.

50. National Institutes of Health and Eunice Kennedy Shriver National Institute of Child Health and Human Development. What are common treatments for Down syndrome? 2014. www.nichd.nih.gov/health/topics/down/conditioninfo/pages/treatments.aspx#drugs. Accessed October 16, 2016.

51. National Institutes of Health and U.S. National Library of Medicine. Autism spectrum disorder. 2016. www.medlineplus.gov/autismspectrumdisorder.html. Accessed October 16, 2016.

52. National Institutes of Health and U.S. National Library of Medicine. Down syndrome. 2016. www.ghr.nlm.nih.gov/condition/down-syndrome#genes. Accessed October 16, 2016.

53. Newschaffer, C, Croen, L, Daniels, J, Giarelli, E, Grether, J, Levy, S, Mandell, D, Miller, L, Pinto-Martin, J, Reaven, J, Reynolds, A, Rice, C, Schendel, D, and Windham, G. The epidemiology of autism spectrum disorders. *Annu Rev Public Health* 28:235-258, 2007.

54. Ogden, C, Carroll, M, and Flegal, K. High body mass index for age among US children and adolescents, 2003-2006. *JAMA* 299:2401-2405, 2008.

55. Pan, C. The efficacy of an aquatic program on physical fitness and aquatic skills in children with and without autism spectrum disorders. *Res Autism Spectr Disord* 5:657-665, 2011.

56. Pan, C and Frey, G. Physical activity patterns in youth with autism spectrum disorders. *J Autism Dev Disord* 36:597-606, 2006.

57. Pardo, C and Eberhart, C. The neurobiology of autism. *Brain Pathol* 17:434-437, 2007.

58. Picker, J and Walsh, C. New innovations: therapeutic opportunities for intellectual disabilities. *Ann Neurol* 74:382-390, 2013.

59. Podgorski, C, Kessler, K, Cacia, B, Peterson, D, and Henderson, C. Physical activity intervention for older adults with intellectual disability: report on a pilot project. *Ment Retard* 42:272-283, 2004.

60. Prupas, A and Reid, G. Effects of exercise frequency on stereotypic behaviors of children with developmental disorders. *Educ Train Ment Ret* 36:196-206, 2001.

61. Rapin, I and Tuchman, R. Autism: definition, neurobiology, screening, diagnosis. *Pediatr Clin North Am* 55:1126-1146, viii, 2008.

62. Rimmer, J, Heller, T, Wang, E, and Valerio, I. Improvements in physical fitness in adults with Down syndrome. *Am J Ment Retard* 109:165-174, 2004.

63. Rosser Sandt, D and Frey, G. Comparison of physical activity levels between children with and without autistic spectrum disorders. *Adapt Phys Activ Q* 27:149-159, 2005.

64. Shields, N, Taylor, N, and Dodd, K. Effects of a community-based progressive resistance training program on muscle performance and physical function in adults with Down syndrome: a randomized controlled trial. *Arch Phys Med Rehabil* 89:1215-1220, 2008.

65. Spiering, B, Kraemer, W, Anderson, J, Armstrong, L, Nindl, B, Volek, J, and Maresh, C. Resistance exercise biology: manipulation of resistance exercise programme variables determines the responses of cellular and molecular signalling pathways. *Sports Med* 38:527-540, 2008.

66. Srinivasan, S, Pescatello, L, and Bhat, A. Current perspectives on physical activity and exercise recommendations for children and adolescents with autism spectrum disorders. *Phys Ther* 94:875-889, 2014.

67. Stratford, B and Ching, E. Responses to music and movement in the development of children with Down's syndrome. *J Ment Def Res* 33:13-24, 1989.

68. Temple, V, Frey, G, and Stanish, H. Physical activity of adults with mental retardation: review and research needs. *Am J Health Promot* 21:2-12, 2006.

69. Tsimaras, V and Fotiadou, E. Effect of training on the muscle strength and dynamic balance ability of adults with Down syndrome. *J Strength Cond Res* 18:343-347, 2004.

70. United States Census Bureau. Survey of Income and Program Participation, 2008 Panel. 2008. www.census.gov/newsroom/cspan/disability/20120726_cspan_disability_slides.pdf. Accessed December 12, 2016.

71. United States Census Bureau. *Americans with Disabilities: Household Economic Studies*. Washington, DC: U.S. Department of Commerce, 2012.

72. United States Department of Health and Human Services. *Physical Activity Guidelines for Americans*. Washington, DC: U.S. Deparment of Health and Human Services, 2008.

73. Varela, A, Sardinha, L, and Pitetti, K. Effects of an aerobic rowing training regimen in young adults with Down syndrome. *Am J Ment Retard* 106:135-144, 2001.

74. Yang, Q, Sherman, S, Hassold, T, Allran, K, Taft, L, Pettay, D, Khoury, M, Erickson, J, and Freeman, S. Risk factors for trisomy 21: maternal cigarette smoking and oral contraceptive use in a population-based case-control study. *Genet Med* 1:80-88, 1999.

75. Zhang, J and Griffin, A. Including children with autism in general physical eduation: eight possible solutions. *JOPERD* 78:33-50, 2007.

Chapter 10 Cancer

1. Adamsen, L, Midtgaard, J, Rorth, M, Borregaard, N, Andersen, C, Quist, M, Møller, T, Zacho, M, Madsen, JK, and Knutsen, L. Feasibility, physical capacity, and health benefits of a multidimensional exercise program for cancer patients undergoing chemotherapy. *Support Care Cancer* 11:707-716, 2003.

2. Alibhai, SMH, Durbano, S, Breunis, H, Brandwein, JM, Timilshina, N, Tomlinson, GA, Oh, PI, and Culos-Reed, SN. A phase II exercise randomized controlled trial for patients with acute myeloid leukemia undergoing induction chemotherapy. *Leuk Res* 39:1178-1186, 2015.

3. American Academy of Pediatrics Committee on Infectious Diseases. *Red Book 2009: Report of the Committee on Infectious Diseases*. 28th ed. Chicago: American Academy of Pediatrics, 2009.

4. American Cancer Society. Cancer Facts & Figures. www.cancer.org. Accessed October 28, 2016.

5. American College of Sports Medicine, Schmitz, KH, Courneya, KS, Matthews, C, Demark-Wahnefried, W, Galvão, DA, Pinto, BM, Irwin, ML, Wolin, KY, Segal, RJ, Lucia, A, Schneider, von Gruenigen, VE, and Schwartz, AL. American College of Sports Medicine roundtable on exercise guidelines for cancer survivors. *Med Sci Sports Exerc* 42:1409-1426, 2010.

6. Aznar, S, Webster, AL, San Juan, AF, Chamorro-Viña, C, Maté-Muñoz, JL, Moral, S, Pérez, M, García-Castro, J, Ramírez, M, Madero, L, and Lucia, A. Physical activity during treatment in children with leukemia: a pilot study. *Appl Physiol Nutr Metab* 31:407-413, 2006.

7. Beesley, V, Janda, M, Eakin, E, Obermair, A, and Battistutta, D. Lymphedema after gynecological cancer treatment: prevalence, correlates, and supportive care needs. *Cancer* 109:2607-2614, 2007.

8. Blair, CK, Morey, MC, Desmond, RA, Cohen, HJ, Sloane, R, Snyder, DC, and Demark-Wahnefried, W. Light-intensity activity attenuates functional decline in older cancer survivors. *Med Sci Sports Exerc* 46:1375-1383, 2014.

9. Bonn, SE, Sjölander, A, Lagerros, YT, Wiklund, F, Stattin, P, Holmberg, E, Grönberg, H, and Bälter, K. Physical activity and survival among men diagnosed with prostate cancer. *Cancer Epidemiol Biomarkers Prev* 24:57-64, 2015.

10. Bonn, SE, Wiklund, F, Sjölander, A, Szulkin, R, Stattin, P, Holmberg, E, Grönberg, H, and Bälter, K. Body mass index and weight change in men with prostate cancer: progression and mortality. *Cancer Causes Control* 25:933-943, 2014.

11. Bradley, WG, Lassman, LP, Pearce, GW, and Walton, JL. The neuromyopathy of vincristine in man: clinical, electrophysiological and pathological studies. *J Neurol Sci* 10:107-131, 1970.

12. Bristow, MR, Billingham, ME, and Mason, JW. Clinical spectrum of anthracycline antibiotic cardiotoxicity. *Cancer Treat Rep* 62, 1978.

13. Brown, JC and Schmitz, KH. Weight lifting and physical function among survivors of breast cancer: a post hoc analysis of a randomized controlled trial. *J Clin Oncol* 1:2184-2189, 2015.

14. Buffart, L, Galvão, D, Chinapaw, M, Brug, J, Taaffe, D, Spry, N, Joseph, D, and Newton, R. Mediators of the resistance and aerobic exercise intervention effect on physical and general health in men undergoing androgen deprivation therapy for prostate cancer. *Cancer* 120:294-301, 2014.

15. Burham, TR and Wilcox, A. Effects of exercise on physiological and psychological variables in cancer survivors. *Med Sci Sports Exerc* 34:1863-1867, 2002.

16. Carlson, L, Beattie, T, Giese-Davis, J, Faris, P, Tamagawa, R, Fick, L, Degelman, E, and Speca, M. Mindfulness-based cancer recovery and supportive-expressive therapy maintain telomere length relative to controls in distressed breast cancer survivors. *Cancer* 121:476-484, 2015.

17. Carlson, L, Smith, D, Russell, J, Fibich, C, and Whittaker, T. Individualized exercise program for the treatment of severe fatigue in patients after allogeneic hematopoietic stem-cell transplant: a pilot study. *Bone Marrow Transplant* 37:945-954, 2006.

18. Celebioglu, F, Perbeck, L, Frisell, J, Gröndal, E, Svensson, L, and Danielsson, R. Lymph drainage studied by lymphoscintigraphy in the arms after sentinel node biopsy compared with axillary lymph node dissection following conservative breast cancer surgery. *Acta Radiol* 48:488-495, 2007.

19. Chamorro-Viña, C, Ruiz, J, Santana-Sosa, E, González Vicent, M, Madero, L, Pérez, M, Fleck, S, Pérez, A, Ramírez, M, and Lucía, A. Exercise during hematopoietic stem cell transplant hospitalization in children. *Med Sci Sports Exerc* 42:1045-1053, 2010.

20. Cheema, B and Gaul, C. Full-body exercise training improves fitness and quality of life in survivors of breast cancer. *J Strength Cond Res* 20:14-21, 2006.

21. Cheema, B, Gaul, C, Lane, K, and Fiatarone Singh, M. Progressive resistance training in breast cancer: a systematic review of clinical trials. *Breast Cancer Res Treat* 109:9-26, 2008.

22. Cormie, P, Galvão, D, Spry, N, Joseph, D, Chee, R, Taaffe, D, Chambers, S, and Newton, R. Can supervised exercise prevent treatment toxicity in patients with prostate cancer initiating androgen-deprivation therapy: a randomised controlled trial. *BJU Int* 115:256-266, 2015.

23. Cormie, P, Newton, R, Spry, N, Joseph, D, Taaffe, D, and Galvão, D. Safety and efficacy of resistance exercise in prostate cancer patients with bone metastases. *Prostate Cancer Prostatic Dis* 16:328-335, 2013.

24. Courneya, K, Friedenreich, C, Quinney, H, Fields, A, Jones, L, and Fairey, A. A randomized trial of exercise and quality of life in colorectal cancer survivors. *Eur J Cancer Care (Engl)* 12:347-357, 2003.

25. Courneya, K, Mackey, J, and Jones, L. Coping with cancer. Can exercise help? *Phys Sportsmed* 28, 2000.

26. Courneya, K, Segal, R, Gelmon, K, Reid, R, Mackey, J, Friedenreich, C, Proulx, C, Lane, K, Ladha, A, Vallance, J, Liu, Q, Yasui, Y, and McKenzie, D. Six-month follow-up of patient-rated outcomes in a randomized controlled trial of exercise training during breast cancer chemotherapy. *Cancer Epidemiol Biomarkers Prev* 16:2572-2578, 2007.

27. Courneya, K, Segal, R, Mackey, J, Gelmon, K, Reid, R, Friedenreich, C, Ladha, A, Proulx, C, Vallance, J, Lane, K, Yasui, Y, and McKenzie, D. Effects of aerobic and resistance exercise in breast cancer patients receiving adjuvant chemotherapy: a multicenter randomized controlled trial. *J Clin Oncol* 25:4396-4404, 2007.

28. Cramp, F and Byron-Daniel, J. Exercise for the management of cancer-related fatigue in adults. *Cochrane Database Syst Rev* 11:CD006145, 2012.

29. Daley, A, Crank, H, Saxton, J, Mutrie, N, Coleman, R, and Roalfe, A. Randomized trial of exercise therapy in women treated for breast cancer. *J Clin Oncol* 25:1713-1721, 2007.

30. Dash, C, Randolph-Jackson, P, Isaacs, C, Mills, M, Makambi, K, Watkins, V, and Adams-Campbell, L. An exercise trial to reduce cancer related fatigue in African American breast cancer patients undergoing radiation therapy: design, rationale, and methods. *Contemp Clin Trials* 47:153-157, 2016.

31. Dimeo, F. Effects of exercise on cancer-related fatigue. *Cancer* 92:1689-1693, 2001.

32. Dimeo, F, Bertz, H, Finke, J, Fetscher, S, Mertelsmann, R, and Keul, J. An aerobic exercise program for patients with haematological malignancies after bone marrow transplantation. *Bone Marrow Transplant* 18:1157-1160, 1996.

33. Dimeo, F, Fetscher, S, Lange, W, Mertelsmann, R, and Keul, J. Effects of aerobic exercise on the physical performance and incidence of treatment-related complications after high-dose chemotherapy. *Blood* 90:3390-3394, 1997.

34. Dimeo, F, Rumberger, B, and Keul, J. Aerobic exercise as therapy for cancer fatigue. *Med Sci Sports Exerc* 30:475-478, 1998.

35. Dimeo, F, Schwartz, S, Fietz, T, Wanjura, T, Böning, D, and Thiel, E. Effects of endurance training on the physical performance of patients with hematological malignancies during chemotherapy. *Support Care Cancer* 11:623-628, 2003.

36. Dimeo, F, Schwartz, S, Wesel, N, Voigt, A, and Thiel, E. Effects of an endurance and resistance exercise program on persistent cancer-related fatigue after treatment. *Ann Oncol* 19:1495-1499, 2008.

37. Dimeo, F, Stieglitz, R, Novelli-Fischer, U, Fetscher, S, and Keul, J. Effects of physical activity on the fatigue and psychologic status of cancer patients during chemotherapy. *Cancer* 85:2273-2277, 1999.

38. Dimeo, F, Stieglitz, R, Novelli-Fischer, U, Fetscher, S, Mertelsmann, R, and Keul, J. Correlation between physical performance and fatigue in cancer patients. *Ann Oncol* 8:1251-1255, 1997.

39. Dimeo, F, Tilmann, M, Bertz, H, Kanz, L, Mertelsmann, R, and Keul, J. Aerobic exercise in the rehabilitation of cancer patients after high dose chemotherapy and autologous peripheral stem cell transplantation. *Cancer* 79:1717-1722, 1997.

40. Esbenshade, A, Friedman, D, Smith, W, Jeha, S, Pui, C, Robison, L, and Ness, K. Feasibility and initial effectiveness of home exercise during maintenance therapy for childhood acute lymphoblastic leukemia. *Pediatr Phys Ther* 26:301-307, 2014.

41. Fairey, A, Courneya, K, Field, C, Bell, G, Jones, L, and Mackey, J. Randomized controlled trial of exercise and blood immune function in postmenopausal breast cancer survivors. *J Appl Physiol* 98:1534-1540, 2005.

42. Fauci, A, Kasper, D, Braunwald, E, Hauser, S, Longo, D, and Jameson, J. *Harrison's Principles of Internal Medicine.* 17th ed. New York: McGraw-Hill Medical, 2008.

43. Francis, W, Abghari, P, Du, W, Rymal, C, Suna, M, and Kosir, M. Improving surgical outcomes: standardizing the reporting of incidence and severity of acute lymphedema after sentinel lymph node biopsy and axillary lymph node dissection. *Am J Surg* 192:636-639, 2006.

44. Friedenreich, C and Orenstein, M. Physical activity and cancer prevention: etiologic evidence and biological mechanisms. *J Nutr* 132:3456S-3464S, 2002.

45. Friedenreich, C, Wang, Q, Neilson, H, Kopciuk, K, McGregor, S, and Courneya, K. Physical activity and survival after prostate cancer. *Eur Urol* 70:576-585, 2016.

46. Galvão, D and Newton, R. Review of exercise intervention studies in cancer patients. *J Clin Oncol* 23:899-909, 2005.

47. Galvão, D, Nosaka, K, Taaffe, D, Spry, N, Kristjanson, L, McGuigan, M, Suzuki, K, Yamaya, K, and Newton, R. Resistance training and reduction of treatment side effects in prostate cancer patients. *Med Sci Sports Exerc* 38:2045-2052, 2006.

48. Galvão, D, Spry, N, Denham, J, Taaffe, D, Cormie, P, Joseph, D, Lamb, D, Chambers, S, and Newton, R. A multicentre year-long randomised controlled trial of exercise training targeting physical functioning in men with prostate cancer previously treated with androgen suppression and radiation from TROG 03.04 RADAR. *Eur Urol* 65:856-864, 2014.

49. Galvão, D, Taaffe, D, Spry, N, and Newton, R. Exercise can prevent and even reverse adverse effects of androgen suppression treatment in men with prostate cancer. *Prostate Cancer Prostatic Dis* 10:340-346, 2007.

50. Gerritsen, J and Vincent, A. Exercise improves quality of life in patients with cancer: a systematic review and meta-analysis of randomized controlled trials. *Br J Sports Med* 50:796-803, 2015.

51. Gil-Rey, E, Quevedo-Jerez, K, Maldonado-Martin, S, and Herrero-Román, F. Exercise intensity guidelines for cancer survivors: a comparison with reference values. *Int J Sports Med*, 2014. [e-pub ahead of print].

52. Haim, N, Barron, S, and Robinson, E. Muscle cramps associated with vincristine therapy. *Acta Oncol* 30:707-711, 1991.

53. Hanahan, D and Weinberg, R. Hallmarks of cancer: the next generation. *Cell* 144:646-674, 2011.

54. Harris, S and Niesen-Vertommen, S. Challenging the myth of exercise-induced lymphedema following breast cancer: a series of case reports. *J Surg Oncol* 74:95-98, 2000.

55. Hauser, M, Gibson, B, and Wilson, N. Diagnosis of anthracycline-induced late cardiomyopathy by exercise-spiroergometry and stress-echocardiography. *Eur J Pediatr* 160:607-610, 2001.

56. Hayes, S, Davies, P, Parker, T, and Bashford, J. Total energy expenditure and body composition changes following peripheral blood stem cell transplantation and participation in an exercise programme. *Bone Marrow Transplant* 31:331-338, 2003.

57. Hayes, S, Davies, P, Parker, T, Bashford, J, and Green, A. Role of a mixed type, moderate intensity exercise programme after peripheral blood stem cell transplantation. *Br J Sports Med* 38:304-309, 2004.

58. Hayes, S, Davies, P, Parker, T, Bashford, J, and Newman, B. Quality of life changes following peripheral blood stem cell transplantation and participation in a mixed-type, moderate-intensity, exercise program. *Bone Marrow Transplant* 33:553-558, 2004.

59. Hayes, S, Rowbottom, D, Davies, P, Parker, T, and Bashford, J. Immunological changes after cancer treatment and participation in an exercise program. *Med Sci Sports Exerc* 35:2-9, 2003.

60. Hayes, S, Spence, R, Galvão, D, and Newton, R. Australian Association for Exercise and Sport Science position stand: optimising cancer outcomes through exercise. *J Sci Med Sport* 12:428-434, 2009.

61. Herrero, F, Balmer, J, San Juan, A, Foster, C, Fleck, S, Pérez, M, Cañete, S, Earnest, C, and Lucía, A. Is cardiorespiratory fitness related to quality of life in survivors of breast cancer? *J Strength Cond Res* 20:535-540, 2006.

62. Herrero, F, San Juan, A, Fleck, S, Balmer, J, Pérez, M, Cañete, S, Earnest, C, Foster, C, and Lucía, A. Combined aerobic and strength training in breast cancer survivors: a randomized, controlled pilot trial. *Int J Sports Med* 27:573-580, 2006.

63. Herrero, F, San Juan, A, Fleck, S, Foster, C, and Lucía, A. Effects of detraining on the functional capacity of previously trained breast cancer survivors. *Int J Sports Med* 28:257-264, 2007.

64. Hojan, K, Kwiatkowska-Borowczyk, E, Leporowska, E, Gorecki, M, Ozga-Majchrzak, O, Milecki, T, and Milecki, P. Physical exercise for functional capacity, blood immune function, fatigue and quality of life in high-risk prostate cancer patients during radiotherapy. A prospective, randomised clinical study. *Eur J Phys Rehabil Med* 52:489-501, 2016.

65. Holmes, M, Chen, W, Feskanich, D, Kroenke, C, and Colditz, G. Physical activity and survival after breast cancer diagnosis. *JAMA* 293:2479-2486, 2005.

66. Hovi, L, Era, P, Rautonen, J, and Siimes, M. Impaired muscle strength in female adolescents and young adults surviving leukemia in childhood. *Cancer* 72:276-281, 1993.

67. Irwin, M, Cartmel, B, Gross, C, Ercolano, E, Li, F, Yao, X, Fiellin, M, Capozza, S, Rothbard, M, Zhou, Y, Harrigan, M, Sanft, T, Schmitz, K, Neogi, T, Hershman, D, and Ligibel, J. Randomized exercise trial of aromatase inhibitor-induced arthralgia in breast cancer survivors. *J Clin Oncol* 33:1104-1111, 2015.

68. Jemal, A, Siegel, R, Ward, E, Hao, Y, Xu, J, Murray, T, and Thun, M. Cancer statistics, 2008. *Cancer J Clin* 58:71-96, 2008.

69. Jones, L, Douglas, P, Khouri, M, Mackey, J, Wojdyla, D, Kraus, W, Whellan, D, and O'Connor, C. Safety and efficacy of aerobic training in patients with cancer who have heart failure: an analysis of the HF-ACTION randomized trial. *J Clin Oncol* 32:2496-2502, 2014.

70. Jones, L, Hornsby, W, Freedland, S, Lane, A, West, M, Moul, J, Ferrandino, M, Allen, J, Kenjale, A, Thomas, S, Herndon, J, Koontz, B, Chan, J, Khouri, M, Douglas, P, and Eves, N. Effects of nonlinear aerobic training on erectile dysfunction and cardiovascular function following radical prostatectomy for clinically localized prostate cancer. *Eur Urol* 65:852-855, 2014.

71. Kent, H. Breast-cancer survivors begin to challenge exercise taboos. *CMAJ* 155:969-971, 1996.

72. Knols, R, Aaronson, N, Uebelhart, D, Fransen, J, and Aufdemkampe, G. Physical exercise in cancer patients during and after medical treatment: a systematic review of randomized and controlled clinical trials. *J Clin Oncol* 23:3830-3842, 2005.

73. Kolden, G, Strauman, T, Ward, A, Kuta, J, Woods, T, Schneider, K, Heerey, E, Sanborn, L, Burt, C, Millbrandt, L, Kalin, N, Stewart, J, and Mullen, B. A pilot study of group exercise training (GET) for women with primary breast cancer: feasibility and health benefits. *Psychooncology* 11:447-456, 2002.

74. Ladha, A, Courneya, K, Bell, G, Field, C, and Grundy, P. Effects of acute exercise on neutrophils in pediatric acute lymphoblastic leukemia survivors: a pilot study. *J Pediatr Hematol Oncol* 28:671-677, 2006.

75. Lane, K, Dolan, L, Worsley, D, and McKenzie, D. Upper extremity lymphatic function at rest and during exercise in breast cancer survivors with and without lymphedema compared with healthy controls. *J Appl Physiol* 103:917-925, 2007.

76. Lane, K, Worsley, D, and McKenzie, D. Exercise and the lymphatic system: implications for breast-cancer survivors. *Sports Med* 35:461-471, 2005.

77. Liu, J, Chen, P, Wang, R, Yuan, Y, Wang, X, and Li, C. Effect of Tai Chi on mononuclear cell functions in patients with non-small cell lung cancer. *BMC Complement Altern Med* 15:3, 2015.

78. Livingston, P, Craike, M, Salmon, J, Courneya, K, Gaskin, C, Fraser, S, Mohebbi, M, Broadbent, S, Botti, M, Kent, B, and ENGAGE Uro-Oncology Clinicians' Group. Effects of a clinician referral and exercise program for men who have completed active treatment for prostate cancer: a multicenter cluster randomized controlled trial (ENGAGE). *Cancer* 121:2646-2654, 2015.

79. Lucia, A, Earnest, C, and Perez, M. Cancer-related fatigue: how can exercise physiology assist oncologists? *Lancet Oncol* 4:616-625, 2003.

80. Lucia, A, Ramírez, M, San Juan, A, Fleck, S, García-Castro, J, and Madero, L. Intra-hospital supervised exercise training: a complementary tool in the therapeutic armamentarium against childhood leukemia. *Leukemia* 19:1334-1337, 2005.

81. MacVicar, M, Winningham, M, and Nickel, J. Effects of aerobic interval training on cancer patients' functional capacity. *Nurs Res* 38:348-351, 1989.

82. Marchese, V, Chiarello, L, and Lange, B. Effects of physical therapy intervention for children with acute lymphoblastic leukemia. *Pediatr Blood Cancer* 42:127-133, 2004.

83. Marx, M, Langer, T, Graf, N, Hausdorf, G, Stöhr, W, Ludwig, R, and Beck, J. Multicentre analysis of anthracycline-induced cardiotoxicity in children following treatment according to the nephroblastoma studies SIOP No.9/GPOH and SIOP 93-01/GPOH. *Med Pediatr Oncol* 39:18-24, 2002.

84. Mattano, LJ, Sather, H, Trigg, M, and Nachman, J. Osteonecrosis as a complication of treating acute lymphoblastic leukemia in children: a report from the Children's Cancer Group. *J Clin Oncol* 18:3262-3272, 2000.

85. Maunsell, E, Brisson, J, and Deschênes, L. Arm problems and psychological distress after surgery for breast cancer. *Can J Surg* 36:315-320, 1993.

86. Mayer, E, Reuter, M, Dopfer, R, and Ranke, M. Energy expenditure, energy intake and prevalence of obesity after therapy for acute lymphoblastic leukemia during childhood. *Horm Res* 53:193-199, 2000.

87. Mazzetti, S, Kraemer, W, Volek, J, Duncan, N, Ratamess, N, Gómez, A, Newton, R, Hakkinen, K, and Fleck, S. The influence of direct supervision of resistance training on strength performance. *Med Sci Sports Exerc* 32:1175-1184, 2000.

88. McKenzie, D. Abreast in a boat—a race against breast cancer. *CMAJ* 159:376-378, 1998.

89. McKenzie, D and Kalda, A. Effect of upper extremity exercise on secondary lymphedema in breast cancer patients: a pilot study. *J Clin Oncol* 21:463-466, 2003.

90. McNeely, M, Campbell, K, Rowe, B, Klassen, T, Mackey, J, and Courneya, K. Effects of exercise on breast cancer patients and survivors: a systematic review and meta-analysis. *CMAJ* 175:34-41, 2006.

91. McNeely, M, Parliament, M, Courneya, K, Seikaly, H, Jha, N, Scrimger, R, and Hanson, J. A pilot study of a randomized controlled trial to evaluate the effects of progressive resistance exercise training on shoulder dysfunction caused by spinal accessory neurapraxia/neurectomy in head and neck cancer survivors. *Head Neck* 26:518-530, 2004.

92. McNeely, M, Parliament, M, Seikaly, H, Jha, N, Magee, D, Haykowsky, M, and Courneya, K. Effect of exercise on upper extremity pain and dysfunction in head and neck cancer survivors: a randomized controlled trial. *Cancer* 113:214-222, 2008.

93. Merino Arribas, J. Quimioterapia del cáncer infantil. In *Hematología y oncología pediátricas*. Madero López, L, and Muñoz Villa, A, eds. Madrid: Ergon, 323-370, 2005.

94. Missel, M, Pedersen, J, Hendriksen, C, Tewes, M, and Adamsen, L. Exercise intervention for patients diagnosed with operable non-small cell lung cancer: a qualitative longitudinal feasibility study. *Support Care Cancer* 23:2311-2318, 2015.

95. Mock, V, Pickett, M, Ropka, M, Muscari Lin, E, Stewart, K, Rhodes, V, McDaniel, R, Grimm, P, Krumm, S, and McCorkle, R. Fatigue and quality of life outcomes of exercise during cancer treatment. *Cancer Pract* 9:119-127, 2001.

96. Moore, G, Durstine, J, Painter, P, and American College of Sports Medicine. *ACSM's Exercise Management for Persons With Chronic Diseases and Disabilities.* 4th ed. Champaign, IL: Human Kinetics, 2016.

97. Mortimer, P. The pathophysiology of lymphedema. *Cancer* 83:2798-2802, 1998.

98. Mortimer, P, Bates, D, Brassington, H, Stanton, A, Strachan, D, and Levick, J. The prevalence of arm oedema following treatment for breast cancer. *Quart J Med* 89:377-380, 1996.

99. Murphy, R and Greenberg, M. Osteonecrosis in pediatric patients with acute lymphoblastic leukemia. *Cancer* 65:1717-1721, 1990.

100. Na, Y, Kim, M, Kim, Y, Ha, Y, and Yoon, D. Exercise therapy effect on natural killer cell cytotoxic activity in stomach cancer patients after curative surgery. *Arch Phys Med Rehabil* 81:777-779, 2000.

101. National Cancer Institute. www.cancer.gov. Accessed December 11, 2016.

102. National Library of Medicine. www.nlm.nih.gov/medlineplus/. Accessed December 11, 2016.

103. Nichols, H, Trentham-Dietz, A, Egan, K, Titus-Ernstoff, L, Holmes, M, Bersch, A, Holick, C, Hampton, J, Stampfer, M, Willett, W, and Newcomb, P. Body mass index before and after breast cancer diagnosis: associations with all-cause, breast cancer, and cardiovascular disease mortality. *Cancer Epidemiol Biomarkers Prev* 18:1403-1409, 2009.

104. Oeffinger, K, Buchanan, G, Eshelman, D, Denke, M, Andrews, T, Germak, J, Tomlinson, G, Snell, L, and Foster, B. Cardiovascular risk factors in young adult survivors of childhood acute lymphoblastic leukemia. *J Pediatr Hematol Oncol* 23:424-430, 2001.

105. Ohira, T, Schmitz, K, Ahmed, R, and Yee, D. Effects of weight training on quality of life in recent breast cancer survivors: the Weight Training for Breast Cancer Survivors (WTBS) study. *Cancer* 106:2076-2083, 2006.

106. Oldervoll, L, Kaasa, S, Knobel, H, and Loge, J. Exercise reduces fatigue in chronically fatigued Hodgkins disease survivors–results from a pilot study. *Eur J Cancer* 39:57-63, 2003.

107. Paramanandam, V and Roberts, D. Weight training is not harmful for women with breast cancer-related lymphoedema: a systematic review. *J Physiother* 60:136-143, 2014.

108. Paskett, E, Naughton, M, McCoy, T, Case, L, and Abbott, J. The epidemiology of arm and hand swelling in premenopausal breast cancer survivors. *Cancer Epidemiol Biomarkers Prev* 16:775-782, 2007.

109. Petrek, J, Senie, R, Peters, M, and Rosen, P. Lymphedema in a cohort of breast carcinoma survivors 20 years after diagnosis. *Cancer* 92:1368-1377, 2001.

110. Porock, D, Kristjanson, L, Tinnelly, K, Duke, T, and Blight, J. An exercise intervention for advanced cancer patients experiencing fatigue: a pilot study. *J Palliat Care* 16:30-36, 2000.

111. Rehman, Y and Rosenberg, J. Abiraterone acetate: oral androgen biosynthesis inhibitor for treatment of castration-resistant prostate cancer. *Drug Des Devel Ther* 6:13-18, 2012.

112. Repka, C, Peterson, B, Brown, J, Lalonde, T, Schneider, C, and Hayward, R. Cancer type does not affect exercise-mediated improvements in cardiorespiratory function and fatigue. *Integr Cancer Ther* 13:473-481, 2014.

113. Rief, H, Petersen, L, Omlor, G, Akbar, M, Bruckner, T, Rieken, S, Haefner, M, Schlampp, I, Förster, R, Debus, J, Welzel, T, and German Bone Research Group. The effect of resistance training during radiotherapy on spinal bone metastases in cancer patients - a randomized trial. *Radiother Oncol* 112:133-139, 2014.

114. Ries, L, Eisner, M, Kosary, C, Hankey, B, Miller, B, Clegg, L, Mariotto, A, Feuer, E, and Edwards, B. *SEER Cancer Statistics Review, 1975-2004.* Bethesda, MD: National Cancer Institute, 2007.

115. Rock, C, Flatt, S, Byers, T, Colditz, G, Demark-Wahnefried, W, Ganz, P, Wolin, K, Elias, A, Krontiras, H, Liu, J, Naughton, M, Pakiz, B, Parker, B, Sedjo, R, and Wyatt, H. Results of the Exercise and Nutrition to Enhance Recovery and Good Health for You (ENERGY) trial: a behavioral weight loss intervention in overweight or obese breast cancer survivors. *J Clin Oncol* 33:3169-3176, 2015.

116. Rove, K and Crawford, E. Androgen annihilation as a new therapeutic paradigm in advanced prostate cancer. *Curr Opin Urol* 23:208-213, 2013.

117. Ryan, J and Emami, A. Vincristine neurotoxicity with residual equinocavus deformity in children with acute leukemia. *Cancer* 51:423-425, 1983.

118. San Juan, A. Cáncer infantile. In *Ejercicio Físico Es Salud*. Izquierdo, M, ed. Spain: Exercycle S.L. BH Group, 2013.

119. San Juan, A, Chamorro-Viña, C, Maté-Muñoz, J, Fernández Del Valle, M, Cardona, C, Hernández, M, Madero, L, Pérez, M, Ramírez, M, and Lucia, A. Functional capacity of children with leukemia. *Int J Sports Med* 29:163-167, 2008.

120. San Juan, A, Chamorro-Viña, C, Moral, S, Fernández Del Valle, M, Madero, L, Ramírez, M, Pérez, M, and Lucia, A. Benefits of intrahospital exercise training after pediatric bone marrow transplantation. *Int J Sports Med* 29:439-446, 2008.

121. San Juan, A, Fleck, S, Chamorro-Viña, C, Maté-Muñoz, J, Moral, S, García-Castro, J, Ramírez, M, Madero, L, and Lucia, A. Early-phase adaptations to intrahospital training in strength and functional mobility of children with leukemia. *J Strength Cond Res* 21:173-177, 2007.

122. San Juan, A, Fleck, S, Chamorro-Viña, C, Maté-Muñoz, J, Moral, S, Pérez, M, Cardona, C, Del Valle, M, Hernández, M, Ramírez, M, Madero, L, and Lucia, A. Effects of an intrahospital exercise program intervention for children with leukemia. *Med Sci Sports Exerc* 39:13-21, 2007.

123. San Juan, A, Wolin, K, and Lucía, A. Physical activity and pediatric cancer survivorship. In *Physical Activity and Cancer*. Berlin, Heidelberg: Springer, 319-347, 2010.

124. Sandler, S, Tobin, W, and Henderson, E. Vincristine-induced neuropathy. *Neurology* 19:367-374, 1969.

125. Schmidt, M, Wiskemann, J, Armbrust, P, Schneeweiss, A, Ulrich, C, and Steindorf, K. Effects of resistance exercise on fatigue and quality of life in breast cancer patients undergoing adjuvant chemotherapy: a randomized controlled trial. *Int J Cancer* 137:471-480, 2015.

126. Schmidt, T, Weisser, B, Dürkop, J, Jonat, W, Van Mackelenbergh, M, Röcken, C, and Mundhenke, C. Comparing endurance and resistance training with standard care during chemotherapy for patients with primary breast cancer. *Anticancer Res* 35:5623-5629, 2015.

127. Schmitz, K, Ahmed, R, Hannan, P, and Yee, D. Safety and efficacy of weight training in recent breast cancer survivors to alter body composition, insulin, and insulin-like growth factor axis proteins. *Cancer Epidemiol Biomarkers Prev* 14:1672-1680, 2005.

128. Schmitz, K, Ahmed, R, Troxel, A, Cheville, A, Lewis-Grant, L, Smith, R, Bryan, C, Williams-Smith, C, and Chittams, J. Weight lifting for women at risk for breast cancer-related lymphedema: a randomized trial. *JAMA* 304:2699-2705, 2010.

129. Schmitz, K, Ahmed, R, Troxel, A, Cheville, A, Smith, R, Lewis-Grant, L, Bryan, C, Williams-Smth, C, and Greene, Q. Weight lifting in women with breast-cancer-related lymphedema. *N Engl J Med* 361:664-673, 2009.

130. Schneider, C, Dennehy, C, and Carter, S. *Exercise and Cancer Recovery*. Champaign, IL: Human Kinetics, 2003.

131. Schneider, C, Hsieh, C, Sprod, L, Carter, S, and Hayward, R. Effects of supervised exercise training on cardiopulmonary function and fatigue in breast cancer survivors during and after treatment. *Cancer* 110:918-925, 2007.

132. Schwartz, A. Daily fatigue patterns and effect of exercise in women with breast cancer. *Cancer Pract* 8:16-24, 2000.

133. Schwartz, A, Mori, M, Gao, R, Nail, L, and King, M. Exercise reduces daily fatigue in women with breast cancer receiving chemotherapy. *Med Sci Sports Exerc* 33:718-723, 2001.

134. Schwartz, A, Mori, M, Gao, R, Nail, L, and King, M. Exercise reduces daily fatigue in women with breast cancer receiving chemotherapy. *Med Sci Sports Exerc* 33:718-723, 2001.

135. Segal, R, Evans, W, Johnson, D, Smith, J, Colletta, S, Gayton, J, Woodard, S, Wells, G, and Reid, R. Structured exercise improves physical functioning in women with stages I and II breast cancer: results of a randomized controlled trial. *J Clin Oncol* 19:657-665, 2001.

136. Segal, R, Reid, R, Courneya, K, Malone, S, Parliament, M, Scott, C, Venner, P, Quinney, H, Jones, L, D'Angelo, M, and Wells, G. Resistance exercise in men receiving androgen deprivation therapy for prostate cancer. *J Clin Oncol* 21:1653-1659, 2003.

137. Shaw, C, Mortimer, P, and Judd, P. Randomized controlled trial comparing a low-fat diet with a weight-reduction diet in breast cancer-related lymphedema. *Cancer* 109:1949-1956, 2007.

138. Silber, J, Cnaan, A, Clark, B, Paridon, S, Chin, A, Rychik, J, Hogarty, A, Cohen, M, Barber, G, Rutkowsky, M, Kimball, T, Delaat, C, Steinherz, L, Zhao, H, and Tartaglione, M. Design and baseline characteristics for the ACE Inhibitor After Anthracycline (AAA) study of cardiac dysfunction in long-term pediatric cancer survivors. *Am Heart J* 142:577-585, 2001.

139. Silverman, L, Gelber, R, Dalton, V, Asselin, B, Barr, R, Clavell, L, Hurwitz, C, Moghrabi, A, Samson, Y, Schorin, M, Arkin, S, Declerck, L, Cohen, H, and Sallan, S. Improved outcome for children with acute lymphoblastic leukemia: results of Dana-Farber Consortium Protocol 91-01. *Blood* 97:1211-1218, 2001.

140. Smets, E, Visser, M, Willems-Groot, A, Garssen, B, Schuster-Uitterhoeve, A, and de Haes, J. Fatigue and

radiotherapy: (B) experience in patients 9 months following treatment. *Br J Cancer* 78:907-912, 1998.

141. Sociedad Española de Oncología Médica. www.seom.org/es/inicio. Accessed October 28, 2016.

142. Thorsen, L, Skovlund, E, Strømme, S, Hornslien, K, Dahl, A, and Fosså, S. Effectiveness of physical activity on cardiorespiratory fitness and health-related quality of life in young and middle-aged cancer patients shortly after chemotherapy. *J Clin Oncol* 23:2378-2388, 2005.

143. Tobin, M, Lacey, H, Meyer, L, and Mortimer, P. The psychological morbidity of breast cancer-related arm swelling. Psychological morbidity of lymphoedema. *Cancer* 72:3248-3252, 1993.

144. Travier, N, Velthuis, M, Steins Bisschop, C, van den Buijs, B, Monninkhof, E, Backx, F, Los, M, Erdkamp, F, Bloemendal, H, Rodenhuis, C, de Roos, M, Verhaar, M, ten Bokkel Huinink, D, van der Wall, E, Peeters, P, and May, A. Effects of an 18-week exercise programme started early during breast cancer treatment: a randomised controlled trial. *BMC Med* 13:121, 2015.

145. U.S. Department of Health and Human Services. Physical Activity Guidelines for Americans. www.health.gov/paguidelines/guidelines. Accessed October 28, 2016.

146. Uth, J, Hornstrup, T, Schmidt, J, Christensen, J, Frandsen, C, Christensen, K, Helge, E, Brasso, K, Rørth, M, Midtgaard, J, and Krustrup, P. Football training improves lean body mass in men with prostate cancer undergoing androgen deprivation therapy. *Scand J Med Sci Sports* 24(suppl 1):105-112, 2014.

147. Vainionpaa, L, Kovala, T, Tolonen, U, and Lanning, M. Vincristine therapy for children with acute lymphoblastic leukemia impairs conduction in the entire peripheral nerve. *Pediatr Neurol* 13:314-318, 1995.

148. Van Brussel, M, Takken, T, Lucia, A, van der Net, J, and Helders, P. Is physical fitness decreased in survivors of childhood leukemia? A systematic review. *Leukemia* 19:13-17, 2005.

149. Van Vulpen, J, Velthuis, M, Steins Bisschop, C, Travier, N, van den Buijs, B, Backx, F, Los, M, Erdkamp, F, Bloemendal, H, Koopman, M, de Roos, M, Verhaar, M, Ten Bokkel-Huinink, D, van der Wall, E, Peeters, P, and May, A. Effects of an exercise program in colon cancer patients undergoing chemotherapy. *Med Sci Sports Exerc* 48:767-775, 2016.

150. van Waart, H, Stuiver, M, van Harten, W, Geleijn, E, Kieffer, J, Buffartm, L, de Maaker-Berkhof, M, Boven, E, Schrama, J, Geenen, M, Meerum Terwogt, J, van Bochove, A, Lustig, V, van den Heiligenberg, S, Smorenburg, C, Hellendoorn-van Vreeswijk, J, Sonke, G, and Aaronson, N. Effect of low-intensity physical activity and moderate- to high-intensity physical exercise during adjuvant chemotherapy on physical fitness, fatigue, and chemotherapy completion rates: results of the PACES randomized clinical trial. *J Clin Oncol* 33:1918-1927, 2015.

151. Wenzel, J, Griffith, K, Shang, J, Thompson, C, Hedlin, H, Stewart, K, DeWeese, T, and Mock, V. Impact of a home-based walking intervention on outcomes of sleep quality, emotional distress, and fatigue in patients undergoing treatment for solid tumors. *Oncologist* 18:476-484, 2013.

152. Wilke, L, McCall, L, Posther, K, Whitworth, P, Reintgen, D, Leitch, A, Gabram, S, Lucci, A, Cox, C, Hunt, K, Herndon, J, and Giuliano, A. Surgical complications associated with sentinel lymph node biopsy: results from a prospective international cooperative group trial. *Ann Surg Oncol* 13:491-500, 2006.

153. Willer, A. Reduction of the individual cancer risk by physical exercise. *Oncol Res Treat* 26:283-289, 2003.

154. Windsor, P, Nicol, K, and Potter, J. A randomized, controlled trial of aerobic exercise for treatment-related fatigue in men receiving radical external beam radiotherapy for localized prostate carcinoma. *Cancer* 101:550-557, 2004.

155. Winningham, M and MacVicar, M. The effect of aerobic exercise on patient reports of nausea. *Oncol Nurs Forum* 15:447-450, 1988.

156. Winningham, M, MacVicar, M, Bondoc, M, Anderson, J, and Minton, J. Effect of aerobic exercise on body weight and composition in patients with breast cancer on adjuvant chemotherapy. *Oncol Nurs Forum* 16:683-689, 1989.

157. Winters-Stone, K, Dobek, J, Bennett, J, Dieckmann, N, Maddalozzo, G, Ryan, C, and Beer, T. Resistance training reduces disability in prostate cancer survivors on androgen deprivation therapy: evidence from a randomized controlled trial. *Arch Phys Med Rehabil* 96:7-14, 2015.

158. Winters-Stone, K, Dobek, J, Bennett, J, Maddalozzo, G, Ryan, C, and Beer, T. Skeletal response to resistance and impact training in prostate cancer survivors. *Med Sci Sports Exerc* 46:1482-1488, 2014.

159. Winzer, B, Paratz, J, Whitehead, J, Whiteman, D, and Reeves, M. The feasibility of an exercise intervention in males at risk of oesophageal adenocarcinoma: a randomized controlled trial. *PLoS One* 10:e0117922, 2015.

160. Wiskemann, J and Huber, G. Physical exercise as adjuvant therapy for patients undergoing hematopoietic stem cell transplantation. *Bone Marrow Transplant* 41:321-329, 2008.

161. Wright, M, Halton, J, and Barr, R. Limitation of ankle range of motion in survivors of acute lymphoblastic leukemia: a cross-sectional study. *Med Pediatr Oncol* 32:279-282, 1999.

162. Wright, M, Halton, J, Martin, R, and Barr, R. Long-term gross motor performance following treatment for acute lymphoblastic leukemia. *Med Pediatr Oncol* 31:86-90, 1998.

163. Yagli, N and Ulger, O. The effects of yoga on the quality of life and depression in elderly breast cancer patients. *Complement Ther Clin Pract* 21:7-10, 2015.

164. Yang, T, Chen, M, and Li, C. Effects of an aerobic exercise programme on fatigue for patients with breast cancer undergoing radiotherapy. *J Clin Nurs* 24:202-211, 2015.

Chapter 11 Children and Adolescents

1. American Academy of Pediatrics. Strength training by children and adolescents. *Pediatrics* 121:835-840, 2008.

2. American College of Sports Medicine. *ACSM's Guidelines for Exercise Testing and Prescription.* Baltimore: Lippincott Williams & Wilkins, 2016.

3. American Dietetic Association. Position of the American Dietetic Association: individual-, family-, school-, and community-based interventions for pediatric overweight. *J Am Diet Assoc* 106:925-945, 2006.

4. Andersen, L and Froberg, K. Advancing the understanding of physical activity and cardiovascular risk factors in children: the European Youth Heart Study (EYHS). *Br J Sports Med* 49:67-68, 2015.

5. Armstrong, L, Casa, D, Millard-Stafford, M, Moran, D, Pyne, S, and Roberts, W. Exertional heat illness during training and competition. *Med Sci Sports Exerc* 39:556-572, 2007.

6. Armstrong, N. *Paediatric Exercise Physiology.* Philadelphia: Elsevier, 2007.

7. Ayers, S and Sariscsany, M, eds. *Physical Education for Lifelong Fitness.* Champaign, IL: Human Kinetics, 2011.

8. Bai, Y, Saint-Maurice, P, Welk, G, Allums-Featherston, K, Candelaria, N, and Anderson, K. Prevalence of youth fitness in the United States: baseline results from the NFL PLAY 60 FITNESSGRAM partnership project. *J Pediatr* 167:662-668, 2015.

9. Bailey, R, Olsen, J, Pepper, S, Porszasz, J, Barstow, T, and Cooper, D. The level and tempo of children's physical activities: an observational study. *Med Sci Sports Exerc* 27:1033-1041, 1995.

10. Baquet, G, Van Praagh, E, and Berthoin, S. Endurance training and aerobic fitness in young people. *Sports Med* 33:1127-1143, 2003.

11. Bar-Or, O and Rowland, T. *Pediatric Exercise Medicine.* Champaign, IL: Human Kinetics, 2004.

12. Behm, D and Chaouachi, A. A review of the acute effects of static and dynamic stretching on performance. *Eur J Appl Physiol* 111:2633-2651, 2011.

13. Behringer, M, Vom Heede, A, Matthews, M, and Mester, J. Effects of strength training on motor performance skills in children and adolescents: a meta-analysis. *Pediatr Exerc Sci* 23:186-206, 2011.

14. Blair, S. Physical inactivity: the biggest public health problem of the 21st century. *Br J Sports Med* 43:1-2, 2009.

15. Bloemers, F, Collard, D, Paw, M, Van Mechelen, W, Twisk, J, and Verhagen, E. Physical inactivity is a risk factor for physical activity-related injuries in children. *Br J Sports Med* 46:669-674, 2012.

16. Boisseau, N and Delamarche, P. Metabolic and hormonal responses to exercise in children and adolescents. *Sports Med* 30:405-422, 2000.

17. Brown, H, Pearson, N, Braithwaite, R, Brown, W, and Biddle, S. Physical activity interventions and depression in children and adolescents: a systematic review and meta-analysis. *Sports Med* 43:195-206, 2013.

18. Bukowsky, M, Faigenbaum, A, and Myer, G. FUNdamental Integrative Training (FIT) for physical education. *JOPERD* 85:23-30, 2014.

19. Calvo-Muñoz, I, Gómez-Conesa, A, and Sánchez-Meca, J. Prevalence of low back pain in children and adolescents: a meta-analysis. *BMC Pediatr* 13:14, 2013.

20. Cattuzzo, M, Dos Santos, HR, Ré, A, de Oliveira, I, Melo, B, de Sousa Moura, M, de Araújo, R, and Stodden, D. Motor competence and health related physical fitness in youth: a systematic review. *J Sci Med Sport,* 2015. [e-pub ahead of print].

21. Centers for Disease Control and Prevention. *The Association Between School Based Physical Activity, Including Physical Education, and Academic Performance.* Atlanta: U.S. Department of Health and Human Services, 2010.

22. Chu, D and Myer, G. *Plyometrics.* Champaign, IL: Human Kinetics, 2013.

23. Clark, J and Metcalfe, J. The mountain of motor development: a metaphor. In *Motor Development: Research and Review.* Clark, E, and Humphrey, H, eds. Reston, VA: National Association for Sports and Physical Education, 62-95, 2002.

24. Cliff, D, Okely, A, Morgan, P, Jones, R, Steele, J, and Baur, L. Proficiency deficiency: mastery of fundamental movement skills and skill components in overweight and obese children. *Obesity (Silver Spring),* 2011. [e-pub ahead of print].

25. Cohen, D, Voss, C, Taylor, M, Delextrat, A, Ogunleye, A, and Sandercock, G. Ten-year secular changes in muscular fitness in English children. *Acta Paediatr* 100:e175-e177, 2011.

26. Costigan, S, Eather, N, Plotnikoff, R, Taaffe, D, and Lubans, D. High-intensity interval training for improving health-related fitness in adolescents: a systematic review and meta-analysis. *Br J Sports Med* 49:1253-1261, 2015.

27. Council on Sports Medicine and Fitness and Council on School Health, Bergeron M., Devore, C, and Rice, S. Policy statement—Climatic heat stress and exercising children and adolescents. *Pediatrics* 128:e741-e747, 2011.

28. Coutts, A, Murphy, A, and Dascombe, B. Effect of direct supervision of a strength coach on measures of muscular strength and power in young rugby league players. *J Strength Cond Res* 18:316-323, 2004.

29. Cunningham, S, Kramer, M, and Venkat Narayan, K. Incidence of childhood obesity in the United States. *N Engl J Med* 370:403-411, 2014.

30. Daniels, S, Hassink, S, and Committee on Nutrition. The role of the pediatrician in primary prevention of obesity. *Pediatrics* 136:e275-e292, 2015.

31. Dencker, M and Andersen, L. Accelerometer measured daily physical activity related to aerobic fitness in children and adolescents. *J Sports Sci* 29:887-895, 2011.

32. Difiori, J, Benjamin, H, Brenner, J, Gregory, A, Jayanthi, N, Landry, G, and Luke, A. Overuse injuries and burnout in youth sports: a position statement from the American Medical Society for Sports Medicine. *Clin J Sport Med* 24:3-20, 2014.

33. Eriksson, B. Muscle metabolism in children: a review. *Acta Physiol Scand* 283:20-28, 1980.

34. Esteban-Cornejo, I, Hallal, P, Mielke, G, Menezes, A, Gonçalves, H, Wehrmeister, F, Ekelund, U, and Rombaldi, A. Physical activity throughout adolescence and cognitive performance at 18 years of age. *Med Sci Sports Exerc* 47:2552-2557, 2015.

35. Faigenbaum, A. Children and adolescents. In *Exercise Physiology*. Porcari, J, Bryant, C, and Comana, F, eds. Philadelphia: Davis, 686-709, 2015.

36. Faigenbaum, A, Bush, J, McLoone, R, Kreckel, M, Farrell, A, Ratamess, N, and Kang, J. Benefits of strength and skill based training during primary school physical education. *J Strength Cond Res* 29:1255-1262, 2015.

37. Faigenbaum, A, Farrell, A, Fabiano, M, Radler, T, Naclerio, F, Ratamess, N, Kang, J, and Myer, G. Effects of integrated neuromuscular training on fitness performance in children. *Pediatr Exerc Sci* 23:573-584, 2011.

38. Faigenbaum, A, Kraemer, W, Blimkie, C, Jeffreys, I, Micheli, L, Nitka, M, and Rowland, T. Youth resistance training: updated position statement paper from the National Strength and Conditioning Association. *J Strength Cond Res* 23:S60-S79, 2009.

39. Faigenbaum, A, Lloyd, R, MacDonald, J, and Myer, G. Citius, Altius, Fortius: beneficial effects of resistance training for young athletes *Br J Sports Med*, 2015. [e-pub ahead of print].

40. Faigenbaum, A, Lloyd, R, and Myer, G. Youth resistance training: past practices, new perspectives and future directions. *Pediatr Exerc Sci* 25:591-604, 2013.

41. Faigenbaum, A, Lloyd, R, Sheehan, D, and Myer, G. The role of the pediatric exercise specialist in treating exercise deficit disorder in youth. *Strength Cond J* 35:34-41, 2013.

42. Faigenbaum, A and McFarland, J. Guidelines for implementing a dynamic warm-up for physical education. *JOPERD* 78:25-28, 2007.

43. Faigenbaum, A, McFarland, J, Herman, R, Naclerio, F, Ratamess, N, Kang, J, and Myer, G. Reliability of the one-repetition-maximum power clean test in adolescent athletes. *J Strength Cond Res* 26:432-437, 2012.

44. Faigenbaum, A, Milliken, L, and Westcott, W. Maximal strength testing in healthy children. *J Strength Cond Res* 17:162-166, 2003.

45. Faigenbaum, A and Myer, G. Resistance training among young athletes: safety, efficacy and injury prevention effects. *Br J Sports Med* 44:56-63, 2010.

46. Faigenbaum, A and Myer, G. Exercise deficit disorder in youth: play now or pay later. *Curr Sports Med Rep* 11:196-200, 2012.

47. Faigenbaum, A, Myer, G, Naclerion, F, and Casas, A. Injury trends and prevention in youth resistance training. *Strength Cond J* 33:36-41, 2011.

48. Faigenbaum, A, Ratamess, N, McFarland, J, Kaczmarek, J, Coraggio, M, Kang, J, and Hoffman, J. Effect of rest interval length on bench press performance in boys, teens, and men. *Pediatr Exerc Sci* 20:457-469, 2008.

49. Faigenbaum, A and Westcott, W. *ACE Youth Fitness Manual*. San Diego: Americn Council on Exercise, 2013.

50. Falk, B and Dotan, R. Child-adult differences in the recovery from high-intensity exercise. *Exerc Sport Sci Rev* 34:107-112, 2006.

51. Gomes, L, Carneiro-Júnior, M, and Marins, J. Thermoregulatory responses of children exercising in a hot environment. *Rev Paul Pediatr* 31:104-110, 2013.

52. Graham, G. *Teaching Children Physical Education*. Champaign, IL: Human Kinetics, 2008.

53. Hardy, L, Barnett, L, Espinel, P, and Okely, A. Thirteen-year trends in child and adolescent fundamental movement skills: 1997-2010. *Med Sci Sports Exerc* 45:1965-1970, 2013.

54. Hillman, C, Pontifex, M, Castelli, D, Khan, N, Raine, L, Scudder, M, Drollette, E, Moore, R, Wu, C, and Kamijo, K. Effects of the FITKids randomized controlled trial on executive control and brain function. *Pediatrics* 134:e1062-e1071, 2014.

55. Institute of Medicine. *Educating the Student Body: Taking Physical Activity and Physical Education to School*. Washington, DC: National Academies Press, 2013.

56. Kelley, G and Kelley, K. Effects of exercise in the treatment of overweight and obese children and adolescents: a systematic review of meta-analyses. *J Obes*, 2013. [e-pub ahead of print].

57. Kohl, H, Craig, C, Lambert, E, Inoue, S, Alkandari, J, Leetongin, G, Kahlmeier, S, and Lancet Physical Activity Series Working Group. The pandemic of physical inactivity: global action for public health. *Lancet* 380:294-305, 2012.

58. Kraus, H and Raab, W. *Hypokinetic Disease*. Springfield, IL: Charles C Thomas, 1961.

59. Lee, S, Bacha, F, Hannon, T, Kuk, J, Boesch, C, and Arslanian, S. Effects of aerobic versus resistance exercise without caloric restriction on abdominal fat, intrahepatic lipid, and insulin sensitivity in obese adolescent boys: a randomized, controlled trial. *Diabetes* 61:2787-2795, 2012.

60. Lephart, SM and Fu, FH. *Proprioception and Neuro-muscular Control in Joint Stability.* Champaign, IL: Human Kinetics, 2000.

61. Lloyd, R, Faigenbaum, A, Stone, M, Oliver, J, Jeffreys, I, Moody, J, Brewer, C, Pierce, K, and Myer, G. Position statement on youth resistance training: the 2014 international consensus. *Br J Sports Med* 48(7):498-505, 2014.

62. Lloyd, R, Oliver, J, Faigenbaum, A, Howard, R, De Ste Croix, M, Williams, C, Best, T, Alvar, B, Micheli, L, Thomas, D, Hatfield, D, Cronin, J, and Myer, G. Long-term athletic development, part 2: barriers to success and potential solutions. *J Strength Cond Res* 29:1451-1464, 2015.

63. Malina, R, Bouchard, C, and Bar-Or, O. *Growth, Maturation and Physical Activity.* Champaign, IL: Human Kinetics, 2004.

64. Malina, R, Cummings, S, Maorano, P, Barron, M, and Miller, S. Maturity status of youth football players: a noninvasive estimate. *Med Sci Sports Exerc* 24:199-209, 2005.

65. Matsudo, S and Matsudo, V. Self-assessment and physician assessment of sexual maturation in Brazilian boys and girls: concordance and reproducibility. *Am J Hum Biol* 6, 451-455, 1994.

66. McDonald, N. Active transportation to school: trends among U.S. schoolchildren, 1969-2001. *Am J Prev Med* 32:509-516, 2007.

67. McPherson, A, Keith, R, and Swift, J. Obesity prevention for children with physical disabilities: a scoping review of physical activity and nutrition interventions. *Disabil Rehabil*, 2014. [e-pub ahead of print].

68. Mediate, P and Faigenbaum, A. *Medicine Ball for All Kids.* Monterey, CA: Healthy Learning, 2007.

69. Myer, G, Faigenbaum, A, Ford, K, Best, T, Bergeron, M, and Hewett, T. When to initiate integrative neuromuscular training to reduce sports-related injuries and enhance health in youth? *Curr Sports Med Rep* 10:155-166, 2011.

70. Myer, G, Faigenbaum, A, Stracciolini, A, Hewett, T, Micheli, L, and Best, T. Exercise deficit disorder in youth: a paradigm shift towards disease prevention and comprehensive care. *Curr Sports Med Rep* 12:248-255, 2013.

71. Myer, G, Jayanthi, N, DiFiori, J, Faigenbaum, A, Kiefer, A, Logerstedt, D, and Micheli, L. Sport specialization, part I: does early sports specialization increase negative outcomes and reduce the opportunity for success in young athletes? *Sports Health* 7:437-442, 2015.

72. Myer, G, Quatman, C, Khoury, J, Wall, E, and Hewett, T. Youth vs. adult "weightlifting" injuries presented to United States emergency rooms: accidental vs. non-accidental injury mechanisms. *J Strength Cond Res* 23:2054-2060, 2009.

73. National Association for Sport and Physical Education. *Physical Education for Lifetime Fitness.* Champaign, IL: Human Kinetics, 2011.

74. Nyberg, G, Nordenfelt, A, Ekelund, U, and Marcus, C. Physical activity patterns measured by accelerometry in 6- to 10-yr-old children. *Med Sci Sports Exerc* 41:1842-1848, 2009.

75. Pedersen, B and Saltin, B. Exercise as medicine – evidence for prescribing exercise as therapy in 26 different chronic diseases. *Scand J Med Sci Sports* 25:1-72, 2015.

76. Pesce, C. Shifting the focus from quantitative to qualitative exercise characteristics in exercise and cognition research. *J Sport Exerc Psychol* 34:766-786, 2012.

77. Pesce, C, Faigenbaum, A, Crova, C, Marchetti, R, and Bellucci, M. Benefits of multi-sports participation in the elementary school context. *Health Educ J* 72:326-336, 2012.

78. Pulgarón, E. Childhood obesity: a review of increased risk for physical and psychological comorbidities. *Clin Ther* 35:A18-A32, 2013.

79. Rasberry, C, Lee, S, Robin, L, Laris, B, Russell, L, Coyle, K, and Nihiser, A. The association between school-based physical activity, including physical education, and academic performance: a systematic review of the literature. *Prev Med* 52:S10-S20, 2011.

80. Robinson, L, Stodden, D, Barnett, L, Lopes, V, Logan, S, Rodrigues, L, and D'Hondt, E. Motor competence and its effect on positive developmental trajectories of health. *Sports Med* 45:1273-1284, 2015.

81. Rowland, T. *Children's Exercise Physiology.* Champaign, IL: Human Kinetics, 2007.

82. Rowland, T. Fluid replacement requirements for child athletes. *Sports Med* 41:279-288, 2011.

83. Salvy, S, Bowker, J, Germeroth, L, and Barkley, J. Influence of peers and friends on overweight/obese youths' physical activity. *Exerc Sport Sci Rev* 40:127-132, 2012.

84. Schranz, N, Tomkinson, G, Parletta, N, Petkov, J, and Olds, T. Can resistance training change the strength, body composition and self-concept of overweight and obese adolescent males? A randomised controlled trial. *Br J Sports Med*, 2013. [e-pub ahead of print].

85. Shrier, I. Does stretching improve performance? A systematic and critical review of the literature. *Clin J Sports Med* 14:267-273, 2004.

86. Sigal, R, Alberga, A, Goldfield, G, Prud'homme, D, Hadjiyannakis, S, Gougeon, R, Phillips, P, Tulloch, H, Malcolm, J, Doucette, S, Wells, G, Ma, J, and Kenny, G. Effects of aerobic training, resistance training, or both on percentage body fat and cardiometabolic risk markers in obese adolescents: the healthy eating aerobic and resistance training in youth randomized clinical trial. *JAMA Pediatr* 168:1006-1014, 2014.

87. Stodden, D, Gao, Z, Goodway, J, and Langendorfer, S. Dynamic relationships between motor skill competence and health-related fitness in youth. *Pediatr Exerc Sci* 26:231-241, 2014.

88. Stodden, D, Goodway, J, Langendorfer, S, Robertson, M, Rudisill, M, and Garcia, C. A developmental perspective on the role of motor skill competence in physical activity: an emergent relationship. *Quest* 60:290-306, 2008.

89. Stracciolini, A, Myer, G, and Faigenbaum, A. Exercise deficit disorder in youth: are we ready to make the diagnosis? *Phys Sportsmed* 41:94-101, 2013.

90. Strong, WB, Malina, RM, Blimkie, CJ, Daniels, SR, Dishman, RK, Gutin, B, Hergenroeder, AC, Must, A, Nixon, PA, Pivarnik, JM, Rowland, T, Trost, S, and Trudeau, F. Evidence based physical activity for school-age youth. *J Pediatr* 146:732-737, 2005.

91. Sugimoto, D, Myer, G, Bush, H, Klugman, M, Medina McKeon, J, and Hewett, T. Compliance with neuromuscular training and anterior cruciate ligament injury risk reduction in female athletes: a meta-analysis. *J Athl Train* 47:714-723, 2012.

92. Tanner, J. *Growth at Adolescence*. Oxford: Blackwell, 1962.

93. Telama, R, Yang, X, Leskinen, E, Kankaanpää, A, Hirvensalo, M, Tammelin, T, Viikari, J, and Raitakari, O. Tracking of physical activity from early childhood through youth into adulthood. *Med Sci Sports Exerc* 46:955-962, 2014.

94. Tremblay, M, Gray, C, Akinroye, K, Harrington, D, Katzmarzyk, P, Lambert, E, Liukkonen, J, Maddison, R, Ocansey, R, Onywera, V, Prista, A, Reilly, J, del Pilar Rodríguez Martínez, M, Sarmiento Duenas, O, Standage, M, and Tomkinson, G. Physical activity of children: a global matrix of grades comparing 15 countries. *J Phys Act Health* 11:S113-S125, 2014.

95. Tudor-Locke, C, Johnson, W, and Katzmarzyk, PT. Accelerometer-determined steps per day in US children and adolescents. *Med Sci Sports Exerc* 42:2244-2250, 2010.

96. Valovich McLeod, T, Decoster, L, Loud, K, Micheli, L, Parker, T, Sandrey, M, and White, C. National Athletic Trainers' Association position statement: prevention of pediatric overuse injuries. *J Athl Train* 46:206-220, 2011.

97. Van der Heijden, G, Wang, Z, Chu, Z, Toffolo, G, Manesso, E, Sauer, PJ, and Sunehag, A. Strength exercise improves muscle mass and hepatic insulin sensitivity in obese youth. *Med Sci Sports Exerc* 11:1973-1980, 2010.

98. Wall, M, Carlson, S, Stein, A, Lee, S, and Fulton, J. Trends by age in youth physical activity: Youth Media Campaign Longitudinal Survey. *Med Sci Sports Exerc* 43:2140-2147, 2011.

99. Whitehead, M. The concept of physical literacy. In *Physical Literacy Through the Lifecourse*. Whitehead, M, ed. London, UK: Routledge, 10-20, 2010.

100. World Health Organization. *Global Recommendations on Physical Activity for Health*. Geneva: WHO Press, 2010.

Chapter 12 Older Adults

1. Ainsworth, B, Haskell, W, Whitt, M, Irwin, M, Swartz, A, Strath, S, O'Brien, W, Bassett, D, Schmitz, K, Emplaincourt, P, and Jacobs, D. Compendium of physical activities: an update of activity codes and MET intensities. *Med Sci Sports Exerc* 32:S498-S504, 2000.

2. Aloia, J, McGowan, D, Vaswani, A, Ross, P, and Cohn, S. Relationship of menopause to skeletal and muscle mass. *Am J Clin Nutr* 53:1378-1383, 1991.

3. American College of Sports Medicine, Chodzko-Zajko, WJ, Proctor, DN, Fiatarone Singh, MA, Minson, CT, Nigg, CR, Salem, GJ, Skinner, JS. American College of Sports Medicine position stand. Exercise and physical activity for older adults. *Med Sci Sports Exerc* 41:1510-1530, 2009.

4. Annesi, J and Westcott, W. Relationship of feeling states after exercise and Total Mood Disturbance over 10 weeks in formerly sedentary women. *Percept Mot Skills* 99:107-115, 2004.

5. Annesi, J and Westcott, W. Relations of physical self-concept and muscular strength with resistance exercise-induced feeling state scores in older women. *Percept Mot Skills* 104:183-190, 2007.

6. Annesi, J, Westcott, W, and Gann, S. Preliminary evaluation of a 10-week resistance and cardiovascular exercise protocol on physiological and psychological measures for a sample of older women. *Percept Mot Skills* 98:163-170, 2004.

7. Annesi, J, Westcott, W, La Rosa Loud, R, and Powers, L. Effects of association and dissociation formats on resistance exercise-induced emotion change and physical self-concept in older women. *J Ment Health Aging* 10:87-98, 2004.

8. Artero, E, Lee, D, Ruiz, J, Sui, X, Ortega, F, Church, T, Lavie, C, Castillo, M, and Blair, S. A prospective study of muscular strength and all-cause mortality in men with hypertension. *J Am Coll Cardiol* 57:1831-1837, 2011.

9. Arthritis Foundation. 2007. Understanding Arthritis. www.arthritis.org/about-arthritis/understanding-arthritis/. Accessed December 12, 2016.

10. Baechle, T and Westcott, W. *Fitness Professional's Guide to Strength Training Older Adults*. Champaign, IL: Human Kinetics, 2010.

11. Balducci, S, Zanuso, S, Fernando, F, Fallucca, S, Fallucca, F, and Pugliese, G. Physical activity/exercise training in type 2 diabetes. The role of the Italian diabetes and exercise study. *Diabetes Metab Res Rev* 25(suppl 1):S29-S33, 2009.

12. Barry, B and Carson, R. The consequences of resistance training for movement control in older adults. *J Gerontol A Biol Sci Med Sci* 59:730-754, 2004.

13. Bemben, D, Fetters, N, Bemben, M, Nabavi, N, and Koh, E. Musculoskeletal response to high and low intensity resistance training in early postmenopausal women. *Med Sci Sports Exerc* 32:1949-1957, 2000.

14. Bevier, W, Wiswell, R, Pyka, G, Kozak, K, Newhall, K, and Marcus, R. Relationship of body composition, muscle strength, and aerobic capacity to bone mineral density in older men and women. *J Bone Miner Res* 4:421-432, 1989.

15. Bircan, C, Karasel, SA, Akgun, B, El, O, and Alper, S. Effects of muscle strengthening versus aerobic exercise program in fibromyalgia. *Rheumatol Int* 28:527-532, 2008.

16. Blessing, D, Stone, M, and Byrd, R. Blood lipid and hormonal changes from jogging and weight training of middle-aged men. *J Strength Cond Res* 1:25-29, 1987.

17. Borg, G. *Borg's Perceived Exertion and Pain Scales.* Champaign, IL: Human Kinetics, 1998.

18. Boyden, T, Pamenter, R, Going, S, Lohman, T, Hall, M, Houtkooper, L, Bunt, J, Ritenbaugh, C, and Aickin, M. Resistance exercise training is associated with decreases in serum low-density lipoprotein cholesterol levels in pre-menopausal women. *Arch Intern Med* 153:97-100, 1993.

19. Boyle, J. Projection of the year 2050 burden of diabetes in the US adult population: dynamic modeling of incidence, mortality, and prediabetes prevalence. *Popul Health Metr* 8:29, 2010.

20. Braith, R and Stewart, K. Resistance exercise training: its role in the prevention of cardiovascular disease. *Circulation* 113:2642-2650, 2006.

21. Broeder, C, Burrhus, K, Svanevik, L, and Wilmore, J. The effects of either high-intensity resistance or endurance training on resting metabolic rate. *Am J Clin Nutr* 55:802-810, 1992.

22. Busse, A, Filho, W, Magaldi, R, Coelho, V, Melo, A, Betoni, R, and Santarem, J. Effects of resistance training exercise on cognitive performance in elderly individuals with memory impairment: results of a controlled trial. *Einstein* 6:402-407, 2008.

23. Bweir, S, Al-Jarrah, M, Almalty, A, Maayah, M, Smirnova, I, Novikova, L, and Stehno-Bittel, L. Resistance exercise training lowers HbA1c more than aerobic training in adults with type 2 diabetes. *Diabetol Metab Syndr* 1:27, 2009.

24. Campbell, W, Crim, M, Young, V, and Evans, W. Increased energy requirements and changes in body composition with resistance training in older adults. *Am J Clin Nutr* 60:167-175, 1994.

25. Carpinelli, R and Otto, R. Strength training: single versus multiple sets. *Sports Med* 26:73-84, 1998.

26. Caserotti, P, Aagaard, P, Buttrup, J, and Puggaard, I. Explosive heavy-resistance training in old and very old adults: changes in rapid muscle force, strength and power. *Scand J Med Sci Sports* 18:773-782, 2008.

27. Cassilhas, R, Viana, V, Grasmann, V, Santos, R, Santos, R, Tufik, S, and Mello, M. The impact of resistance exercise on the cognitive function of the elderly. *Med Sci Sports Exerc* 39:1401-1407, 2007.

28. Castaneda, C, Layne, J, Munez-Orians, L, Gordon, P, Walsmith, J, Foldvari, M, Roubenoff, R, Tucker, K, and Nelson, M. A randomized controlled trial of resistance exercise training to improve glycemic control in older adults with type 2 diabetes. *Diabetes Care* 25:2335-2341, 2002.

29. Cauza, E, Hanusch-Enserer, U, Strasser, B, Ludvik, B, Metz-Schimmerl, S, Pacini, G, Wagner, O, Georg, P, Prager, R, Kostner, K, Dunky, A, and Haber, P. The relative benefits of endurance and strength training on metabolic factors and muscle function of people with type 2 diabetes. *Arch Phys Med Rehabil* 86:1527-1533, 2005.

30. Chestnut, I and Docherty, D. The effects of 4 and 10 repetition maximum weight training protocols on neuromuscular adaptations in untrained men. *J Strength Cond Res* 13:353-359, 1999.

31. Chilibeck, P, Calder, A, Sale, D, and Webber, C. Twenty weeks of weight training increases lean tissue mass but not bone mineral mass or density in healthy, active women. *Can J Physiol Pharmacol* 74:1180-1185, 1996.

32. Chilibeck, P, Calder, A, Sale, D, and Webber, C. A comparison of strength and muscle mass increases during resistance training in young women. *Eur J Appl Physiol Occup Physiol* 77:170-175, 1997.

33. Clark, D, Hunt, M, and Dotson, C. Muscular strength and endurance as a function of age and activity level. *Res Q* 63:302-310, 1992.

34. Colcombe, S and Kramer, A. Fitness effects on the cognitive function of older adults: a meta-analytic study. *Psychol Sci* 14:125-130, 2003.

35. Coon, P, Rogus, E, Drinkwater, D, Muller, D, and Goldberg, A. Role of body fat distribution in the decline in insulin sensitivity and glucose tolerance with age. *J Clin Endocrinol Metab* 75:1125-1132, 1992.

36. Cornelissen, V and Fagard, R. Effect of resistance training on resting blood pressure: a meta-analysis of randomized controlled trials. *J Hypertens* 23:251-259, 2005.

37. Crapo, R. The aging lung. In *Pulmonary Disease in the Elderly.* Mahier, D, ed. New York: Marcel Dekker, 1-25, 1993.

38. Cussler, E, Lohman, T, Going, S, Houtkooper, L, Metcalfe, L, Flint-Wagner, H, Harris, R, and Teixeira, P. Weight lifted in strength training predicts bone change in postmenopausal women. *Med Sci Sports Exerc* 35:10-17, 2003.

39. de Morais Barbosa, C, Bértolo, M, Neto, J, Coimbra, I, Davitt, M, and de Paiva Magalhães, E. The effect of foot orthoses on balance, foot pain and disability in elderly women with osteoporosis: a randomized clinical trial. *Rheumatology* 52:515-522, 2013.

40. DeMichele, P, Pollock, M, Graves, J, Foster, D, Carpenter, D, Garzarella, L, Brechue, W, and Fulton, M. Isometric torso rotation strength: effect of training frequency on its development. *Arch Phys Med Rehabil* 78:64-69, 1997.

41. Dornemann, T, McMurray, R, Renner, J, and Anderson, J. Effects of high intensity resistance exercise on bone mineral density and muscle strength of 40-50 year-old women. *J Sports Med Phys Fitness* 37:246-251, 1997.

42. Dunstan, D, Daly, R, Owen, N, Jolley, D, De Courten, M, Shaw, J, and Zimmet, P. High-intensity resistance training improves glycemic control in older patients with type 2 diabetes. *Diabetes Care* 25:1729-1736, 2002.

43. Dustman, R, Emmerson, R, Ruhling, R, Shearer, D, Steinhaus, L, Johnson, S, Bonekat, H, and Shigeoka, J. Age and fitness effects on EEG, ERPs, visual sensitivity, and cognition. *Neurobiol Aging* 11:193-200, 1990.

44. Dutta, C and Hadley, E. The significance of sarcopenia in old age. *J Gerontol A Biol Sci Med Sci* 50:1-4, 1995.

45. Eichmann, B and GieBing, J. Effects of ten weeks of either multiple-set training or single-set training on strength and muscle mass. *Br J Sports Med* 10:e3, 2013.

46. Engle, W. Selective and nonselective susceptibility of muscle fiber types: a new approach to human neuromuscular diseases. *Arch Neurol* 22:97-117, 1970.

47. Eves, N and Plotnikoff, R. Resistance training and type 2 diabetes: considerations for implementation at the population level. *Diabetes Care* 29:1933-1941, 2006.

48. Evetovich, T and Hinnerichs, K. Client consultation and health appraisal. In *NSCA's Essentials of Personal Training.* 2nd ed. Coburn, J, and Malek, M, eds. Champaign, IL: Human Kinetics, 147-178, 2012.

49. Fahlman, M, Boardly, D, Lambert, C, and Flynn, M. Effects of endurance training and resistance training on plasma lipoprotein profiles in elderly women. *J Gerontol A Biol Sci Med Sci* 57:B54-B60, 2002.

50. Ferrini, A and Ferrini, R. *Health in the Later Years.* 3rd ed. Boston: McGraw-Hill, 2000.

51. Fiatarone, M, Marks, E, Ryan, N, Meredith, C, Lipsitz, L, and Evans, W. High-intensity strength training in nonagenarians. *JAMA* 263:3029-3034, 1990.

52. Flack, K, Davy, K, Hulver, M, Winett, R, Frisard, M, and Davy, B. Aging, resistance training, and diabetes prevention. *J Aging Res* 2011:127315, 2011.

53. Fleg, J. Alterations in cardiovascular structure and function with advancing age. *Am J Cardiol* 57:33-44, 1986.

54. Flegal, K, Carroll, M, Ogden, C, and Curtin, L. Prevalence and trends in obesity among US adults, 1999-2008. *JAMA* 303:235-241, 2010.

55. Focht, B. Effectiveness of exercise interventions in reducing pain symptoms among older adults with knee osteoarthritis: a review. *J Aging Phys Act* 14:212-235, 2006.

56. Forbes, G and Halloran, E. The adult decline in lean body mass. *Hum Biol* 48:161-173, 1976.

57. Frontera, W, Hughes, V, Fiatarone, M, Fielding, R, Evans, W, and Roubenoff, R. Aging of skeletal muscle: a 12-yr longitudinal study. *J Appl Physiol* 88:1321-1326, 2000.

58. Frontera, W, Meredith, C, O'Reilly, K, Knuttgen, H, and Evans, W. Strength conditioning in older men: skeletal muscle hypertrophy and improved function. *J Appl Physiol* 64:1038-1044, 1988.

59. Frontera, W, Reid, K, Phillips, E, Krivickas, L, Hughes, V, Roubenoff, R, and Fielding, R. Muscle fiber size and function in elderly humans: a longitudinal study. *J Appl Physiol* 105:637-642, 2008.

60. Going, S and Laudermilk, M. Osteoporosis and strength training. *Am J Lifestyle Med* 3:310-319, 2009.

61. Going, S, Lohman, T, Houtkooper, L, Metcalfe, L, Flint-Wagner, H, Blew, R, Stanford, V, Cussler, E, Martin, J, Teixeira, P, Harris, M, Milliken, L, Figueroa-Galvez, A, and Weber, J. Effects of exercise on BMD in calcium replete postmenopausal women with and without hormone replacement therapy. *Osteoporos Int* 14:637-643, 2003.

62. Gordon, B, Benson, A, Bird, S, and Fraser, S. Resistance training improves metabolic health in type 2 diabetes: a systematic review. *Diabetes Res Clin Pract* 83:157-175, 2009.

63. Graafmans, W, Ooms, M, Hofstee, H, Bezemer, P, Bouter, L, and Lips, P. Falls in the elderly: a prospective study of risk factors and risk profiles. *Am J Epidemiol* 143:1129-1136, 1996.

64. Graham, J. Resistance training exercise technique. In *NSCA's Essentials of Personal Training.* 2nd ed. Coburn, J, and Malek, M, eds. Champaign, IL: Human Kinetics, 289, 2012.

65. Graves, J, Pollock, M, Jones, A, Colvin, A, and Leggett, S. Specificity of limited range of motion variable resistance training. *Med Sci Sports Exerc* 21:84-89, 1989.

66. Guan, J and Wade, M. The effect of aging on adaptive eye-hand coordination. *J Gerontol B Psychol Sci Soc Sci* 55:151-162, 2000.

67. Gutin, B and Kasper, M. Can exercise play a role in osteoporosis prevention? A review. *Osteoporos Int* 2:55-69, 1992.

68. Hackney, K, Engels, H, and Gretebeck, R. Resting energy expenditure and delayed-onset muscle soreness after full-body resistance training with an eccentric concentration. *J Strength Cond Res* 22:1602-1609, 2008.

69. Hagerman, F, Walsh, S, Staron, R, Hikida, R, Gilders, R, Murray, T, Toma, K, and Ragg, K. Effects of high-intensity resistance training on untrained older men: strength, cardiovascular, and metabolic responses. *J Gerontol A Biol Sci Med Sci* 55:B336-B346, 2000.

70. Häkkinen, A, Häkkinen, K, Hannonen, P, and Alen, M. Strength training induced adaptations in neuromuscular function of premenopausal women and fibromyalgia: comparison with healthy women. *Ann Rheum Dis* 60:21-26, 2001.

71. Haltom, R, Kraemer, R, Sloan, R, Hebert, E, Frank, K, and Tryniecki, J. Circuit weight training and its effects on excess post-exercise oxygen consumption. *Med Sci Sports Exerc* 31:1613-1618, 1999.

72. Harris, C, DeBeliso, M, Spitzer-Gibson, T, and Adams, K. The effect of resistance training intensity on strength gain response in the older adult. *J Strength Cond Res* 18:833-838, 2004.

73. Riebe, D, Franklin, BA, Thompson, PD, Garber, CE, Whitfield, GP, Magal, M, and Pescatello, LS. Updating ACSM's recommendations for exercise preparticipation health screening. *Med Sci Sports Exerc* 47:2473-2479, 2015.

74. Hatfield, B and Kaplan, P. Exercise psychology for the personal trainer. In *NSCA's Essentials of Personal Training*. 2nd ed. Coburn, J, and Malek, M, eds. Champaign, IL: Human Kinetics, 125-144, 2012.

75. Hayden, J, von Tulder, M, and Tomlinson, G. Systematic review: strategies for using exercise therapy to improve outcomes in chronic low back pain. *Ann Intern Med* 142:776-785, 2005.

76. Heden, T, Lox, C, Rose, P, Reid, S, and Kirk, E. One-set resistance training elevates energy expenditure for 72 hours similar to three sets. *Eur J Appl Physiol* 111:477-484, 2011.

77. Henwood, T and Taaffe, D. Improved physical performance in older adults undertaking a short-term programme of high-velocity resistance training. *Gerontology* 51:108-115, 2005.

78. Hiraoka, M. Oral beta-blockers. *Card Electrophysiol Rev* 2:215-217, 1998.

79. Holten, M, Zacho, M, Gaster, C, Juel, C, Wojaszewskil, J, and Dela, F. Strength training increases insulin-mediated glucose uptake, GLUT4 content, and insulin signaling in skeletal muscle in patients with type 2 diabetes. *Diabetes* 53:294-305, 2004.

80. Holviala, J, Sallinen, J, Kraemer, W, Alen, M, and Häkkinen, K. Effects of strength training on muscle strength characteristics, functional capabilities, and balance in middle-aged and older woman. *J Strength Cond Res* 20:336-344, 2006.

81. Hsu, W, Chen, C, Tsauo, J, and Yang, R. Balance control in elderly people with osteoporosis. *J Formos Med Assoc* 113:334-339, 2014.

82. Hunter, G, Bickel, C, Fisher, G, Neumeier, W, and McCarthy, J. Combined aerobic and strength training and energy expenditure in older women. *Med Sci Sports Exerc* 45:1386-1393, 2013.

83. Hunter, G, Bryan, D, Wetzstein, C, Zuckerman, P, and Bamman, M. Resistance training and intra-abdominal adipose tissue in older men and women. *Med Sci Sports Exerc* 34:1025-1028, 2002.

84. Hunter, G, Wetzstein, C, Fields, D, Brown, A, and Bamman, M. Resistance training increases total energy expenditure and free-living physical activity in older adults. *J Appl Physiol* 89:977-984, 2000.

85. Hurley, B. Strength training in the elderly to enhance health status. *Med Exerc Nutr Health* 4:217-229, 1995.

86. Hurley, B, Hanson, E, and Sheaff, A. Strength training as a countermeasure to aging muscle and chronic disease. *Sports Med* 41:289-306, 2011.

87. Hurley, B and Roth, S. Strength training in the elderly: effects on risk factors for age-related diseases. *Sports Med* 30:249-268, 2000.

88. Ibanez, J, Izquierdo, M, Arguelles, I, Forga, L, Larrion, J, Garcia-Unciti, M, Idoate, F, and Gorostiaga, E. Twice weekly progressive resistance training decreases abdominal fat and improves insulin sensitivity in older men with type 2 diabetes. *Diabetes Care* 28:662-667, 2005.

89. Izquierdo, M, Ibanez, J, Gorostiaga, E, Garrues, M, Zuniga, A, Anton, A, Larrion, J, and Häkkinen, K. Maximal strength and power characteristics in isometric and dynamic actions of the upper and lower extremities in middle-aged and older men. *Acta Physiol Scand* 167:57-68, 1999.

90. Jan, M, Lin, J, Liau, J, Lin, Y, and Lin, D. Investigation of clinical effects of high- and low-resistance training for patients with knee osteoarthritis: a randomized controlled trial. *Phys Ther* 88:427-436, 2008.

91. Joseph, L, Davey, S, Evans, W, and Campbell, W. Differential effect of resistance training on the body composition and lipoprotein-lipid profile in older men and women. *Metabolism* 48:1474-1480, 1999.

92. Jurca, R, Lamonte, M, Church, T, Ernest, C, Fitzgerald, S, Barlow, C, Jordan, A, Kampert, J, and Blaire, S. Associations of muscle strength and fitness with metabolic syndrome in men. *Med Sci Sports Exerc* 36:1301-1307, 2004.

93. Kaido, M, Toda, I, Ishida, R, Konagai, M, Dogru, M, and Tsubota, K. Age-related changes in functional visual acuity in healthy individuals. *Jpn J Ophthalmol* 55:183-189, 2011.

94. Kalapotharakos, V, Michalopoulos, M, Tokmakidis, S, Godolias, G, and Gourgoulis, V. Effects of heavy and moderate resistance training on functional performance in older adults. *J Strength Cond Res* 19:652-657, 2005.

95. Kasch, V, Boyer, J, Van Camp, S, Verity, L, and Wallace, J. The effects of physical activity and inactivity on aerobic power in older men: a longitudinal study. *Phys Sportsmed* 18:73-83, 1990.

96. Kelemen, M and Effron, M. Exercise training combined with antihypertensive drug therapy. *JAMA* 263:2766-2771, 1990.

97. Kelley, G. Dynamic resistance exercise and resting blood pressure in healthy adults: a meta-analysis. *J Appl Physiol* 82:1559-1565, 1997.

98. Kelley, G and Kelley, K. Progressive resistance exercise and resting blood pressure: a meta-analysis of randomized controlled trials. *Hypertension* 35:838-843, 2000.

99. Kelley, G and Kelley, K. Impact of progressive resistance training on lipids and lipoproteins in adults: a meta-analysis of randomized controlled trials. *Prev Med* 48:9-19, 2009.

100. Kemmler, W, Von Stengel, S, Weineck, J, Lauber, D, Kalender, W, and Engelke, K. Exercise effects on menopausal risk factors of early postmenopausal women: 3-yr Erlanger fitness osteoporosis prevention study results. *Med Sci Sports Exerc* 37:194-203, 2005.

101. Kerr, D, Ackland, T, Maslen, B, Morton, A, and Prince, R. Resistance training over 2 years increases bone mass in calcium-replete postmenopausal women. *J Bone Miner Res* 16:175-181, 2001.

102. Kerr, D, Morton, A, Dick, I, and Prince, R. Exercise effects on bone mass in post-menopausal women are site-specific and load-dependent. *J Bone Miner Res* 11:218-225, 1996.

103. Keys, A, Taylor, H, and Grande, F. Basal metabolism and age of adult man. *Metabolism* 22:579-587, 1973.

104. Klein, C, March, G, Petrella, R, and Rice, C. Muscle fiber number in the biceps brachii muscle of young and old men. *Muscle Nerve* 28:62-68, 2003.

105. Koffler, K, Menkes, A, Redmond, A, Whitehead, W, Pratley, R, and Hurley, B. Strength training accelerates gastrointestinal transit in middle-aged and older men. *Med Sci Sports Exerc* 24:415-419, 1992.

106. Kohrt, W, Kirwan, J, Staten, M, Bourey, R, King, D, and Holloszy, J. Insulin resistance in aging is related to abdominal obesity. *Diabetes* 42:273-281, 1993.

107. Kokkinos, P, Hurley, B, Vaccaro, P, Patterson, J, Gardner, L, Ostrove, S, and Goldberg, A. Effects of low and high repetition resistive training on lipoprotein-lipid profiles. *Med Sci Sports Exerc* 29:50-54, 1998.

108. Krieger, J. Single versus multiple sets of resistance exercise: a meta-regression. *J Strength Cond Res* 23:1890-1901, 2009.

109. Lackmann, M, Neupert, S, Betrand, R, and Jette, A. The effects of strength training on memory of older adults. *J Aging Phys Act* 14:59-73, 2006.

110. LaForest, S, St-Pierre, D, Cyr, J, and Gayton, D. Effects of age and regular exercise on muscle strength and endurance. *Eur J Appl Physiol* 60:104-111, 1990.

111. Lakatta, A. Changes in cardiovascular function with aging. *Eur Heart J* 11:22-29, 1990.

112. Lange, A, Vanwanseele, B, and Fiatarone Singh, M. Strength training for treatment of osteoarthritis of the knee: a systematic review. *Arthritis Rheum* 59:1488-1494, 2008.

113. Layne, J and Nelson, M. The effects of progressive resistance training on bone density: a review. *Med Sci Sports Exerc* 31:25-30, 1999.

114. Lemmer, J, Ivey, F, Ryan, A, Martel, G, Hurlbut, D, Metter, J, Fozard, J, Fleg, J, and Hurley, B. Effect of strength training on resting metabolic rate and physical activity. *Med Sci Sports Exerc* 33:532-541, 2001.

115. Liddle, S, Baxter, G, and Gracey, J. Exercise and chronic low back pain: what works? *Pain* 107:176-190, 2004.

116. Lloyd-Jones, D, Adams, R, Carnethon, M, De Simone, G, Ferguson, T, Flegal, K, Ford, E, Furie, K, Go, A, Greenlund, K, Haase, N, Hailpern, S, Ho, M, Howard, V, Kissela, B, Kitner, S, Lackland, D, Lisabeth, L, Marelli, A, McDermott, M, Meigs, J, Mozaffarian, D, Nickol, G, O'Donnell, C, Roger, V, Rosamond, W, Sacco, R, Sorlie, P, Stafford, R, Steinberger, J, Thom, T, Wasserthiel-Smoller, S, Wong, N, Wylie-Rosett, J, and Hong, Y. Heart disease and stroke statistics: 2009 update. A report from the American Heart Association Statistics Committee and Stroke Statistics Subcommittee. *Circulation* 119:480-486, 2009.

117. Lohman, T, Going, S, Pamenter, R, Hall, M, Boyden, T, Houtkooper, L, Ritenbaugh, C, Bare, L, Hill, A, and Aickin, M. Effects of resistance training on regional and total BMD in premenopausal women: a randomized prospective study. *J Bone Miner Res* 10:1015-1024, 1995.

118. Maden-Wilkinson, T, McPhee, J, Jones, D, and Degens, H. Age-related loss of muscle mass, strength, and power and their association with mobility in recreationally-active older adults in the United Kingdom. *J Aging Phys Act* 23:352-360, 2015.

119. Maggio, C and Pi-Sunyer, F. Obesity and type 2 diabetes. *Endocrinol Metab Clin North Am* 32:805-822, 2003.

120. Malek, M. *NSCA's Essentials of Personal Training.* 2nd ed. Champaign, IL: Human Kinetics, 17-28, 521-533, 2012.

121. Marcell, T. Sarcopenia: causes, consequences, and preventions. *J Gerontol A Biol Sci Med Sci* 58:M911-M916, 2003.

122. McCarthy, J and Roy, L. Physiological responses and adaptations to aerobic endurance training. In *NSCA's Essentials of Personal Training.* 2nd ed. Coburn, J, and Malek, M, eds. Champaign, IL: Human Kinetics, 89-106, 2012.

123. McKinnon, N, Connelly, D, Rice, C, Hunter, S, and Doherty, T. Neuromuscular contributions to the age-related reduction in muscle power: mechanisms and potential role of high velocity power training. *Ageing Res Rev*, 2016. [e-pub ahead of print].

124. McKinnon, N, Montero-Odasso, M, and Doherty, T. Motor unit loss is accompanied by decreased peak muscle power in the lower limb of older adults. *Exp Gerontol* 70:111-118, 2015.

125. McMahon, G, Morse, C, Burden, A, Winwood, K, and Onambelle, G. Impact of range of motion during ecologically valid resistance training protocols on muscle size, subcutaneous fat, and strength. *J Strength Cond Res* 28:245-255, 2014.

126. Melov, S, Tarnopolsky, M, Beckman, K, Felkey, K, and Hubbard, A. Resistance exercise reverses aging in human skeletal muscle. *PLoS One* 2:e465, 2007.

127. Menkes, A, Mazel, S, Redmond, R, Koffler, K, Libanati, C, Gunberg, C, Zizic, T, Hagberg, J, Pratley, R, and Hurley, B. Strength training increases regional bone mineral density and bone remodeling in middle-aged and older men. *J Appl Physiol* 74:2478-2484, 1993.

128. Metter, E, Conwit, R, Tobin, J, and Fozard, J. Age-associated loss of power and strength in the upper extremities in women and men. *J Gerontol A Biol Sci Med Sci* 52:B267-B276, 1997.

129. Milliken, L, Going, S, Houtkooper, L, Flint-Wagner, H, Figueroa, A, Metcalfe, L, Blew, R, Sharp, S, and Lohman, T. Effects of exercise training on bone remodeling, insulin-like growth factors, and BMD in post-menopausal women with and without hormone replacement therapy. *Calcif Tissue Int* 72:478-484, 2003.

130. Miranda, H, Fleck, S, Simão, R, Barreto, A, Dantas, E, and Novaes, J. Effect of two different rest period lengths on the number of repetitions performed during resistance training. *J Strength Cond Res* 21:1032-1036, 2007.

131. Munn, J, Herbert, R, Hancock, M, and Gandevia, S. Resistance training for strength: effect of number of sets and contraction speed. *Med Sci Sports Exerc* 37:1622-1626, 2005.

132. National Council on Patient Information and Education. MUST for Seniors Fact Sheet: Medicine Use and Older Adults. www.mustforseniors.org/documents/must_factsheet.pdf. Accessed November 1, 2016.

133. National Institutes of Health and National Heart, Lung, and Blood Institute. Clinical Guidelines on the Identification, Evaluation, and Treatment of Overweight and Obesity in Adults. 1998. www.nhlbi.nih.gov/guidelines/obesity/ob_gdlns.pdf. Accessed January 13, 2003.

134. National Osteoporosis Foundation. Fast Facts. 2009. www.nof.org/osteoporosis/diseasefacts.htm.

135. Nelson, M, Fiatarone, M, Morganti, C, Trice, I, Greenberg, R, and Evans, W. Effects of high-intensity strength training on multiple risk factors for osteoporotic fractures. *JAMA* 272:1909-1914, 1994.

136. Nichols, J, Nelson, K, Peterson, K, and Sartoris, D. BMD responses to high intensity strength training in active older women. *J Aging Phys Act* 3:26-28, 1995.

137. O'Connor, P, Herring, M, and Caravalho, A. Mental health benefits of strength training in adults. *Am J Lifestyle Med* 4:377-396, 2010.

138. Ong, K, Cheung, B, Man, Y, Lau, C, and Lam, K. Hypertension treatment and control: prevalence, awareness, treatment, and control of hypertension among United States adults 1999-2004. *Hypertension* 49:69-75, 2007.

139. Parise, G, Brose, A, and Tarnopolsky, M. Resistance exercise training decreases oxidative damage to DNA and increases cytochrome oxidase activity in older adults. *Exp Gerontol* 40:173-180, 2005.

140. Pate, R, Pratt, M, Blair, S, Haskell, W, Macera, C, Bouchard, C, Buchner, D, Ettinger, W, Heath, G, and King, A. Physical activity and public health: a recommendation from the Centers for Disease Control and Prevention and the American College of Sports Medicine. *JAMA* 273:402-407, 1995.

141. Pedersen, B. Muscles and their myokines. *J Exp Biol* 214:337-346, 2011.

142. Pedersen, B, Åkerström, T, Nielsen, A, and Fischer, C. Role of myokines in exercise and metabolism. *J Appl Physiol* 103:1093-1098, 2007.

143. Phillips, S. Resistance exercise: good for more than just Grandma and Grandpa's muscles. *Appl Physiol Nutr Metab* 32:1198-1205, 2007.

144. Phillips, S and Winett, R. Uncomplicated resistance training and health-related outcomes: evidence for a public health mandate. *Curr Sports Med Rep* 9:208-213, 2010.

145. Pinto, R, Gomes, N, Radaelli, R, Botton, C, Brown, L, and Bottaro, M. Effect of range of motion on muscle strength and thickness. *J Strength Cond Res* 26:2140-2145, 2012.

146. Pitsavos, C, Panagiotakos, D, Tambalis, K, Chrysohoou, C, Sidossis, L, Skouas, J, and Stefanadis, C. Resistance exercise plus aerobic activities is associated with better lipids profile among healthy individuals: the ATTIICA study. *QJM* 102:609-616, 2009.

147. Porter, C, Reidy, P, Bhattarai, N, Sidossis, L, and Rasmussen, B. Resistance exercise training alters mitochondrial function in human skeletal muscle. *Med Sci Sports Exerc* 47:1922-1931, 2015.

148. Pratley, R, Nicklas, B, Rubin, M, Miller, J, Smith, A, Smith, M, Hurley, B, and Goldberg, A. Strength training increases resting metabolic rate and norepinephrine levels in healthy 50- to 65-year-old men. *J Appl Physiol* 76:133-137, 1994.

149. Profant, O, Tintěra, J, Balogová, Z, Ibrahim, I, Jilek, M, and Syka, J. Functional changes in the human auditory cortex in ageing. *PLoS One* 10:e0116692, 2015.

150. Rhea, M, Alvar, B, and Burkett, L. A meta-analysis to determine the dose response for strength development. *Med Sci Sports Exerc* 35:456-464, 2003.

151. Risch, S, Norvell, N, Polock, M, Risch, E, Langer, H, Fulton, M, Graves, M, and Leggett, S. Lumbar strengthening in chronic low back pain patients. *Spine* 18:232-238, 1993.

152. Rochon, P, Schmader, K, and Sokol, H. Drug prescribing for older adults. 2013. www.uptodate.com/contents/drug-prescribing-for-older-adults. Accessed December 12, 2016.

153. Roubenoff, R. Sarcopenia and its implications for the elderly. *Eur J Clin Nutr* 54:S40-S47, 2000.

154. Salvi, S, Akhtar, S, and Currie, Z. Ageing changes in the eye. *Postgrad Med J* 82:581-587, 2006.

155. Schlicht, J, Camaione, D, and Owen, S. Effect of intense strength training on standing balance, walk-

ing speed, and sit-to-stand performance in older adults. *J Gerontol A Biol Sci Med Sci* 56:M281-M286, 2001.

156. Shephard, R. *Aging, Physical Activity, and Health.* Champaign, IL: Human Kinetics, 1997.

157. Singh, M. Exercise and aging. *Clin Geriatr Med* 20:201-221, 2004.

158. Singh, N, Clements, K, and Fiatarone, M. A randomized controlled trial of progressive resistance exercise in depressed elders. *J Gerontol A Biol Sci Med Sci* 52:M27-M35, 1997.

159. Smutok, M, Reece, C, Kokkinos, P, Farmer, C, Dawson, P, Shulman, R, De Vane-Bell, J, Patterson, J, Charabogos, C, and Goldberg, A. Aerobic vs. strength training for risk factor intervention in middle-aged men at high risk for coronary heart disease. *Metabolism* 42:177-184, 1993.

160. Spirduso, W, Francis, K, and MacRae, P. *Physical Dimensions of Aging.* Champaign, IL: Human Kinetics, 2005.

161. Strasser, B and Schobersberger, W. Evidence of resistance training as a treatment therapy in obesity. *J Obes* 2011:482564, 2011.

162. Strasser, B, Siebert, U, and Schobersberger, W. Resistance training in the treatment of metabolic syndrome. *Sports Med* 40:397-415, 2010.

163. Taaffe, D, Pruitt, L, Pyka, G, Guido, D, and Marcus, R. Comparative effects of high and low intensity resistance training on thigh muscle strength, fiber area, and tissue composition in elderly women. *Clin Physiol* 16:381-392, 1996.

164. Tambalis, K, Panagiotakos, D, Kavouras, S, and Sidossis, L. Responses of blood lipids to aerobic, resistance and combined aerobic with resistance exercise training: a systematic review of current evidence. *Angiology* 60:614-632, 2009.

165. Tang, J, Hartman, J, and Phillips, S. Increased muscle oxidative potential following resistance training induced fiber hypertrophy in young men. *Appl Physiol Nutr Metab* 31:495-501, 2006.

166. Trappe, S, Gallagher, P, Harber, M, Carrithers, J, Fluckey, J, and Trappe, T. Single muscle fibre contractile properties in young and old men and women. *J Physiol* 552:47-58, 2003.

167. Trappe, S, Williamson, D, Godard, M, and Gallagher, P. Maintenance of whole muscle strength and size following resistance training in older men. *Med Sci Sports Exerc* 33:S147, 2001.

168. Treuth, M, Hunter, G, Kekes-Szabo, T, Weinsier, R, Goran, M, and Berland, L. Reduction in intra-abdominal adipose tissue after strength training in older women. *J Appl Physiol* 78:1425-1431, 1995.

169. Treuth, M, Ryan, A, Pratley, R, Rubin, M, Miller, J, Nicklas, B, Sorkin, J, Harman, S, Goldberg, A, and Hurley, B. Effects of strength training on total and regional body composition in older men. *J Appl Physiol* 77:614-620, 1994.

170. Troiano, R, Berrigan, D, Dodd, K, Masse, L, Tilert, T, and McDowell, M. Physical activity in the United States measured by accelerometer. *Med Sci Sports Exerc* 40:181-188, 2008.

171. Tucker, L and Silvester, L. Strength training and hypercholesterolemia: an epidemiologic study of 8499 employed men. *Am J Health Promot* 11:35-41, 1996.

172. U.S. Department of Health and Human Services. Historical background, terminology, evolution of recommendations, and measurement, Appendix B, NIH consensus conference statement. In *Physical Activity and Health: A Report of the Surgeon General.* Atlanta: U.S. Department of Health and Human Services, Centers for Disease Control and Prevention, National Center for Chronic Disease Prevention and Health Promotion, 47, 1996.

173. U.S. Department of Health and Human Services. Bone health and osteoporosis. In *A Report of the Surgeon General.* Rockville, MD: U.S. Department of Health and Human Services, Public Health Service, Office of the Surgeon General, 2004.

174. Ulrich, I, Reid, C, and Yeater, R. Increased HDL-cholesterol levels with a weight training program. *South Med J* 80:328-331, 1987.

175. Van Etten, L, Westerterp, K, Verstappen, F, Boon, B, and Saris, W. Effect of an 18-week weight-training program on energy expenditure and physical activity. *J Appl Physiol* 82:298-304, 1997.

176. Von Stengel, S, Kemmler, W, Kalender, W, Engelke, K, and Lauber, D. Differential effects of strength versus power training on bone mineral density in postmenopausal women: a 2-year longitudinal study. *Br J Sports Med* 41:649-655, 2007.

177. Warren, M, Petit, A, Hannan, P, and Schmitz, K. Strength training effects on bone mineral content and density in premenopausal women. *Med Sci Sports Exerc* 40:1282-1288, 2008.

178. Westcott, W. How to take them from sedentary to active. *IDEA Today* 13:46-54, 1995.

179. Westcott, W. Strength training for frail older adults. *J Act Aging* 8:52-59, 2009.

180. Westcott, W, Apovian, C, Puhala, K, Corina, L, LaRosa Loud, R, Whitehead, S, Blum, K, and DiNubile, N. Nutrition programs enhance exercise effects on body composition and resting blood pressure. *Phys Sportsmed* 41:85-91, 2013.

181. Westcott, W and Faigenbaum, A. Clients who are preadolescent, older, or pregnant. In *NSCA's Essentials of Personal Training.* 2nd ed. Coburn, J, and Malek, M, eds. Champaign, IL: Human Kinetics, 2012.

182. Westcott, W, Winett, R, Annesi, J, Wojcik, J, Anderson, E, and Madden, P. Prescribing physical activity: applying the ACSM protocols for exercise type, intensity, and duration across 3 training frequencies. *Phys Sportsmed* 2:51-58, 2009.

183. Wilson, G, Newton, R, Murphy, A, and Humphries, B. The optimal training load for the development of dynamic athletic performance. *Med Sci Sports Exerc* 25:1279-1286, 1993.

184. Wilson, I, Schoen, C, Neuman, P, Strollo, M, Rogers, W, Chang, H, and Safran, D. Physician–patient communication about prescription medication nonadherence: a 50-state study of America's seniors. *J Gen Intern Med* 22:6-12, 2007.

185. Wilson, P, D'Agostino, R, Sullivan, L, Parise, H, and Kannel, W. Overweight and obesity as determinants of cardiovascular risk: the Framingham experience. *Arch Intern Med* 162:1867-1872, 2002.

186. Winjdaele, K, Duvigneaud, N, Matton, L, Duquet, W, Thomis, M, Beunen, G, Lefevre, J, and Phillippaerts, R. Muscular strength, aerobic fitness, and metabolic syndrome risk in Flemish adults. *Med Sci Sports Exerc* 39:233-240, 2007.

187. Wolfe, R. The unappreciated role of muscle in health and disease. *Am J Clin Nutr* 84:475-482, 2006.

188. Wolff, I, Van Croonenborg, J, Kemper, H, Kostense, P, and Twisk, J. The effect of exercise training programs on bone mass: a meta-analysis of published controlled trials in pre and post-menopausal women. *Osteoporos Int* 9:1-12, 1999.

189. Yarasheski, K, Campbell, J, and Kohrt, W. Effect of resistance exercise and growth hormone on bone density in older men. *Clin Endocrinol* 47:223-229, 1997.

Chapter 13 Female-Specific Conditions

1. Ackerman, K and Misra, M. Bone health in adolescent athletes with a focus on female athlete triad. *Phys Sportsmed* 39:131-141, 2013.

2. Ağıl, A, Abıke, F, Daşkapan, A, Alaca, R, and Tüzün, H. Short-term exercise approaches on menopausal symptoms, psychological health, and quality of life in postmenopausal women. *Obstet Gynecol Int* 274261, 2010.

3. Ahlborg Jr, G, Bodin, L, and Hogstedt, C. Heavy lifting during pregnancy-a hazard to the fetus? A prospective study. *Int J Epidemiol* 19:90-97, 1990.

4. Allison, KC, Lundgren, JD, O'Reardon, JP, Martino, NS, Sarwer, DB, Wadden, TA, and Stunkard, AJ. The Night Eating Questionnaire (NEQ): psychometric properties of a measure of severity of the night eating syndrome. *Eat Behav* 9:62-72, 2008.

5. American College of Obstetricians and Gynecologists. Weight Gain During Pregnancy. 2013. www.acog.org/ Resources-And-Publications/Committee-Opinions/ Committee-on-Obstetric-Practice/Weight-Gain-During-Pregnancy. Accessed December 24, 2016.

6. American College of Obstetricians and Gynecologists. Physical Activity and Exercise During Pregnancy and the Postpartum Period. 2015. www.acog.org/ Resources-And-Publications/Committee-Opinions/ Committee-on-Obstetric-Practice/Physical-Activity-and-Exercise-During-Pregnancy-and-the-Postpartum-Period. Accessed December 24, 2016.

7. American College of Obstetricians and Gynecologists. Exercise During Pregnancy. 2016. www.acog.org/ Patients/FAQs/Exercise-During-Pregnancy. Accessed December 24, 2016.

8. American College of Sports Medicine. ACSM Current Comment: exercise during pregnancy. 2015. www.acsm.org/docs/current-comments/exerciseduring-pregnancy.pdf. Accessed December 24, 2016.

9. American Psychiatric Association. DSM-5 task force. In *Diagnostic and Statistical Manual of Mental Disorders* (DSM-5). Washington, DC: American Psychiatric Association, 2013.

10. Artal, R, Fortunato, V, Welton, A, Constantino, N, Khodiguian, N, Villalobos, L, and Wiswell, R. A comparison of cardiopulmonary adaptations to exercise in pregnancy at sea level and altitude. *Am J Obstet Gynceol* 172:1170-1180, 1995.

11. Ashrafinia, F, Mirmohammadali, M, Rajabi, H, van-Kazemnejad, A, Sadeghniiathaghighi, K, Amelvaliza-deh, M, and Chen, H. The effects of Pilates exercise on sleep quality in postpartum women. *J Bodyw Mov Ther* 18:190-199, 2013.

12. Avery, ND, Stocking, K, Tranmer, J, Davies, G, and Wolfe, L. Fetal responses to maternal strength conditioning in late gestation. *Can J Appl Physiol* 24:362-376, 1999.

13. Barrack, MT, Ackerman, K, and Gibbs, J. Update on the female athlete triad. *Curr Rev Musculoskelet Med* 6:195-204, 2013.

14. Barrack, MT, Gibbs, JC, de Souza, MJ, Williams, NI, Nichols, JF, Rauh, MJ, and Nattiv, A. Higher incidence of bone stress injuries with increasing female athlete triad-related risk factors: a prospective multisite study of exercising girls and women. *Am J Sports Med* 42:949-958, 2014.

15. Bauer, PW, Broman, C, and Pivarnik, J. Exercise and pregnancy knowledge among healthcare providers. *J Womens Health (Larchmt)* 19:335-341, 2010.

16. Bayliss, DA and Millhorn, D. Central neural mechanisms of progesterone action: application to the respiratory system. *J Appl Physiol* 73:393-404, 1992.

17. Beals, KA. *Disordered Eating among Athletes: A Comprehensive Guide for Health Professionals.* Champaign, IL: Human Kinetics, 2004.

18. Bonci, CM, Bonci, L, Granger, L, Johnson, C, Malina, R, Milne, L, Ryan, R, and Vanderbunt, E. National athletic trainers' association position statement: preventing, detecting, and managing disordered eating in athletes. *J Athl Train* 43:80-108, 2008.

19. Bratland-Sanda, S and Sundgot-Borgen, J. Eating disorders in athletes: overview of prevalence, risk factors and recommendations for prevention and treatment. *Eur J Sport Sci* 13:499-508, 2013.

20. Brearley, AL, Sherburn, M, Galea, MP, and Clarke, SJ. Pregnant women maintain body temperatures within safe limits during moderate-intensity aqua-aerobic classes conducted in pools heated up to 33 degrees

Celsius: an observational study. *J Physiother* 61:199-203, 2015.

21. Bump, RC and Norton, P. Epidemiology and natural history of pelvic floor dysfunction. *Obstet Gynecol Clin North Am* 25:723-746, 1998.

22. Burbos, N and Morris, E. Menopausal symptoms. 2011. www.clinicalevidence.bmj.com/x/systematic-review/0804/overview.html. Accessed December 24, 2016.

23. Burger, HG. Androgen production in women. *Fertil Steril* 77(suppl 4):S3-S5, 2002.

24. Burtscher, M, Gatterer, J, Philippe, M, Krössmann, P, Kernbeiss, S, Frontull, V, and Kofler, P. Effects of a single low-dose acetaminophen on body temperature and running performance in the heat: a pilot project. *Int J Physiol Pathophysiol Pharmacol* 5:190-193, 2013.

25. Calatayud, J, Borreani, S, Moya, D, Colado, J, and Triplett, N. Exercise to improve bone mineral density. *Strength Cond J* 35:70-74, 2013.

26. Cedergren, M. Effects of gestational weight gain and body mass index on obstetric outcome in Sweden. *Int J Gynaecol Obstet* 93:269-274, 2006.

27. Centers for Disease Control and Prevention. Recommendation regarding elected conditions affecting women's health. *MMWR* 49(No. RR-2), 2000.

28. Centers for Disease Control and Prevention. Healthy Pregnant or Postpartum Women. 2014. www.cdc.gov/physicalactivity/everyone/guidelines/pregnancy.html. Accessed December 24, 2016.

29. Chaconas, EJ, Olivencia, O, and Russ, B. Exercise interventions for the individual with osteoporosis. *Strength Cond J* 35:49-55, 2013.

30. Chen, Y, Tenforde, A, and Fredericson, M. Update on stress fractures in female athletes: epidemiology, treatment, and prevention. *Curr Rev Musculoskelet Med* 6:173-181, 2013.

31. Clark, S, Cotton, D, Pivarnik, J, Lee, W, Hankins, G, Benedetti, T, and Phelan, J. Position change and central hemohynamic profile during normal third-trimester pregnancy and postpartum. *Am J Obstet Gynecol* 164:883-887, 1991.

32. Coelho, G, de Farias, M, de Mendonça, L, de Mello, D, Lanzillotti, H, Ribeiro, B, and Soares, E. The prevalence of disordered eating and possible health consequences in adolescent female tennis players from Rio de Janeiro, Brazil. *Appetite* 64:39-47, 2013.

33. Coelho, G, Soares Ede, A, and Ribeiro, B. Are female athletes at increased risk for disordered eating and its complications? *Appetite* 55:379-387, 2010.

34. Copeland, J, Chu, S, and Tremblay, M. Aging, physical activity, and hormones in women–a review. *J Aging Phys Act* 12:101-116, 2004.

35. Cummings, S, Black, D, Nevitt, M, Browner, W, Cauley, J, Ensrud, K, Genant, H, Palermo, L, Scott, J, and Vogt, T. Bone density at various sites for prediction of hip fractures. *Lancet* 341:72-75, 1993.

36. da Costa, N, Schtscherbyna, A, Soares, E, and Ribeiro, B. Disordered eating among adolescent female swimmers: dietary, biochemical, and body composition factors. *Nutrition* 29:172-177, 2013.

37. Daley, A, Stokes-Lampard, H, and MacArthur, C. Exercise for vasomotor menopausal symptoms (Review). *Cochrane Database Syst Rev* 5:1-39, 2011.

38. Dawes, J. The role of exercise in the prevention and treatment of gestational diabetes mellitus. *Strength Cond J* 2:66-68, 2006.

39. de Souza, M, Nattiv, A, Joy, E, Misra, M, Williams, N, Mallinson, R, Gibbs, J, Olmsted, M, Goolsby, M, and Matheson, G. 2014 Female Athlete Triad Coalition Consensus Statement on Treatment and Return to Play of the Female Athlete Triad: 1st international conference held in San Francisco, CA, May 2012, and 2nd international conference held in Indianapolis, IN, May 2013. *Clin J Sport Med* 24:96-119, 2014.

40. de Souza Santos, CA, Dantas, E, and Moreira, M. Correlation of physical aptitude: functional capacity, corporal balance and quality of life (QoL) among elderly women submitted to a post-menopausal physical activities program. *Arch Gerontol Geriatr* 53:344-349, 2011.

41. Dempsey, J, Butler, C, and Williams, M. No need for a pregnant pause: physical activity may reduce the occurrence of gestational diabetes mellitus and preeclampsia. *Exerc Sport Sci Rev* 33:141-149, 2005.

42. Dewey, K, Lovelady, C, Nommsen-Rivers, L, McCrory, M, and Lonnerdal, B. A randomized study of the effects of aerobic exercise by lactating women on breast-milk volume and composition. *N Engl J Med* 330:449-453, 1994.

43. Donnelly, J, Blair, S, Jakicic, J, Manore, M, Rankin, J, and Smith, B. American College of Sports Medicine position stand. Appropriate physical activity intervention strategies for weight loss and prevention of weight regain for adults. *Med Sci Sports Exerc* 41:459-471, 2009.

44. Drug Enforcement Agency. Drugs of Abuse. 2015. www.dea.gov/pr/multimedia-library/publications/drug_of_abuse.pdf. Accessed December 24, 2016.

45. Elavsky, S and McAuley, E. Lack of perceived sleep improvement after 4-month structured exercise programs. *Menopause* 14:535-540, 2007.

46. Elavsky, S and McAuley, E. Personality, menopausal symptoms, and physical activity outcomes in middle-aged women. *Pers Individ Dif* 46:123-128, 2009.

47. Entin, P and Munhall, K. Recommendations regarding exercise during pregnancy made by private small group practice obstetricians in the USA. *J Sports Sci Med* 5:449-458, 2006.

48. Food and Drug Administration. Pregnancy and Lactation Labeling (Drugs) Final Rule. 2016. www.fda.gov/Drugs/DevelopmentApprovalProcess/DevelopmentResources/Labeling/ucm093307.htm. Accessed December 24, 2016.

49. Freeman, E, Guthrie, K, Caan, B, Sternfeld, B, Cohen, L, Joffe, H, Carpenter, J, Anderson, G, Larson, J, Ensrud, K, and Reed, S. Efficacy of escitalopram for hot flashes in healthy menopausal women: a randomized controlled trial. *JAMA* 305:267-274, 2011.

50. Freeman, E and Sherif, K. Prevalence of hot flashes and night sweats around the world: a systematic review. *Climacteric* 10:197-214, 2007.

51. Gibbs, J, Nattiv, A, Barrack, M, Williams, N, Rauh, M, Nichols, J, and de Souza, M. Low bone density risk is higher in exercising women with multiple triad risk factors. *Med Sci Sports Exerc* 46:167-176, 2014.

52. Gunderson, E and Abrams, B. Epidemiology of gestational weight gain and body weight changes after pregnancy. *Epidemiol Rev* 21:167-176, 1999.

53. Harman, S, Vittinghoff, E, Brinton, E, Budoff, M, Cedars, M, Lobo, R, Merriam, G, Miller, V, Naftolin, F, Pal, L, and Santoro, N. Timing and duration of menopausal hormone treatment may affect cardiovascular outcomes. *Am J Med* 124:199-205, 2011.

54. Hausenblas, H and Symons Downs, D. Prospective examination of leisure-time exercise during pregnancy. *J Applied Sport Psychol* 17:240-246, 2005.

55. Hinman, S, Smith, K, Quillen, D, and Smith, M. Exercise in pregnancy: a clinical review. *Sports Health* 7:527-537, 2015.

56. Hoogenboom, B, Morris, J, Morris, C, and Schaefer, K. Nutritional knowledge and eating behaviors of female, collegiate swimmers. *N Am J Sports Phys Ther* 4:139-148, 2009.

57. Howe, T, Shea, B, Dawson, L, Downie, F, Murray, A, Ross, C, Harbour, R, Caldwell, L, and Creed, G. Exercise for preventing and treating osteoporosis in postmenopausal women. *Cochrane Database Syst Rev* 6:CD000333, 2011.

58. Hunter, G and Treuth, M. Relative training intensity and increases in strength in older women. *J Strength Cond Res* 9:188-191, 1995.

59. Hunter, G, Wetzstein, C, McLafferty, C, Zuckerman, P, Landers, K, and Bamman, M. High resistance versus variable-resistance training in older adults. *Med Sci Sports Exerc* 33:1759-1764, 2001.

60. Jaque-Fortunato, V, Wiswell, R, Khodiguian, N, and Artal, R. A comparison of the ventilatory responses to exercise in pregnant, postpartum, and nonpregnant women. *Semin Perinatol* 20:263-276, 1996.

61. Javed, A, Tebben, P, Fischer, P, and Lteif, A. Female athlete triad and its components: toward improved screening and management. *Mayo Clin Proc* 88:996-1009, 2013.

62. Kac, G, D'Aquino Benicio, M, Valente, J, and Velasquez-Melendez, G. Postpartum weight retention among women in Rio de Janeiro: a follow-up study. *Rep Public Health* 19:S149-S161, 2003.

63. Kelley, G, Kelley, K, and Kohrt, W. Exercise and bone mineral density in premenopausal women: a meta-analysis of randomized controlled trials. *Int J Endocrinol* 2013:741639, 2013.

64. Kemmler, K, Engelke, K, Von Stengel, S, Weineck, J, Lauber, D, and Kalender, W. Long-term four-year exercise has a positive effect on menopausal risk factors: the Erlangen fitness osteoporosis prevention study. *J Strength Cond Res* 21:232-239, 2007.

65. Kemmler, W, Weineck, J, Kalender, W, and Engelke, K. The effect of habitual physical activity, non-athletic exercise, muscle strength, and VO2max on bone mineral density is rather low in early postmenopausal osteopenic women. *J Musculoskelet Neuronal Interact* 4:325-334, 2004.

66. Kraemer, W, Adams, K, Cafarelli, E, Dudley, G, Dooly, C, Feigenbaum, M, Fleck, S, Franklin, B, Fry, A, Hoffman, J, Newton, R, Potteiger, J, Stone, M, Ratamess, N, and Triplett-McBride, T. American College of Sports Medicine position stand: progression models in resistance training for healthy adults. *Med Sci Sports Exerc* 34:364-380, 2002.

67. Kransdorf, L, Vegunta, S, and Files, J. Everything in moderation: what the female athlete triad teaches us about energy balance. *J Womens Health (Larchmt)* 22:790-792, 2013.

68. Lambrinoudaki, I and Papadimitriou, D. Pathophysiology of bone loss in the female athlete. *Ann N Y Acad Sci* 1205:45-50, 2010.

69. Liddle, D and Connor, D. Nutritional supplements and ergogenic aids. *Prim Care* 40:487-505, 2013.

70. Liu, M, Wang, Y, Li, X, Liu, P, Yao, C, Ding, Y, Zhu, S, Bai, W, and Liu, J. A health survey of Beijing middle-aged registered nurses during menopause. *Maturitas* 74:84-88, 2013.

71. Loucks, A, Stachenfeld, N, and DiPietro, L. The female athlete triad: do female athletes need to take special care to avoid low energy availability? *Med Sci Sports Exerc* 38:1694-1700, 2006.

72. Loud, K, Gordon, C, Micheli, L, and Field, A. Correlates of stress fractures among preadolescent and adolescent girls. *Pediatrics* 115:e399-e406, 2005.

73. Lovejoy, J, Champagne, C, deJonge, L, Xie, H, and Smith, S. Increased visceral fat and decreased energy expenditure during the menopausal transition. *Int J Obesity* 32:949-958, 2008.

74. Lovelady, C, Garner, K, Moreno, K, and Williams, J. The effect of weight loss in overweight, lactating women on the growth of their infants. *N Engl J Med* 342:449-453, 2000.

75. Lovelady, C, Lonnerdal, B, and Dewey, K. Lactation performance of exercising women. *Am J Clin Nutr* 52:103-109, 1990.

76. Mallinson, R, Williams, N, Olmsted, M, Scheid, J, Riddle, E, and de Souza, M. A case report of recovery of menstrual function following a nutritional intervention in two exercising women with amenorrhea of varying duration. *J Int Soc Sports Nutr* 10:34, 2013.

77. Manore, M. Dietary recommendations and athletic menstrual dysfunction. *Sports Med* 32:887-901, 2012.

78. Manore, M, Kam, L, Loucks, A, and International Association of Athletics Federations. The female athlete triad: components, nutrition issues, and health consequences. *J Sports Sci* 25:S61-S71, 2007.

79. Martens, D, Hernandez, B, Strickland, G, and Boatwright, D. Pregnancy and exercise: physiological changes and effects on the mother and fetus. *Strength Cond J* 28:78-82, 2006.

80. Martyn-St James, M and Carroll, S. Meta-analysis of walking for preservation of bone density in postmenopausal women. *Bone* 43:521-531, 2008.

81. Mauger, A, Jones, A, and Williams, C. Influence of acetaminophen on performance during time trial cycling. *J Appl Physiol* 108:98-104, 2010.

82. Melin, A, Tornberg, Å, Skouby, S, Faber, J, Ritz, C, Sjödin, A, and Sundgot-Borgen, J. The LEAF questionnaire: a screening tool for the identification of female athletes at risk for the female athlete triad. *Br J Sports Med* 48:540-545, 2014.

83. Mencias, T, Noon, M, and Hoch, A. Female athlete triad screening in National Collegiate Athletic Association Division I athletes: is the preparticipation evaluation form effective? *Clin J Sport Med* 22:122-125, 2012.

84. Mendelsohn, F and Warren, M. Anorexia, bulimia, and the female athlete triad: evaluation and management. *Endocrinol Metab Clin North Am* 39:155-167, 2010.

85. Metcalfe, L, Lohman, T, Going, S, Houtkooper, L, Ferreira, D, Flint-Wagner, H, Guido, T, Martin, J, Wright, J, and Cussler, E. Post-menopausal women and exercise for prevention of osteoporosis. *ACSMs Health Fit J* 5:6-14, 2001.

86. Mirror Mirror. Purging Disorder. 2016. www.mirror-mirror.org/purging-disorder.htm. Accessed December 24, 2016.

87. Mørkved, S and Bø, K. The effect of postpartum pelvic floor muscle exercise in the prevention and treatment of urinary incontinence. *Int Urogynecol J* 8:217-222, 1997.

88. National Institute of Mental Health. Eating Disorders. 2016. www.nimh.nih.gov/health/topics/eating-disorders/index.shtml. Accessed December 24, 2016.

89. National Osteoporosis Foundation. What Women Need to Know. 2016. www.nof.org/prevention/general-facts/what-women-need-to-know/. Accessed December 24, 2016.

90. Nattiv, A, Loucks, A, Manore, M, Sanborn, C, Sundgot-Borgen, J, and Warren, M. American College of Sports Medicine position stand. The female athlete triad. *Med Sci Sports Exerc* 39:1867-1882, 2007.

91. Nehring, I, Schmoll, S, Beyerlein, A, Hauner, H, and vonKries, R. Gestational weight gain and long-term postpartum weight retention: a meta-analysis. *Am J Clin Nutr* 94:1225-1231, 2011.

92. Neumaker, K. Morality rates and causes of death. *Eur Eat Disord Rev* 8:181-187, 2000.

93. Newton, K, Reed, S, Guthrie, K, Sherman, K, Booth-LaForce, C, Caan, B, Sternfeld, B, Carpenter, J, Learman, L, Freeman, E, and Cohen, L. Efficacy of yoga for vasomotor symptoms: a randomized controlled trial. *Menopause* 21:339, 2014.

94. Office of the Surgeon General. Bone Health and Osteoporosis: A Report of the Surgeon General. 2004. www.ncbi.nlm.nih.gov/books/NBK45513/. Accessed December 24, 2016.

95. Oken, E, Taveras, E, Popoola, F, Rich-Edwards, J, and Gillman, M. Television, walking, and diet. Association with postpartum weight retention. *Am J Prev Med* 32:305-311, 2007.

96. Omo-Aghoja, L. Maternal and fetal acid-base chemistry: a major determinant of perinatal outcome. *Ann Med Health Sci Res* 4:8-17, 2014.

97. Parise, G, Bosman, M, Boecker, D, Barry, M, and Tarnopolsky, M. Selective serotonin reuptake inhibitors: their effect on high-intensity exercise performance. *Arch Phys Med Rehabil* 82:867-871, 2001.

98. Pedersen, S, Kristensen, K, Hermann, P, Katzenellenbogen, J, and Richelsen, B. Estrogen controls lipolysis by up-regulating α2A-adrenergic receptors directly in human adipose tissue through the estrogen receptor α. Implications for the female fat distribution. *J Clin Endocrinol Metab* 89:1869-1878, 2004.

99. Pereira, M, Rifas-Shiman, S, Kleinman, K, Rich-Edwards, J, Peterson, K, and Gillman, M. Predictors of change in physical activity during and after pregnancy: Project Viva. *Am J Prev Med* 32:312-319, 2007.

100. Pettee, K, Brach, J, Kriska, A, Boudreau, R, Richardson, C, Colbert, L, Satterfield, S, Visser, M, Harris, T, Ayonayon, N, and Newman, A. Influence of marital status on physical activity levels among older adults. *Med Sci Sports Exerc* 38:541-546, 2006.

101. Philp, H. Hot flashes—a review of the literature on alternative and complementary treatment approaches. *Altern Med Rev* 8:284-302, 2003.

102. Pinna, F, Sanna, L, and Carpiniello, B. Alexithymia in eating disorders: therapeutic implications. *Psychol Res Behav Manag* 8:1-15, 2015.

103. Piper, T, Jacobs, E, Haiduke, M, Waller, M, and McMillan, C. Core training exercise selection during pregnancy. *Strength Cond J* 34:55-62, 2012.

104. Pivarnik, J, Chambliss, H, Clapp, J, Dugan, S, Hatch, M, Lovelady, C, Mottola, M, and Williams, M. Impact of physical activity during pregnancy and postpartum on chronic disease risk: an ACSM Roundtable consensus statement. *Med Sci Sports Exerc* 38:989-1005, 2006.

105. Pruett, M and Caputo, J. Exercise guidelines for pregnant and postpartum women. *Strength Cond J* 33:100-103, 2011.

106. Pujol, T, Barnes, J, and Elder, C. Resistance training during pregnancy. *Strength Cond J* 29:44-46, 2007.

107. Rasmussen, K and Yaktine, A. *Weight Gain During Pregnancy: Reexamining the Guidelines.* Washington, DC: National Academy Press, 2009.

108. Ratamess, N, Alvar, B, Evetoch, T, Housh, T, Kibler, W, Kraemer, W, and Triplett, N. Progression models in resistance exercise training for healthy adults. *Med Sci Sports Exerc* 41:687-708, 2009.

109. Reed, J, de Souza, M, and Williams, N. Changes in energy availability across the season in Division I female soccer players. *J Sports Sci* 31:314-324, 2013.

110. Rossner, S and Ohlin, A. Pregnancy as a risk factor for obesity: lessons from the Stockholm Pregnancy and Weight Development Study. *Obes Res* 3:267S-275S, 1995.

111. Sangenis, P, Drinkwater, BL, Loucks, A, Sherman, RT, Sundgot-Borgen, J, and Thompson, RA. International Olympic Committee Medical Commission Working Group Women in Sport. Position Stand on the Female Athlete Triad. International Olympic Committee. 2005. https://stillmed.olympic.org/media/Document%20Library/OlympicOrg/IOC/Who-We-Are/Commissions/Medical-and-Scientific-Commission/EN-Position-Stand-on-the-Female-Athlete-Triad.pdf#_ga=1.118851721.1640999716.1482507714. Accessed December 23, 2016.

112. Satariano, W, Haight, T, and Tager, I. Living arrangements and participation in leisure-time physical activities in an older population. *J Aging Health* 14:427-451, 2002.

113. Schierbeck, L, Rejnmark, L, Tofteng, C, Stilgren, L, Eiken, P, Mosekilde, L, Køber, L, and Jensen, J. Effect of hormone replacement therapy on cardiovascular events in recently postmenopausal women: randomised trial. *BMJ* 345:e6409, 2012.

114. Schiff, I. Invited reviews: a new addition to menopause. *Menopause* 20:243, 2013.

115. Schoenfeld, B. Resistance training during pregnancy: safe and effective program design. *Strength Cond J* 33:67-75, 2011.

116. Setji, T, Brown, A, and Feniglos, M. Gestational diabetes mellitus. *Clin Diabetes* 23:17-24, 2005.

117. Smink, F, van Hoeken, D, and Hoek, H. Epidemiology of eating disorders: incidence, prevalence and mortality rates. *Curr Psychiatry Rep* 14:406-414, 2012.

118. Smink, F, van Hoeken, D, and Hoek, H. Epidemiology, course, and outcome of eating disorders. *Curr Opin Psychiatry* 26:543-548, 2013.

119. Sorensen, T, Williams, M, Lee, I, Dashow, E, Thompson, M, and Luthy, D. Recreational physical activity during pregnancy and risk of preeclampsia. *Hypertension* 41:1273-1280, 2003.

120. Sourel-Cubizolles, M and Kaminski, M. Pregnancy women's working conditions and their changes during pregnancy; a national study in France. *Br J Ind Med* 44:236-243, 1987.

121. Steinmuller, P, Meyer, N, Kruskall, L, Manore, M, Rodriguez, N, Macedonio, M, Bird, R, Berning, J, and American Dietetic Association Dietitians in Sports Cardiovascular, and Wellness Nutrition Dietetic Practice Group, ADA Quality Management Committee. American Dietetic Association Standards of Practice and Standards of Professional Performance for registered dietitians (generalist, specialty, advanced) in sports dietetics. *J Am Diet Assoc* 109:544-552, 2009.

122. Stengel, S, Kemmler, W, Pintag, R, Beeskow, C, Weineck, J, Lauber, D, Kalender, W, and Engelke, K. Power training is more effective than strength training for maintaining bone mineral density in postmenopausal women. *J Appl Physiol* 99:181-188, 2005.

123. Sternfeld, B, Guthrie, K, Ensrud, K, Lacroix, A, Larson, J, Dunn, A, Anderson, G, Seguin, R, Carpenter, J, Newton, K, Reed, S, Greeman, E, Cohen, L, Joffer, H, Roberts, M, and Cann, B. Efficacy of exercise for menopausal symptoms: a randomized controlled trial. *Menopause* 21:330-338, 2014.

124. Stetka, B and Correll, C. A Guide to DSM-5: Binge Eating Disorder. 2013. www.medscape.com/viewarticle/803884_5. Accessed January 1, 2016.

125. Stojanovskaa, L, Apostolopoulosa, V, Polmanb, R, and Borkolesb, E. To exercise, or, not to exercise, during menopause and beyond. *Maturitas* 77:318-323, 2014.

126. Sundgot-Borden, J. Weight and eating disorders in elite athletes. *Scand J Med Sci Sports* 12:259-260, 2002.

127. Sundgot-Borgen, J and Torstveit, M. Aspects of disordered eating continuum in elite high-intensity sports. *Scand J Med Sci Sports* 20:112-121, 2010.

128. Szymanski, L and Satin, A. Exercise during pregnancy: fetal responses to current public health guidelines. *Obstet Gynceol* 119:603-610, 2006.

129. Szymanski, L and Satin, A. Strenuous exercise during pregnancy: is there a limit? *Am J Obstet Gynecol* 207:179, 2012.

130. Talmadge, A, Kravitz, L, and Robergs, R. Exercise during pregnancy: research and application. *IDEA Health Fitness Source* 18:28-35, 2000.

131. Teixeira-Coelho, F, Uendeles-Pinto, J, Serafim, A, Wanner, S, de Matos Coelho, M, and Soares, D. The paroxetine effect on exercise performance depends on the aerobic capacity of exercising individuals. *J Sports Sci Med* 13:232-243, 2014.

132. Temme, K and Hoch, A. Recognition and rehabilitation of the female athlete triad/tetrad: a multidisciplinary approach. *Curr Sports Med Rep* 12:190-199, 2013.

133. *The Medical Letter.* Drugs for postmenopausal osteoporosis. Issue 1452, 2014.

134. Thurston, R, Joffe, H, Soares, C, and Harlow, B. Physical activity and risk of vasomotor symptoms in women with and without a history of depression: results from the Harvard study of moods and cycles. *Menopause* 213:553-560, 2006.

135. U.S. Department of Health and Human Services. *2008 Physical Activity Guidelines for Americans.* Washington, DC: Department of Health and Human Services, 2008.

136. van der Wijden, C, Kleijnen, J, and Van den Berk, T. Lactational amenorrhea for family planning. *Cochrane Database Syst Rev* CD001329, 2003.

137. Van Poppel, M and Brown, W. "It's my hormones, doctor"–does physical activity help with menopausal symptoms? *Menopause* 15:78-85, 2008.

138. Villaverde-Gutierrez, C, Araujo, E, Cruz, F, Roa, J, Barbosa, W, and Ruiz-Villaverde, G. Quality of life of rural menopausal women in response to a customized exercise programme. *J Adv Nurs* 54:11-19, 2006.

139. Warr, B and Woolf, K. The female athlete triad: patients do best with a team approach to care. *J Am Acad Physician Assist* 24:50-55, 2011.

140. WebMD. Menopause and Hot Flashes. 2016. www.webmd.com/menopause/guide/menopause-hot-flashes. Accessed December 24, 2016.

141. Wolfe, L. Pregnancy. In *Exercise Testing and Exercise Prescription for Special Cases: Theoretical Basis and Clinical Application.* Skinner, J, ed. Philadelphia: Lippincott Williams & Wilkins, 1993.

142. Woo, S, Hellstein, J, and Kalmar, J. Systematic review: bisphosphonates and osteonecrosis of the jaw. *Ann Intern Med* 144:753-761, 2006.

143. World Health Organization. Assessment of fracture risk and its application to screening for postmenopausal osteoporosis. Report of a WHO Study Group. *World Health Organ Tech Rep Ser* 843:1-129, 1994.

144. Writing Group for the Women's Health Initiative Investigators. Risks and benefits of estrogen plus progestin in healthy postmenopausal women: principal results from the Women's Health Initiative randomized controlled trial. *JAMA* 288:321-333, 2002.

Index

Note: The italicized *f* and *t* following page numbers refer to figures and tables, respectively.

About the Editor

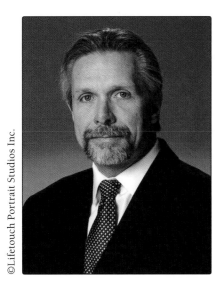

©Lifetouch Portrait Studios Inc.

Patrick L. Jacobs, PhD, CSCS,*D, earned his doctorate in Exercise Physiology from the University of Miami and is the owner and head coach at Superior Performance. He is a Fellow of the National Strength and Conditioning Association, American College of Sports Medicine, and the International Society of Sports Nutrition. He is a licensed Athletic Trainer (Florida) and a Certified Strength and Conditioning Specialist.

Jacobs has published many peer-reviewed scientific articles on exercise and nutritional interventions in populations ranging from people with spinal cord injuries to the elite athletic competitor. He has coordinated the performance programs of collegiate and professional championship athletes including football, baseball, powerlifting, bodybuilding, auto racing, and sailing. He is also an inventor whose name appears on several exercise device patents.

About the Editor

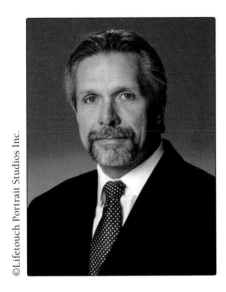

Patrick L. Jacobs, PhD, CSCS,*D, earned his doctorate in Exercise Physiology from the University of Miami and is the owner and head coach at Superior Performance. He is a Fellow of the National Strength and Conditioning Association, American College of Sports Medicine, and the International Society of Sports Nutrition. He is a licensed Athletic Trainer (Florida) and a Certified Strength and Conditioning Specialist.

Jacobs has published many peer-reviewed scientific articles on exercise and nutritional interventions in populations ranging from people with spinal cord injuries to the elite athletic competitor. He has coordinated the performance programs of collegiate and professional championship athletes including football, baseball, powerlifting, bodybuilding, auto racing, and sailing. He is also an inventor whose name appears on several exercise device patents.

Contributors

Jill A. Bush, PhD, CSCS,*D
The College of New Jersey, Ewing

James E. Clark, MS, CSCS
Manchester Community College, CT

Brett A. Comstock, PhD, CSCS
Bloomsburg University, Bloomsburg, PA

Jay Dawes, PhD, CSCS,*D, NSCA-CPT,*D, FNSCA
University of Colorado, Colorado Springs

Avery D. Faigenbaum, EdD, CSCS, CSPS, FNSCA
The College of New Jersey, Ewing

Steven J. Fleck, PhD, CSCS, FNSCA
Andrews Research & Education Foundation, Gulf Breeze, FL

John F. Graham, MS, CSCS,*D, RSCC*E, FNSCA
St Luke's University Health Network, Pennsylvania/New Jersey

Patrick L. Jacobs, PhD, CSCS,*D, FNSCA
Superior Performance, LLC

Misty Kesterson, EdD, CSCS
Texas A&M University—Corpus Christi

William J. Kraemer, PhD, CSCS,*D, FNSCA
The Ohio State University, Columbus

Thomas P. LaFontaine, PhD, CSCS, NSCA-CPT
Optimus: The Center for Health and Performance, Columbia, MO

Anna Lepeley, PhD, CSCS, CISSN

Don Melrose, PhD, CSCS,*D
Texas A&M University—Corpus Christi

Alejandro Lucia, MD, PhD
Universidad Europea de Madrid (Polideportivo)

Benjamin Reuter, PhD, ATC, CSCS,*D
California University of Pennsylvania, California, PA

Jeffrey L. Roitman, EdD
Rockhurst University (Retired)

Kenneth W. Rundell, PhD
Geisinger Commonwealth School of Medicine, Scranton, PA

Alejandro F. San Juan, PhD, PT
Department of Health Sciences, Public University of Navarre (Spain)

Carwyn Sharp, PhD, CSCS,*D
National Strength and Conditioning Association, Colorado Springs

James M. Smoliga, DVM, PhD, CSCS
High Point University, High Point, NC

Paul Sorace, MS, CSCS
Hackensack Meridian Health, Hackensack, NJ

Stephanie M. Svoboda, MS, DPT, CSCS, CISSN
Superior Performance, LLC and Nicklaus Children's Hospital, Miami, FL

Ann Marie Swank, PhD, CSCS
University of Louisville, KY

Pnina Weiss, MD, FAAP
Yale University School of Medicine, New Haven, CT

Wayne L. Westcott, PhD, CSCS
Quincy College, MA

Malcolm T. Whitehead, PhD, CSCS, FMS
Stephen F. Austin State University, Nacogdoches, TX

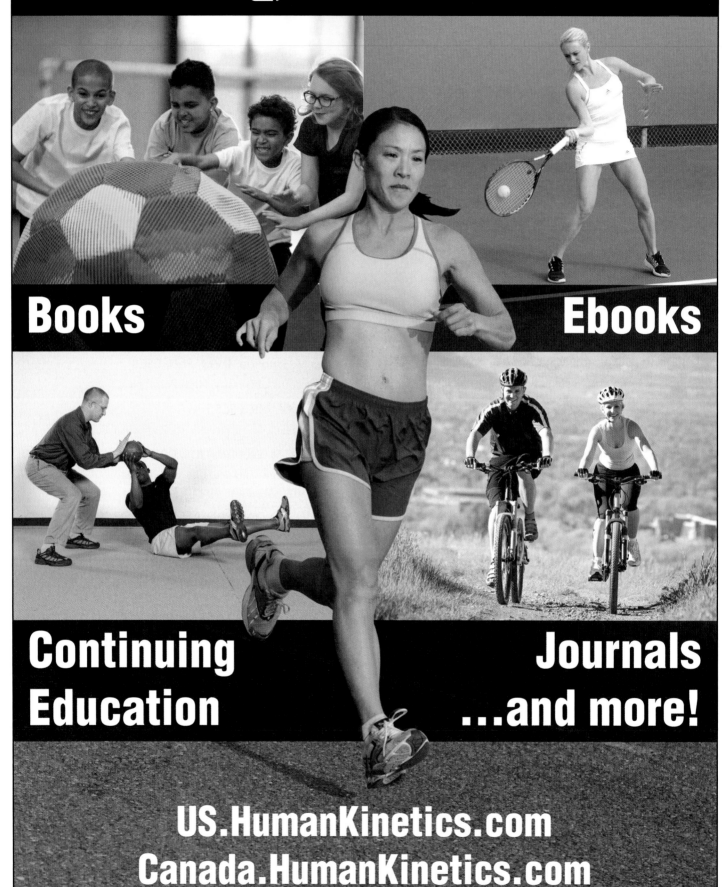